T0140377

NUTRITION AND HEALTH

Adrianne Bendich, Ph.D., FACN, FASN,
Connie W. Bales, Ph.D., R.D., SERIES EDITORS

More information about this series at http://www.springer.com/series/7659

Rajkumar Rajendram • Victor R. Preedy
Vinood B. Patel

Editors

Diet, Nutrition, and Fetal Programming

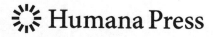 Humana Press

Editors
Rajkumar Rajendram
Department of Internal Medicine
King Abdulaziz Medical City
Riyadh Ministry of National Guard Health Affairs
Saudi Arabia

King's College London, Department of Nutrition
and Dietetics
Nutritional Sciences Division
School of Biomedical & Health Sciences
London, UK

Vinood B. Patel
University of Westminster
Faculty of Science & Technology
Department of Biomedical Sciences
London, UK

Victor R. Preedy
Department of Nutrition and Dietetics
Nutritional Sciences Division
School of Biomedical & Health Sciences
King's College London
London, UK

Nutrition and Health
ISBN 978-3-319-86826-4   ISBN 978-3-319-60289-9   (eBook)
DOI 10.1007/978-3-319-60289-9

Printed on acid-free paper

This Humana Press imprint is published by Springer Nature
The registered company is Springer International Publishing AG
The registered company address is: Gewerbestrasse 11, 6330 Cham, Switzerland

Preface

The exposure of the fetus to adverse nutritional conditions has long-term effects, which can then extend into adulthood. These include increased rates of cardiovascular disease, diabetes, and metabolic syndrome. Some cancer rates are also reported to increase, and there is evidence that neurological deficiencies occur in adults who were previously exposed to nutritional inadequacies in utero.

There are complex interrelationships between these aforementioned conditions and their causative mechanisms. These include deficient receptor-post-receptor signaling, endocrine imbalance, defective DNA methylation, and alterations in other pathways. It is highly probable that many scientific processes are intertwined in a multifaceted way, impacting on the fetus and then the adult. Understanding these causative events, effects, and long-term outcomes means that there are windows of opportunity throughout the life cycle where diet and nutrition can be monitored, controlled, or rectified where necessary. However, presently there is no coherent text that reviews the wide-ranging effects of adverse fetal nutrition and beyond. This is addressed in the present book *Diet, Nutrition, and Fetal Programming*, which has over 40 detailed chapters ranging from molecular biochemistry to epidemiology. Coverage includes international aspects, ethnicity, famines, malnutrition (general and specific), maternal stress, fetal growth restriction, birth weights, biomarkers, myogenesis, fibrogenesis, adipogenesis, gametogenesis, nephrogenesis, food preferences, physiology, immunology, endocrinology, neuroendocrinology, hepatology, the pancreas, the cardiovascular system, obesity, metabolic syndrome, neuropsychiatric disorders, cognition, sleep, food preferences, high-fat diets, junk food diets, fish and fish oil, n-3 fatty acids, taurine, caffeine, telomere biology, knockouts, microRNAs, and many other areas too numerous to list here.

Contributors are authors of international and national standing, leaders in the field, and trendsetters. Emerging fields of science and important discoveries are also incorporated in *Diet, Nutrition, and Fetal Programming*.

This book is designed for nutritionists and dietitians, public health scientists, medical doctors, midwives, obstetricians, pediatricians, epidemiologists, health-care professionals of various disciplines, and policy makers. It is designed for teachers and lecturers, undergraduates and graduates, researchers, and professors.

London, UK

Rajkumar Rajendram
Victor R. Preedy
Vinood B. Patel

Series Editor Page

The great success of the Nutrition and Health Series is the result of the consistent overriding mission of providing health professionals with texts that are essential because each includes (1) a synthesis of the state of the science; (2) timely, in-depth reviews by the leading researchers and clinicians in their respective fields; (3) extensive, up-to-date fully annotated reference lists; (4) a detailed index; (5) relevant tables and figures; (6) identification of paradigm shifts and the consequences; (7) virtually no overlap of information between chapters but targeted, interchapter referrals; (8) suggestions of areas for future research; and (9) balanced, data-driven answers to patients' as well as health professionals' questions which are based upon the totality of evidence rather than the findings of any single study.

The series volumes are not the outcome of a symposium. Rather, each editor has the potential to examine a chosen area with a broad perspective, both in subject matter and in the choice of chapter authors. The international perspective, especially with regard to public health initiatives, is emphasized where appropriate. The editors, whose trainings are both research and practice oriented, have the opportunity to develop a primary objective for their book, define the scope and focus, and then invite the leading and emerging authorities from around the world to be part of their initiative. The authors are encouraged to provide an overview of the field, discuss their own research, and relate the research findings to potential human health consequences. Because each book is developed de novo, the chapters are coordinated so that the resulting volume imparts greater knowledge than the sum of the information contained in the individual chapters.

Diet, Nutrition, and Fetal Programming, edited by Rajkumar Rajendram, Victor R. Preedy, and Vinood B. Patel, is a most timely and very welcome addition to the Nutrition and Health Series and fully exemplifies the series' goals. The term "fetal programming" was first proposed by Drs. David Barker and Charles N. Hales in 2001 following their in-depth examination of epidemiological data that pointed to poor maternal nutrition during fetal development increasing the risk of a number of chronic diseases in the offspring over their lifetime. Subsequently, the topic of fetal programming and the mechanisms that result in this phenomenon has been linked to another field of research called epigenetics; this volume brings together these two fields, and thus an objective, up-to-date volume on these topics is very timely. There is new attention being given to developmental biology, including embryology, that has contributed to the fetal programming hypothesis, also known as the fetal origins hypothesis, or the developmental origins of health and disease (DOHaD). The hypothesis suggests that conditions very early in development in utero can, through epigenesis, leave lasting alterations on the fetus that may affect its susceptibility to diseases with onsets that may occur many decades later.

The editors of this volume are experts in their respective fields and represent the medical profession as well as the academic research community. Dr. Rajkumar Rajendram is an intensive care physician, anesthetist, and perioperative physician. He was trained in general medicine and intensive care in Oxford, and he attained membership in the Royal College of Physicians (MRCP) in 2004. Dr. Rajendram then trained in anesthesia and intensive care in the Central School of Anesthesia, London Deanery, and became a fellow of the Royal College of Anaesthetists (FRCA) in 2009. He is one of the first intensivists to become a fellow of the faculty of intensive care medicine (FFICM). Dr. Rajendram recognized that nutritional support was a fundamental aspect of critical care, and, as a visiting lecturer in the Nutritional Sciences Research Division of King's College London, he has published over 150 textbook chapters, review articles, peer-reviewed papers, and abstracts. Professor Victor R. Preedy is a senior member of King's College London where he is a professor of nutritional biochemistry. He is also director of the Genomics Centre and a member of the School of Medicine. He is a member of the Royal College of Pathologists and a fellow of the Royal Society of Biology, the Royal College of Pathologists, the Royal Society for Public Health, and, in 2012, the Royal Society of Chemistry. Dr. Vinood B. Patel is a senior lecturer in clinical biochemistry at the University of Westminster and honorary fellow at King's College London. Dr. Patel obtained his degree in pharmacology from the University of Portsmouth and his Ph.D. in protein metabolism from King's College London and completed postdoctoral research at Wake Forest University School of Medicine. Dr. Patel is a recognized leader in alcohol research and was involved in several NIH-funded biomedical grants related to alcoholic liver disease. Dr. Patel has edited biomedical books in the area of nutrition and health and disease prevention and has published over 160 articles.

The 42 chapters within this clinically important as well as basic research-oriented volume provide the reader with a comprehensive examination of the growing acknowledgment that environmental exposures during the fetal period can affect the fetus' health throughout life. The global prevalence and consequences of maternal malnutrition and primary fetal environmental exposure affect the health of the mother, the length of the pregnancy, as well as the health and growth of the fetus. One critical example, which is captured in the recent book edited by this volume's editors, entitled *Nutrition and Diet in Maternal Diabetes*, shows that gestational diabetes (GDM), and in fact, any maternal hyperglycemia, is associated with complications such as increased birth weight, macrosomia, cesarean birth, and preterm birth. Women who are diagnosed with GDM have a significantly increased risk of developing type 2 diabetes within 10 years, and the offspring also have an increased risk of diabetes. GDM also increases the risk of preeclampsia and other adverse birth outcomes.

This comprehensive volume is organized into eight sections that include chapters on general considerations of maternal diet and health and the fetus followed by an in-depth examination of the effects of maternal undernutrition and protein restriction. Part III reviews the effects of obesity, high-fat diet, and junk food on fetal outcomes, and Part IV includes chapters on specific dietary components including fish and its fatty acids, folate, taurine, and tryptophan. The fifth part contains chapters that look at data on fetal programming effects in different countries, and the sixth part looks at the data with respect to effects seen in childhood and adolescence. New research that describes the biochemical and genetic mechanisms involved in fetal programming is discussed in the seventh part, and the last part provides readers with relevant resources.

Part I: Maternal Diet, Health, and the Fetus – General Considerations

The first section, containing six chapters, begins with two chapters that examine associations between maternal stress, nutritional status, and fetal responses to these critical environmental factors. The first chapter informs us that there is a large literature and active research area that suggests that certain exposures in the prenatal period may have lasting effects on the behavior and physiology of the child. Prenatal diet and nutrition is one area of focus, and another area of research includes the examination of the role of prenatal stress and its effects on fetal and infant health and development. Chapter 1 describes the well-researched historical events where both maternal stress and poor nutrition occurred together. In the Dutch Hunger Winter of 1944–1945, the women who were pregnant during that period have been followed for many decades to understand the long-term effects on their physiology and that of subsequent generations. Gestational exposure to the Dutch famine has been linked to psychological and metabolic changes in the offspring later in life. Similar findings have been reported in studies of pregnancies during the Great Leap Forward Famine in China from 1959 to 1961. In both cases, the physiological changes observed in offspring are frequently attributed to the substantial caloric and micronutrient deficiencies that fetuses experienced during these natural experiments. However, we learn that, in addition to nutritional status, maternal stress and stress physiology are an important coexisting factor. The constant military threat, limited food rations, displacement, and general upheaval would have placed a serious psychological burden on the pregnant woman and affected fetal programming. The chapter provides many examples where low socioeconomic status is adversely associated with nutritionally poor diets, food insecurity, and heightened psychosocial stress, and the authors suggest that poor diet may serve as a proxy for stress exposure and vice versa. Poor diet and nutritional deficiencies may confound the negative effects of exposure to psychosocial stress but may also interact with or modify the effects of stress. Chapter 2 examines the effects of modern diets and maternal nutritional status on the fetus' ability to cope with stressful environments during growth and maturation and into adulthood. Poor prenatal metabolic/nutritional environments can lead to altered fetal programming of neural circuitry that may result in adverse adult stress responses The chapter reviews the effects of epigenetic alterations during fetal development and the altered roles of the limbic system and the hypothalamic-pituitary-adrenal (HPA) axis. The strong relationship between stress and heart disease, high blood pressure, and the development of affective disorders, such as anxiety and depression, and the new data on the effects of maternal obesity are also examined.

Chapter 3 links fetal nutritional status with brain development and cognition as these can be modified by nutrient and gene interactions through epigenetics. Cognition refers to the mental ability to process and retrieve new information using functions which include attention, memory, thinking, learning, and perception. DNA methylation is an epigenetic mechanism that requires dietary nutrients, including folate, vitamin B12, and vitamin B6, that are needed for biochemical reactions whereby methyl groups are donated to DNA nucleotides and thus modify the regulation of gene expression. The chapter, which includes nearly 100 relevant references and 7 informative figures and tables, reviews the epigenetic modifications that mediate DNA methylation, disrupt cell-signaling molecules, and increase neurotoxins in the brain which may adversely affect cognitive function.

The next three chapters examine the effects of maternal nutritional status before and during pregnancy on fetal programming. Chapter 4 looks at the importance of exercise, normal maternal body mass index (BMI), and strength on the development of the fetus as well as the beneficial effects of exercise on maternal health before, during, and after pregnancy. Physical activity and cardiorespiratory fitness both produce significant cardiovascular health benefits. During pregnancy, regular physical activity has been shown to help maintain physical fitness, decrease gestational weight gain, and reduce the risk of developing gestational diabetes and potentially preeclampsia. The chapter examines the research linking infant birth weight and subsequent child weight from exercising mothers versus sedentary mothers. Chapter 5 describes the factors that influence the development of fetal growth retardation. We learn that fetal growth restriction (FGR) affects up to 10% of live-born infants worldwide. Using global norms, approximately 10% of term infants in developed countries are small for gestational age (SGA) compared to 23% of term infants in developing countries. Normal fetal growth is a multifactorial process that is dependent on genetic background, endocrine milieu, and appropriate placental function. FGR is defined as the failure of a fetus to reach its growth potential according to gestational age and gender. FGR is a risk factor for hypertension, hyperlipidemia, coronary heart disease, and diabetes mellitus in adulthood. The chapter reviews the maternal factors, such as age, alcohol consumption, smoking, diastolic blood pressure, and diet, that strongly modify embryonic growth trajectories early in pregnancy. First trimester embryonic growth has been related to subsequent fetal growth in the second and third trimesters of pregnancy, as well as to adverse pregnancy outcomes including preterm delivery and SGA infants. With regard to fetal programming and epigenetic factors, the genome-wide differential DNA methylation of all known imprinted genes in normal and FGR placentas has been analyzed. The data point to differential methylation changes that occur in FGR throughout the genomic regions, including genes actively expressed in the placenta. Analyses of genome-wide methylation patterns in normal, SGA, and FGR human placentas show that certain methylation patterns are associated with infant growth. The final chapter in this section examines the importance of fetal brain sensitivity to insulin. Chapter 6 describes the use of a new technology, fetal magnetoencephalography (fMEG), which is a noninvasive technique which enables a direct measurement of fetal neuronal activity in utero. Maternal postprandial exposure to insulin showed a direct effect on fetal brain responses. This is an important new area of fetal programming research.

Part II: Maternal Undernutrition and Protein Restriction – Effects on Fetus

Part II also contains six chapters, and the first three chapters examine the effects of overall maternal undernutrition, and the last three chapters look at specific protein restriction and the effects on fetal programming. Chapters 7, 8, and 9 review the importance of the cascade of events that follow fetal exposure to maternal undernutrition. Undernutrition can alter both maternal and fetal concentrations of many hormones including insulin, insulin-like growth factors, thyroid hormones, leptin, cortisol, and glucocorticoids. Because some maternal hormones can cross the placenta, the fetal endocrine response to undernutrition reflects the activity of both maternal and fetal endocrine glands, as reviewed in Chap. 7. Reduction in availability of nutrients during fetal development programs the endocrine pancreas and insulin-sensitive tissues, and the malnourished offspring may be born with defects in their β-cell and insulin-sensitive tissues. Chapter 8 continues to explore the effects of maternal undernutrition during critical periods of fetal development that affects the development of visceral obesity later in life. Prenatal undernutrition particularly during the later stages of gestation can induce differential signals in adipose tissue in such a way that lipid storing capacity is increased. The consequent increased adiposity can result in elevated inflammatory responses and associated metabolic disturbances during gestation and throughout the infant's lifespan. Chapter 9 examines the direct epigenetic mechanisms underlying the aberrant expression of hepatic genes in malnourished offspring that persist into adulthood. The neonatal liver is sensitive to oxidative stress associated with maternal undernutrition and this can result in epigenetic changes. Thus the liver is another tissue that is adversely affected by maternal undernutrition and can also result in metabolic dysfunctions that last throughout the lifetime of the child.

Chapters 10, 11, and 12 concentrate on the effects of maternal protein malnutrition on fetal programming of the heart, kidney, and brain. Protein malnutrition in utero is strongly associated with intrauterine growth retardation. Reduced growth in fetal life and small birth weight, along with accelerated growth in childhood, are associated with a greater risk of coronary heart disease in adult life and increased risk of hypertension and type 2 diabetes. Chapter 10 reviews the studies that indicate that exposure to low protein in utero adversely affects heart cell number (cardiomyocyte number). Additionally, neonate's fetal growth restriction is associated with an increase in aortic intima-media thickness, which can hinder the movement of blood through the heart. The chapter reviews the data from animal models and human survey studies that show an increased risk of cardiovascular disease and direct heart effects that are associated with epigenetic changes that were initiated under an environment of maternal protein malnutrition. Related to the changes in the cardiovascular system are the effects of low maternal protein on the kidneys. Chapter 11 provides compelling evidence of the association of maternal low-protein ingestion with low nephron number in the fetus that is directly related to the development of arterial hypertension and kidney dysfunction in adulthood and aging. Chapter 12 looks at the effects of maternal protein deficiency on the brain. Protein restriction during the prenatal period that is followed by low birth weight is associated with the development of neurological and psychiatric diseases. Substantial evidence from studies in animals and in humans shows that gestational and early postnatal dietary protein restriction influence cognitive performance and can lead to behavioral abnormalities and disorders in memory and learning. The chapter clearly explains that, in humans, the greatest time period of vulnerability of the brain and other components of the CNS occurs from the second third of pregnancy through the first year of life; the peak of brain growth occurs during pregnancy, and over 25% of the brain's weight at birth is attained during this time period. Thus, maternal protein deficiency can have an irreversible impact on the brain development of the fetus.

Part III: Effects of Obesity, High-Fat Diet, and Junk Food on Fetal Outcomes

As indicated in earlier chapters, there is a growing awareness of the negative impact of maternal obesity and overweight on fetal programming. The six chapters in Part III examine some of these impacts and the effects of certain dietary components on fetal health. The first two chapters, Chaps. 13 and 14, provide an overview of the effects of obesity during pregnancy. Maternal obesity increases the risk of many adverse events including, but not limited to, thromboembolic complications, gestational diabetes, hypertension, maternal hemorrhage, and infection. There is also increased risk for spontaneous miscarriage, fetal malformations, fetal macrosomia, stillbirth, and preterm delivery. Other complications that are associated with maternal obesity are reviewed including greater need for cesarean delivery and respiratory risks with anesthesia. Chapter 13 also examines the potential opportunities to reduce these risks with diet, exercise, and bariatric surgery prior to pregnancy and reviews the inconsistent data from the USA and UK. With regard to fetal programming, maternal obesity is associated with infants who have an increased risk of overweight and obesity, insulin resistance, and diabetes in childhood and adulthood. Chapter 14 describes the molecular effects of maternal obesity and its many consequences. Maternal obesity further increases inflammatory cytokines, insulin, and lipids compared to that found in normal pregnancy. Maternal obesity also affects placental vascularity, metabolism, and/or nutrient transport function leading to alterations in fetal growth, metabolism, and organ development. Maternal obesity is linked to an increased incidence of offspring metabolic dysregulation including obesity, hyperglycemia, hyperinsulinemia, hyperlipidemia, type 2 diabetes, and cardiovascular disease. These changes are due to gene-environment interactions in utero which produce epigenetically induced changes in gene expression. The chapter reviews the current research using small and large animal models including sheep that suggest that maternal obesity can initiate fetal programming events that have adverse effects on her offspring as well as her offspring's children.

Chapter 15 reviews the role of ethnicity on the development of maternal obesity and its consequences. The chapter tabulates the prevalence rates of many chronic diseases and links these to the risk of maternal obesity, gestational diabetes, and many of the other adverse effects noted above. The chapter indicates that cardiovascular disease, diabetes, and asthma all occur at differing prevalence rates among people of different ethnicities. Coronary artery disease is up to two times more common among South Asians compared to Europeans, and type 2 diabetes is almost four times more common in South Asians. Diabetes is also more common in Filipinos, Hispanics, Chinese, Middle Easterners, North Africans, South and Central Americans, and people from the western Pacific region than seen in Europeans. Black individuals have a consistently higher prevalence of hypertension, diabetes, and stroke compared to white populations. The authors note that the etiology of stroke differs according to ethnicity. Western populations are more likely to experience emboli originating from the heart or extracranial large arteries compared to Asian populations where small-vessel occlusion or intracranial atherosclerosis occurs more frequently. Emerging evidence suggests that the associations between obesity and adverse pregnancy outcomes may also be additive in some ethnicities. Obesity is a stronger risk factor for maternal gestational diabetes in Asian compared to Caucasian women. Obesity is also more strongly associated with preeclampsia in Latino compared to Caucasian women. This unique chapter, with 100 important references and 4 excellent figures, provides valuable data to help in assessing the role of fetal programming balanced against ethnic and country environmental factors.

Chapter 16 looks at the molecular mechanisms involved in the liver's metabolism during fetal development and points out the main and recent findings on the role of microRNAs in modulating hepatic metabolism in the offspring of obese mothers or mothers consuming a high-fat diet during important periods of fetal and neonatal development including pregnancy and lactation. The liver regulates many vital physiological processes. The functions are reviewed including processing nutrients after intestinal absorption, synthesis and excretion of metabolites, detoxification of xenobiotics, modulation of lipid and glucose metabolism, and energy homeostasis. The eight figures and tables help to explain the findings from the recent animal model studies.

Chapters 17 and 18 describe the findings from animal models that examine the mechanism and potential for diets that are high in fats and carbohydrates to affect fetal programming events and life-long outcomes. Chapter 17 reviews the effects of maternal high-fat diet during gestation and/or lactation on the mother and on stress-related neurodevelopment and behavior in her offspring. The chapter includes descriptions of animal models using maternal high-fat diet exposure and their impacts on physiological, behavioral, and epigenetic outcomes observed in offspring. Chapter 18 looks at the impact of maternal junk food diets during pregnancy and/or lactation on the developing offspring in well-described animal models. Maternal junk food diets have been shown to result in increased fat mass and heighted preference for fat and sugar intake through the offspring's life course. More recent studies focus on defining the biological mechanisms driving these effects and have identified the developing fat cell, or adipocyte, and the central neural network that regulates the response to reward as major targets. It has been demonstrated that maternal junk food intake results in an activation of lipogenic pathways in fetal and neonatal fat depots, which leads to early accumulation of excess fat tissue and persistently increases the capacity of the fat depots to store fat. In parallel, exposure to maternal junk diets also leads to permanent alterations in the structure and function of the reward pathways in the brain that appear to differ between males and females.

Part IV: Specific Dietary Components

Seven chapters review specific components of the maternal diet including fish; fish oil; n-3 fatty acids; folate, vitamin B12, choline, and other methyl donors; taurine; tryptophan; and caffeine. Chapters 19, 20, and 21 look at a number of the functions that have been attributed to the consumption of fish that are the major source of long-chain n-3 fatty acids. Chapter 19 presents a balanced perspective on the plusses and minuses of fish consumption during pregnancy and provides the reader with four comprehensive tables that outline the relevant studies. We learn that fish is the primary dietary source of n-3 long-chain polyunsaturated fatty acids and a rich source of protein, selenium, iodine, and vitamin D but is also a major source of exposure to methylmercury (MeHg) and other environmental pollutants. In utero exposure to nutrients and toxicants found in the same fish might act on the exact same end points with opposite effects. Overall, evidence on the association of maternal fish consumption during pregnancy with child health outcomes has been largely inconsistent. However, in 2014, the US FDA and Environmental Protection Agency updated their advice on fish consumption for women of child-bearing age, encouraging women who are pregnant, breastfeeding, or likely to become pregnant to consume more fish but no more than three servings per week to limit fetal exposure to MeHg. The European Food Safety Authority (EFSA) has also reported recently that the benefits from fish consumption of up to three to four servings per week during pregnancy could outweigh the risks associated with MeHg exposure. Chapter 19 looks at fish oil supplementation during pregnancy and outcomes. The supplements contain no or very low levels of the contaminants found in whole fish. The chapter describes the evidence that fatty acids may alter the epigenome, although studies in healthy humans and experiments in animals have shown variable long-term metabolic and gene function responses to fish oil supplementation during pregnancy. Detailed descriptions of models showing the potential effects of fish oil on epigenetic alterations of RNAs especially with regard to insulin resistance are included. Chapter 20 describes the clinical data that show that n-3 fatty acid consumption in adults reduces systolic and diastolic blood pressure as well as resting heart rate. The reduced heart rate is thought to be due to direct effects on cardiac electrophysiology as well as indirect pathways involving the heart muscle. The n-3 fatty acids also may be involved in programming the fetus' blood pressure as maternal docosahexaenoic acid (DHA), a major long-chain n-3 fatty acid, is readily transferred via the placenta to the fetus and later is an important component of breast milk and is rapidly accumulated in the synapses during fetal development and early postnatal life. DHA comprises 30% of the phospholipid fatty acids within the brain's cortex and 15% within the hypothalamus, a key brain center that controls blood pressure. Relevant survey and intervention studies are tabulated. Chapter 21 reviews the experimental and clinical studies that point to the intrauterine environment as a predictor of neonatal blood pressure. Underlying mechanisms include alterations in fetal kidney function and damage to the nephron's vasculature. Maternal malnutrition can reduce nitric oxide-dependent vasodilatation and microvascular density as well as total peripheral resistance. The n-3 fatty acids have the potential to lower blood pressure in offspring of supplemented mothers during pregnancy and lactation. The laboratory animal studies as well as human survey and intervention studies are discussed and tabulated.

Chapter 22 looks closely at the role of one carbon metabolism, maternal deficiencies, and fetal programming via DNA methylation and regulation of gene expression. This complex metabolic network is regulated by a number of genes and requires micronutrients including folate; vitamins B12, B6, and B2; and choline. Folate, vitamin B12, and choline are methyl donors, which are involved in the synthesis of the precursor of S-adenosylmethionine, the universal donor of methyl groups needed for DNA methylation. Deficiencies in these nutrients can alter the epigenetic regulation of gene expression. The chapter highlights animal studies, human association studies, and interventional studies and finds consistent evidence that maternal status of nutrients required for efficient one carbon metabolism affects many metabolic factors in the offspring including low B12 and increased homocysteine related to adverse cardiovascular outcomes, low folate status and reduced cognitive performance in offspring, and low folate status and significant increased risk of neural tube defects.

The next two chapters examine the effects of two different amino acids, taurine and tryptophan. We learn in Chap. 23 that taurine is a sulfur-containing amino acid that has multiple cellular and molecular functions mainly associated with the conjugation of bile acids, cellular osmoregulation, energy storage, the absorption of intestinal fat, glucose metabolism, antioxidant function, neurotransmission, and cytoprotective effects during cell development and survival. In adults, taurine is nonessential and is synthesized in the liver and adipose tissue from ingested methionine and cysteine. In humans, taurine is the most abundant amino acid found in the developing brain, skeletal muscle, liver, spinal cord, retina, pancreas, heart, white blood cells, platelets, and placenta and is found in breast milk as well. The fetus cannot synthesize taurine and maternal taurine deficiency, either from protein restriction or, as seen in the animal models described, by maternal diabetes, affects fetal development of the endocrine pancreas. The pancreatic changes during fetal and neonatal life increase the risk of the offspring developing diabetes, obesity, and hypertension. The chapter includes 92 relevant references and important figures that help the reader understand the findings in this unique chapter. Chapter 24 describes the role of nutrition, with emphasis on tryptophan, in fetal development. Tryptophan is an essential amino acid and therefore cannot be synthesized within the body and must be consumed as part of the normal dietary intake. Tryptophan is the precursor of serotonin, a neurotransmitter synthesized mainly in the central nervous system and, as discussed below, also in the endocrine pancreas. Tryptophan is involved in the regulation of several body functions including the growth and maturation of specific developing brain regions and secretion of hormones such as growth hormone and gonadotropins.

The final chapter in this part, Chap. 25, discusses the data linking caffeine consumption with fetal programming. Caffeine is a methylxanthine alkaloid that is widely present in coffee, tea, soft drinks, foods, and some prescription drugs. Many studies have reported that caffeine ingestion can enhance mood and alertness, awareness, attention, and reaction time. The chapter, containing over 120 references, objectively reviews the correlation between prenatal caffeine ingestion and intrauterine growth retardation (IUGR) and agrees that the data are inconsistent and many human survey findings remain controversial. Different doses of caffeine ingested, clinically insignificant magnitudes of IUGR, and other confounding factors including the age and health condition of the pregnant woman may be possible reasons for the conflicting results. Therefore, the chapter concentrates on data from animal experiments that suggest an association between certain adverse developmental events and prenatal caffeine ingestion.

Part V: International Aspects and Policies

Five chapters examine the contrasting effects of maternal malnutrition in different countries around the world including India and Africa as well as Ireland and Japan. Chapter 26 posits that famine or severe maternal malnutrition does not provide molecular evidence that epigenetic changes caused by starvation or other environmental influences are part of an ordered predictable (or programmed) response. The environmental influence could cause random and nonspecific stochastic effects on individual cells within the organism. Somatic and germ cells with favorable epigenotypes and/or genotypes could then be selected on the basis of their ability to survive and proliferate in the mother in the prevailing negative environmental circumstances. The chapter reviews the survey data linking famines in Europe and China with adverse health outcomes in males born during these times and examines data from animal studies where embryonic loss can be documented. However, at present, there are no definitive findings of an effect on the genome of the offspring born during a famine and limited data of an epigenetic effect.

Chapter 27 describes strategies reducing pregnancy risks in malnourished women in India. The chapter authors emphasize that appropriate nutrition, in particular, during adolescence, pregnancy, and lactation, affects the growth and development of the fetus, thereby translating into healthy statistics for birth outcomes, childhood health, and long-term health and economic benefits, and concentrate their review on the dual issues of under- and overnutrition seen in today's population of Indian women of childbearing potential. According to the Indian National Family Health Survey in 2005–2006, the prevalence of undernourished women, based on a body mass index (BMI) less than 18.5 kg/m^2, was 36.5%, and nearly half of the women had a BMI less than 17 kg/m^2, pointing to the widespread prevalence of moderate to severe undernutrition. Moreover, the prevalence of anemia among women in their childbearing years, aged 15–49 years, ranges from 32.7% to 76.3% that is indicative of the wide variation across states in India. The overall prevalence of overweight women aged 15–49 years was 13%, with about 3% falling in the obese category (BMI greater than 30 kg/m^2). The chapter reviews over 40 years of national programs designed to provide key nutrients to malnourished women especially during pregnancy, taking into account cultural changes associated with urbanization and the research into fetal programming. Chapter 28 sensitively reviews the nutritional status of women in many of Africa's nations. Africa, like India, is also experiencing the paradox of escalating maternal hunger and obesity. The consequence is the birth of small, low-birth weight (LBW) neonates as well as large babies with fetal macrosomia. However, unlike India, the authors note that Africa is saddled with food insecurity arising from huge humanitarian crises, refugee and poverty situations, and emerging African cities where there is a growing risk of maternal obesity with micronutrient deficiencies as a result of overconsumption of fast foods. Babies adapt to maternal undernutrition by slowing their growth velocity, which leads to LBW, whereas babies of obese mothers adjust in favor of high growth trajectory giving rise to macrosomia. Other critical issues include maternal infection with HIV, malaria, and other common infectious agents that can adversely affect fetal growth directly or through placental infection. Major factors that affect food availability include political instabilities and wars, poverty, lack of electricity and refrigeration, as well as sanitation issues, cultural factors including religions and tribal factors, and rural versus city life; all of these and other relevant factors are considered within the chapter.

Chapter 29 objectively examines the current status of birth outcomes in Ireland and describes the major nutrition-related issues of current public health concern; the chapter includes six informative tables and figure. The critical issues include maternal obesity; excessive gestational weight gain; increased risk of gestational diabetes; inadequate intake of folate before and during pregnancy; lower than recommended intakes of vitamin D, iron, and long-chain polyunsaturated acids; and higher than recommended intake of alcohol prior to and during pregnancy. For each issue, the chapter describes the extent of the problem and any Irish-based interventions to improve the situation. National policies and clinical guidelines relating to each issue are also discussed. Chapter 30 objectively describes current issues in Japan. In contrast to Ireland, female obesity does not appear to be a significant issue during pregnancy in Japan. However, over the last 20 years, the proportion of low-birth weight infants in Japan has exceeded that of other developed countries. The desire of young Japanese women to be thin has been identified as an underlying cause. The chapter reports on the literature review of 50 relevant Japanese studies of pregnancy outcomes. A recent review in 2014 reported that the proportion of LBW (1500–2499 g) babies in Japan is consistently increasing. The National Health Survey in 2013 reported that both men and women at childbearing age (20–39 years) had a higher energy intake but a lower vitamin intake than in 2003. These data substantiate the increasing concern about the components of the diets of teenagers especially young women and highlight the importance of education about nutrition and health in early life. Several vitamin deficiencies are reviewed, and there is an in-depth review of studies involving exposure to mercury, PCBs, and other contaminants and their effects on pregnancy outcomes. Research on fetal programming in Japanese populations is in its infancy.

Part VI: Effects of Fetal Programming in Childhood and Adulthood

Five chapters examine specific aspects of fetal programming during childhood and beyond. Chapter 31 reviews the classical growth curves that are based on population studies of gestational age and gender and have been in use for many decades. The chapter then looks at the more recent, new customized growth criteria that incorporate variables, such as mother's height, parity, and initial weight, in addition to gender and gestational age, with the aim of better assessing a child's true growth potential. However, we learn that the baby's gender and mother's parity, height, weight, and ethnicity can predict only about 20–35% of the neonate's birth weight. Since the 1990s, a number of customized growth curves have been developed including certain maternal biomarkers that appear to be better predictors of adverse fetal growth and development. Chapter 32 looks at the recent epidemiological and animal studies that have examined the effects of overnutrition during fetal development and subsequent offspring's risk of developing aspects of the metabolic syndrome including elevated blood pressure, hyperglycemia and excess adiposity, impaired insulin signaling and resistance, glucose intolerance, and hypertriglyceridemia. The chapter examines the associations between both under- and overnutrition during fetal development as well as maternal factors including gestational diabetes and subsequent metabolic diseases that may go beyond the first generation exposed to hyperglycemia in pregnancy. The chapter delves into the specific eating habits of children undernourished in utero and at increased risk for metabolic diseases. Chapter 33 examines both clinical and experimental data that indicate that exposure to fetal undernutrition may have programming effects on feeding preferences and behaviors that can contribute to the development of diseases. Individuals born small for gestational age (SGA) have preferences toward highly caloric and palatable foods such as carbohydrates and fats and display altered eating behaviors. These behaviors can lead to small but persistent nutrient imbalances across the lifespan, increasing the risk of metabolic diseases in adult life. The chapter includes a detailed description of the parts of the brain that are involved in food choices. The hypothalamus is the central brain region involved in regulating appetite and guaranteeing the energy intake needed for survival. The pleasurable sensations associated with the intake of highly palatable foods that are usually rich in sugar and fat are controlled mostly by the mesocorticolimbic dopaminergic pathway, with inputs from other brain systems such as the opioids. Impulse control and decision-making processes, largely based on the prefrontal cortex, are important determinants of food choices. Adding to this complexity, the brain areas are enriched with receptors for peripheral hormones involved in energy intake and expenditure, such as insulin, leptin, and ghrelin, and therefore signals from the gastrointestinal tract and adipose tissue depots are able to modulate the central responses from the brain in a finely regulated fashion.

Chapter 34 provides a careful review of the relatively new data linking fetal undernutrition with alterations in bone and muscle structure and function. In the 1990s, researchers developed the theory that changes in early stages of bone development due to starvation and reduced provision of nutrition, minerals, and growth factors would lead to bone metabolic changes in adults. This theory was further elaborated in the following decade, when the pathogenesis of osteoporosis was described and a role was attributed to intrauterine programming, confirming the earlier analysis of growth in infancy and bone mass in adult life. Important connections were shown to exist between maternal life style, maternal body mass, and vitamin D dependence, which could predict bone mass in offspring and the risk of future fracture. In 2015, research confirmed that bone metabolic aberrations resulted from intrauterine macro- and micro-nutritional deprivation. The nine tables and figures provide evidence of the role of overall nutrition, specific nutrients, and timing of fetal exposures on bone development that affects bone growth and loss throughout life and may affect the next generation's bones as well.

Chapter 35 describes the unique consequences of fetal growth retardation (FGR) on the development of sleep patterns that begin in utero and continue to be programmed through early childhood. FGR is associated with increased risks of preterm birth, perinatal mortality, and short- and long-term morbidity. FGR is associated with a high risk of neurodevelopmental impairment, including motor and sensory deficits, cognitive and learning difficulties, and cerebral palsy. Underpinning these deficits, FGR is associated with altered brain structure with reduced total brain and cortical gray matter volume. Poor sleep in childhood is related to neurocognitive impairment and in adulthood to metabolic disorders and cardiovascular disease. The chapter examines the development of the phases of sleep from its origins in the fetus though childhood and the relevance of sleep patterns to cognition and other brain functions.

Part VII: Mechanisms of Programming

The final part of this comprehensive volume, containing six chapters, reviews the major laboratory studies, including in vivo models and in vitro findings that delve into the genetic and other molecular factors that are considered to have key roles in fetal programming involved in the development of metabolic diseases. Chapter 36 describes the new high-throughput experimental and computational technologies from the fields of genomics, transcriptomics, proteomics, and metabolomics and how these methodologies may provide potential predictive biomarkers of abnormal birth weight and also biomarkers of maternal diseases that can affect neonatal birth weight. This technical chapter describes the data linking specific genes with abnormal birth weight: IGF-I, IGF-II, ADCY5, CDKAL1, ADRB1, HMGA2, LCORL, CMPXM2, CLDN1, TXNDC5, LRP2, PHLDB2, LEP, and GCH1.

Proteins that have been proposed as abnormal birth weight biomarkers include IL-8, TNF-alpha, IFN-gamma, IL-10, alpha fetoprotein, free beta hCG, PAPP-A, MMP-9, VEGF, endothelin peptides, and A-FABP. Additionally, phospholipids, monoglycerides, and vitamin D3 metabolites are potential metabolic biomarkers of abnormal birth weight.

Chapters 37 and 38 look at pancreatic functions linked to fetal programming. Chapter 37 concentrates on the endocrine pancreas. The endocrine pancreas is impaired by nutritional restriction during the perinatal phase. The pancreatic islets are a key target of metabolic programming. Fetal and neonatal insulin secretion and insulin sensitivity are altered by maternal under- or overnutrition prior to and during pregnancy and lactation. The chapter reviews the well-characterized animal models and genes, transcription factors, and other bioactives that affect pancreatic islet cell function. Chapter 38 further provides insights into the complexity of pancreatic cells' functions. Pancreatic beta-cell development and function are influenced by locally produced GABA and serotonin. GABA has a direct inhibitory action on insulin secretion and a stimulatory action on glucagon secretion. During pregnancies associated with reduced fetal growth, long-term changes to beta-cell GABA receptors can persist in the offspring into adulthood, compromising normal glucose homeostasis. Serotonin receptors are also abundant on beta cells throughout life, and serotonin can promote glucose-stimulated insulin release. Intrauterine growth retardation results in altered serotonin receptor gene expression in the offspring due to epigenetic modifications. This could contribute to the increased risk of metabolic disease in offspring. The chapter reviews the major animal models and links these data to human functions of the pancreatic islets of Langerhans and the beta cells that synthesize neurotransmitter molecules including GABA and serotonin. These molecules have both autocrine and paracrine actions within individual islets that include beta-cell proliferation, survival, and glucose-stimulated insulin secretion. IUGR significantly increases the risk of metabolic diseases including type 2 diabetes that results from disturbances in pancreatic beta-cell functions in utero.

Chapter 39 examines the critical role of glucocorticoids in the transfer of nutrients through the placenta to the fetus and how untimely overexposure to this hormone can alter normal fetal programming. Maternal malnutrition invokes a stress response in the mother and fetus and that stress may further reduce food intake and expose the developing fetus to excess glucocorticoids. The chapter reviews the processes that could result in inappropriate timing of glucocorticoid exposure or excessive exposure that can restrict fetal growth and cause permanent structural, functional, and behavioral changes with adverse consequences later in life including, but not limited to, metabolic diseases. Chapter 40 discusses the role of gene knockouts in animal models in helping to elucidate the effects of maternal high-fat diets on fetal development. The chapter describes the removal of a mammalian gerontogene involved in the regulation of oxidative stress and in fat storage. Knocking out this gene in mice protected them from oxidative stress and from maternal diet-induced obesity resulting in overall improved health in the offspring.

Chapter 41 introduces the reader to the field of telomere biology and examines the effects of the fetal environment on telomere length that is associated with longevity. We learn that telomere biology is a highly evolutionarily conserved system that plays a central role in maintaining the integrity of the genome and cell. Telomere biology refers to the structure and function of two entities – telomeres, non-coding double-stranded repeats of guanine-rich tandem DNA sequences and shelterin protein structures that cap the ends of linear chromosomes, and telomerase, the reverse transcriptase enzyme that adds telomeric DNA to telomeres. Telomeres protect chromosomes from mistaken recognition by the DNA damage-repair system. As telomere length shortens, cells become senescent and die. Telomerase maintains telomere length and preserves healthy cell function. The chapter examines the hypothesis that a reduction in the initial (newborn) setting of telomere length and telomerase expression capacity confers greater susceptibility for earlier onset and faster progression of age-related disorders that manifest in later life. New data suggest that maternal nutritional status of folate, as an example, had a programming effect on fetal telomere length during pregnancy. The chapter includes over 130 references and important tables and figures that help the reader to better understand this new area of fetal programming research.

Part VIII: Resources

The final chapter in this comprehensive volume, Chap. 42, contains a compilation of important resources for health professionals who are interested in learning more about nutritional aspects and consequences of fetal programming. The chapter includes lists of relevant journals, books, and references as well as websites of interest.

Conclusions

The above descriptions of the volume's 42 chapters attest to the depth of information provided by the 95 well-recognized and respected editors and chapter authors who come from more than 20 countries around the world and provide a unique perspective on the value of adequate nutritional status during the female's reproductive years, pregnancy, and lactation to help assure normal fetal programming of all aspects of fetal organ and systems development. The volume presents compelling evidence that inadequate maternal nutrition, both under- and overnutrition, as well as inadequate intake of vitamins, minerals, and other bioactive dietary components, can adversely affect the offspring throughout the lifespan and may even adversely affect the next generation. As many of the chapters reflect new findings in this area of research, each chapter includes fully defined abbreviations for the reader and consistent use of terms between chapters. Key features of this comprehensive volume include over 200 detailed tables and informative figures; an extensive, detailed index; and more than 2700 up-to-date references that provide the reader with excellent sources of worthwhile information. Moreover, the final chapter contains a comprehensive list of web-based resources that will be of great value to the health provider as well as graduate and medical students.

In conclusion, *Diet, Nutrition, and Fetal Programming*, edited by Rajendram Rajkumar, Victor R. Preedy, and Vinood B. Patel, provides health professionals in many areas of research and practice with the most up-to-date, well-referenced volume on the importance of maintaining optimal nutritional status for individuals during their reproductive years to help reduce the risk of the adverse effects of inadequate nutrition on the fetus that is manifest in damage to the fetal programming processes. Negative effects of fetal programming not only affect the fetus, neonate, and child but continue throughout life and may affect the next generation as well. The volume serves the reader as the benchmark in this complex area of interrelationships between maternal nutrition, be it undernutrition or more recently, with the increasing prevalence of obesity during reproductive years, overnutrition and the development of obesity, metabolic diseases, and many of the other chronic diseases of aging. The importance of diet quality including types and quantity of carbohydrates, dietary protein intakes and long-chain fatty acids, essential micronutrients, and other relevant dietary bioactive factors is reviewed in depth. The areas of genomics, proteomics, placental health, stress effects on glucocorticoid production, novel animal models including knockout models, and nutrients' and toxic dietary components' effects on cognition and other higher brain functions are clearly discussed so that students as well as practitioners can better understand the complexities of these issues as well as learn about the newest research in developing more sensitive and earlier diagnostic tools. The editors are applauded for their efforts to develop the most up-to-date, unique resource in the area of fetal programming and its effects on the health of the fetus and potentially their offspring. The volume authors aim to identify factors and mechanisms that have the potential to reduce the risk of the adverse effects associated with maternal malnutrition that predispose the fetus to increased risk of chronic diseases during their life. The editors are to be congratulated on developing this volume that provides the reader with the most comprehensive compilation on fetal programming to date, and this excellent text is a very welcome addition to the Nutrition and Health Series.

Series Editor Bio

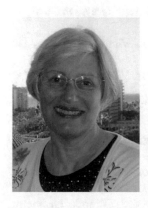

Dr. Adrianne Bendich, PhD, FASN, FACN, has served as the *Nutrition and Health Series Editor* for more than 20 years and has provided leadership and guidance to more than 200 editors that have developed the 80+ well-respected and highly recommended volumes in the Series.

In addition to *Diet, Nutrition, and Fetal Programming, edited by Rajkumar Rajendram, Victor R. Preedy, and Vinood B. Patel*, major new editions published in 2012–2017 include:

1. *Dietary Patterns and Whole Plant Foods in Aging and Disease*, edited as well as written by Mark L. Dreher, Ph.D., 2017
2. *Dietary Fiber in Health and Disease*, edited as well as written by Mark L. Dreher, Ph.D., 2017
3. *Clinical Aspects of Natural and Added Phosphorus in Foods*, edited by Orlando M. Gutierrez, Kamyar Kalantar-Zadenh, and Rajnish Mehrotra, 2017
4. *Nutrition and Diet in Maternal Diabetes*, edited by Rajendram Rajkumar, Victor R. Preedy, and Vinood B. Patel, 2017
5. *Nitrite and Nitrate in Human Health and Disease, Second Edition*, edited by Nathan S. Bryan and Joseph Loscalzo, 2017
6. *Nutrition in Lifestyle Medicine*, edited by James M. Rippe, 2017
7. *Nutrition Guide for Physicians and Related Healthcare Professionals, Second Edition*, edited by Norman J. Temple, Ted Wilson, and George A. Bray, 2016
8. *Clinical Aspects of Natural and Added Phosphorus in Foods*, edited by Orlando M. Gutiérrez, Kamyar Kalantar-Zadeh, and Rajnish Mehrotra, 2016
9. *L-Arginine in Clinical Nutrition*, edited by Vinood B. Patel, Victor R. Preedy, and Rajkumar Rajendram, 2016
10. *Mediterranean Diet: Impact on Health and Disease*, edited by Donato F. Romagnolo, Ph.D. and Ornella Selmin, Ph.D., 2016
11. *Nutrition Support for the Critically Ill*, edited by David S. Seres, MD and Charles W. Van Way, III, MD, 2016
12. *Nutrition in Cystic Fibrosis: A Guide for Clinicians*, edited by Elizabeth H. Yen, M.D. and Amanda R. Leonard, MPH, RD, CDE, 2016
13. *Preventive Nutrition: The Comprehensive Guide For Health Professionals, Fifth Edition*, edited by Adrianne Bendich, Ph.D. and Richard J. Deckelbaum, M.D., 2016
14. *Glutamine in Clinical Nutrition*, edited by Rajkumar Rajendram, Victor R. Preedy, and Vinood B. Patel, 2015
15. *Nutrition and Bone Health, Second Edition*, edited by Michael F. Holick and Jeri W. Nieves, 2015

16. *Branched Chain Amino Acids in Clinical Nutrition, Volume II*, edited by Rajkumar Rajendram, Victor R. Preedy, and Vinood B. Patel, 2015

17. *Branched Chain Amino Acids in Clinical Nutrition, Volume I*, edited by Rajkumar Rajendram, Victor R. Preedy, and Vinood B. Patel, 2015

18. *Fructose, High Fructose Corn Syrup, Sucrose and Health*, edited by James M. Rippe, 2014

19. *Handbook of Clinical Nutrition and Aging, Third Edition*, edited by Connie Watkins Bales, Julie L. Locher, and Edward Saltzman, 2014

20. *Nutrition and Pediatric Pulmonary Disease*, edited by Dr. Youngran Chung and Dr. Robert Dumont, 2014

21. *Integrative Weight Management*, edited by Dr. Gerald E. Mullin, Dr. Lawrence J. Cheskin, and Dr. Laura E. Matarese, 2014

22. *Nutrition in Kidney Disease, Second Edition*, edited by Dr. Laura D. Byham-Gray, Dr. Jerrilynn D. Burrowes, and Dr. Glenn M. Chertow, 2014

23. *Handbook of Food Fortification and Health, Volume I*, edited by Dr. Victor R. Preedy, Dr. Rajaventhan Srirajaskanthan, Dr. Vinood B. Patel, 2013

24. *Handbook of Food Fortification and Health, Volume II*, edited by Dr. Victor R. Preedy, Dr. Rajaventhan Srirajaskanthan, Dr. Vinood B. Patel, 2013

25. *Diet Quality: An Evidence-Based Approach, Volume I*, edited by Dr. Victor R. Preedy, Dr. Lan-Ahn Hunter, and Dr. Vinood B. Patel, 2013

26. *Diet Quality: An Evidence-Based Approach, Volume II*, edited by Dr. Victor R. Preedy, Dr. Lan-Ahn Hunter, and Dr. Vinood B. Patel, 2013

27. *The Handbook of Clinical Nutrition and Stroke*, edited by Mandy L. Corrigan, MPH, RD Arlene A. Escuro, MS, RD, and Donald F. Kirby, MD, FACP, FACN, FACG, 2013

28. *Nutrition in Infancy, Volume I*, edited by Dr. Ronald Ross Watson, Dr. George Grimble, Dr. Victor Preedy, and Dr. Sherma Zibadi, 2013

29. *Nutrition in Infancy, Volume II*, edited by Dr. Ronald Ross Watson, Dr. George Grimble, Dr. Victor Preedy, and Dr. Sherma Zibadi, 2013

30. *Carotenoids and Human Health*, edited by Dr. Sherry A. Tanumihardjo, 2013

31. *Bioactive Dietary Factors and Plant Extracts in Dermatology*, edited by Dr. Ronald Ross Watson and Dr. Sherma Zibadi, 2013

32. *Omega 6/3 Fatty Acids*, edited by Dr. Fabien De Meester, Dr. Ronald Ross Watson, and Dr. Sherma Zibadi, 2013

33. *Nutrition in Pediatric Pulmonary Disease*, edited by Dr. Robert Dumont and Dr. Youngran Chung, 2013

34. *Nutrition and Diet in Menopause*, edited by Dr. Caroline J. Hollins Martin, Dr. Ronald Ross Watson, and Dr. Victor R. Preedy, 2013.

35. *Magnesium and Health*, edited by Dr. Ronald Ross Watson and Dr. Victor R. Preedy, 2012.

36. *Alcohol, Nutrition and Health Consequences*, edited by Dr. Ronald Ross Watson, Dr. Victor R. Preedy, and Dr. Sherma Zibadi, 2012

37. *Nutritional Health, Strategies for Disease Prevention, Third Edition*, edited by Norman J. Temple, Ted Wilson, and David R. Jacobs, Jr., 2012

38. *Chocolate in Health and Nutrition*, edited by Dr. Ronald Ross Watson, Dr. Victor R. Preedy, and Dr. Sherma Zibadi, 2012

39. *Iron Physiology and Pathophysiology in Humans*, edited by Dr. Gregory J. Anderson and Dr. Gordon D. McLaren, 2012

Earlier books included *Vitamin D, Second Edition*, edited by Dr. Michael Holick; *Dietary Components and Immune Function* edited by Dr. Ronald Ross Watson, Dr. Sherma Zibadi, and Dr. Victor R. Preedy; *Bioactive Compounds and Cancer* edited by Dr. John A. Milner and Dr. Donato F. Romagnolo; *Modern Dietary Fat Intakes in Disease Promotion* edited by Dr. Fabien De Meester, Dr. Sherma Zibadi, and Dr. Ronald Ross Watson; *Iron Deficiency and Overload* edited by Dr. Shlomo

Yehuda and Dr. David Mostofsky; *Nutrition Guide for Physicians* edited by Dr. Edward Wilson, Dr. George A. Bray, Dr. Norman Temple, and Dr. Mary Struble; *Nutrition and Metabolism* edited by Dr. Christos Mantzoros; and *Fluid and Electrolytes in Pediatrics* edited by Leonard Feld and Dr. Frederick Kaskel. Recent volumes include: *Handbook of Drug-Nutrient Interactions* edited by Dr. Joseph Boullata and Dr. Vincent Armenti; *Probiotics in Pediatric Medicine* edited by Dr. Sonia Michail and Dr. Philip Sherman; *Handbook of Nutrition and Pregnancy* edited by Dr. Carol Lammi-Keefe, Dr. Sarah Couch, and Dr. Elliot Philipson; *Nutrition and Rheumatic Disease* edited by Dr. Laura Coleman; *Nutrition and Kidney Disease* edited by Dr. Laura Byham-Grey, Dr. Jerrilynn Burrowes, and Dr. Glenn Chertow; *Nutrition and Health in Developing Countries* edited by Dr. Richard Semba and Dr. Martin Bloem; *Calcium in Human Health* edited by Dr. Robert Heaney and Dr. Connie Weaver; and *Nutrition and Bone Health* edited by Dr. Michael Holick and Dr. Bess Dawson-Hughes.

Dr. Bendich is President of Consultants in Consumer Healthcare LLC and is the editor of ten books including *Preventive Nutrition: The Comprehensive Guide for Health Professionals, Fifth Edition*, co-edited with Dr. Richard Deckelbaum (www.springer.com/series/7659). Dr. Bendich serves on the Editorial Boards of the *Journal of Nutrition in Gerontology and Geriatrics*, and *Antioxidants*, and has served as Associate Editor for *Nutrition*, the International Journal; served on the Editorial Board of the *Journal of Women's Health and Gender-Based Medicine*; and served on the Board of Directors of the American College of Nutrition.

Dr. Bendich was Director of Medical Affairs at GlaxoSmithKline (GSK) Consumer Healthcare and provided medical leadership for many well-known brands including TUMS and Os-Cal. Dr. Bendich had primary responsibility for GSK's support for the Women's Health Initiative (WHI) intervention study. Prior to joining GSK, Dr. Bendich was at Roche Vitamins Inc. and was involved with the groundbreaking clinical studies showing that folic acid-containing multivitamins significantly reduced major classes of birth defects. Dr. Bendich has co-authored over 100 major clinical research studies in the area of preventive nutrition. She is recognized as a leading authority on antioxidants, nutrition and immunity and pregnancy outcomes, vitamin safety, and the cost-effectiveness of vitamin/mineral supplementation.

Dr. Bendich received the Roche Research Award, is a *Tribute to Women and Industry* Awardee, and was a recipient of the Burroughs Wellcome Visiting Professorship in Basic Medical Sciences. Dr. Bendich was given the Council for Responsible Nutrition (CRN) Apple Award in recognition of her many contributions to the scientific understanding of dietary supplements. In 2012, she was recognized for her contributions to the field of clinical nutrition by the American Society for Nutrition and was elected a Fellow of ASN. Dr. Bendich is Adjunct Professor at Rutgers University. She is listed in *Who's Who of American Women*.

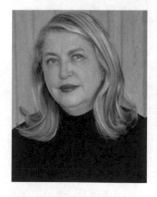 **Connie W. Bales, PhD, RD** is Professor of Medicine in the Division of Geriatrics, Department of Medicine, at the Duke School of Medicine and Senior Fellow in the Center for the Study of Aging and Human Development at Duke University Medical Center. She is also Associate Director for Education/Evaluation of the Geriatrics Research, Education, and Clinical Center at the Durham VA Medical Center. Dr. Bales is a well-recognized expert in the field of nutrition, chronic disease, function, and aging. Over the past two decades her laboratory at Duke has explored many different aspects of diet and activity as determinants of health during the latter half of the adult life course. Her current research focuses primarily on the impact of protein-enhanced meals on muscle quality, function, and other health indicators during obesity reduction in older adults with functional limitations. Dr. Bales has served on NIH and USDA grant review panels and is a member of the American Society for Nutrition's Medical Nutrition Council. Dr. Bales has edited three editions of the *Handbook of Clinical Nutrition in Aging and is Editor-in-Chief of the Journal of Nutrition in Gerontology and Geriatrics*.

Editors Bio

Dr. Rajkumar Rajendram, AKC, BSc. (Hons), MBBS (Dist), MRCP (UK), FRCA, EDIC, FFICM

Consultant in Internal Medicine
King Abdulaziz Medical City
Riyadh
Saudi Arabia

Visiting Lecturer
Division of Diabetes and Nutritional Sciences
King's College London

Dr. Rajkumar Rajendram is a clinician scientist whose focus is on perioperative medicine, anesthesia, and intensive care. One of the many aspects of his role is fetal nutritional support through the management of maternal diabetes and nutrition. Dr. Rajendram graduated in 2001 with a distinction from Guy's, King's and St. Thomas Medical School in London. As an undergraduate, he was awarded several prizes, merits, and distinctions in preclinical and clinical subjects.

Dr. Rajendram began his postgraduate medical training in general medicine and intensive care in Oxford. He attained membership of the Royal College of Physicians (MRCP) in 2004 and completed specialist training in acute and general medicine in Oxford in 2010. Dr. Rajendram also trained in anesthesia and intensive care in London and became a fellow of the Royal College of Anaesthetists (FRCA) in 2009. He has completed advanced training in regional anesthesia and intensive care. He became a fellow of the Faculty of Intensive Care Medicine (FFICM) in 2013 and obtained the European diploma of intensive care medicine (EDIC) in 2014.

Dr. Rajendram returned to Oxford as a consultant in general medicine at the John Radcliffe Hospital, Oxford, before moving to the Royal Free London Hospitals as a consultant in intensive care, anesthesia, and perioperative medicine. He is currently a consultant in internal and perioperative medicine at King Abdulaziz Medical City, Riyadh, Saudi Arabia.

Dr. Rajendram recognizes that nutritional support is a fundamental aspect of perioperative medicine. As a clinician scientist, he has therefore devoted significant time and effort into nutritional science research. As a visiting lecturer in the Division of Diabetes and Nutritional Sciences, King's College London, he has published over 100 textbook chapters, review articles, peer-reviewed papers, and abstracts.

Victor R. Preedy, BSc, PhD, DSc, FRSB, FRSPH, FRCPath, FRSC, is a senior staff member of the Faculty of Life Sciences and Medicine within King's College London. He is a member of the Division of Diabetes and Nutritional Sciences (research) and the Department of Nutrition and Dietetics (teaching). Additionally, Professor Preedy is the director of the Genomics Centre of King's College London.

Professor Preedy graduated in 1974 with an honors degree in biology and physiology with pharmacology. He gained his University of London Ph.D. in 1981. In 1992, he received his membership of the Royal College of Pathologists, and in 1993, he gained his second doctorate (D.Sc.), for his outstanding contribution to protein metabolism in health and disease. Professor Preedy was elected as a fellow to the Institute of Biology in 1995 and to the Royal College of Pathologists in 2000. Since then, he has been elected as a fellow to the Royal Society for the Promotion of Health (2004) and the Royal Institute of Public Health (2004). In 2009, Professor Preedy became a fellow of the Royal Society for Public Health and, in 2012, a fellow of the Royal Society of Chemistry. Professor Preedy has carried out research at the National Heart Hospital (part of Imperial College London), the School of Pharmacy (now part of University College London), and the MRC Centre at Northwick Park Hospital. He has collaborated with research groups in Finland, Japan, Australia, the USA, and Germany. Professor Preedy has a long-standing interest in the science of health including the impact of nutrition on the various life stages. To his credit, Professor Preedy has published over 600 articles, which include peer-reviewed manuscripts based on original research, abstracts and symposium presentations, reviews, and numerous books and volumes.

Dr. **Vinood B. Patel, BSc**, **PhD**, **FRSC**, is a reader in clinical biochemistry at the University of Westminster and honorary fellow at King's College London. Dr. Patel graduated from the University of Portsmouth with a degree in pharmacology and completed his Ph.D. in protein metabolism from King's College London in 1997. His postdoctoral work was carried out at Wake Forest University Baptist Medical School studying structural-functional alterations to mitochondrial ribosomes, where he developed novel techniques to characterize their biophysical properties. Dr. Patel is a nationally and internationally recognized scientist, and in 2014, he was elected as a fellow to the Royal Society of Chemistry. He presently directs studies on metabolic pathways involved in tissue pathology particularly related to mitochondrial energy regulation and cell death. Research is being undertaken to study the role of nutrients, antioxidants, phytochemicals, iron, alcohol, and fatty acids in tissue pathology. Other areas of interest are identifying new biomarkers that can be used for diagnosis and prognosis of liver disease and understanding mitochondrial oxidative stress in Alzheimer's disease and gastrointestinal dysfunction in autism. Dr. Patel has edited biomedical books in the area of nutrition and health, disease prevention, autism, and biomarkers and has published over 150 articles.

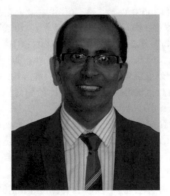

Dr. Vinood Patel
Reader in Clinical Biochemistry
Course Leader for M.Sc Biomedical Sciences (Clinical Biochemistry)

Acknowledgments

The development of this book is built upon the foundation of the excellent work provided by the staff of Humana and Springer Nature. In particular, we wish to acknowledge the outstanding support, advice, and great patience of the series editor, Dr. Adrianne Bendich; the developmental editor, Michael Griffin; and assistant editor, Samantha Lonuzzi.

Contents

Part I Maternal Diet, Health and the Fetus: General Considerations

1 Prenatal Maternal Stress in Context: Maternal Stress Physiology, Immunology,
Neuroendocrinology, Nutrition and Infant Development 3
Emily S. Barrett, Ana Vallejo Sefair, and Thomas G. O'Connor

2 The Effects of Parental Diet on Fetal Programming
of Stress-Related Brain Regions and Behaviours: Implications for Development
of Neuropsychiatric Disorders 15
Austin C. Korgan and Tara S. Perrot

3 Maternal Nutrition and Cognition 29
Rachael M. Taylor, Roger Smith, Clare E. Collins, and Alexis J. Hure

4 Maternal Fitness and Infant Birth Weight 43
Michèle Bisson and Isabelle Marc

5 Maternal Characteristics Predisposing to Fetal Growth Restriction 55
Irene Cetin, Chiara Mandò, and Francesca Parisi

6 Maternal Insulin Sensitivity and Fetal Brain Activity 67
Franziska Schleger, Katarzyna Linder, Andreas Fritsche, and Hubert Preissl

Part II Maternal Undernutrition and Protein Restriction: Effects on Fetus

7 Dietary Restriction and the Endocrine Profiles in Offspring and Adults 81
Young Ju Kim

8 Maternal Undernutrition and Visceral Adiposity 91
Prabhat Khanal and Mette Olaf Nielsen

9 Maternal Undernutrition and Long-Term Effects on Hepatic Function 107
Daniel B. Hardy

10 Maternal Protein Restriction and Its Effects on Heart 121
Heloisa Balan Assalin, José Antonio Rocha Gontijo, and Patrícia Aline Boer

11 Effects of Maternal Protein Restriction on Nephrogenesis and Adult
and Aging Kidney 131
Patrícia Aline Boer, Ana Tereza Barufi Franco, and José Antonio Rocha Gontijo

12 Maternal Protein Restriction and Effects on Behavior and Memory in Offspring 145
Agnes da Silva Lopes Oliveira, José Antonio Rocha Gontijo, and Patrícia Aline Boer

Part III Effects of Obesity, High Fat Diet and Junk Food on Fetal Outcomes

13 **Trends in Obesity and Implications for the Fetus**.. 159
Jamie O. Lo and Antonio E. Frias

14 **Maternal Obesity and Implications for Fetal Programming**............................... 171
Stephen P. Ford and John F. Odhiambo

15 **Ethnicity, Obesity, and Pregnancy Outcomes on Fetal Programming**.............. 185
Miranda Davies-Tuck, Mary-Ann Davey, Joel A. Fernandez, Maya Reddy,
Marina G. Caulfield, and Euan Wallace

16 **Obesogenic Programming of Foetal Hepatic Metabolism by microRNAs**.......... 199
Laís Angélica de Paula Simino, Marcio Alberto Torsoni, and Adriana Souza Torsoni

17 **Impacts of Maternal High-Fat Diet on Stress-Related Behaviour
and the Endocrine Response to Stress in Offspring**.. 213
Sameera Abuaish and Patrick O. McGowan

18 **Maternal Junk Food Diets: The Effects on Offspring Fat Mass and Food
Preferences**... 227
Beverly S. Muhlhausler, Jessica R. Gugusheff, and Simon C. Langley-Evans

Part IV Specific Dietary Components

19 **Maternal Fish Intake During Pregnancy and Effects on the Offspring**.............. 241
Leda Chatzi and Nikos Stratakis

20 **Maternal Fish Oil Intake and Insulin Resistance in the Offspring**................... 261
Emilio Herrera, Patricia Casas-Agustench, and Alberto Dávalos

21 **Maternal n-3 Fatty Acids and Blood Pressure in Children**................................ 279
Hasthi U.W. Dissanayake, Melinda Phang, and Michael R. Skilton

22 **Maternal Folate, Methyl Donors, One-Carbon Metabolism, Vitamin B12
and Choline in Foetal Programming**.. 293
Jean-Louis Guéant and Rosa-Maria Guéant-Rodriguez

23 **Maternal Taurine Supplementation Prevents Misprogramming**........................ 309
Edith Arany

24 **Fetal Programming: Maternal Diets, Tryptophan, and Postnatal Development**......... 325
Giuseppe Musumeci, Paola Castrogiovanni, Francesca Maria Trovato,
Marta Anna Szychlinska, and Rosa Imbesi

25 **Intrauterine Programming and Effects of Caffeine**.. 339
Zhexiao Jiao, Hao Kou, Dan Xu, Hanwen Luo, and Hui Wang

Part V International Aspects and Policies

26 **Famines, Pregnancy and Effect on the Adults**... 357
Matthew Edwards

27 **Maternal Malnutrition, Foetal Programming, Outcomes and Strategies in India**...... 371
Poornima Prabhakaran and Prabhakaran Dorairaj

28 **Maternal Nutritional Factors Dictating Birth Weights: African Perspectives**........... 385
Baba Usman Ahmadu

Contents

29 Maternal Nutrition in Ireland: Issues of Public Health Concern.................................. 393
John M. Kearney and Elizabeth J. O'Sullivan

30 Maternal Malnutrition, Fetal Programming, Outcomes, and Implications
of Environmental Factors in Japan... 411
Hideko Sone and Tin-Tin Win-Shwe

Part VI Effects of Fetal Programming in Childhood and Adulthood

31 Growth Criteria and Predictors of Fetal Programming.............................. 431
Sandra da Silva Mattos and Felipe Alves Mourato

32 Effects of Fetal Programming on Metabolic Syndrome 439
Renata Pereira Alambert and Marcelo Lima de Gusmão Correia

33 Fetal Programming of Food Preferences and Feeding Behavior.................. 453
Adrianne Rahde Bischoff, Roberta DalleMolle, and Patrícia Pelufo Silveira

34 Effects of Fetal Programming on Osteoporosis.. 471
George M. Weisz and William Randall Albury

35 Childhood Sleep After Fetal Growth Restriction...................................... 487
Stephanie R. Yiallourou

Part VII Mechanisms of Programming

36 Biomarkers of Abnormal Birth Weight in Pregnancy.............................. 503
Beata Anna Raczkowska, Monika Zbucka-Kretowska, Adam Kretowski,
and Michal Ciborowski

37 Mechanisms of Programming: Pancreatic Islets and Fetal Programming.................. 517
Luiz F. Barella, Paulo C. F. Mathias, and Júlio C. de Oliveira

38 Pancreatic GABA and Serotonin Actions in the Pancreas
and Fetal Programming of Metabolism.. 529
David J. Hill

39 Maternal Malnutrition, Glucocorticoids, and Fetal Programming: A Role
for Placental 11β-Hydroxysteroid Dehydrogenase Type 2.......................... 543
Emily K. Chivers and Caitlin S. Wyrwoll

40 High-Fat Diet and Foetal Programming: Use of P66Shc Knockouts
and Implications for Human Kind.. 557
Alessandra Berry and Francesca Cirulli

41 Fetal Programming of Telomere Biology: Role of Maternal Nutrition,
Obstetric Risk Factors, and Suboptimal
Birth Outcomes 569
Sonja Entringer, Karin de Punder, Glenn Verner, and Pathik D. Wadhwa

Part VIII Resources

42 Current Research and Recommended Resources on Fetal Nutrition 597
Rajkumar Rajendram, Vinood B. Patel, and Victor R. Preedy

Index.. 605

Contributors

Sameera Abuaish, MSc Department of Biological Sciences and Center for Environmental Epigenetics and Development, University of Toronto Scarborough, Toronto, ON, Canada

Departments of Cell and Systems Biology, University of Toronto, Toronto, ON, Canada

Baba Usman Ahmadu, MBBS, MHPM, FMCPaed Fellow National Postgraduate Medical College Nigeria, Paediatrics (FMCPaed), Member Paediatric Association of Nigeria (PAN), Member Medical and Dental Consultant Association of Nigeria (MDCAN), Member Nigerian Medical Association (NMA). Paediatrician and Visiting Paediatrician at Federal Medical Centre Yola, Abubakar Tafawa Balewa Teaching Hospital Bauchi and Federal Medical Centre Jalingo. Chair, Co-Chair and Member of Committees, Yola, Adamawa State, Nigeria

Renata Pereira Alambert, PhD Department of Internal Medicine – Endocrinology and Metabolism, FOE Diabetes Research Center, University of Iowa, Iowa City, IA, USA

William Randall Albury, BA, PhD School of Humanities, University of New England, Armidale, NSW, Australia

Edith Arany, MD, PhD Schulich School of Medicine and Dentistry, Department of Pathology and Laboratory Medicine, Lawson Health Research Institute & the Children Health Institute, University of Western Ontario, London, ON, Canada

Heloisa Balan Assalin, BSc, PhD Department of Internal Medicine, Faculty of Medical Sciences, University of Campinas, Campinas, SP, Brazil

Luiz F. Barella, PhD Laboratory of Secretion Cell Biology, Department of Biotechnology, Genetics and Cell Biology, State University of Maringa, Maringa, PR, Brazil

Molecular Signaling Section, Laboratory of Bioorganic Chemistry, National Institute of Diabetes and Digestive and Kidney Diseases, National Institutes of Health (NIDDK/NIH), Bethesda, MD, USA

Emily S. Barrett, PhD Department of Epidemiology, Rutgers University School of Public Health, Piscataway, NY, USA

Department of Obstetrics and Gynecology, University of Rochester School of Medicine and Dentistry, Rochester, NY, USA

Alessandra Berry, PhD Center for Behavioral Sciences and Mental Health, Istituto Superiore di Sanità, Rome, Italy

Adrianne Rahde Bischoff, MD Division of Neonatology in the Department of Pediatrics, University of Toronto and the Hospital for Sick Children, Toronto, ON, Canada

Michèle Bisson, PhD Department of Pediatrics, Centre Hospitalier Universitaire de Québec-Université Laval, Québec City, PQ, Canada

Patrícia Aline Boer, BSc, PhD Department of Internal Medicine, Faculty of Medical Sciences, University of Campinas, Campinas, SP, Brazil

Patricia Casas-Agustench, PhD Laboratory of Disorders of Lipid Metabolism and Molecular Nutrition, IMDEA Food Institute, Madrid, Spain

Paola Castrogiovanni, PhD Department of Biomedical and Biotechnological Sciences, Human Anatomy and Histology Section, School of Medicine, University of Catania, Catania, Italy

Marina G. Caulfield, MBBS (Hons), BMedSc (Hons) Department of Obstetrics and Gynecology, Monash University, Clayton, VIC, Australia

Irene Cetin, MD, PhD Department of Biomedical and Clinical Sciences "L. Sacco" and Centro di Ricerche Fetali Giorgio Pardi, University of Milan, Milan, Italy

Leda Chatzi, MD, PhD Keck School of Medicine, Division of Environmental Health, University of Southern California, Los Angeles, California, USA

Department of Social Medicine, Faculty of Medicine, University of Crete, Heraklion, Crete, Greece

Department of Genetics & Cell Biology Faculty of Health, Medicine and Life Sciences Maastricht University, The Netherlands

Emily K. Chivers, BSc School of Human Sciences, The University of Western Australia, Crawley, WA, Australia

Michal Ciborowski, PhD Clinical Research Centre, Medical University of Bialystok, Bialystok, Poland

Francesca Cirulli, PhD Center for Behavioral Sciences and Mental Health, Istituto Superiore di Sanità, Rome, Italy

Clare E. Collins Priority Research Centre for Physical Activity and Nutrition, University of Newcastle, Newcastle, NSW, Australia

Marcelo Lima de Gusmão Correia, MD, PhD Department of Internal Medicine – Endocrinology and Metabolism, FOE Diabetes Research Center, University of Iowa, Iowa City, IA, USA

Roberta DalleMolle, MSc, PhD McGill Center for the Convergence of Health and Economics and Montreal Neurological Institute McGill University, Montreal, QC, Canada

Alberto Dávalos, PhD Laboratory of Disorders of Lipid Metabolism and Molecular Nutrition, IMDEA Food Institute, Madrid, Spain

Mary-Ann Davey Department of Obstetrics and Gynaecology, School of Clinical Sciences, Monash University, Clayton, VIC, Australia

Miranda Davies-Tuck The Ritchie Centre, Hudson Institute of Medical Research, Clayton, VIC, Australia

Júlio C. de Oliveira, PhD Institute of Health Sciences, Federal University of Mato Grosso, Sinop, MT, Brazil

Hasthi U.W. Dissanayake, BSc, MPhil Boden Institute of Obesity, Nutrition, Exercise and Eating Disorders, Charles Perkins Centre, Sydney Medical School, University of Sydney, Camperdown, NSW, Australia

Prabhakaran Dorairaj, MD, DM(Cardiology), MSc, FRCP, FNASc Professor, Chronic Disease Epidemiology and Vice-President, Research & Policy, Public Health Foundation of India, Gurgaon, Haryana, India

Matthew Edwards Department of Paediatrics, School of Medicine, Western Sydney University, Penrith, NSW, Australia

Sonja Entringer, PhD Department of Medical Psychology, Charité – Universitätsmedizin Berlin, corporate member of Freie Universität Berlin, Humboldt-Universität zu Berlin, and Berlin Institute of Health (BIH), Institute of Medical Psychology, Berlin, Germany

Department of Pediatric, Development, Health and Disease Research Program University of California, Irvine, School of Medicine, Irvine, CA, USA

Joel A. Fernandez, BMedSc (Hons) Department of Obstetrics and Gynaecology, Monash Medical Centre, Melbourne, VIC, Australia

Stephen P. Ford, PhD Center for the Study of Fetal Programming, Department of Animal Science, University of Wyoming, Laramie, WY, USA

Ana Tereza Barufi Franco, BSc, MSc Department of Internal Medicine, Faculty of Medical Sciences, University of Campinas, Campinas, SP, Brazil

Antonio E. Frias Department of Obstetrics and Gynecology, Oregon Health & Science University, Portland, OR, USA

Andreas Fritsche, MD Institute for Diabetes Research and Metabolic Diseases of the Helmholtz Center Munich, University of Tübingen, Tübingen, Germany

Department of Internal Medicine, Division of Endocrinology, Diabetology, Angiology, Nephrology and Clinical Chemistry, University of Tübingen, Tübingen, Germany

José Antonio Rocha Gontijo, MD, PhD Department of Internal Medicine, Faculty of Medical Sciences, University of Campinas, Campinas, SP, Brazil

Jessica R. Gugusheff, PhD FOODplus Research Centre, School of Agriculture Food and Wine, The University of Adelaide, Urrbrae, SA, Australia

Jean-Louis Guéant, MD, DSc University Hospital Nancy and Inserm 954 Research Unity, N-GERE, (Nutrition-Genetics-Environmental Risks), Institute of Medical Research (Pôle BMS), University of Lorraine, Vandoeuvre-les-Nancy, France

Rosa-Maria Guéant-Rodriguez, MD, PhD University Hospital Nancy and Inserm 954 Research Unity, N-GERE, (Nutrition-Genetics-Environmental Risks), Institute of Medical Research (Pôle BMS), University of Lorraine, Vandoeuvre-les-Nancy, France

Daniel B. Hardy, PhD The Departments of Obstetrics & Gynecology and Physiology & Pharmacology, The Children's Health Research Institute and the Lawson Health Research Institute, The University of Western Ontario, London, ON, Canada

Emilio Herrera, PhD Department of Biochemistry and Chemistry, University CEU San Pablo, Madrid, Spain

David J. Hill, BSc, DPhil Lawson Health Research Institute, St. Joseph's Health Care London, London Health Sciences Centre, and Western University, London, ON, Canada

Alexis J. Hure, PhD, BND (Hons I) Priority Research Centre for Gender, Health and Ageing, University of Newcastle, Newcastle, NSW, Australia

Rosa Imbesi, MD Department of Biomedical and Biotechnological Sciences, Human Anatomy and Histology Section, School of Medicine, University of Catania, Catania, Italy

Zhexiao Jiao, PhD pending Department of Pharmacology, Basic Medical School, Wuhan University, Wuhan, China

John M. Kearney, BSc (Ag), PgDip, PhD Dublin Institute of Technology (DIT), Biological Sciences, Dublin, Ireland

Prabhat Khanal, PhD Department of Veterinary and Animal Sciences, Faculty of Health and Medical Sciences, University of Copenhagen, Frederiksberg, Denmark

Institute of Basic Medical Sciences, Department of Nutrition, Faculty of Medicine, Norwegian Transgenic Centre, University of Oslo, Oslo, Norway

Young Ju Kim, MD, PhD Department of Obstetrics and Gynecology, College of Medicine, Ewha Womans University, Seoul, South Korea

Austin C. Korgan, MSc Department of Psychology and Neuroscience, Dalhousie University, Halifax, Nova Scotia, Canada

Hao Kou, PhD Department of Pharmacology, Basic Medical School, Wuhan University, Wuhan, China

Adam Kretowski, MD, PhD Clinical Research Centre, Medical University of Bialystok, Bialystok, Poland

Simon C. Langley-Evans, PhD School of Biosciences, University of Nottingham, Loughborough, UK

Katarzyna Linder, MD Institute for Diabetes Research and Metabolic Diseases of the Helmholtz Center Munich, University of Tübingen, Tübingen, Germany

Department of Internal Medicine, Division of Endocrinology, Diabetology, Angiology, Nephrology and Clinical Chemistry, University of Tübingen, Tübingen, Germany

Jamie O. Lo, MD Department of Obstetrics and Gynecology, Oregon Health & Science University, Portland, OR, USA

Hanwen Luo, MD Department of Pharmacology, Basic Medical School, Wuhan University, Wuhan, China

Chiara Mandò, PhD Department of Biomedical and Clinical Sciences "L. Sacco" and Centro di Ricerche Fetali Giorgio Pardi, University of Milan, Milan, Italy

Isabelle Marc, MD, PhD Department of Pediatrics, Centre Hospitalier Universitaire de Québec-Université Laval, Québec City, PQ, Canada

Paulo C.F. Mathias, PhD Laboratory of Secretion Cell Biology, Department of Biotechnology, Genetics and Cell Biology, State University of Maringa, Maringa, PR, Brazil

Sandra da Silva Mattos, MD, PhD Royal Portuguese Hospital, Maternal Fetal Cardiac Unit, Recife, PE, Brazil

Patrick O. McGowan, PhD Department of Biological Sciences and Center for Environmental Epigenetics and Development, University of Toronto Scarborough, Toronto, ON, Canada

Departments of Cell and Systems Biology, University of Toronto, Toronto, ON, Canada

Felipe Alves Mourato, MD, MSc Royal Portuguese Hospital, Maternal Fetal Cardiac Unit, Recife, PE, Brazil

Beverly S. Muhlhausler, PhD FOODplus Research Centre, School of Agriculture Food and Wine, The University of Adelaide, Urrbrae, SA, Australia

Giuseppe Musumeci, PhD Department of Biomedical and Biotechnological Sciences, Human Anatomy and Histology Section, School of Medicine, University of Catania, Catania, Italy

Mette Olaf Nielsen, PhD Department of Large Animal Sciences, Faculty of Health and Medical Sciences, University of Copenhagen, Frederiksberg, Denmark

John F. Odhiambo, PhD Center for the Study of Fetal Programming, Department of Animal Science, University of Wyoming, Laramie, WY, USA

Thomas G. O'Connor, PhD Department of Psychiatry, University of Rochester Medical Center, Rochester, NY, USA

Elizabeth J. O'Sullivan, BA, BSc, PgDip, PhD Dublin Institute of Technology (DIT), School of Biological Sciences, Dublin, Ireland

Agnes da Silva Lopes Oliveira, BSc, PhD Department of Internal Medicine, School of Medicine, State University of Campinas, Campinas, SP, Brazil

Francesca Parisi, MD Department of Biomedical and Clinical Sciences "L. Sacco" and Centro di Ricerche Fetali Giorgio Pardi, University of Milan, Milan, Italy

Vinood B. Patel University of Westminster, Faculty of Science & Technology, Department of Biomedical Sciences, London, UK

Tara S. Perrot, PhD Department of Psychology and Neuroscience, Dalhousie University, Halifax, Nova Scotia, Canada

Melinda Phang Boden Institute of Obesity, Nutrition, Exercise and Eating Disorders, Charles Perkins Centre, Sydney Medical School, University of Sydney, Camperdown, NSW, Australia

Poornima Prabhakaran, MBBS, MSc(Epidemiology), PhD(Social Medicine) Associate Professor and Senior Research Scientist, Chronic Disease Epidemiology and Fellow, Centre for Environmental Health, Public Health Foundation of India, Gurgaon, Haryana, India

Hubert Preissl, PhD Institute for Diabetes Research and Metabolic Diseases of the Helmholtz Center Munich, University of Tübingen, Tübingen, Germany

Victor R. Preedy Department of Nutrition and Dietetics, Nutritional Sciences Division, School of Biomedical & Health Sciences, King's College London, London, UK

Karin de Punder, MSc Charité – Universitätsmedizin Berlin, corporate member of Freie Universität Berlin, Humboldt-Universität zu Berlin, and Berlin Institute of Health (BIH), Institute of Medical Psychology, Laramie, WY, USA

Beata Anna Raczkowska, MSc Department of Endocrinology, Diabetology and Internal Medicine, Medical University of Bialystok, Bialystok, Poland

Rajkumar Rajendram, AKC BSc. (hons) MBBS (dist) EDIC FRCP Edin Department of Internal Medicine, King Abdulaziz Medical City, Riyadh, Ministry of National Guard Health Affairs, Saudi Arabia

King's College London, Department of Nutrition and Dietetics, Nutritional Sciences Division, School of Biomedical & Health Sciences, London, UK

Maya Reddy Monash Health, Monash Medical Centre, Clayton, Australia

Franziska Schleger, PhD Institute for Diabetes Research and Metabolic Diseases of the Helmholtz Center Munich, University of Tübingen, Tübingen, Germany

Ana Vallejo Sefair, BA Department of Clinical and Social Sciences in Psychology, University of Rochester, Rochester, NY, USA

Patrícia Pelufo Silveira, MD, PhD Departamento de Pediatria – FAMED – Universidade Federal do Rio Grande do Sul, Porto Alegre, RS, Brazil

Ludmer Centre for Neuroinformatics and Mental Health, Douglas Mental Health University Institute, McGill University, Montreal, QC, Canada

Lais Angélica de Paula Simino, MSc Laboratory of Metabolic Disorders, School of Applied Sciences, University of Campinas, Limeira, SP, Brazil

Michael R. Skilton, BSc, PhD Boden Institute of Obesity, Nutrition, Exercise and Eating Disorders, Charles Perkins Centre, Sydney Medical School, University of Sydney, NSW, Australia

Roger Smith, MB, BS (Hons) PhD Department of Endocrinology, John Hunter Hospital, Mothers and Babies Research Centre, University of Newcastle, Newcastle, NSW, Australia

Hideko Sone, PhD Center for Health and Environmental Risk Research National Institute for Environmental Studies 16-2 Onogawa, Tsukuba, Ibaraki, Japan

Nikos Stratakis, MSc NUTRIM School of Nutrition and Translational Research in Metabolism, Faculty of Health, Medicine and Life Sciences, Maastricht University Medical Centre, Maastricht, The Netherlands

Marta Anna Szychlinska, PhD Department of Biomedical and Biotechnological Sciences, Human Anatomy and Histology Section, School of Medicine, University of Catania, University Hospital Vittorio Emanuele, Catania, Italy

Rachael M. Taylor, BND Mothers and Babies Research Centre, University of Newcastle, Newcastle, NSW, Australia

Adriana Souza Torsoni, PhD Laboratory of Metabolic Disorders, School of Applied Sciences, University of Campinas, Limeira, SP, Brazil

Marcio Alberto Torsoni, PhD Laboratory of Metabolic Disorders, School of Applied Sciences, University of Campinas, Limeira, SP, Brazil

Francesca Maria Trovato, MD Department of Clinical and Experimental Medicine, Internal Medicine Division, School of Medicine, University of Catania, Catania, Italy

Department of Clinical and Experimental Medicine, Internal Medicine Division, School of Medicine, University of Catania, Catania, Italy

Glenn Verner, MSc Charité – Universitätsmedizin Berlin, corporate member of Freie Universität Berlin, Humboldt-Universität zu Berlin, and Berlin Institute of Health (BIH), Institute of Medical Psychology, Berlin, Germany

École des Hautes Études en Santé Publique, Paris, France

Pathik D. Wadhwa, MD Departments of Psychiatry & Human Behavior, Obstetrics & Gynecology, Pediatrics, Epidemiology, Development, Health and Disease Research Program, University of California, Irvine, School of Medicine, Irvine, CA, USA

Euan Wallace Department of Obstetrics and Gynecology, Monash University, Clayton, VIC, Australia

George M. Weisz, MD, BA, MA, DR, FRACS (Ortho) School of Humanities and Languages, University of New South Wales, Sydney, NSW, Australia

School of Humanities, University of New England, Armidale, NSW, Australia

Tin-Tin Win-Shwe, MD, PhD Center for Health and Environmental Risk Research National Institute for Environmental Studies 16-2 Onogawa, Tsukuba, Ibaraki, Japan

Hui Wang, PhD Department of Pharmacology, Basic Medical School, Wuhan University, Wuhan, China

Caitlin S. Wyrwoll, PhD School of Human Sciences, The University of Western Australia, Crawley, WA, Australia

Dan Xu, PhD Department of Pharmacology, Basic Medical School, Wuhan University, Wuhan, China

Stephanie R. Yiallourou, BSc (Hons), PhD Centre for Primary Care and Prevention, Mary MacKillop Institute for Health Research, Australian Catholic University, Melbourne, VIC, Australia

Monika Zbucka-Kretowska Department of Reproduction and Gynecological Endocrinology, Medical University of Bialystok, Bialystok, Poland

Part I
Maternal Diet, Health and the Fetus: General Considerations

Chapter 1
Prenatal Maternal Stress in Context: Maternal Stress Physiology, Immunology, Neuroendocrinology, Nutrition and Infant Development

Emily S. Barrett, Ana Vallejo Sefair, and Thomas G. O'Connor

Key Points

- Although typically studied individually, prenatal stress and dietary factors often covary and may affect the same developing body systems.
- There is an extensive body of literature on prenatal stress and infant development, with a heavy emphasis on the role of the hypothalamic-pituitary-adrenal axis.
- Prenatal stress has been linked to impaired prenatal growth followed by rapid postnatal catch-up growth.
- Stress may alter maternal prenatal immune function with downstream effects on the child's development.
- Children born to stressed mothers show long-lasting changes in brain activity, behavior, and temperament.
- Additional research is needed to explore the overlapping contributions of diet and stress in shaping infant developmental trajectories.

Keywords Prenatal stress • Anxiety • Pregnancy • Infant development • Fetal programming • HPA axis • Immune function • Neurodevelopment

Abbreviations

BBB   Blood brain barrier
CRH   Corticotropin releasing hormone
DoHaD   Developmental origins of health and disease
HPA   Hypothalamic-pituitary-adrenal

E.S. Barrett, PhD (✉)
Department of Epidemiology, Rutgers University School of Public Health, Piscataway, NJ, USA

Department of Obstetrics and Gynecology, University of Rochester School of Medicine and Dentistry, Rochester, NY, USA
e-mail: emily.barrett@eohsi.rutgers.edu

A.V. Sefair, BA
Department of Clinical and Social Sciences in Psychology, University of Rochester, Rochester, NY, USA

T.G. O'Connor, PhD
Department of Psychiatry, University of Rochester Medical Center, Rochester, NY, USA

© Springer International Publishing AG 2017
R. Rajendram et al. (eds.), *Diet, Nutrition, and Fetal Programming*,
Nutrition and Health, DOI 10.1007/978-3-319-60289-9_1

Introduction

As evidenced by the current volume, there is a large and rapidly growing literature indicating that certain exposures in the prenatal period may have lasting effects on the behavior and biology of the child. Prenatal diet and nutrition is a particular focus of this volume. We seek to build upon and connect that literature to an equally large, but thus far largely separate, line of research suggesting that prenatal stress can also alter fetal and infant health and development in a manner consistent with a fetal programming hypothesis.

To date, surprisingly little research has explored the relationship between prenatal nutrition and stress in the context of infant development [1], however several lines of evidence suggest that this is an important future direction. First, maternal stress and poor nutrition often occur together. This overlap is most clearly illustrated in extreme cases such as the Dutch Hunger Winter of 1944–1945. The famine, which occurred due to military blockades during World War II, has been well-described, and individuals who gestated during that period have been followed for many decades to understand the long-term effects on their physiology (as well as that of subsequent generations) [2]. Gestational exposure to the Dutch famine has been linked to psychological [3] and metabolic [4] changes in the offspring later in life. Similar findings have been reported in studies of those who gestated during the Great Leap Forward Famine in China (1959–1961) [5, 6]. In both cases, the physiological changes observed in offspring are frequently attributed to the substantial caloric and micronutrient deficiencies that fetuses experienced during these tragic "natural experiments", however the role of stress (and stress physiology) is an important alternative explanation. With the constant military threat, limited food rations, displacement, and general upheaval, the psychological burden on the population, including pregnant women, is incontrovertible. The profound psychological distress suffered by mothers during these events could contribute to altered development in their gestating offspring; indeed, some of the earliest evidence suggesting a role of prenatal maternal stress on child health outcomes examined war as the source of psychological stress and ignored the associated nutritional deficiencies [7]. Similarly, animal models that examine fetal programming by extreme caloric restriction cannot rule out the possibility that psychological stress due to starvation confounds interpretation of the impact of diet on offspring outcomes.

It is not only in these extreme cases that stress and nutrition will likely be confounded. In daily life, under normative stressful circumstances, women may be less likely to choose healthy, nutrient rich foods [8]. Similarly, low socioeconomic status populations are disproportionately exposed to nutritionally poor (albeit often calorically rich) diets, food insecurity, and heightened psychosocial stress – suggesting that poor diet may serve as a proxy for stress exposure and vice versa. Furthermore, poor diet and nutritional deficiencies may not only be confounded by exposure to psychosocial stress, but may also interact with or modify the effects of stress. While we await the advent of multidisciplinary research that considers these exposures together [1], understanding the ways in which maternal stress may affect fetal development can inform studies of programming by diet and nutrition and vice versa can move both fields forward (Fig. 1.1). In this chapter, we review the ways in which prenatal stress (and associated constructs) alters infant behavioral and biological development; we highlight those areas for which there are particular parallels in the nutrition and stress literatures, with the goal of stimulating future research that adopts a more integrative, ecologically relevant model for human development.

Stressful situations can evoke a physiological cascade of hormone and neurotransmitter release, preparing the individual for "fight or flight". As part of this response, hypothalamic-pituitary-adrenal (HPA) axis activity is temporarily upregulated and levels of stress hormones, such as cortisol, rise to better respond to a stressor or challenge. This model applies also to pregnancy – accounting for the dominant role of HPA axis-related research on prenatal stress – although changes in the hormonal, endocrine, metabolic and immune systems in pregnancy complicate the model, especially in late pregnancy [9]. Understanding how and if maternal stress physiology alters fetal and child development

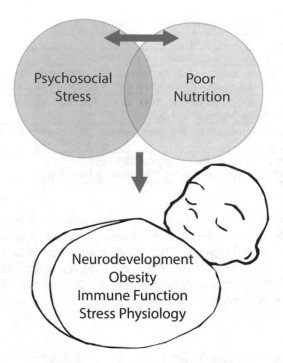

Fig. 1.1 Nutrition and stress may co-occur and interact to affect child outcomes

presents notable challenges. For example, normally during pregnancy, the placental barrier enzyme 11βHSD2 buffers the fetus from maternal stress hormones. This barrier is not impermeable, however, and there is evidence that in the face of heightened maternal stress, the enzyme may be down-regulated, allowing more cortisol to reach the fetus [10]. Accordingly, research on maternal prenatal stress physiology and fetal programming has broadened to incorporate factors that regulate this barrier enzyme. The extent to which 11βHSD2 is affected by diet and nutrition, in broad terms, is not yet evident, but one interesting example is liquorice which contains glycyrrhizin, an inhibitor of 11βHSD2. There is now evidence suggesting that liquorice consumption in pregnancy is associated with poorer cognitive development and elevated cortisol levels in the child [11] – the same outcomes that have been linked with prenatal maternal stress and will be discussed in this chapter. Although liquorice consumption may have limited relevance for the diet and nutrition of most women, this example illustrates parallels and confounds between research on prenatal maternal stress and prenatal diet and nutrition. In addition to placental mechanisms, the blood-brain barrier (BBB) of the fetus is also a reasonable target for research on prenatal maternal stress, as well as diet and nutrition. The BBB is not fully developed in the fetus and may be particularly susceptible to maternal insults including stress and inflammation [12].

Even if the mechanisms are not yet resolved, what is abundantly clear from hundreds of studies in animal models and humans is that prenatal stress can have an impact on the development of nearly every body system in the fetus. For this reason, it is impossible to comprehensively review the large body of research on stress and infant development in a single chapter. Therefore in this chapter we have selected four particular aspects of infant physiology that may have particular relevance for our aim of identifying overlap and congruence in research on prenatal maternal stress and diet and nutrition: stress physiology, growth and metabolism, immune function, and neurodevelopment.

We offer an important caveat in interpreting the research on maternal stress and child outcomes. Integrating and interpreting research on "stress" in pregnancy is complicated by the number of different (but related) terms and concepts have been used (Table 1.1). It is helpful that evidence of a prenatal

Table 1.1 Some common ways to assess psychosocial stress and related constructs during pregnancy

Construct	Description	Sample publication
Anxiety	Excessive and uncontrolled intense worry or concern	O'Donnell et al. (2012)
Life events stress	Major events such as illness, job loss, death or illness to friend or family member, or divorce that affects subjective well-being during pregnancy	Barrett et al. (2013)
Natural disasters	Acute environmental stressor (e.g., flood, ice storm) in subject's immediate environment during pregnancy	Liu et al. (2016)
Trauma	Ongoing mental or emotional response to extreme adverse events, often occurring much earlier	Moog et al. (2016)
Pregnancy-related distress	Symptoms of anxiety related to the pregnancy itself (e.g. worry about pain during labor, fears about health of fetus)	DiPietro et al. (2006)

"stress" effect on child outcomes is not confined to one measure or type of measure – and it is unlikely that these different but moderately overlapping measures differentially reflect maternal stress-related biology (neuroendocrine, immune, hormonal systems) that may alter fetal and child development. Therefore in this review, "stress" is used as a generic term, recognizing that there are multiple distinct, but over-lapping constructs that are likely to influence fetal physiology in similar ways and through similar mechanisms.

Prenatal Maternal Stress and Infant Stress Physiology

A basic tenet of and one of the most extensively tested hypotheses in this field proposes that prenatal maternal stress alters or "programs" infant stress physiology, represented most commonly by the HPA axis, including corticotropin releasing hormone [CRH] and cortisol (Fig. 1.2). These HPA axis alterations are then hypothesized to drive changes in infant behavior and biology that underlie a range of health outcomes. Animal models overwhelmingly support this hypothesis [13, 14] and such a mechanism could account for the widespread behavioral and biological effects that have been linked to prenatal maternal psychosocial stress across studies in numerous species. The basic physiological model proposes that prenatal maternal stress activates the mother's HPA axis, leading to elevated maternal cortisol levels. As discussed, maternal cortisol can crosses the placenta (in a limited manner) [15] and may also modify 11βHSD2 production, making the placenta more permeable to glucocorticoids and increasing fetal exposure to cortisol [10]. This elevated fetal exposure to cortisol is then hypothesized to program subsequent developmental trajectories, leading to a wide range of generally averse outcomes. Although well-articulated and substantiated by extensive animal data, the model is only partly confirmed by data from human studies. There is evidence that prenatal stress is associated with altered maternal cortisol profiles [16] and placental 11βHSD2 activity, with the net effect being greater prenatal exposure of the fetus to glucocorticoids [10] and altered HPA axis function in the offspring. At birth, placental expression of mitochondrial genes involved in the stress response is predicted from maternal prenatal stress levels [17]. These alterations in HPA axis activity may persist long-term. In fact, studies have found that following maternal prenatal stress, HPA axis activity is altered among offspring not only during the neonatal period and infancy [18], but even up to 15 years of age [19], suggesting the downstream sequelae of prenatal stress may be "programmed" .

Notably, there is not yet strong direct evidence that alterations in HPA axis function mediate the relationship between maternal distress during pregnancy and subsequent behavioral and biological outcomes in the child. The implication is that there may be an over-emphasis on HPA axis-mediated pathways and too little attention to alternative explanations including immune systems changes and inflammation. In addition, until recently, genetic and epigenetic changes were also under-studied. It is in this context that we reiterate an organizing theme of this chapter, that is, the current lack of integration

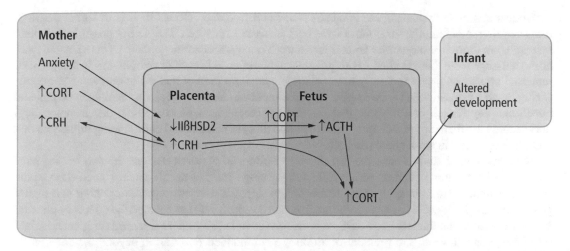

Fig. 1.2 A schematic model for understanding maternal stress, HPA axis activity, and infant development

between research on prenatal maternal stress and diet and nutrition and related factors, such as exercise. The need for integrative research is especially underscored when discussing glucocorticoids, which have, by design, a fundamental connection to stress response and diet and metabolism. Although we discuss glucocorticoids in the context of stress in this chapter, their important role in glucose metabolism and more generally, energetics should not be forgotten.

Prenatal Maternal Stress and Infant Growth and Metabolism

The hypothesis that maternal prenatal diet and nutrition can have significant and potentially lasting effects on infant growth and metabolism is strongly supported [20] and the clinical applications of this research are well-developed. Many kinds of controlled trials that manipulate prenatal diet have demonstrated that there can be beneficial effects on subsequent child outcomes; prenatal zinc is just one example [21]. What may be less familiar is the growing evidence base indicating that prenatal stress can also predict physical growth and metabolism in the baby, with potentially lasting effects and in a manner consistent with the programming hypothesis that underlies the Developmental Origins of Health and Disease (DOHaD) model. A starting point for this literature is the number of studies linking prenatal maternal stress with birth weight, gestational age, and the likelihood of being born small for dates [22, 23]. Several mechanisms have been explored. Placental concentration of CRH in late pregnancy is associated with infant birthweight (adjusting for gestational age) as well as patterns of weight gain in infancy [24]. Additionally, prenatal anxiety is associated with altered methylation of genes involved in fetal growth (IGF2 and H19), particularly in female fetuses [25].

The association between prenatal stress and fetal growth has obvious public health significance given the wealth of data linking low birth weight to endocrine and metabolic dysfunction – and ultimately cardiovascular disease and diabetes – in adulthood [26, 27]. One plausible pathway linking size at birth to adult metabolic disease is that the postnatal "catch-up growth" typical of low birth weight babies leads to the increased subsequent metabolic risk. Indeed, change in infant fat mass from birth to 6 months is among the strongest predictors of childhood obesity [28]. More recently, several studies have directly implicated maternal stress in pregnancy as a potential causal factor underlying growth patterns and body composition later in childhood; for example, neuroendocrine correlates of maternal prenatal distress such as cortisol and CRH have been associated with child adiposity and obesity [29], as well as levels of adiponectin (a protein involved in glucose regulation) at age 3 [30].

Understanding how prenatal maternal stress and nutrition may interact to alter offspring development requires manipulation or control over both of these exposures. That is not possible in human research, but there is a substantial animal literature that may offer some guidance. One valuable take-home message from these studies – with potential application to human development – is that prenatal maternal stress and prenatal dietary manipulations may both predict metabolic outcomes in the offspring, such as obesity [31]. The implication that prenatal stress may mimic the effects of prenatal nutritional deprivation or a high fat diet (or perhaps other forms of suboptimal diet in pregnancy) underscores the theme of this chapter that stress and diet are parallel and confounding influences that require integration in subsequent research.

Whereas animal studies have the benefit of experimental research designs, human studies have relied on observational studies, which offer less leverage for causal inference. Nonetheless, some intriguing findings are emerging. One interesting example is a recent report suggesting that higher polyunsaturated fatty acid intake (operationalized as the n3:n6 ratio) attenuated the effects of prenatal stress on infant temperament in an African-American sample [32]. There is a need for greater insight into how prenatal stress and prenatal nutrition are confounded that moves beyond the covariation between stress and obesity, for example, and which stress-related constructs may modify or be modified by specific nutrients in predicting infant growth and metabolism.

Prenatal Maternal Stress and Immune Function

There are many reasons for considering the maternal and infant immune systems mechanisms in the context of prenatal maternal stress. For example, the immune system is a stress-responsive system and pregnancy is itself a significant immunological stressor characterized by sizable changes in levels of pro- and anti-inflammatory cytokines [33]. In humans, the infant immune system develops prenatally and may therefore be influenced by in utero exposures, including maternal stress. In mid-gestation (approximately 20–24 weeks), the fetal immune system begins to develop in response to in utero and exogenous antigens, such as maternal antibodies and inflammatory cytokines [34]. Following this immunoregulatory response, the maternal system establishes an active immunological tolerance against placental antigens released by the fetus. The fetal and maternal tissue are not in direct contact, but the placenta functions as an important intermediary for maternal-fetal immune system communication [35]. This bi-directional communication is critical to a healthy pregnancy, and leaves the fetal immune system vulnerable to environmental disruptions and exposures in the maternal system [36]. Psychosocial stress during pregnancy can lead to immune dysregulation in the maternal environment, which in turn may alter brain development and immune function in the child [12, 37].

Research on the impact of prenatal maternal stress on maternal and child immune function, and the potentially complicating role of diet and nutrition, is just beginning. This line of research has the important disadvantage that there is a less well-developed animal model, and the animal data reported may be a less than adequate guide. That is, although there are many studies of prenatal stress and the immune system in the mouse, [38], humans and rodents are born at different points in ontogeny and at differing points in immune development [39]. Non-human primates provide a more suitable model system with findings likely to be more relevant to human health, but that research base is more limited. Nonetheless, studies have shown that, for example, pregnant rhesus macaques who are stressed during the second or third trimester have offspring who displayed blunted immune responses to antigens. Compared to controls, these prenatally stressed infants demonstrated a blunted IL-6 and TNF-alpha response following lipopolysaccharide stimulation [40], as well as reduced T-cell response to antigens [41].

In women, stress during pregnancy is associated with elevated levels of pro-inflammatory cytokines [42]. Alterations in maternal cytokine levels have, in turn, been associated with higher risk of allergies in infants [43]. Prenatal anxiety and stress have also been linked to illness and antibiotic use in infancy [44]. It is also worth considering that some of the other infant outcomes linked to maternal stress, such as somatic illnesses [45], and higher BMI and obesity prevalence [46], may well be immune-mediated rather than strictly HPA axis mediated, as is often assumed. The potential effects of maternal stress on the child's immune system may continue throughout adulthood. A recent study found that that young women whose mothers experienced major negative life events during their pregnancy demonstrated over-production of IL-4, IL-6 and IL-10, a cytokine profile consistent with asthma and autoimmune disorders [47]. Furthermore, these women were also found to have higher BMIs, percentage body fat, and primary insulin resistance [48]. In a recent, large-scale Danish cohort study, young men whose mothers had experienced a major life stressor (death of a close relative) during pregnancy were more likely to be overweight and obese in adulthood [49]. Collectively, these findings suggest reliable associations between – and confounds among – prenatal maternal stress physiology, immunology, and diet and nutrition that may predict child health outcomes.

Prenatal Maternal Stress and Child Neurodevelopment

One of the most commonly studied areas of research related to prenatal diet and nutrition is child cognitive and neurodevelopment. There is an equally well-developed literature examining prenatal maternal stress as the exposure of interest. Dozens of studies in various animal models have linked prenatal stressors to neurodevelopmental outcomes spanning many domains, including memory, cognition, and social behavior. That the offspring of stressed dams show concomitant anatomical and cellular changes in key brain regions offers further support for a programming model [50]. Not surprisingly, studying these phenomena in humans once again presents a challenge for many reasons. One major complications is the potential for confounding by socioeconomic factors and parenting behaviors as well as postnatal maternal stress and depression.

Nevertheless, even after adjusting for these confounding factors, there is robust evidence that maternal stress is associated with neurodevelopmental changes in children that are evident at birth. Maternal anxiety during pregnancy is associated with changes in orientation, self-regulation, and reactivity among neonates [51]. Temperamental changes have been reported later in infancy. Prenatal stress and anxiety have been linked to a "difficult" infant temperament (according to maternal report), and heightened fearfulness in a structured experimental setting [52, 53]. Furthermore, motor and mental development may be delayed in such infants [52, 54].

Biological evidence further supports this behavioral and observational data and mirrors results from animal models. Ultrasound and heart rate data during pregnancy suggest relative developmental immaturity among fetuses carried by stressed mothers, with particularly acute delays among female fetuses [55]. Postnally, children of mothers who exhibited depressed symptoms during pregnancy also have different patterns of brain activity as measured by electroencephalogram starting as early as 1 week of age and extending into later infancy [56]. Finally, functional magnetic resonance imaging shows further changes in the brains of prenatally stressed children, including changes in functional connectivity (particularly in the amygdala) and brain volumes of key regions such as the hippocampus [57, 58].

To further underscore the impact of maternal prenatal stress on resulting child development, it is worth noting that like many other aspects of fetal programming, effects may be long-lasting. Stress-related neurodevelopmental changes in the brain and neuroendocrine systems may be still apparent in behavior and cognition in mid-to-late childhood. For example, anxiety during pregnancy predicts poorer executive function (including working memory, inhibitory control, and externalizing problems) at age 6–9 [59, 60]. As teenagers, the offspring of women who suffered from perinatal anxiety and/or depression are at increased risk of themselves developing anxiety disorders and more likely to have academic problems [61, 62].

It will again be evident that the above findings connecting prenatal maternal stress and child neurodevelopment resemble what has been reported for prenatal nutrition and child outcomes. There is, for example, a sizable literature linking prenatal obesity and child neurodevelopment [63, 64]. A focus on child neurodevelopment therefore provides a further illustration of the confounded and parallel literatures on prenatal stress and prenatal nutrition for child health and development.

Conclusions

In summary, although they are typically studied individually, prenatal stress and dietary factors often covary, may act upon the same developing body systems, and predict parallel and overlapping child outcomes. Adopting a multidisciplinary model, incorporating both exposures in relation to infant outcomes, is needed before deriving clear conclusions about the effects of either type of exposure. Of course that would not resolve the matter completely because of the myriad concurrent other exposures that may be relevant for child health and development also including, but not limited to: physical activity, environmental exposures, and medication use. Nevertheless, by integrating concurrent assessments of diet and stress (through standardized questionnaires or biospecimens) into study designs, we can improve our current understanding of how these exposures affect infant development. This approach will allow us to move away from overly simplified "main effects" models to interaction models that may more accurately approximate the complex and confounded patterns of prenatal exposures relevant for child health.

Future Directions

There remain a number of unanswered questions regarding prenatal stress and infant development. Additional directions that warrant future research include: (1) further elucidating the biological and molecular mechanisms by which maternal stress is transmitted to the fetus, including the role of the placenta and immune pathways; (2) examining the extent to which male and female fetuses respond differently to maternal stress, as has been suggested by several lines of research in this field; (3) identifying critical windows of exposure during pregnancy; (4) exploring whether developmental changes in the offspring of stressed mothers may sometimes represent adaptations to prepare for a harsh postnatal environment, rather than pathologies; and (5) developing interventions to reduce prenatal stress in order to improve infant health and developmental trajectories, particularly in at-risk populations.

References

1. Monk C, Georgieff MK, Osterholm EA. Research review: maternal prenatal distress and poor nutrition – mutually influencing risk factors affecting infant neurocognitive development. J Child Psychol Psychiatry. 2013;54(2):115–30. PubMed PMID: 23039359. Pubmed Central PMCID: PMC3547137. Epub 2012/10/09. eng.
2. Lumey LH, Stein AD, Kahn HS, van der Pal-de Bruin KM, Blauw GJ, Zybert PA, et al. Cohort profile: the Dutch hunger winter families study. Int J Epidemiol. 2007;36(6):1196–204. PubMed PMID: 17591638. Epub 2007/06/27. eng.
3. Brown AS, Susser ES. Prenatal nutritional deficiency and risk of adult schizophrenia. Schizophr Bull. 2008;34(6):1054–63. PubMed PMID: 18682377. Pubmed Central PMCID: PMC2632499. Epub 2008/08/07. eng.
4. de Rooij SR, Painter RC, Phillips DI, Osmond C, Michels RP, Godsland IF, et al. Impaired insulin secretion after prenatal exposure to the Dutch famine. Diabetes Care. 2006;29(8):1897–901. PubMed PMID: 16873799. Epub 2006/07/29. eng.

5. Li Y, He Y, Qi L, Jaddoe VW, Feskens EJ, Yang X, et al. Exposure to the Chinese famine in early life and the risk of hyperglycemia and type 2 diabetes in adulthood. Diabetes. 2010;59(10):2400–6. PubMed PMID: 20622161. Pubmed Central PMCID: PMC3279550. Epub 2010/07/14. eng.

6. St Clair D, Xu M, Wang P, Yu Y, Fang Y, Zhang F, et al. Rates of adult schizophrenia following prenatal exposure to the Chinese famine of 1959–1961. JAMA. 2005;294(5):557–62. PubMed PMID: 16077049. Epub 2005/08/04. eng.

7. Meijer A. Child psychiatric sequelae of maternal war stress. Acta Psychiatr Scand. 1985;72(6):505–11. PubMed PMID: 2417452. Epub 1985/12/01. eng.

8. Barrington WE, Beresford SA, McGregor BA, White E. Perceived stress and eating behaviors by sex, obesity status, and stress vulnerability: findings from the vitamins and lifestyle (VITAL) study. J Acad Nutr Diet. 2014;114(11):1791–9. PubMed PMID: 24828150. Pubmed Central PMCID: PMC4229482. Epub 2014/05/16. eng.

9. Glynn LM, Wadhwa PD, Dunkel-Schetter C, Chicz-Demet A, Sandman CA. When stress happens matters: effects of earthquake timing on stress responsivity in pregnancy. Am J Obstet Gynecol. 2001;184(4):637–42. PubMed PMID: 11262465. Epub 2001/03/23. eng.

10. O'Donnell KJ, Bugge Jensen A, Freeman L, Khalife N, O'Connor TG, Glover V. Maternal prenatal anxiety and downregulation of placental 11beta-HSD2. Psychoneuroendocrinology. 2012;37(6):818–26. PubMed PMID: 22001010. Epub 2011/10/18. eng.

11. Raikkonen K, Seckl JR, Pesonen AK, Simons A, Van den Bergh BR. Stress, glucocorticoids and liquorice in human pregnancy: programmers of the offspring brain. Stress. 2011;14(6):590–603. PubMed PMID: 21875300. Epub 2011/08/31. eng.

12. Wadhwa PD. Psychoneuroendocrine processes in human pregnancy influence fetal development and health. Psychoneuroendocrinology. 2005;30:724–43. PubMed PMID: 15919579.

13. Barbazanges A, Piazza PV, Le Moal M, Maccari S. Maternal glucocorticoid secretion mediates long-term effects of prenatal stress. J Neurosci. 1996;16(12):3943–9. PubMed PMID: 8656288. Epub 1996/06/15. eng.

14. Maccari S, Darnaudery M, Morley-Fletcher S, Zuena AR, Cinque C, Van Reeth O. Prenatal stress and long-term consequences: implications of glucocorticoid hormones. Neurosci Biobehav Rev. 2003;27(1–2):119–27. PubMed PMID: 12732228. Epub 2003/05/07. eng.

15. Seckl JR, Meaney MJ. Glucocorticoid programming. Ann N Y Acad Sci. 2004;1032:63–84. PubMed PMID: 15677396. Epub 2005/01/29. eng.

16. Kivlighan KT, DiPietro JA, Costigan KA, Laudenslager ML. Diurnal rhythm of cortisol during late pregnancy: associations with maternal psychological well-being and fetal growth. Psychoneuroendocrinology. 2008;33(9):1225–35. PubMed PMID: 18692319. Pubmed Central PMCID: 2806090. Epub 2008/08/12. eng.

17. Lambertini L, Chen J, Nomura Y. Mitochondrial gene expression profiles are associated with maternal psychosocial stress in pregnancy and infant temperament. PLoS One. 2015;10(9):e0138929. PubMed PMID: 26418562. Pubmed Central PMCID: PMC4587925. Epub 2015/09/30. eng.

18. O'Connor TG, Bergman K, Sarkar P, Glover V. Prenatal cortisol exposure predicts infant cortisol response to acute stress. Dev Psychobiol. 2013;55(2):145–55. PubMed PMID: 22315044. Pubmed Central PMCID: 3398188. Epub 2012/02/09. eng.

19. O'Donnell KJ, Glover V, Jenkins J, Browne D, Ben-Shlomo Y, Golding J, et al. Prenatal maternal mood is associated with altered diurnal cortisol in adolescence. Psychoneuroendocrinology. 2013;38(9):1630–8. PubMed PMID: 23433748. Pubmed Central PMCID: 3695029. Epub 2013/02/26. eng.

20. Uauy R, Kain J, Mericq V, Rojas J, Corvalan C. Nutrition, child growth, and chronic disease prevention. Ann Med. 2008;40(1):11–20. PubMed PMID: 18246473. Epub 2008/02/05. eng.

21. Merialdi M, Caulfield LE, Zavaleta N, Figueroa A, Costigan KA, Dominici F, et al. Randomized controlled trial of prenatal zinc supplementation and fetal bone growth. Am J Clin Nutr. 2004;79(5):826–30. PubMed PMID: 15113721. Epub 2004/04/29. eng.

22. Wadhwa PD, Sandman CA, Porto M, Dunkel-Schetter C, Garite TJ. The association between prenatal stress and infant birth weight and gestational age at birth: a prospective investigation. Am J Obstet Gynecol. 1993;169(4):858–65. PubMed PMID: 8238139. Epub 1993/10/01. eng.

23. Edwards CH, Cole OJ, Oyemade UJ, Knight EM, Johnson AA, Westney OE, et al. Maternal stress and pregnancy outcomes in a prenatal clinic population. J Nutr. 1994;124(6 Suppl):1006S–21S. PubMed PMID: 8201440. Epub 1994/06/01. eng.

24. Stout SA, Espel EV, Sandman CA, Glynn LM, Davis EP. Fetal programming of children's obesity risk. Psychoneuroendocrinology. 2015;53:29–39. PubMed PMID: 25591114. Pubmed Central PMCID: PMC4350576. Epub 2015/01/16. eng.

25. Mansell T, Novakovic B, Meyer B, Rzehak P, Vuillermin P, Ponsonby AL, et al. The effects of maternal anxiety during pregnancy on IGF2/H19 methylation in cord blood. Transl Psychiatry. 2016;6:e765. PubMed PMID: 27023171. Pubmed Central PMCID: PMC4872456. Epub 2016/03/31. eng.

26. Hales CN, Barker DJ. The thrifty phenotype hypothesis. Br Med Bull. 2001;60:5–20. PubMed PMID: 11809615. Epub 2002/01/26. eng.

27. Barker DJ. Fetal origins of cardiovascular disease. Ann Med. 1999;31(Suppl 1):3–6. PubMed PMID: 10342493. Epub 1999/05/26. eng.

28. Koontz MB, Gunzler DD, Presley L, Catalano PM. Longitudinal changes in infant body composition: association with childhood obesity. Pediatr Obes. 2014;9(6):e141–4. PubMed PMID: 25267097. Pubmed Central PMCID: 4702488.

29. Gillman MW, Rich-Edwards JW, Huh S, Majzoub JA, Oken E, Taveras EM, et al. Maternal corticotropin-releasing hormone levels during pregnancy and offspring adiposity. Obesity (Silver Spring). 2006;14(9):1647–53. PubMed PMID: 17030976. Pubmed Central PMCID: 1899091.

30. Fasting MH, Oken E, Mantzoros CS, Rich-Edwards JW, Majzoub JA, Kleinman K, et al. Maternal levels of corticotropin-releasing hormone during pregnancy in relation to adiponectin and leptin in early childhood. J Clin Endocrinol Metab. 2009;94(4):1409–15. PubMed PMID: 19190112. Pubmed Central PMCID: PMC2682476. Epub 2009/02/05. eng.

31. Tamashiro KL, Terrillion CE, Hyun J, Koenig JI, Moran TH. Prenatal stress or high-fat diet increases susceptibility to diet-induced obesity in rat offspring. Diabetes. 2009;58(5):1116–25. PubMed PMID: 19188431. Pubmed Central PMCID: 2671057. Epub 2009/02/04. eng.

32. Brunst KJ, Enlow MB, Kannan S, Carroll KN, Coull BA, Wright RJ. Effects of prenatal social stress and maternal dietary fatty acid ratio on infant temperament: does race matter? Epidemiology (Sunnyvale). 2014;4(4.) PubMed PMID: 25328835. Pubmed Central PMCID: 4197958.

33. Christian LM. Psychoneuroimmunology in pregnancy: immune pathways linking stress with maternal health, adverse birth outcomes, and fetal development. Neurosci Biobehav Rev. 2012;36(1):350–61. PubMed PMID: 21787802. Pubmed Central PMCID: 3203997. Epub 2011/07/27. eng.

34. Coussons-Read ME, Okun ML, Nettles CD. Psychosocial stress increases inflammatory markers and alters cytokine production across pregnancy. Brain Behav Immun. 2007;21:343–50. PubMed PMID: 17029703.

35. Beijers R, Jansen J, Riksen-Walraven M, de Weerth C. Maternal prenatal anxiety and stress predict infant illnesses and health complaints. Pediatrics. 2010;126:e401–e9. PubMed PMID: 20643724.

36. Prescott SL. Early origins of allergic disease: a review of processes and influences during early immune development. Curr Opin Allergy Clin Immunol. 2003;3(2):125–32. PubMed PMID: 12750609. Epub 2003/05/17. eng.

37. Marques AH, O'Connor TG, Roth C, Susser E, Bjørke-Monsen A-L. The influence of maternal prenatal and early childhood nutrition and maternal prenatal stress on offspring immune system development and neurodevelopmental disorders. Front Neurosci. 2013;7:1–17.

38. Merlot E, Couret D, Otten W. Prenatal stress, fetal imprinting and immunity. Brain Behav Immun. 2008;22:42–51. PubMed PMID: 17716859.

39. Dent GW, Ma S, Levine S. Rapid induction of corticotropin-releasing hormone gene transcription in the paraventricular nucleus of the developing rat. Endocrinology. 2000;141:1593–8. PubMed PMID: 10803566.

40. Coe CL, Kramer M, Kirschbaum C, Netter P, Fuchs E. Prenatal stress diminshes the cytokine response of leukocytes to endotoxin stimulation in juvenil rhesus monkeys. J Clin Endocrinol Metab. 2002;87:675–81. PubMed PMID: 11836303.

41. Coe C, Lubach G, Karaszewski J. Prenatal stress and immune recognition of self and nonself in the primate neonate. Neonatology. 1999;76:301–10.

42. Mold J, McCune J. Immunological tolerance during fetal development: from mouse to man. Adv Immunol. 2012;115:73–111.

43. Breckler LA, Hale J, Jung W, Westcott L, Dunstan JA, Thornton CA, et al. Modulation of in vivo and in vitro cytokine production over the course of pregnancy in allergic and non-allergic mothers. Pediatr Allergy Immunol. 2010;21:14–21. PubMed PMID: 19490478.

44. Buss C, Entringer S, Wadhwa PD. Fetal programming of brain development: intrauterine stress and susceptibility to psychopathology. Sci Signal. 2012;5:7. PubMed PMID: 23047922.

45. Tegethoff M, Greene N, Olsen J, Schaffner E, Meinlschmidt G. Stress during pregnancy and offspring pediatric disease: a National Cohort Study. Environ Health Perspect. 2011;119(11):1647–52. PubMed PMID: 21775267. Pubmed Central PMCID: 3226491. Epub 2011/07/22. eng.

46. Li J, Olsen J, Vestergaard M, Obel C, Baker JL, Sorensen TI. Prenatal stress exposure related to maternal bereavement and risk of childhood overweight. PLoS One. 2010;5(7):e11896. PubMed PMID: 20689593. Pubmed Central PMCID: PMC2912844.

47. Entringer S, Buss C, Wadhwa PD. Prenatal stress, development, health and disease risk: a psychobiological perspective-2015 Curt Richter award paper. Psychoneuroendocrinology. 2015;62:366–75. PubMed PMID: 26372770.

48. Entringer S, Wust S, Kumsta R, Layes IM, Nelson EL, Hellhammer DH, et al. Prenatal psychosocial stress exposure is associated with insulin resistance in young adults. Am J Obstet Gynecol. 2008;199(5):498. e1-7. PubMed PMID: 18448080. Epub 2008/05/02. eng.

49. Hohwu L, Li J, Olsen J, Sorensen TI, Obel C. Severe maternal stress exposure due to bereavement before, during and after pregnancy and risk of overweight and obesity in young adult men: a Danish National Cohort Study. PLoS One. 2014;9(5):e97490. PubMed PMID: 24828434. Pubmed Central PMCID: PMC4020839.

50. Weinstock M. Sex-dependent changes induced by prenatal stress in cortical and hippocampal morphology and behaviour in rats: an update. Stress. 2011;14(6):604–13. PubMed PMID: 21790452. Epub 2011/07/28. eng.

51. Hernandez-Martinez C, Arija V, Balaguer A, Cavalle P, Canals J. Do the emotional states of pregnant women affect neonatal behaviour? Early Hum Dev. 2008;84(11):745–50. PubMed PMID: 18571345. Epub 2008/06/24. eng.

52. Bergman K, Sarkar P, O'Connor TG, Modi N, Glover V. Maternal stress during pregnancy predicts cognitive ability and fearfulness in infancy. J Am Acad Child Adolesc Psychiatry. 2007;46(11):1454–63. PubMed PMID: 18049295. Epub 2007/12/01. eng.

53. Austin MP, Hadzi-Pavlovic D, Leader L, Saint K, Parker G. Maternal trait anxiety, depression and life event stress in pregnancy: relationships with infant temperament. Early Hum Dev. 2005;81(2):183–90. PubMed PMID: 15748973. Epub 2005/03/08. eng.

54. Huizink AC, Robles de Medina PG, Mulder EJ, Visser GH, Buitelaar JK. Stress during pregnancy is associated with developmental outcome in infancy. J Child Psychol Psychiatry. 2003;44(6):810–8. PubMed PMID: 12959490. Epub 2003/09/10. eng.

55. Doyle C, Werner E, Feng T, Lee S, Altemus M, Isler JR, et al. Pregnancy distress gets under fetal skin: maternal ambulatory assessment & sex differences in prenatal development. Dev Psychobiol. 2015;57(5):607–25. PubMed PMID: 25945698. Pubmed Central PMCID: PMC4549003. Epub 2015/05/07. eng.

56. Diego MA, Jones NA, Field T. EEG in 1-week, 1-month and 3-month-old infants of depressed and non-depressed mothers. Biol Psychol. 2010;83(1):7–14. PubMed PMID: 19782119. Pubmed Central PMCID: PMC2838453. Epub 2009/09/29.. eng

57. Qiu A, Anh TT, Li Y, Chen H, Rifkin-Graboi A, Broekman BF, et al. Prenatal maternal depression alters amygdala functional connectivity in 6-month-old infants. Transl Psychiatry. 2015;5:e508. PubMed PMID: 25689569. Pubmed Central PMCID: PMC4445753. Epub 2015/02/18. eng.

58. Qiu A, Rifkin-Graboi A, Chen H, Chong YS, Kwek K, Gluckman PD, et al. Maternal anxiety and infants' hippocampal development: timing matters. Transl Psychiatry. 2013;3:e306. PubMed PMID: 24064710. Pubmed Central PMCID: PMC3784768. Epub 2013/09/26. eng.

59. Buss C, Davis EP, Hobel CJ, Sandman CA. Maternal pregnancy-specific anxiety is associated with child executive function at 6–9 years age. Stress. 2011;14(6):665–76. PubMed PMID: 21995526. Pubmed Central PMCID: PMC3222921. Epub 2011/10/15. eng.

60. Van den Bergh BR, Marcoen A. High antenatal maternal anxiety is related to ADHD symptoms, externalizing problems, and anxiety in 8- and 9-year-olds. Child Dev. 2004;75(4):1085–97. PubMed PMID: 15260866. Epub 2004/07/21. eng.

61. Capron LE, Glover V, Pearson RM, Evans J, O'Connor TG, Stein A, et al. Associations of maternal and paternal antenatal mood with offspring anxiety disorder at age 18 years. J Affect Disord. 2015;187:20–6. PubMed PMID: 26301478. Pubmed Central PMCID: PMC4595479. Epub 2015/08/25. eng.

62. Pearson RM, Bornstein MH, Cordero M, Scerif G, Mahedy L, Evans J, et al. Maternal perinatal mental health and offspring academic achievement at age 16: the mediating role of childhood executive function. J Child Psychol Psychiatry. 2015;29:491–501. PubMed PMID: 26616637. Epub 2015/12/01. Eng.

63. Krakowiak P, Walker CK, Bremer AA, Baker AS, Ozonoff S, Hansen RL, et al. Maternal metabolic conditions and risk for autism and other neurodevelopmental disorders. Pediatrics. 2012;129(5):e1121–8. PubMed PMID: 22492772. Pubmed Central PMCID: 3340592.

64. Tanda R, Salsberry PJ. Racial differences in the association between maternal prepregnancy obesity and children's behavior problems. J Dev Behav Pediatr. 2014;35(2):118–27. PubMed PMID: 24509056. Pubmed Central PMCID: 3920306.

Chapter 2
The Effects of Parental Diet on Fetal Programming of Stress-Related Brain Regions and Behaviours: Implications for Development of Neuropsychiatric Disorders

Austin C. Korgan and Tara S. Perrot

Key Points

- The early environment programs adult brain and behavior during sensitive/critical periods via epigenetic mechanisms
- Stress-related brain regions that underlie adult coping behavior are programmed during development by maternal stress
- Many of the same brain regions are affected in offspring of mothers exposed to stress during pregnancy and those that are obese during pregnancy
- Stress-related neuropsychiatric disorders, such as anxiety and depression are increased by maternal stress, providing a solid foundation for examining the effects of maternal diet
- Gestational under-nutrition, over-nutrition, and high-fat consumption alter development of the fetus, including stress-related brain regions
- Neuropsychiatric disorders, included those related to stress, are associated with maternal obesity

Keywords Maternal diet • Paternal diet • HPA axis • Stress • Mood disorders • Neurodevelopment

Abbreviations

ACTH   Adrenocorticotrophin hormone
AVP   Arginine-vasopressin
BDNF   Brain-derived neurotrophic factor
BMI   Body mass index
CPT   Cold pressor test
CRH   Corticotrophin-releasing hormone
DNMTs   DNA methyltransferases
GCs   Glucocorticoids
GR   Glucocorticoid receptors
GWG   Gestational weight gain

A.C. Korgan, MSc, PhD • T.S. Perrot, PhD (✉)
Department of Psychology and Neuroscience, Dalhousie University, Halifax, Nova Scotia, Canada
e-mail: akorgan@dal.ca; tara.perrot@dal.ca

© Springer International Publishing AG 2017
R. Rajendram et al. (eds.), *Diet, Nutrition, and Fetal Programming*,
Nutrition and Health, DOI 10.1007/978-3-319-60289-9_2

HFD   High fat diet
HPA   Hypothalamic-pituitary-adrenal
KO   Knock-out
MR   Mineralocorticoid receptors
NPY   Neuropeptide Y
NSFT   Novelty-suppressed feeding test
PS   Prenatal stress
PVN   Hypothalamic paraventricular nucleus
TSST   Trier social stress test

Introduction

In this chapter, we review the latest studies reporting on developmental programming of stress responding by parental diet. We discuss this literature within the broader context of developmental programming, particularly of adult stress responding by early life adversity. It appears that many of the same brain regions are affected in offspring of mothers exposed to stress during pregnancy and those that are obese during pregnancy. The incidence of the same neuropsychiatric disorders is increased by stress and obesity during pregnancy, likely being mediated by similar mechanisms.

Much of the work on the effects of maternal diet has focused on the gestational period, but more recent work has shown the importance of *pre*-pregnancy metabolic markers as well as the postnatal period for shaping offspring stress-related programming. While we focus here on the maternal environment, we include reference to the importance of the father's diet also.

Throughout the chapter, inclusion of non-human animal studies serves to provide evidence for cause and effect relationships between parental diet and offspring outcomes. This work complements the correlational evidence provided by human studies for these relationships.

Finally, whenever possible, differences in outcomes for male and female offspring are discussed. Sex differences in effects of maternal stress on offspring are well-characterized. However, the reports of effects of maternal obesity are fewer and most do not include separate reference to male and female offspring. This will hopefully change as the field matures.

The Role of the Early Environment in Shaping Adult Brain and Behavior

Neurodevelopment is orchestrated by both genetic and environmental influences, and for the fetus, the environment is dictated by maternal factors. Events that occur during the prenatal and early postnatal periods exert strong programming effects on the mammalian brain and resulting behavior. During critical periods in development, environmental events can produce stable alterations in brain and behavior that manifest throughout life. In this way, transgenerational transmission of traits can occur. Indeed, modifications to regulatory DNA sequences provide the mechanism by which environmental events affect the brain, and since some of these modifications are permanent, a molecular means for passing on those events to future generations (see Fig. 2.1; [1]).

Epigenetic changes are critical to development, guiding cellular phenotypes via heritable and persistent changes in gene expression without altering DNA sequence. Three key molecular events have been identified which appear to drive these changes in gene expression. First, DNA methylation is the process by which methyl groups are attached to the DNA at CpG islands (i.e., regions of the DNA containing higher than normal levels of the base pairs, cytosine (C) – guanine (G), held together by a phosphodiester (p) bond). The process is mediated by enzymes known as DNA methyltransferases (DNMTs), generally resulting in a downregulation of gene expression. Second, chromatin modification

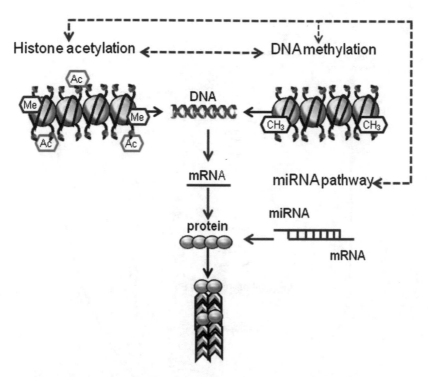

Fig. 2.1 Summary of three distinct but interrelated epigenetic mechanisms (Adapted from: Fig. 2 from Desai et al. [1])

is the repackaging or folding of the DNA around the histones, proteins responsible for arranging DNA into chromatin. Histones can be modified in various ways, allowing for both upregulation (acetylation) and downregulation (deacetylation) of gene transcription. Finally, non-coding RNA (ncRNA) are transcribed from DNA but not translated into proteins. Instead, they act to regulate gene expression at the transcriptional and post-transcriptional level. Short ncRNAs (<30 nts) include microRNAs (miRNAs), short inhibitory RNAs (shRNAs), and piwi-interacting RNAs (piRNAs). These are usually responsible for downregulation of gene expression. Long ncRNAs (>200 nts) are crucial during development and have been associated with adipogenesis [1].

It is becoming evident from both human and animal research that these mechanisms are involved in the development of HPA-axis dysfunction, obesity, and diabetes (for review [1]).

Overview of Stress Responding and Stress-Related Behavior

The effects associated with prenatal stress (PS) have been studied widely and provide a useful comparison for the effects of prenatal diet. Thus, for the purposes of this chapter, we will summarize the effects of PS on stress related outcomes (particularly, behavioral) to provide context for our main goal of reviewing the effects of prenatal diet on these same endpoints.

The limbic system is involved in regulating motivational/emotional behavior. It is a set of integrated brain structures that allow an organism to engage in motivated behavior, such as feeding, mating, and predator avoidance. The hypothalamic-pituitary-adrenal (HPA) axis (see Fig. 2.2) is the main system in mammals involved in coordination of the physiological and behavioral responses needed to deal with stimuli that pose a threat to homeostasis. As such, it is widely conserved across vertebrate species, but amenable to environmental programming [2]; also see section "Effects of PS on Adult Stress Responding and Stress-Related Disease").

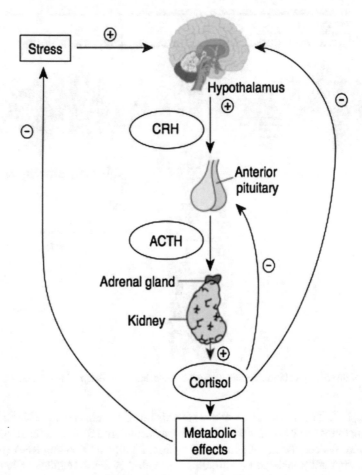

Fig. 2.2 Simplified depiction of the hypothalamic-pituitary-adrenal (HPA) axis. *Plus signs* indicate positive feedforward, while *minus signs* indicate negative feedback, between individual brain regions (Reprinted with permission from Hiller-Sturmhöfel [50])

Upon perception of a stressor (real or only perceived), activation of the HPA axis results in increased circulating corticotrophin-releasing hormone (CRH) and arginine-vasopressin (AVP), adrenocorticotrophin hormone (ACTH), glucocorticoids (GCs), as well as other neurosteroids and peptides (reviewed in [3]). While activation of this system is necessary for adaptive responses to the stressor, including orchestrating effective behavioral strategies, the damaging effects of prolonged and/or heightened exposure to GCs such as corticosterone or cortisol are well known. GCs typically bind to one of two cytoplasmic receptor proteins: type I mineralocorticoid (MR), and type 2 glucocorticoid (GR) receptors. Both MR and GR are ligand-gated transcriptional regulators, and are expressed in various regions of brain including the hippocampus, amygdala, medial prefrontal cortex, hypothalamic paraventricular nucleus (PVN), and others (reviewed in [3, 4]).

HPA activation is very useful in the short-term under conditions of acute stress. However, elevated and prolonged GC exposure may alter later HPA axis regulation through cell loss in key areas, permanent sensitization of regulatory structures to one or more of the stress hormones, and by altered cortical and limbic neurobiology [5]. The strong relationship between stress (and excess GC release) and circulatory/immune-related diseases (ex. heart disease, high blood pressure) and the development of affective disorders, such as anxiety and depression (as reviewed in [6]) exact a huge financial and social toll.

In humans, acute stress is typically measured via behavioral and molecular endpoints. The effects of laboratory manipulations, such as the Trier social stress test (TSST) or the cold pressor test (CPT), can be monitored with salivary or blood assays for cortisol and self-report stress questionnaires. Studies of naturalistic stress are inherently more difficult in humans, but can offer insights into the long-term effects that chronic stress has on development. One ongoing series of studies is measuring the long-term impact of a severe ice storm that resulted in power outages for many days, leading to profound levels of stress. By enlisting pregnant women that survived this experience, as well as age/gestation-matched controls, the researchers are able to test and observe the effects of natural prenatal maternal stress on development. To date, they have identified effects of maternal stress on birth outcomes, infant temperament, motor function, cognitive and linguistic function, body composition, eating disorders, autism traits, as well as identifying DNA methylation patterns on specific genes, elucidating the mechanism for the diverse set of physical/behavioral symptoms [7–9].

Effects of PS on Adult Stress Responding and Stress-Related Disease

Although the stress response shows characteristic features across individuals, such as release of GCs, it is highly individualistic in terms of precipitation factors and the magnitude of the response. In fact, we know that adult stress responding is shaped during prenatal, postnatal, through to adolescent, periods of development. Individuality in stress responding is due, in part, to the nature in which maternal events influence the neurodevelopment of key brain structures such as the hippocampus and prefrontal cortex [10–13] compromising the regulation of the HPA axis across the lifespan, and increasing development of mood disorders such as anxiety and depression (as reviewed in [14]). Figure 2.3 illustrates some of the negative effects of early life stress with respect to HPA programming. While adverse events during early life, such as trauma or abuse, generally increase susceptibility of those affected to develop stress-related disorders [15], a moderate amount of stress during development can actually lead to inoculation to stress later in life, resulting in coping and resilience to future stressors [16]. Thus, the relationship between early life stress and future stress responding is an inverted U-shaped function.

While anything that affects the mother (e.g., drug use, malnutrition, metabolic conditions) can have effects on offspring neurodevelopment, stress exposure is somewhat unique, because it is ubiquitous, prevalent, and intrinsic to adaptation and survival. Both animal and human studies have shown that maternal stress has a significant effect on neurological and general development [5, 6]; see Fig. 2.4). Human epidemiological evidence clearly associates maternal distress during pregnancy with prenatally

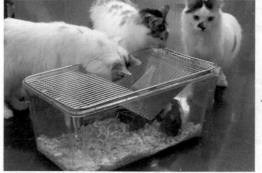

Prenatal or Early Life Stress
↓ Birth weight
↓ Gestational time

↑ Anxiety, depression & mood disorders
↑ Cardiovascular disease & metabolic disorders

Fig. 2.3 Some general effects of early life stress on offspring that result from using a model such as that depicted on the *left*, in which pregnant rats are exposed repeatedly during the last week of gestation to a predatory threat (Adapted from: Korgan et al. [51])

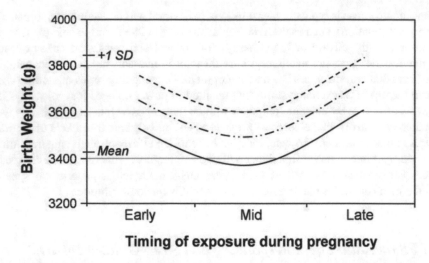

Fig. 2.4 Mean birth weight as a function of perceived maternal stress (*dotted line* = low stress, *dashed/dotted line* = medium stress, *solid line* = high stress) experienced during early, mid-, and late gestation (Reprinted with permission from Dancause et al. [9])

stressed infants that have an increased predisposition to develop psychopathologies such as anxiety and depression [14, 17]. These findings are complemented by results from animal research showing long-term behavioral and associated neurobiological effects of PS (as reviewed in [15]).

The concept of a developmental origin for various chronic illnesses (e.g., type II diabetes, cardio-metabolic disease, obesity), and importantly, affective disorders (reviewed in [6]) is now well-accepted, although the exact mechanisms are complex and not fully known. What has become clear is that these mechanisms involve environmentally induced epigenetic modulation of gene expression (see section "The Role of the Early Environment in Shaping Adult Brain and Behavior"; [18]). Epigenetic modifications, such as DNA methylation, are well described in neuronal development and in association with altered HPA axis functioning as a result of early life events [18]. Thus, environmental influences on fetal programming of brain development may be facilitated through epigenetic modulation of specific targets and determining these targets may lead to new treatment/intervention strategies for affective disorders. One potential target is the neurotrophin, brain-derived neurotrophic factor (BDNF), which is affected by stress in an age-, sex-, and stressor type-dependent manner (as reviewed in [19]) and is critical for normal regulation and development of neural circuits. Altered BDNF promoter methylation has been noted in patients suffering from major depressive disorder [20], but more importantly for the present review, maternal diet programs BDNF levels in offspring brain, and through this mechanism, significantly influences adult offspring cerebrovascular health [21].

Developmental Programming of Limbic System Function by Prenatal Diet

Developmental programming of the limbic system, and in particular the HPA axis, underlies metabolic homeostasis, as well as future responses to stressors in offspring.

Similar to the U-shaped function that describes the relationship between early life stress and adult brain function, both under-nutrition and over-nutrition during gestation produce adverse outcomes with respect to metabolic and stress-related markers in adult offspring (reviewed in [22]). For example, imbalances in maternal nutrition program hyperphagia in offspring, no matter whether the imbalance is too much or too little (see Fig. 2.5).

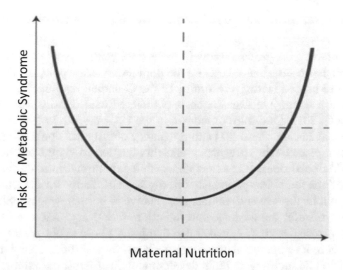

Fig. 2.5 A U-shaped function describes the relationship between maternal nutrition and various offspring outcomes, such as development of metabolic syndrome

The Effects of Gestational Under-Nutrition

Epidemiological studies have consistently demonstrated a robust connection between the early nutritional environment and adult metabolic outcomes. For example, low birthweight predisposes individuals to a host of adverse health conditions, including obesity, hypertension, and diabetes. This was first documented in adult offspring of mothers that had been exposed to famine conditions during the last 2 months of pregnancy at the end of the World War II [23, 24]. These offspring grew up to be obese and the hypothesis was generated that the lack of nutrition during gestation and resulting low birth weight resulted in a situation of 'catch-up' growth once offspring became adults living in non-famine conditions.

Mechanisms are best gleaned with animal models in which gestational diet can be manipulated. Female sheep fed a 50% nutrient-restricted diet for the first third of pregnancy gave birth to lambs that showed higher ACTH and cortisol levels in response to CRH challenge at 2 months of age and higher basal cortisol levels at 5.5 months [25], both suggesting altered hypothalamic function. In rats, under-nutrition of mothers resulted in increased basal corticosterone levels, but lower levels relative to control offspring in response to challenge with the synthetic GC, dexamethasone. The authors speculate that the low sensitivity of the HPA axis may be due to low expression of GC receptors in hypothalamus and/or pituitary gland [26]. More recent examinations indicate that protein restriction in rats during pregnancy interferes with normal molecular development of nutrient sensing cells in offspring hypothalamus [27], specifically by delaying the maturation of the K_{atp} inhibitory response in orexigenic neuropeptide Y (NPY) neurons [28]. When provided with a high-fat diet, male and female offspring from even a moderately calorie restricted (20%) mom showed an altered amount of NPY mRNA, and female offspring also showed lower leptin receptor mRNA in hypothalamus [29]. This study shows the potential for different outcomes in male and female offspring.

Interestingly, effects of under-nutrition on leptin and other metabolic markers can be reversed by cross-fostering pups to normal weight dams after birth [30], demonstrating the importance of hormones in milk and/or maternal behavior during lactation.

The Effects of Gestational Over-Nutrition and High-Fat Consumption

The prevalence of obesity has grown rapidly in the last 20 years, especially in developed nations. While this epidemic has deleterious effects on the population as a whole, for the developing fetus it has the potential to be devastating. According to the Canadian Institute for Health Information and the Public Health Agency of Canada, costs associated with obesity were between $4.6 and $7.1 billion dollars in 2011. One-third of women in the US, one-fifth in the UK (reviewed in [1]) and one quarter in Canada are obese [31] and pregnancy obesity has doubled since 1993. Obesity has become commonplace during pregnancy and this has led to significant health risks for the developing fetus. Maternal obesity is associated with a suboptimal intrauterine environment for both the mother and the fetus. Pre-pregnancy obesity is a risk factor for diabetes mellitus, hypertension, thromboembolic disease and asthma, and relative to normal weight mothers, obese mothers are more likely to suffer hemorrhage and infection at delivery, and less likely to breastfeed (reviewed in [32]). A recent review demonstrated that infants born to obese mothers suffered more frequently from neurodevelopmental disorders such as spina bifida, neural tube defects, and hydrocephaly [32]. While such severe brain development disorders are troubling and make maternal obesity worthy of further study, the impact of maternal diet on more general neural developmental processes is equally compelling, having implications for offspring stress-related mood disorders, cognitive disorders, and even psychotic disorders. A multitude of brain regions are likely affected in such disorders; however, the core circuitry of the HPA axis is undoubtedly affected and will be our focus below.

Non-human Animal Models of High Fat Diet (HFD)

Non-human animal studies have been used to gain insight into the mechanisms by which gestational diet programs key brain structures that are at the intersection for stress responding and feeding, such as the hypothalamus. In rats, gestational HFD stimulated the proliferation and differentiation of hypothalamic neuronal precursor cells, resulting in a greater proportion of these new neurons expressing orexigenic peptides [33]. Such a basic alteration, that shifts the balance of appetite more toward stimulation, and away from suppression, may be involved in programming obesity in offspring.

In addition to programming obesity in offspring, maternal diet can program hypothalamic responses to stressors. In ewes, maternal over-nutrition and obesity, before and during gestation, affected HPA axis sensitivity of offspring, but did not affect HPA responses to an acute stressor [34]. This is in contrast to work using rats, in which it was shown that maternal HFD throughout pregnancy and lactation resulted in attenuated HPA axis habituation in response to both acute [35] and repeated stressors [36] in adult offspring. Basal levels of GCs were found to be lower in adult offspring exposed to maternal HFD, and sex-specific alterations in GC receptors and inflammatory markers were noted [35]. More work is needed to resolve species differences, enabling more concrete conclusions, but it is clear that maternal HFD sets the stage for altered development of hypothalamic and stress-related circuitry, having implications for adult stress responding in offspring.

Importantly, alterations in markers of the HPA axis were accompanied by increased stress-induced depressive behavior [36] as well as increased anxiety-related behavior [35] in adult offspring that were exposed to maternal HFD. Interestingly, the effects of maternal HFD on adolescent offspring were opposite with respect to anxiety-related behavior, with HFD-offspring showing less anxiety than controls [37]. Clearly, more studies are needed that track changes across postnatal development.

Genetic Models of HFD

The mechanisms of early programming by HFD can be explored at a molecular level by utilizing genetic knockout (KO) models. These models allow for the homo- or heterozygous deletion of specific genes involved in development, stress responding, and/or metabolism. The classic example of a KO is the *ob/ob* mouse, which carries a recessive stop codon for the leptin gene. A heterozygous *ob/ob* mouse is mildly obese, while the homozygous genotype presents a classic obese phenotype. These phenotypes are related to the reduced quantity of circulating leptin, compared to wildtype animals [38]. Other genetic models of metabolic effects provide evidence that both maternal and postnatal diet are critical for developmental programming. For example, *p66^Shc* gene is involved in metabolism and oxidative stress. A KO model reveals a HFD resistance and increased lifespan. However, administration of HFD to pregnant *p66^Shc−/−* females produces differences in offspring weight, development, metabolic function, and emotionality, particularly in male offspring [39]. While these models are useful for identifying molecular pathways, they are less practical for translational science/medicine as the number of loss-of-function mutations in humans is relatively uncommon (for review [38]).

The Importance of Maternal Care

While effects of maternal diet during gestation can have profound effects on offspring metabolism, postnatal maternal care is equally critical for shaping the developing metabolic and stress pathways [40].

HFD fed dams display reductions in overall activity, which is associated with decreased pup survival [41]. However, despite showing reduced licking and grooming behavior toward offspring, the offspring of HFD fed dams show metabolic effects independent of maternal care behavior, at least in the first generation [42]. Thus, altered maternal behavior is likely driven by differences in circulating reproductive hormones, such as progestins, estrogens, and prolactin, in addition to altered GC levels. In studies of gestational stress, maternal GC levels are increased which, in turn, have a deleterious effect on maternal care [43]. However, in maternal HFD models, GC levels are maintained (compared to controls), indicating a divergent mechanism driving differences in maternal care behavior [42]. Though specific mechanisms have yet to be described, it is important to note that, in humans, both early maternal stress [9] and diet [44] have the potential to disrupt maternal care and impact the development of obesity in children.

Paternal Transmission of HPA-Axis and Metabolic Disruption

The father's role in offspring development, adaptability, and survival has received significantly less attention than maternal effects. However, recent advances in understanding and application of epigenetic techniques have inspired investigation into the potential for non-genomic influences of the male germline. Animal models have shown an impact on offspring following preconception changes in paternal stress, age, obesity, and environmental exposure [45].

Rodent models suggest that paternal obesity is a risk factor for offspring development. Similar to studies of maternal stress and nutritional disruption, first-generation offspring develop metabolic syndrome. However, in this model penetrance to the second generation is sex-dependent [46]. Decreased penetrance of inherited phenotypes has also been described in humans, though a theoretical model suggests that societal factors prevent the decreasing penetrance seen in animal models [47].

Multi-generational human studies have also found paternal nutrition effects in offspring and grand-offspring. As previously mentioned, the Dutch famine studies provided rare insight into the transgenerational inheritance of metabolic phenotypes. Veenendaal et al. [48] recently showed that grand-offspring of fathers that where in utero during the famine had higher BMI. These studies further demonstrate the importance of understanding transgenerational epigenetic inheritance, especially as it pertains to potential treatments.

Prenatal Diet Programming of Neuropsychiatric Disorders

The inability to manage the duration and/or amount of stress in one's life, accompanied (or not) by inadequate coping behaviors in the face of stress, can be precipitating factors in the development of a host of neuropsychiatric disorders. As discussed throughout this review, a healthy stress response system in adults begins in the womb, where programming of various aspects of the HPA axis, and accompanying limbic circuitry begins. The increased levels of hormones (e.g., leptin, insulin) and nutrients (e.g., glucose, fatty acids), among other things, that a fetus of an obese mother is exposed to permanently alter development of neural circuits that are critical in the regulation of stress-related behavior, which directly increases the risk of stress-related mental health disorders, such as anxiety and depression. Moreover, there is evidence that the increased hormones, excess nutrients, and elevated inflammatory and metabolic markers that the fetus of an obese woman is exposed to have direct programming effects on the developing brain, altering underlying circuitry, and increasing the risk for disorders such as ADHD, ASD, and schizophrenia.

An excellent recent review summarizes the work showing a relationship between maternal obesity and mental health disorders [49]. Here, we will summarize the findings and refer readers to Rivera et al. (2015) for details.

Cognitive Impairments Associated with Maternal Obesity

Pre-pregnancy BMI has been associated with an increased risk of cognitive impairments in six separate studies using varied designs [49]. The results of earlier studies linking maternal obesity and IQ are somewhat suspect as sampling was highly selective, there was little control for maternal or paternal IQ or SES, and retrospective maternal self-report of weight was used. A more recent study, one in which maternal, family, and child factors were controlled, confirmed an association between maternal obesity and reduced reading and math scores on standardized tests. However, this finding has not been consistently reported, with other studies failing to find relationships between maternal obesity and cognitive deficits, despite finding reduced language skills in 8-year old children of obese mothers.

More work is definitely warranted to investigate the relationship between maternal obesity and cognitive deficits. Work from non-human animal models supports the idea that maternal obesity is linked to cognitive deficits as offspring of mothers exposed to HFD showed reduced spatial learning [49]. Cognitive deficits in rat offspring of HFD mothers would be consistent with the finding discussed in section "Effects of PS on Adult Stress Responding and Stress-Related Disease", in which BDNF levels in hippocampus are reduced in these offspring [36].

ADHD and ASD Associated with Maternal Obesity

The strongest evidence for a link between maternal obesity and neurodevelopmental disorders comes from the studies on ADHD symptomology and risk, and ASD risk and severity of symptoms. Increased pre-pregnancy BMI and GWG have been associated with ADHD and ASD in nine separate studies since 2008 (reviewed in Rivera et al. [49]). In ASD in particular, maternal complications such as diabetes, hypertension or pre-eclampsia were also positively associated with diagnosis, making it difficult without further study to tease apart BMI, GWG, and complications as causal factors.

Non-human animal studies generally support the idea that maternal HFD increases hyperactivity and decreases sociality in offspring [49].

Anxiety and Depression Associated with Maternal Obesity

Anxiety and depression are among the most commonly diagnosed neuropsychiatric disorders, not only in adults, but also in children and adolescents. Maternal pre-pregnancy BMI has been associated with an increased risk for disrupted emotions (i.e., fear and sadness) and increased behaviors associated with withdrawal and depression in children [49]. This finding has been supported by other, less direct work, but has also been shown to exhibit sexual dimorphism, with the association being stronger in females than males. This may not be that surprising, given the higher incidence of anxiety and depression in women relative to men.

As alluded to above (particularly, section "Non-human Animal Models of High Fat Diet (HFD)"), evidence exists from studies using non-human animal models to suggest that maternal HFD increases emotionality, and alters anxiety and depressive-like behaviors in offspring. A review of the available studies [49] indicates that, although not a lot of work has been performed to date, it is consistent with the human literature in suggesting that maternal HFD increases anxiety-like behavior in rats. Unfortunately, most of this work has been performed only in males, despite the sex differences found in incidence of these disorders in humans, and the findings of sexual dimorphism in the link between obesity and anxiety. Studies that have used both sexes have produced inconsistent results [49], indicating a critical need for more work in this area.

Pilot data from our lab examining anxiety behavior in rats using the novelty-suppressed feeding test (NSFT) revealed that an increased number of center crosses (i.e., lower anxiety) was negatively correlated with adrenal weight in maternal HFD offspring ($r = -0.526$, $p = 0.036$), but not control offspring (see Fig. 2.6). In other words, in HFD offspring, heavier adrenal glands (associated with higher stress) were associated with higher anxiety behavior. This association was not observed in offspring from moms fed a normal diet, suggesting that the HFD altered the relationship between physiology and behavior with respect to stress.

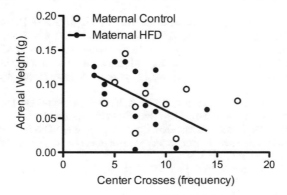

Fig. 2.6 Scatterplot depicting the negative correlation between adrenal gland weight and center crosses (increased center crosses = lower anxiety). This correlation was significant only in the offspring from HFD-fed moms, not in offspring from control diet-fed moms

Psychosis Associated with Maternal Obesity

The prevalence of the neurodevelopmental disorder, schizophrenia, is on the rise, and in Western countries, obesity is believed to impact the risk [49]. As first discussed in section "The Effects of Gestational Under-Nutrition", malnutrition can have similar effects as too many nutrients during gestation. The link between schizophrenia and the nutritional environment during development first came to light with an increased incidence of the disorder in those who had suffered during the Dutch Hunger Winter. To date, six human studies have demonstrated an association between maternal obesity and schizophrenia. The most compelling was a case-controlled study that showed a 24% increase in schizophrenia risk for every BMI unit increase during early pregnancy, that dropping to 19% during later gestation [49].

Concluding Remarks

Developed nations face a number of challenges in the years to come. Significant health risks are associated with being overweight and obese; yet, the incidence of both continues to rise. Unfortunately, the problem is compounded by the transgenerational nature of obesity, as we have discussed in this chapter. Gestational, and even pre-pregnancy, obesity alters development of the brain regions involved in feeding and stress responding, perpetuating a number of health risks, including diabetes, hypertension, and a number of neuropsychiatric disorders. Dedicated research into the mechanisms underlying this altered developmental programming is essential to provide possibilities for intervention and treatment to break the cycle.

References

1. Desai M, Jellyman JK, Ross MG. Epigenomics, gestational programming and risk of metabolic syndrome. Int J Obes. 2015;39(4):633–41.
2. Buschdorf JP, Meaney MJ. Epigenetics/programming in the HPA axis. Compr Physiol. 2015;6:87–110.
3. Joels M, Baram TZ. The neuro-symphony of stress. Nat Rev Neurosci. 2009;10:459–66.
4. Oitzl MS, Champagne DL, van der Veen R, de Kloet ER. Brain development under stress: hypotheses of glucocorticoid actions revisited. Neurosci Biobehav Rev. 2010;34(6):853–66.
5. Weinstock M. Alterations induced by gestational stress in brain morphology and behaviour of the offspring. Prog Neurobiol. 2001;65:427–51.
6. Harris A, Seckl J. Glucocorticoids, prenatal stress and the programming of disease. Horm Behav. 2011;59(3):279–89.
7. Cao-Lei L, Massart R, Suderman MJ, Machnes Z, Elgbeili G, Laplante DP, et al. DNA methylation signatures triggered by prenatal maternal stress exposure to a natural disaster: project ice storm. PLoS One. 2014;9(9):e107653-e.
8. Cao-Lei L, Dancause KN, Elgbeili G, Massart R, Szyf M, Liu A, et al. DNA methylation mediates the impact of exposure to prenatal maternal stress on BMI and central adiposity in children at age 13(1/2) years: project ice storm. Epigenetics. 2015;10(8):749–61.
9. Dancause KN, Laplante DP, Oremus C, Fraser S, Brunet A, King S. Disaster-related prenatal maternal stress influences birth outcomes: project ice storm. Early Hum Dev. 2011;87(12):813–20.
10. Van den Hove DL, Leibold NK, Strackx E, Martinez-Claros M, Lesch KP, HWM S, et al. Prenatal stress and subsequent exposure to chronic mild stress in rats; interdependent effects on emotional behavior and the serotonergic system. Eur Neuropsychopharmacol. 2013;24:1–13.
11. Kolb B, Mychasiuk R, Muhammad A, Li Y, Frost DO, Gibb R. Experience and the developing prefrontal cortex. Proc Natl Acad Sci U S A. 2012;109(Suppl):17186–93.
12. Markham J, Mullins SE, Koenig JI. Periadolescent maturation of the prefrontal cortex is sex-specific and is disrupted by prenatal stress. J Comp Neurol. 2013;521(8):1828–43.
13. Mychasiuk R, Gibb R, Kolb B. Prenatal stress alters dendritic morphology and synaptic connectivity in the prefrontal cortex and hippocampus of developing offspring. Synapse. 2012;66(4):308–14.

14. Weir JM, Zakama A, Rao U. Developmental risk I: depression and the developing brain. Child Adolesc Psychiatr Clin N Am. 2012;21(2):237–59. vii.
15. Cirulli F, Francia N, Berry A, Aloe L, Alleva E, Suomi SJ. Early life stress as a risk factor for mental health: role of neurotrophins from rodents to non-human primates. Neurosci Biobehav Rev. 2009;33(4):573–85.
16. Ashokan A, Sivasubramanian M, Mitra R. Seeding stress resilience through inoculation. Neural Plast. 2016;2016:1–6.
17. Pawlby S, Hay DF, Sharp D, Waters CS, O'Keane V. Antenatal depression predicts depression in adolescent offspring: prospective longitudinal community-based study. J Affect Disord. 2009;113(3):236–43.
18. Meaney MJ, Szyf M, Seckl JR. Epigenetic mechanisms of perinatal programming of hypothalamic-pituitary-adrenal function and health. Trends Mol Med. 2007;13(7):269–77.
19. Bath KG, Schilit A, Lee FS. Stress effects on BDNF expression: effects of age, sex, and form of stress. Neuroscience. 2013;239:149–56.
20. D'Addario C, Dell'Osso B, Galimberti D, Palazzo MC, Benatti B, Di Francesco A, et al. Epigenetic modulation of BDNF gene in patients with major depressive disorder. Biol Psychiatry. 2013;73(2):e6–7.
21. Lin C, Shao B, Zhou Y, Niu X, Lin Y. Maternal high-fat diet influences stroke outcome in adult rat offspring. J Mol Endocrinol. 2016;56(2):101–12.
22. Ross MG, Desai M. Developmental programming of appetite/satiety. Ann Nutr Metab. 2014;64(Suppl 1):36–44.
23. Roseboom TJ, van der Meulen JHP, Ravelli ACJ, Osmond C, Barker DJ, Bleker OP. Effects of prenatal exposure to the Dutch famine on adult disease in later life – an overview. Mol Cell Endocrinol. 2001;185:93–8.
24. Hoek HW, Brown AS, Susser E. The Dutch famine and schizophrenia spectrum disorders. Soc Psychiatry Psychiatr Epidemiol. 1998;33:373–9.
25. Chadio SE, Kotsampasi B, Papadomichelakis G, Deligeorgis S, Kalogiannis D, Menegatos I, et al. Impact of maternal undernutrition on the hypothalamic-pituitary-adrenal axis responsiveness in sheep at different ages postnatal. J Endocrinol. 2007;192(3):495–503.
26. Navarrete M, Nunez H, Ruiz S, Soto-Moyano R, Valladares L, White A, et al. Prenatal undernutrition decreases the sensitivity of the hypothalamo-pituitary-adrenal axis in rat, as revealed by subcutaneous and intra-paraventricular dexamethasone challenges. Neurosci Lett. 2007;419(2):99–103.
27. Guzman-Quevedo O, Da Silva AR, Perez Garcia G, Matos RJ, de Sa Braga Oliveira A, Manhaes de Castro R, et al. Impaired hypothalamic mTOR activation in the adult rat offspring born to mothers fed a low-protein diet. PLoS One. 2013;8(9):e74990.
28. Juan De Solis A, Baquero AF, Bennett CM, Grove KL, Zeltser LM. Postnatal undernutrition delays a key step in the maturation of hypothalamic feeding circuits. Mol Metab. 2016;5(3):198–209.
29. Palou M, Picó C, Ja MK, Sánchez J, Priego T, Mathers JC, et al. Protective effects of leptin during the suckling period against later obesity may be associated with changes in promoter methylation of the hypothalamic pro-opiomelanocortin gene. Br J Nutr. 2011;106(5):769–78.
30. Wattez JS, Delahaye F, Barella LF, Dickes-Coopman a, Montel V, Breton C, et al. Short- and long-term effects of maternal perinatal undernutrition are lowered by cross-fostering during lactation in the male rat. J Dev Orig Health Dis. 2014;5(2):109–20.
31. Gotay CC, Katzmarzyk PT, Janssen I, Dawson MY, Aminoltejari K, Bartley NL. Updating the Canadian obesity maps: an epidemic in progress. Can J Public Health. 2013;104:64–8.
32. Van Lieshout RJ, Taylor VH, Boyle MH. Pre-pregnancy and pregnancy obesity and neurodevelopmental outcomes in offspring: a systematic review. Obes Reviews Off J Int Assoc Study Obes. 2011;12(5):e548–59.
33. Chang GQ, Gaysinskaya V, Karatayev O, Leibowitz SF. Maternal high-fat diet and fetal programming: increased proliferation of hypothalamic peptide-producing neurons that increase risk for overeating and obesity. J Neurosci. 2008;28(46):12107–19.
34. Long NM, Nathanielsz PW, Ford SP. The impact of maternal overnutrition and obesity on hypothalamic-pituitary-adrenal axis response of offspring to stress. Domest Anim Endocrinol. 2012;42(4):195–202.
35. Sasaki a, de Vega WC, St-Cyr S, Pan P, McGowan PO. Perinatal high fat diet alters glucocorticoid signaling and anxiety behavior in adulthood. Neuroscience. 2013;240:1–12.
36. Lin C, Shao B, Huang H, Zhou Y, Lin Y. Maternal high fat diet programs stress-induced behavioral disorder in adult offspring. Physiol Behav. 2015;152:119–27.
37. Sasaki A, Vega WD, Sivanathan S, St-Cyr S, McGowan P. Maternal high fat diet alters anxiety behavior and glucocorticoid signaling in adolescent offspring. Neuroscience. 2014;272:92.
38. Speakman J, Hambly C, Mitchell S, Krol E. Animal models of obesity. Obes Rev. 2007;8(s1):55–61.
39. Bellisario V, Berry A, Capoccia S, Raggi C, Panetta P, Branchi I, et al. Gender-dependent resiliency to stressful and metabolic challenges following prenatal exposure to high-fat diet in the p66Shcâ⁻/â⁻ mouse. Front Behav Neurosci. 2014;8(August):1–12.
40. McGowan PO, Meaney MJ, Szyf M. Diet and the epigenetic (re)programming of phenotypic differences in behavior. Brain Res. 2008;1237:12–24.
41. Bellisario V, Panetta P, Balsevich G, Baumann V, Noble J, Raggi C, et al. Maternal high-fat diet acts as a stressor increasing maternal glucocorticoids' signaling to the fetus and disrupting maternal behavior and brain activation in C57BL/6J mice. Psychoneuroendocrinology. 2015;60:138–50.

42. Connor KL, Vickers MH, Beltrand J, Meaney MJ, Sloboda DM. Nature, nurture or nutrition? Impact of maternal nutrition on maternal care, offspring development and reproductive function. J Physiol. 2012;590(9):2167–80.
43. Champagne FA, Meaney MJ. Stress during gestation alters postpartum maternal care and the development of the offspring in a rodent model. Biol Psychiatry. 2006;59(12):1227–35.
44. Lissau I, Sorensen TIA. Parental neglect during childhood and increased risk of obesity in young adulthood. Lancet. 1994;343(8893):324–7.
45. Curley JP, Mashoodh R, Champagne F. Epigenetics and the origins of paternal effects. Horm Behav. 2011;59(3):306–14.
46. Fullston T, Ohlsson Teague EMC, Palmer NO, DeBlasio MJ, Mitchell M, Corbett M, et al. Paternal obesity initiates metabolic disturbances in two generations of mice with incomplete penetrance to the F2 generation and alters the transcriptional profile of testis and sperm microRNA content. FASEB J Off Publ Fed Am Soc Exp Biol. 2013;27(10):4226–43.
47. Vickers MH. Developmental programming and transgenerational transmission of obesity. Ann Nutr Metab. 2014;64:26–34.
48. Veenendaal MV, Painter RC, de Rooij SR, Bossuyt PM, van der Post JA, Gluckman PD, et al. Transgenerational effects of prenatal exposure to the 1944–1945 Dutch famine. BJOG. 2013;120(5):548–53.
49. Rivera HM, Christiansen KJ, Sullivan EL. The role of maternal obesity in the risk of neuropsychiatric disorders. Front Neurosci. 2015;9:194.
50. Hiller-Sturmhofel S. The endocrine system: an overview. Alcohol Health Res World. 1998;22(3):153–65.
51. Korgan AC, Green AD, Perrot TS, Esser MJ. Limbic system activation is affected by prenatal predator exposure and postnatal environmental enrichment and further moderated by dam and sex. Behav Brain Res. 2014;259:106–18.

Chapter 3
Maternal Nutrition and Cognition

Rachael M. Taylor, Roger Smith, Clare E. Collins, and Alexis J. Hure

Key Points

- Cognition refers to the mental ability to process and retrieve new information using functions which include attention, memory, thinking, learning and perception
- The neural basis for cognition is largely unknown, however cognition is associated with brain maturation and the efficiency and connectivity of synapses in the neural circuit
- During the third trimester of pregnancy until the first years of life the brain is vulnerable epigenetic modifications which are a predictor of long-term brain function
- Epigenetics refers to the processes that occur 'on top of genetics' and encompasses the changes that occur to the genome that do not alter the DNA sequence
- DNA methylation is an epigenetic mechanism in which dietary nutrients (folate, methionine, vitamin B_2, B_6, B_{12}, choline and betaine) transfer methyl groups to DNA nucleotide bases and regulate gene transcription
- Epigenetic mechanisms can modify brain structure and function by the following mechanisms: (1) changing brain growth and development; (2) disturbing cell signalling molecules; and (3) increasing the toxic effects of neurotoxins

Keywords Child • Brain • Cognition • Development • DNA methylation • Epigenetics • Infant • Nutrition • Pregnancy • Supplement

R.M. Taylor, BND (✉)
Mothers and Babies Research Centre, University of Newcastle, Newcastle, NSW, Australia
e-mail: rachael.m.taylor@uon.edu.au

R. Smith, MB, BS (Hons) PhD
Department of Endocrinology, John Hunter Hospital, Mothers and Babies Research Centre,
University of Newcastle, Newcastle, NSW, Australia

C.E. Collins
Priority Research Centre for Physical Activity and Nutrition, University of Newcastle, Newcastle, NSW, Australia

A.J. Hure, PhD, BND (Hons I)
Priority Research Centre for Gender, Health and Ageing, University of Newcastle, Newcastle, NSW, Australia

© Springer International Publishing AG 2017
R. Rajendram et al. (eds.), *Diet, Nutrition, and Fetal Programming*,
Nutrition and Health, DOI 10.1007/978-3-319-60289-9_3

Abbreviations

5-MTHF	5-methyltetrahydrofolate
5,10-MeTH	Methylenetetrahydrofolate
ACh	Acetylcholine
ATP	Adenosine triphosphate
BER	Base excision repair
CHT	Choline transporter
DHF	Dihydrofolate
DHFR	Dihydrofolate reductase
DTI	Diffusion tensor imaging
DMG	Dimethylglycine
Dnmts	DNA methyltransferase
g	Grams
HDAC	Histone deacetylase complexes
HM	High methionine
HM/LF	High methionine/low folate
IAP	Intracisternal A-type particle
IGF-2	Insulin-like growth factor-2
Kg	Kilograms
LF	Low folate
MECPs	Methyl-CpG-binding proteins
mg	Milligrams
MRI	Magnetic resonance imaging
mmol/l	Millimoles per litre
MTHF	Methyltetrahydrofolate
MTHFR	Methyltetrahydrofolate reductase
SAH	S-adenosylhomocysteine
SAM	S-adenosylmethionine
SNPs	Single nucleotide polymorphisms
THF	Tetrahydrofolate
μg	Micrograms

Introduction

Adequate nutrition during early life is essential for optimal foetal brain development. The prenatal and postnatal periods are characterised by rapid changes in neuronal organisation, this is a critical period in which the nutrition environment can have a profound influence on the long-term function of the brain [1]. Increasing evidence suggests that nutrient-gene interactions, a process called epigenetics, can modify the genetic programming required for brain development [2–4]. DNA methylation is an epigenetic mechanism that requires dietary nutrients to allow the donation of methyl groups to DNA nucleotides and modify gene structure or gene expression. DNA methylation has been correlated with brain plasticity which is important for cognitive function including memory and learning [5]. This chapter focuses largely on the methyl donors and cofactors involved in DNA methylation, as a potential pathway for nutrition to affect cognition. The key points of this chapter are summarised in Table 3.1.

Table 3.1 Key points of early life nutrition and cognition

1. Cognition refers to the mental ability to process and retrieve new information using functions which include attention, memory, thinking, learning and perception
2. The neural basis for cognition is largely unknown, however cognition is associated with brain maturation and the efficiency and connectivity of synapses in the neural circuit
3. During the third trimester of pregnancy until the first years of life the brain is vulnerable epigenetic modifications which are a predictor of long-term brain function
4. Epigenetics refers to the processes that occur 'on top of genetics' and encompasses the changes that occur to the genome that do not alter the DNA sequence
5. DNA methylation is an epigenetic mechanism in which dietary nutrients (folate, methionine, vitamin B_2, B_6, B_{12}, choline and betaine) transfer methyl groups to DNA nucleotide bases and regulate gene transcription
6. Epigenetic mechanisms can modify brain structure and function by the following mechanisms: (1) changing brain growth and development; (2) disturbing cell signalling molecules; and (3) increasing the toxic effects of neurotoxins

Optimising Cognitive Development

Suboptimal cognition has major long-term consequences for individuals and societies. Grantham-McGregor et al. [6] estimated that more than 200 million children under the age of 5 years in developing countries fail to reach their cognitive potential due to many factors including nutrition. Children with suboptimal cognition are less likely to lead productive adult lives due to fewer years of schooling and less learning per school year [6]. Data from 51 developing countries demonstrates that each year of schooling increased annual income by 9.7% [7]. Suboptimal cognition during childhood has been associated with an increased risk for adolescent delinquency leading to adult violent criminality [8–12]. Strategies that aim to maximise child cognition are important for public health and optimising nutrition during pregnancy and infancy is a good place to start.

Brain Development

The development of the brain follows a series of lifelong neurological processes (Fig. 3.1). The human brain originates from the fertilized ovum that undergoes cell division, resulting in a cluster of proliferating cells, called a blastocyst [13]. The cells of the blastocyst then differentiate into the trophoblast and also a three-layer structure, called the embryonic disk, of which the outer layer or the ectoderm gives rise to the central nervous system [13]. Strategies (including nutrition) that aim to optimise brain development are essential given that neuroanatomical maturation is correlated with cognitive development [14–16].

Cognition refers to the mental ability to process and retrieve new information using functions which include attention, memory, thinking, learning and perception [18]. The neural mechanisms that underlie cognition remain largely unknown, however the prefrontal cortex is thought to play a prominent [19–21]. Evidence from adults and primates has shown that prefrontal lesions are associated with impairments in cognitive functions [22, 23]. In addition, frontal lobe maturation (decrease in grey matter) was associated with increased verbal memory functioning in healthy children aged 7–16 years [16].

Emerging evidence suggests that cognitive function requires integrated brain systems rather the prefrontal cortex in isolation [24, 25]. One neuroimaging study demonstrated that the maturation of the prefrontal cortex is associated with the development of the uncinate fasciculus and superior longitudinal fasciculus, responsible for establishing connectivity between frontal and limbic structures (including amygdala and hippocampus) that regulate mood and emotions (Fig. 3.2) [26]. Nagy et al.

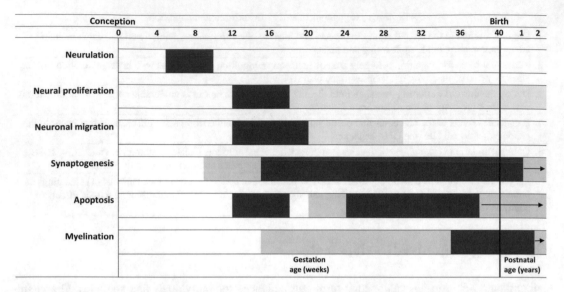

Fig. 3.1 A timeline of the neurological processes required for human brain development during fetal and postnatal life. Neurulation: formation of neural tube. Neural proliferation: production of neurons and glial cells. Neuronal migration: neurons migrate to specific brain regions. Synaptogenesis: neurons form synapses. Apoptosis: programmed cell death. Myelination: myelin surround neuron axons. Peak neurological activity is indicated in *red* and low or medium activity is indicated in *grey*. The *arrows* indicate that synaptogenesis, apoptosis and myelination are lifelong processes (Adapted from Linderkamp et al. [17])

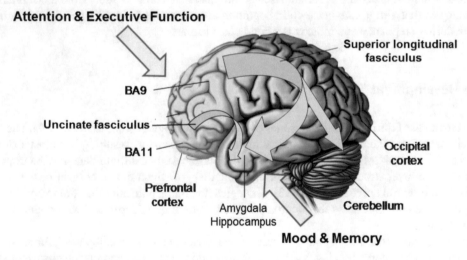

Fig. 3.2 Frontal lobe connectivity with limbic structures is mediated in the uncinate fasciculus and superior longitudinal fasciculus which matures during childhood and adolescence (Reprinted with permission from McNamara et al. [26])

[27] used diffusion tensor imaging (DTI) in children aged 8–18 years and found that the prefrontal-parietal connectivity is associated with memory capacity. Liston and colleagues [28] demonstrated that DTI-based connectivity in frontostriatal and posterior fibres was associated with age but also working memory capacity, measured using the Go/No Go task which requires subjects to press the go or no-go button in response to a different set of stimuli. These findings highlight that the underlying connectivity of the prefrontal cortex is more important for cognition compared to region specific

maturation. Further evidence also suggests that cognitive development during childhood coincides with the gradual elimination of synapses which strengthens the connectivity and communication of the neural circuit [14, 16, 29].

Child cognitive function is influenced by genetic, biomedical, nutrition, social and environmental factors. Recent evidence suggests that 50% of individual variation in cognitive ability is attributed to genetic factors, including the expression of specific genes, single nucleotide polymorphisms (SNPs) and inheritable phenotypes [30]. Biomedical risk factors that contribute to child cognition include time of birth, maternal age, gravidity, maternal physical condition, intrauterine growth and prematurity [31]. Suboptimal cognition is associated with a shorter childhood stature and lower weight for age related to postnatal nutritional status [32, 33]. Parental social position, parental education, maternal intelligence and home environment are all considered to be significant predictors of child cognitive function [34, 35].

Nutrition and Brain Development

Lipids, protein, carbohydrates, vitamins and minerals are required for the structural composition of the developing foetal brain. The composition of the brain (Table 3.2) changes throughout life due to ongoing neurological processes including neural differentiation, apoptosis, synaptogenesis and myelination. Lipids are highly prevalent in the structural matrix of cell membranes, as well as myelin [36]. Protein is required for neurotransmitters, enzymes, cell membranes and myelin [36]. A constant supply of glucose is required to support the energy demand of the brain.

The human brain is vulnerable to nutritional insults during periods of rapid growth, particularly during the third trimester of pregnancy and the first 2 years of infant life [39]. This is a critical period for nutrient-gene interactions to affect the expression of multiple genes involved in cell development, signalling and function [40–42] in the brain. Although nutrient-gene interactions continue to occur across the lifespan, the potential for nutrition to influence brain function is much greater during early life than in adulthood [43].

Epigenetics

Epigenetics refers to the processes that occur 'on top of genetics' and encompasses the changes that occur to the genome that do not alter the DNA sequence [44]. The major processes involved in epigenetics are DNA methylation, histone modification and noncoding RNA. Most studies that have examined the effects of nutrition on epigenetics have focused on DNA methylation [44].

Table 3.2 Composition of the human brain during development

	Pregnancy 13–14 weeks	Pregnancy 20–22 weeks	Birth	Adult
Brain weight (g)	4.65	34	365	1438
Water (ml)	914	922	897	774
Lipids (%) total brain weight	[a]	[a]	4	12
Proteins (%) total brain weight	[a]	[a]	6	11
Carbohydrates (%) total brain weight	[a]	[a]	[a]	1

Adapted from: Widdowson et al. [37] and Turner et al. [38]
[a]Unquantified value

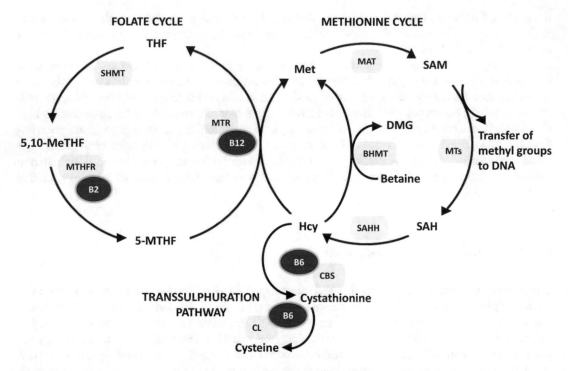

Fig. 3.3 Methionine/homocysteine metabolic pathway (Adapted from Refsum et al. [48])

DNA methylation involves the transfer of methyl groups between substrates via the methionine/ homocysteine metabolic pathway (Fig. 3.3). Methyl groups are obtained from dietary nutrients including, folate, methionine, vitamin B_2, B_6, B_{12}, choline and betaine. The methionine/homocysteine metabolic pathway is facilitated by the folate dependent cycle; 5,10 methylenetetrahydrofolate (5,10-MeTHF) is reduced to 5-methyltetrahydrofolate (5-MTHF) by methyltetrahydrofolate reductase (MTHFR) with vitamin B_2 serving as a cofactor [45]. 5-methyltetrahydrofolate (MTHF) serves as the methyl donor in the conversion of the amino acid, homocysteine to methionine [45]. This reaction is catalyzed by methionine synthase (methyltetrahydrofolate-homocysteine methyltransferase) and vitamin B_{12} serves as a cofactor. Alternatively, betaine (derived from choline) converts homocysteine to dimethylglycine (DMG) and methionine, via the methionine cycle [46]. Methionine is activated by the addition of an adenosyl group from adenosine triphosphate (ATP) to form S-adenosylmethionine (SAM), which serves as a methyl donor to form S-adenosylhomocysteine (SAH) [47]. Through the removal of the adenosine group, SAH is converted to homocysteine by S-adenosylhomocysteine hydrolase [47]. A family of enzymes called DNA methyltransferase (Dnmts) catalyses the transfer of methyl groups from SAM to DNA cytosine bases that are followed by a guanosine (5′-CpG-3′ sites) [46].

Most CpG sites in the human genome are methylated (90–98%) [49] however, there are CpG-rich areas (or CpG islands) located at the 5′ end of the regulatory region of genes that are not methylated [50]. When CpG islands are methylated, gene expression is usually repressed [50, 51]. The mechanisms that underlie the repression of transcription by DNA methylation are not well understood, however several mechanisms have been hypothesised [52]. Firstly, methylated cytosines interfere with the binding of RNA polymerase and transcriptions factors required for DNA transcription. However DNA methylation does not inhibit the binding of all transcription factors and not every methylated DNA site will contain a CpG dinucleotide, therefore regulation by this mechanism is rare [52]. DNA methylation can also repress gene expression via methyl-CpG-binding proteins (MECPs)

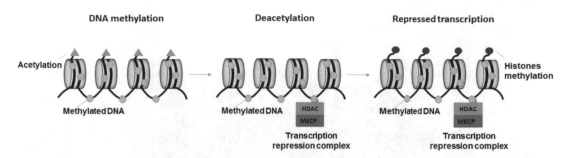

Fig. 3.4 DNA methylation and histone modification mechanisms interact in synergy to repress gene transcription. Methyl-CpG-binding proteins (MECPs) and histone deacetylase (HDAC) complexes are recruited to methylated DNA and induce histone deacetylation. These complexes catalyse the methylation of specific lysine residues on the histones and represses transcription (Adapted from Li et al. [56])

which interact with histone modification mechanisms (Fig. 3.4) [53]. MECP forms a complex with histone deacetylase complexes (HDAC), which induces histone deacetylation and catalyses the methylation of specific lysine residues [54]. These modifications prevent the binding of transcription factors and RNA polymerase to the DNA which silences gene expression [55]. This process highlights that interactions can occur between DNA methylation and histone modification mechanisms to prevent DNA transcription.

Maternal Diet and Epigenetics

The Agouti mouse model [57–59] is the most widely cited example of the effects of maternal nutrition on the epigenome of the offspring. Supplementing the maternal diet with methyl donor nutrients increased DNA methylation of an intracisternal A-type particle (IAP) retrotransposon inserted near the agouti gene and shifted the offspring's coat colour from yellow to brown (pseudoagouti) (Fig. 3.5) [57, 60]. The agouti phenotype, associated with a yellow coat colour [57, 60], predisposes mice to overeating, obesity, diabetes, tumorigenesis and reduced longevity [59, 61, 62]. The findings demonstrate that maternal nutrition can be associated with epigenetic modifications, which have long-term consequences for the health of the offspring.

A recent human study in The Gambia found that maternal diet related to the season of conception can produce differences in the methylation of metastable epialleles (loci) [64]. This study demonstrated that children who were conceived during the nutritionally disadvantageous, 'hungry', rainy season had increased DNA methylation at these loci, compared to children who were conceived during the nutritionally advantageous dry season. These findings illustrate that subtle dietary changes during conception can result in significant epigenetic modifications in the offspring.

Epigenetics and Brain Development

Epigenetic mechanisms are known to modify brain structure and function by at least three mechanisms: (1) changing brain growth and development; (2) disturbing cell signalling molecules; (3) increasing the toxic effects of neurotoxins [65–67] . The following section reviews the literature on the effects of maternal nutrition on epigenetics in the brain of the offspring.

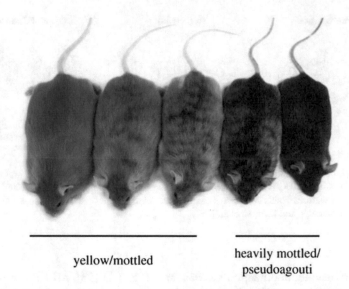

yellow/mottled

heavily mottled/
pseudoagouti

Fig. 3.5 Genetically identical 3-months-old Avy mice representing the five coat colour phenotypes. Yellow mice are hypomethylated at the transposable element upstream of the Agouti gene allowing maximal ectopic expression, whereas hypermethylation of this site silences ectopic Agouti expression in the pseudoagouti animals (Reprinted with permission from Cropley et al. [63])

Methyl Donor Nutrients and Brain Development

Folate

Dietary folate is the most extensively studied micronutrient in DNA methylation research. A major driver of this interest is the strong evidence from a randomised control trial that demonstrated that taking folic acid supplementation taken before and during early pregnancy could prevent 72% of neural tube defect affected pregnancies [68]. Since this publication 70 countries have introduced mandatory food fortification with folate added into grain or flour and women are advised to consume 400 µg folic acid supplement from preconception until the end of the first trimester [69]. Folic acid is the form of vitamin provided from food fortification and supplements, whereas folate is predominantly the form of vitamin that naturally occurs in food. The utilisation of folic acid in the methionine/homocysteine pathway differs from that of dietary folate primarily because the synthetic form needs be reduced to tetrahydrofolate (THF) via dihydrofolate (DHF) by DHF reductase (DHFR) [70].

The epigenetic effects of folic acid on cell signalling pathways via the growth hormone, insulin-like growth factor-2 (IGF-2) have been analysed in three human studies [71–73]. Growth hormones are believed to affect cognitive function via their actions on the excitatory circuits involved in synaptic plasticity [74]. Steegers-Theunissen et al. [71] found that maternal folic acid supplementation (400 mg/day) was associated with a 4.5% increase in IGF-2 methylation (49.5% vs. 47.4%) in their children (*n* = 120) at 18 months, as measured by bisulphite sequencing using whole blood samples. However a cross-sectional study did not support these findings, as IGF-2 methylation patterns in the cord blood of their offspring (*n* = 99) was not associated with maternal serum folate [72]. Although these findings may not be externally valid considering that none of the women took folic acid supplements before or during pregnancy and serum folate concentrations were comparable to populations without access to fortified foods. Hoyo et al. [73] also demonstrated that maternal folic acid supplementation (400 mg/day) was associated with lower methylated levels within the IGF-2 promoter of blood leukocytes located in the umbilical cord [73]. The heterogeneity of the methodologies used in these studies may account for the varied findings. For example, DNA methylation patterns are tissue specific, therefore maternal whole blood samples versus cord blood samples are likely to vary in their methylation profile. Due to the lack of comparability between these studies it is difficult to determine the real effects of dietary folate on methylation patterns of IGF-2 and cognitive function.

Folate is responsible for donating a methyl group to the nucleobase uracil to form thymine, which is required for of DNA maintenance and repair [75]. A folate deficiency may result in the misincorporation of uracil in the place of thymine [75] which can cause DNA instability [76, 77] and neurological disorders. Langie et al. [78] tested the effect of maternal folate depletion in mice during pregnancy and lactation and high-fat feeding from weaning on DNA methylation and the expression of selected base excision repair (BER) related genes [79]. The analysis of DNA methylation using pyrosequencing of bisulfite-converted DNA revealed that maternal folate depletion increased BER activity in the offspring at weaning [79]. High-fat feeding from weaning as well as folate depletion was associated with a significant decrease in BER activity in the cortex, cerebellum, hippocampus and subcortical regions in the offspring at 6 months [79]. The expression of BER related genes was also correlated with a decrease in BER activity [79]. This evidence an animal model indicates that folate deficiencies during both pregnancy and lactation compromises DNA repair mechanisms which may predispose the brain to nutritional insults and neurological disorders.

Choline and Betaine

Choline is a major source of methyl groups in the diet, the nutrient can be oxidised to betaine in the methionine/homocysteine pathway [80]. Foods rich in choline include beef and chicken liver, eggs, wheat germ, bacon, dried soybeans and pork [80]. During pregnancy the synthesis of choline is upregulated, however due to the high demand for this nutrient, the maternal choline stores become depleted [81, 82]. Therefore, an adequate intake of choline during pregnancy is essential to meet the high physiological demands for this nutrient.

Choline is a precursor of the neurotransmitter acetylcholine (ACh) which is required for cell signalling pathways which are known to be important for cognitive processes. There is convincing evidence that cortical cholinergic transmission is essential for mediating attention functions and capacities [82, 83]. Previous studies have shown that the maternal choline status influences the mechanisms that control ACh synthesis. Prenatally choline-supplemented rats are known to derived a high proportion of choline for ACh synthesis from phosphatidylcholine [84, 85], whereas choline deficient rats are reliant on the upregulation of choline transport by the high-affinity choline transporter (CHT) [84]. Evidence suggests that epigenetic mechanisms trigger the over-expression of the CHT gene which causes the upregulation of the choline transport [86]. This evidence highlights that the epigenome is responsive to changes in the availability of prenatal choline, however it is unclear how long this mechanism will compensate for a choline deficiency.

Recent studies have analysed whether epigenetic mechanisms are involved in release of synthesised ACh [86–88]. It is known that the IGF-2 receptor is involved in the release of ACh in response to the binding of IGF-2 in the hippocampus [88]. Given this knowledge, Mellot et al. [86] found that prenatal choline supplementation (35.6 mmol/kg) in rodents, increased the expression of the IGF-2 receptor gene in the frontal cortex of the offspring at embryonic day 18, as analysed using oligonucleotide microarrays. Another study of newborn piglets confirmed that IGF-2 receptor gene was upregulated following prenatal betaine supplementation [89]. Napoli et al. [87] extended on the findings on the previous studies demonstrating that IGF-2/depolarization-evoked ACh release from hippocampal slices and frontal cortex was enhanced by prenatal choline supplementation [87]. These early findings emphasise that choline availability affects the synthesis and release of ACh via epigenetic modifications which is important for attention functions and capacities.

Vitamins B_2, B_6 and B_{12}

Vitamins B_2, B_6 and B_{12} are important for catalysing the reactions involved in the methionine/homocysteine metabolic pathway. The epigenetic effects of these nutrients on brain development has not been well explored in the literature. Most studies have investigated the effects of administrating folic acid supplements alone or in combination with other B-vitamins during pregnancy. This is a concern considering that biochemical pathways of vitamin B_2, B_6 and B_{12} are interrelated in the one-carbon metabolism, therefore increasing the level of one vitamin could mask the effects of another vitamin deficiency. For example, Morris et al. [90] demonstrated that a low vitamin B_{12} status was associated with significant cognitive decline over an 8 year period and this effect was exacerbated in those taking folate supplements. In addition, Min et al. [91] analysed the effects of folate supplementation on one-carbon metabolism in vitamin B_{12} deficient rats with elevated plasma homocysteine. This study found that folate supplementation did normalise plasma homocysteine but also changed SAM and SAH concentrations in the brain which may affect DNA methylation levels. Based on this evidence it is important that future studies focus on understanding the effects of vitamin B_2, B_6 and B_{12} in isolation and combination. This knowledge will be important for understanding the synergistic effects of B-vitamins on DNA methylation and brain development.

Methionine

Methionine is an essential amino acid acquired from dietary protein and is required for homocysteine metabolism. Excess dietary methionine will disrupt DNA methylation by inhibiting remethylation of homocysteine which is expected to cause hyperhomocysteinemia [92]. It is known that high levels of homocysteine are neurotoxic causing oxidative stress, the inhibition of methylation reactions, DNA damage and apoptosis [93]. The effects of hyperhomocysteinemia on the brain in the aging population has been extensively studied [94–96]. However, few studies have examined the effects in the developing brain. Devlin et al. [97] compared brain SAM, SAH and genome-wide DNA methylation in wildtype and heterozygous methylenetetrahydrofolate reductase knockout mice (hyperhomocysteinemia). The mice of different genotypes were fed one of four diets: control, high methionine (HM), low folate (LF) or high methionine/low folate (HM/LF), starting at weaning for 7–15 weeks. This study reported that methionine supplementation significantly reduced the SAM:SAH ratio in the brain of the heterozygous methylenetetrahydrofolate reductase knockout mice, the SAM:SAH ratio was further reduced in both phenotypes that were fed the LF or LF/HM diet [97]. Methionine supplementation did not significantly affect the brain genome-wide DNA methylation [97]. Further evidence is required to clarify if any epigenetic changes occurred at a gene-specific level. Based on the limited evidence available it is yet to be determined how excessive dietary methionine affects the epigenome and brain function.

Conclusion

Early life is a critical window for establishing epigenetic marks that modify brain structure and function by altering neuroanatomical development, disturbing cell signalling molecules and increasing neurotoxins, these key events may be modified by variations in maternal and child nutrition. Considerable more research is needed in this area to determine the effects of methyl donor nutrients during the pre and postnatal period on brain function and cognition. This evidence will be important for informing dietary recommendations for pregnant women in order to optimise foetal brain development and long-term cognitive function and child outcomes.

References

1. Fagiolini M, Jensen CL, Champagne FA. Epigenetic influences on brain development and plasticity. Curr Opin Neurobiol. 2009;19(2):207–12. PubMed PMID: 19545993. Pubmed Central PMCID: PMC2745597. Epub 2009/06/24. eng.
2. Bryan J, Osendarp S, Hughes D, Calvaresi E, Baghurst K, van Klinken JW. Nutrients for cognitive development in school-aged children. Nutr Rev. 2004;62(8):295–306. PubMed PMID: WOS:000227435000001. English.
3. Toga AW, Thompson PM, Sowell ER. Mapping brain maturation. Trends Neurosci. 2006;29(3):148–59.
4. Giedd JN, Blumenthal J, Jeffries NO, Castellanos FX, Liu H, Zijdenbos A, et al. Brain development during childhood and adolescence: a longitudinal MRI study. Nat Neurosci. 1999;2(10):861. PubMed PMID: 8829982.
5. Lister R, Mukamel EA, Nery JR, Urich M, Puddifoot CA, Johnson ND, et al. Global epigenomic reconfiguration during mammalian brain development. Science. 2013;341(6146):1237905. PubMed PMID: 23828890. Pubmed Central PMCID: PMC3785061. Epub 2013/07/06. eng.
6. Grantham-McGregor S, Cheung YB, Cueto S, Glewwe P, Richter L, Strupp B. Developmental potential in the first 5 years for children in developing countries. Lancet. 2007;369(9555):60–70. PubMed PMID: 17208643. Pubmed Central PMCID: PMC2270351. Epub 2007/01/09. eng.
7. Psacharopoulos G, Patrinos HA. Returns to investment in education: a further update. Educ Econ. 2004;12(2):111–34.
8. Farrington DP. Early predictors of adolescent aggression and adult violence. Violence Vict. 1989;4(2):79–100. PubMed PMID: 2487131. Epub 1989/01/01. eng.
9. Kaslow FW, Lipsitt PD, Buka SL, Lipsitt LP. Family law issues in family therapy practice: early intelligence scores and subsequent delinquency: a prospective study. Am J Fam Ther. 1990;18(2):197–208.
10. Fergusson DM, Horwood LJ, Ridder EM. Show me the child at seven II: childhood intelligence and later outcomes in adolescence and young adulthood. J Child Psychol Psychiatry. 2005;46(8):850–8. PubMed PMID: 16033633. Epub 2005/07/22. eng.
11. Stattin H, Klackenberg-Larsson I. Early language and intelligence development and their relationship to future criminal behavior. J Abnorm Psychol. 1993;102(3):369–78. PubMed PMID: 8408948. Epub 1993/08/01. eng.
12. Frisell T, Pawitan Y, Långström N. Is the association between general cognitive ability and violent crime caused by family-level confounders? PLoS One. 2012;7(7):e41783.
13. Johnson MH. Developmental cognitive neuroscience. 3rd ed. Hoboken: Wiley-Blackwell; 2010.
14. Casey BJ, Giedd JN, Thomas KM. Structural and functional brain development and its relation to cognitive development. Biol Psychol. 2000;54(1–3):241–57. PubMed PMID: 11035225. Epub 2000/10/18. eng.
15. Spear LP. The adolescent brain and age-related behavioral manifestations. Neurosci Biobehav Rev. 2000;24(4):417–63. PubMed PMID: 10817843. Epub 2000/05/19. eng.
16. Sowell ER, Delis D, Stiles J, Jernigan TL. Improved memory functioning and frontal lobe maturation between childhood and adolescence: a structural MRI study. J Int Neuropsychol Soc: JINS. 2001;7(3):312–22. PubMed PMID: 11311032. Epub 2001/04/20. eng.
17. Linderkamp O, Ludwig J, Rupert L, Dagmar BS. Time table of normal foetal brain development. Int J Prenat Perinatal Psychol Med. 2009;21:4–16.
18. Bhatnagar S, Taneja S. Zinc and cognitive development. Br J Nutr. 2001;85(SUPPL. 2):S139–S45. PubMed PMID: 2001227169. English.
19. Goldman-Rakic PS. Circuitry of primate prefrontal cortex and regulation of behavior by representational memory. Comprehensive physiology. Maryland, United States: Wiley; 2011.
20. Diamond A. Abilities and neural mechanisms underlying $\overline{AB}$ performance. Child Dev. 1988;59(2):523–7.
21. Dempster FN. The rise and fall of the inhibitory mechanism: toward a unified theory of cognitive development and aging. Dev Rev. 1992;12(1):45–75.
22. Miller EK, Cohen JD. An integrative theory of prefrontal function. Annu Rev Neurosci. 2001;24(1):167–202.
23. Luria AR. Higher cognitive functions. New York: ManBasic Books; 1966.
24. Goldman-Rakic PS. Topography of cognition: parallel distributed networks in primate association cortex. Annu Rev Neurosci. 1988;11:137–56. PubMed PMID: 3284439. Epub 1988/01/01. eng.
25. Luna B, Thulborn KR, Munoz DP, Merriam EP, Garver KE, Minshew NJ, et al. Maturation of widely distributed brain function subserves cognitive development. NeuroImage. 2001;13(5):786–93. PubMed PMID: 11304075. Epub 2001/04/17. eng.
26. McNamara RK, Vannest JJ, Valentine CJ. Role of perinatal long-chain omega-3 fatty acids in cortical circuit maturation: mechanisms and implications for psychopathology. World J Psychiatr. 2015;5(1):15–34.
27. Nagy Z, Westerberg H, Klingberg T. Maturation of white matter is associated with the development of cognitive functions during childhood. J Cogn Neurosci. 2004;16(7):1227–33. PubMed PMID: 15453975. Epub 2004/09/30. eng.
28. Liston C, Watts R, Tottenham N, Davidson MC, Niogi S, Ulug A, et al. Developmental differences in diffusion measures of cortical fiber tracts. J Cogn Neurosci. 2003;15:S57–S8.

29. Tau GZ, Peterson BS. Normal development of brain circuits. Neuropsychopharmacology. 2010;35(1):147–68. PubMed PMID: 19794405. Pubmed Central PMCID: PMC3055433. Epub 2009/10/02. eng.

30. Deary IJ, Johnson W, Houlihan LM. Genetic foundations of human intelligence. Hum Genet. 2009;126(1):215–32.

31. Lawlor DA, Batty GD, Morton SM, Deary IJ, Macintyre S, Ronalds G, et al. Early life predictors of childhood intelligence: evidence from the Aberdeen children of the 1950s study. J Epidemiol Community Health. 2005;59(8):656–63. PubMed PMID: 16020642. Pubmed Central PMCID: PMC1733112. Epub 2005/07/16. eng.

32. Stabler B, Clopper RR, Siegel PT, Stoppani C, Compton PG, Underwood LE. Academic achievement and psychological adjustment in short children. The National Cooperative Growth Study. J Dev Behav Pediatr: JDBP. 1994;15(1):1–6. PubMed PMID: 8195431. Epub 1994/02/01. eng.

33. Stathis SL, O'Callaghan MJ, Williams GM, Najman JM, Andersen MJ, Bor W. Behavioural and cognitive associations of short stature at 5 years. J Paediatr Child Health. 1999;35(6):562–7. PubMed PMID: 10634984. Epub 2000/01/15. eng.

34. Tong S, Baghurst P, Vimpani G, McMichael A. Socioeconomic position, maternal IQ, home environment, and cognitive development. J Pediatr. 2007;151(3):284–8. 8 e1. PubMed PMID: 17719939. Epub 2007/08/28. eng.

35. Bacharach VR, Baumeister AA. Direct and indirect effects of maternal intelligence, maternal age, income, and home environment on intelligence of preterm, low-birth-weight children. J Appl Dev Psychol. 1998;19(3):361–75.

36. Bourre JM. Effects of nutrients (in food) on the structure and function of the nervous system: update on dietary requirements for brain. Part 1: micronutrients. J Nutr Health Aging. 2006;10(5):377–85. PubMed PMID: 17066209. Epub 2006/10/27. eng.

37. Widdowson EM, Dickerson JWT. The effect of growth and function on the chemical composition of soft tissues. Biochem J. 1960;77(1):30–43. PubMed PMID: PMC1204895.

38. Turner AJ. In: McIlwain H, Bachelard HS, editors. Biochemistry and the central nervous system. 5th ed. Edinburgh: Churchill Livingstone; 1985. p. 660. £40 ISBN 0-443-01961-4. Biochemical Education. 1986;14(1):46.

39. Nyaradi A, Jiang Hong L, Hickling S, Foster J, Oddy WH. The role of nutrition in children's neurocognitive development, from pregnancy through childhood. Front Hum Neurosci. 2013;7:97.

40. Qureshi IA, Mehler MF. Epigenetic mechanisms governing the process of neurodegeneration. Mol Asp Med. 2013;34(4):875–82.

41. Dauncey MJ, White P, Burton KA, Katsumata M. Nutrition-hormone receptor-gene interactions: implications for development and disease. Proc Nutr Soc. 2001;60(1):63–72. PubMed PMID: 11310425. Epub 2001/04/20. eng.

42. Dauncey M. Genomic and epigenomic insights into nutrition and brain disorders. Forum Nutr. 2013;5(3):887. PubMed PMID: doi:10.3390/nu5030887.

43. Georgieff MK, Brunette KE, Tran PV. Early life nutrition and neural plasticity. Dev Psychopathol. 2015;27(Special Issue 02):411–23.

44. Burdgea GC, Hoilea SP, Lillycropb KA. Epigenetics: are there implications for personalised nutrition. Curr Opin Clin Nutr Metab Care. 2012;15(5):442–7.

45. Tibbetts AS, Appling DR. Compartmentalization of mammalian folate-mediated one-carbon metabolism. Annu Rev Nutr. 2010;30:57–81.

46. Zeisel SH. Epigenetic mechanisms for nutrition determinants of later health outcomes. Am J Clin Nutr. 2009;89(5):1488S–93S. PubMed PMID: PMC2677001.

47. Stipanuk MH. Sulfur amino acid metabolism pathways for production and removal of homocysteine and cysteine. Annu Rev Nutr. 2004;24:539–77.

48. Refsum H, Grindflek AW, Ueland PM, Fredriksen Å, Meyer K, Ulvik A, et al. Screening for serum total homocysteine in newborn children. Clin Chem. 2004;50(10):1769–84.

49. Suzuki MM, Bird A. DNA methylation landscapes: provocative insights from epigenomics. Nat Rev Genet. 2008;9(6):465–76. PubMed PMID: 18463664. Epub 2008/05/09. eng.

50. Jeltsch A. Beyond Watson and Crick: DNA methylation and molecular enzymology of DNA methyltransferases. Chembiochem: Eur J Chem Biol. 2002;3(4):274–93. PubMed PMID: 11933228. Epub 2002/04/05. eng.

51. Bird AP. CpG-rich islands and the function of DNA methylation. Nature. 1986;321(6067):209–13. PubMed PMID: 2423876. Epub 1986/05/15. eng.

52. Crider KS, Yang TP, Berry RJ, Bailey LB. Folate and DNA methylation: a review of molecular mechanisms and the evidence for folate's role. Adv Nutr (Bethesda, Md). 2012;3(1):21–38. PubMed PMID: 22332098. Pubmed Central PMCID: PMC3262611. Epub 2012/02/15. eng.

53. Dhasarathy A, Wade PA. The MBD protein family-reading an epigenetic mark? Mutat Res. 2008;647(1–2):39–43. PubMed PMID: 18692077. Pubmed Central PMCID: PMC2670759. Epub 2008/08/12. eng.

54. Nan X, Ng HH, Johnson CA, Laherty CD, Turner BM, Eisenman RN, et al. Transcriptional repression by the methyl-CpG-binding protein MeCP2 involves a histone deacetylase complex. Nature. 1998;393(6683):386–9. PubMed PMID: 9620804. Epub 1998/06/10. eng.

55. Gluckman PD, Hanson MA, Buklijas T, Low FM, Beedle AS. Epigenetic mechanisms that underpin metabolic and cardiovascular diseases. Nat Rev Endocrinol. 2009;5(7):401–8. PubMed PMID: 19488075. Epub 2009/06/03. eng.

56. Li E. Chromatin modification and epigenetic reprogramming in mammalian development. Nat Rev Genet. 2002;3(9):662–73.
57. Wolff GL, Kodell RL, Moore SR, Cooney CA. Maternal epigenetics and methyl supplements affect agouti gene expression in Avy/a mice. FASEB J. 1998;12(11):949–57.
58. Waterland RA, Jirtle RL. Transposable elements: targets for early nutritional effects on epigenetic gene regulation. Mol Cell Biol. 2003;23(15):5293–300. PubMed PMID: 12861015. Pubmed Central PMCID: PMC165709. Epub 2003/07/16. eng.
59. Morgan HD, Sutherland HG, Martin DI, Whitelaw E. Epigenetic inheritance at the agouti locus in the mouse. Nat Genet. 1999;23(3):314–8. PubMed PMID: 10545949. Epub 1999/11/05. eng.
60. Cooney CA, Dave AA, Wolff GL. Maternal methyl supplements in mice affect epigenetic variation and DNA methylation of offspring. J Nutr. 2002;132(8 Suppl):2393S–400S. PubMed PMID: 12163699. Epub 2002/08/07. eng.
61. Wolff GL, Roberts DW, Galbraith DB. Prenatal determination of obesity, tumor susceptibility, and coat color pattern in viable yellow (Avy/a) mice. The yellow mouse syndrome. J Hered. 1986;77(3):151–8. PubMed PMID: 3734404. Epub 1986/05/01. eng.
62. Wolff GL, Roberts DW, Mountjoy KG. Physiological consequences of ectopic agouti gene expression: the yellow obese mouse syndrome. Physiol Genomics. 1999;1(3):151–63. PubMed PMID: 11015573. Epub 2000/10/04. eng.
63. Cropley JE, Dang TH, Martin DI, Suter CM. The penetrance of an epigenetic trait in mice is progressively yet reversibly increased by selection and environment. Proc Biol Sci/Royal Soc. 2012;279(1737):2347–53. PubMed PMID: 22319121. Pubmed Central PMCID: PMC3350677. Epub 2012/02/10. eng.
64. Waterland RA, Kellermayer R, Laritsky E, Rayco-Solon P, Harris RA, Travisano M, et al. Season of conception in rural gambia affects DNA methylation at putative human metastable epialleles. PLoS Genet. 2010;6(12):e1001252. PubMed PMID: 21203497. Pubmed Central PMCID: PMC3009670. Epub 2011/01/05. eng.
65. Gallagher EA, Newman JP, Green LR, Hanson MA. The effect of low protein diet in pregnancy on the development of brain metabolism in rat offspring. J Physiol. 2005;568(Pt 2):553–8. PubMed PMID: 16081486. Pubmed Central PMCID: PMC1474740. Epub 2005/08/06. eng.
66. Rubia K, Lee F, Cleare AJ, Tunstall N, Fu CH, Brammer M, et al. Tryptophan depletion reduces right inferior prefrontal activation during response inhibition in fast, event-related fMRI. Psychopharmacology. 2005;179(4):791–803. PubMed PMID: 15887056. Epub 2005/05/12. eng.
67. Liu J, Zhao S, Reyes T. Neurological and epigenetic implications of nutritional deficiencies on psychopathology: conceptualization and review of evidence. Int J Mol Sci. 2015;16(8):18129. PubMed PMID: doi:10.3390/ijms160818129.
68. Wald N, Sneddon J. Prevention of neural tube defects: results of the Medical Research Council vitamin study. Lancet. 1991;338(8760):131. PubMed PMID: 9108192209.
69. WHO. Guideline: daily iron and folic acid supplementation in pregnant women. Geneva: World Health Organization; 2012.
70. Bailey LB, Stover PJ, McNulty H, Fenech MF, Gregory JF, Mills JL, et al. Biomarkers of nutrition for development—folate review. J Nutr. 2015;3:2015.
71. Steegers-Theunissen RP, Obermann-Borst SA, Kremer D, Lindemans J, Siebel C, Steegers EA, et al. Periconceptional maternal folic acid use of 400 μg per day is related to increased methylation of the *IGF2* gene in the very young child. PLoS One. 2009;4(11):e7845.
72. Ba Y, Yu H, Liu F, Geng X, Zhu C, Zhu Q, et al. Relationship of folate, vitamin B12 and methylation of insulin-like growth factor-II in maternal and cord blood. Eur J Clin Nutr. 2011;65(4):480–5. PubMed PMID: 21245875. Pubmed Central PMCID: PMC3071883. Epub 2011/01/20. eng.
73. Hoyo C, Murtha AP, Schildkraut JM, Jirtle RL, Demark-Wahnefried W, Forman MR, et al. Methylation variation at IGF2 differentially methylated regions and maternal folic acid use before and during pregnancy. Epigenetics. 2011;6(7):928–36. PubMed PMID: 21636975. Pubmed Central PMCID: PMC3154433. Epub 2011/06/04. eng.
74. Nyberg F, Hallberg M. Growth hormone and cognitive function. Nat Rev Endocrinol. 2013;9(6):357–65.
75. Duthie SJ, Narayanan S, Brand GM, Pirie L, Grant G. Impact of folate deficiency on DNA stability. J Nutr. 2002;132(8):2444S–9S.
76. Fang JY, Zhu SS, Xiao SD, Jiang SJ, Shi Y, Chen XY, et al. Studies on the hypomethylation of c-myc, c-Ha-ras oncogenes and histopathological changes in human gastric carcinoma. J Gastroenterol Hepatol. 1996;11(11):1079–82. PubMed PMID: 8985834. Epub 1996/11/01. eng.
77. Beetstra S, Thomas P, Salisbury C, Turner J, Fenech M. Folic acid deficiency increases chromosomal instability, chromosome 21 aneuploidy and sensitivity to radiation-induced micronuclei. Mutat Res/Fundam Mol Mech Mutagen. 2005;578(1–2):317–26.
78. SAS L, Achterfeldt S, Gorniak JP, KJA H-H, Oxley D, van Schooten FJ, et al. Maternal folate depletion and high-fat feeding from weaning affects DNA methylation and DNA repair in brain of adult offspring. FASEB J. 2013;27(8):3323–34.
79. Langie SA, Achterfeldt S, Gorniak JP, Halley-Hogg KJ, Oxley D, van Schooten FJ, et al. Maternal folate depletion and high-fat feeding from weaning affects DNA methylation and DNA repair in brain of adult offspring. FASEB J: Off Publ Fed Am Soc Exp Biol. 2013;27(8):3323–34. PubMed PMID: 23603834. Epub 2013/04/23. eng.

80. Zeisel SH. Nutritional importance of choline for brain development. J Am Coll Nutr. 2004;23(6 Suppl): 621S–6S. PubMed PMID: 15640516. Epub 2005/01/11. eng.
81. Craciunescu CN, Albright CD, Mar MH, Song J, Zeisel SH. Choline availability during embryonic development alters progenitor cell mitosis in developing mouse hippocampus. J Nutr. 2003;133(11):3614–8. PubMed PMID: 14608083. Pubmed Central PMCID: PMC1592525. Epub 2003/11/11. eng.
82. Arnold H, Burk J, Hodgson E, Sarter M, Bruno J. Differential cortical acetylcholine release in rats performing a sustained attention task versus behavioral control tasks that do not explicitly tax attention. Neuroscience. 2002;114(2):451–60.
83. Himmelheber AM, Sarter M, Bruno JP. Increases in cortical acetylcholine release during sustained attention performance in rats. Cogn Brain Res. 2000;9(3):313–25.
84. Cermak JM, Holler T, Jackson DA, Blusztajn JK. Prenatal availability of choline modifies development of the hippocampal cholinergic system. FASEB J. 1998;12(3):349–57.
85. Holler T, Cermak JM, Blusztajn JK. Dietary choline supplementation in pregnant rats increases hippocampal phospholipase D activity of the offspring. FASEB J: Off Publ Fed Am Soc Exp Biol. 1996;10(14):1653–9. PubMed PMID: 9002559. Epub 1996/12/01. eng.
86. Mellott TJ, Kowall NW, Lopez-Coviella I, Blusztajn JK. Prenatal choline deficiency increases choline transporter expression in the septum and hippocampus during postnatal development and in adulthood in rats. Brain Res. 2007;1151:1–11. PubMed PMID: PMC1952662.
87. Napoli I, Blusztajn JK, Mellott TJ. Prenatal choline supplementation in rats increases the expression of IGF2 and its receptor IGF2R and enhances IGF2-induced acetylcholine release in hippocampus and frontal cortex. Brain Res. 2008;1237:124–35. PubMed PMID: 18786520. Epub 2008/09/13. eng.
88. Hawkes C, Jhamandas JH, Harris KH, Fu W, MacDonald RG, Kar S. Single transmembrane domain insulin-like growth factor-II/mannose-6-phosphate receptor regulates central cholinergic function by activating a G-protein-sensitive, protein kinase C-dependent pathway. J Neurosci: Off J Soc Neurosci. 2006;26(2):585–96. PubMed PMID: 16407557. Epub 2006/01/13. eng.
89. Li X, Sun Q, Li X, Cai D, Sui S, Jia Y, et al. Dietary betaine supplementation to gestational sows enhances hippocampal IGF2 expression in newborn piglets with modified DNA methylation of the differentially methylated regions. Eur J Nutr. 2015;54(7):1201–10. PubMed PMID: 25410747. Epub 2014/11/21. eng.
90. Morris MS, Selhub J, Jacques PF. Vitamin B-12 and folate status in relation to decline in scores on the mini-mental state examination in the framingham heart study. J Am Geriatr Soc. 2012;60(8):1457–64. PubMed PMID: 22788704. Pubmed Central PMCID: PMC3419282. Epub 2012/07/14. eng.
91. Min H. Effects of dietary supplementation of high-dose folic acid on biomarkers of methylating reaction in vitamin B(12)-deficient rats. Nutrition research and practice. 2009;3(2):122–7. PubMed PMID: 20016712. Pubmed Central PMCID: PMC2788180. Epub 2009/12/18. eng.
92. Hirche F, Schroder A, Knoth B, Stangl GI, Eder K. Methionine-induced elevation of plasma homocysteine concentration is associated with an increase of plasma cholesterol in adult rats. Ann Nutr Metab. 2006;50(2):139–46. PubMed PMID: 16391469. Epub 2006/01/05. eng.
93. Obeid R, Herrmann W. Mechanisms of homocysteine neurotoxicity in neurodegenerative diseases with special reference to dementia. FEBS Lett. 2006;580(13):2994–3005.
94. Sharma M, Tiwari M, Tiwari RK. Hyperhomocysteinemia: impact on neurodegenerative diseases. Basic Clin Pharmacol Toxicol. 2015;117(5):287–96.
95. Kamat PK, Vacek JC, Kalani A, Tyagi N. Homocysteine induced cerebrovascular dysfunction: a link to Alzheimer's disease etiology. Open Neurol J. 2015;9:9–14. PubMed PMID: PMC4485324.
96. Petras M, Tatarkova Z, Kovalska M, Mokra D, Dobrota D, Lehotsky J, et al. Hyperhomocysteinemia as a risk factor for the neuronal system disorders. J Physiol Pharmacol: Off J Polish Physiol Soc. 2014;65(1):15–23. PubMed PMID: 24622826. Epub 2014/03/14. eng.
97. Devlin AM, Arning E, Bottiglieri T, Faraci FM, Rozen R, Lentz SR. Effect of Mthfr genotype on diet-induced hyperhomocysteinemia and vascular function in mice. Blood. 2003;103(7):2624–9.

Chapter 4
Maternal Fitness and Infant Birth Weight

Michèle Bisson and Isabelle Marc

Key Points

- Moderate intensity physical activity is recommended and safe in low-risk pregnancy
- Physical activity interventions during pregnancy slightly reduce infant birth weight without increasing the risk of delivering a small infant, but the influence of exercise on fetal growth in high-risk pregnancy remains unknown
- Physical activity volume and intensity modulate the influence of maternal physical activity on fetal growth, with high levels of physical activity associated with a decreased birth weight and adiposity
- Although some observational studies have found long-lasting benefits of maternal exercise during pregnancy on the child's obesity risk, more studies are needed before definitive conclusions regarding the child's long term health can be drawn
- The mechanisms responsible for the effect of maternal physical activity on infant birth weight remain partly understood but are thought to include the modulation of blood flow, nutrients and oxygen delivery to the fetus, placental adaptations, epigenetic modifications and gestational weight gain regulation

Keywords Birth weight • Exercise • Fitness • Neonatal body composition • Physical activity • Pregnancy

Abbreviations

BMC   Bone mineral content
BMD   Bone mineral density
BMI   Body mass index
CI   Confidence interval
DXA   Dual energy x-ray absorptiometry
Hb   Hemoglobin
HDL   High density lipoprotein
OR   Odds ratio

M. Bisson, PhD • I. Marc, MD, PhD (✉)
Department of Pediatrics, Centre Hospitalier Universitaire de Québec-Université Laval, Québec City, PQ, Canada
e-mail: isabelle.marc@crchudequebec.ulaval.ca

© Springer International Publishing AG 2017
R. Rajendram et al. (eds.), *Diet, Nutrition, and Fetal Programming*,
Nutrition and Health, DOI 10.1007/978-3-319-60289-9_4

Introduction

Physical activity and cardiorespiratory fitness both produce significant cardiovascular health benefits [1]. During pregnancy, regular physical activity has been shown to help maintain physical fitness [2], decrease gestational weight gain [3] and reduce the risk of developing gestational diabetes [4] and potentially preeclampsia [5].

Regarding the child, birth weight is a marker of fetal growth and an important determinant of later body composition [6], fitness [7, 8], cardiovascular disease risk and metabolic disturbances [9, 10], and also appears to be influenced by maternal physical activity during pregnancy. Several mechanisms have been proposed, including the modulation of nutrient availability and blood flow [11], and a reduced weight gain during pregnancy. In response to physical activity interventions during pregnancy, infant birth weight has been shown to be slightly reduced, as suggested by the results of a recent meta-analysis [3]. Yet, discrepant findings have been observed between individual studies, suggesting that physical activity type, intensity, volume and timing during pregnancy, in addition to maternal characteristics, might exert different fetal growth adaptations [11].

The present chapter will review evidence regarding the influence of maternal physical activity and fitness on infant birth weight and other markers of fetal growth, with a specific focus on the different growth responses elicited by different physical activity stimuli. Implications of such effects on later child growth and development will also be discussed.

Physical Activity Recommendations

Given the recognized benefits and safety of moderate intensity physical activity, numerous medical associations including the American Congress of Obstetricians and Gynecologists, the Society of Obstetricians and Gynaecologists of Canada and the Royal College of Obstetricians and Gynaecologists encourage pregnant women with a low-risk, uncomplicated pregnancy to engage regularly in such activity [12–14]. Some conditions constitute absolute (e.g. ruptured membranes, preeclampsia) or relative (e.g. history of spontaneous abortion/premature labour, anemia, eating disorder) contraindications to physical activity during pregnancy [15]. Historically, women with these conditions were excluded from physical activity studies and accordingly, the impact of exercise on such conditions and on perinatal outcomes remains to be established [13]. While women with absolute contraindications should refrain from doing physical activity, those with a relative contraindication could be allowed to exercise following medical evaluation.

According to the exercise guidelines, previously inactive women should begin physical activity progressively, with a goal of achieving eventually 30 min of moderate intensity physical activity on most days of the week. As for previously active women, they are encouraged to pursue an active lifestyle during pregnancy, while adapting their exercise practice in order to aim for a good conditioning level without focusing on reaching high performances [13, 14].

Physical Fitness and Birth Weight

Physical fitness refers to "a set of attributes that people have or achieve that relates to the ability to perform physical activity" [16]. While individual responses exist regarding gains in cardiorespiratory fitness following regular physical activity practice [17], most evidence suggests that pregnant women can maintain or improve their cardiorespiratory fitness through exercise during pregnancy [2].

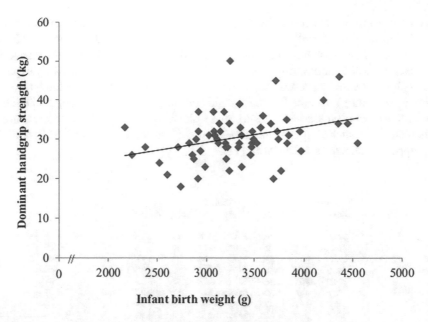

Fig. 4.1 Correlation between infant birth weight and maternal handgrip strength measured in early second trimester of pregnancy. Legend: $r = 0.34$, $P = 0.007$ (Reproduced with permission from Bisson et al. [18])

However, physical activity levels usually tend to decline throughout pregnancy [18, 19], which could hamper cardiorespiratory fitness benefits.

Only a few studies have directly evaluated the association between maternal physical fitness and infant birth weight, with most of them being performed more than 40 years ago. Using a cycling exercise test, Pomerance et al. found no association between maternal fitness score in late pregnancy and birth weight [20]. Similarly, Erkkola found no difference in birth weight between women with various physical work capacities [21]. However, the proportion of infants with a birth weight >3500 g was higher in women with a work capacity above 100% of the predicted value, based on reference values obtained from non-pregnant women of similar age and weight [21]. In a randomised trial, Erkkola and Mäkelä found no difference in birth weight between infants of women following an exercise regimen throughout pregnancy, resulting in improved fitness, compared with women of the control group [22]. More recently, our group found a positive association between maternal muscular fitness, as assessed by handgrip strength, and infant birth weight (Fig. 4.1). This association was independent of maternal body mass index (BMI), age, smoking status, gestational age at delivery, gestational weight gain, parity and infant sex [18]. As seen in previous studies, we did not find a significant association between maternal cardiorespiratory fitness and infant birth weight.

As fitness is not only dependent upon physical activity levels but also upon genetic and nutritional factors [23], measuring the association between physical activity and birth weight might be more relevant regarding public health recommendations. The next section will thus specifically review studies evaluating the impact of physical activity levels on infant birth weight.

Physical Activity and Birth Weight

Numerous observational and randomized studies have evaluated the association between maternal physical activity practice and infant birth weight. In 2015, Wiebe and colleagues have summarized results from randomized physical activity trials including direct exercise supervision in a meta-analysis [3]. Compared with standard care, physical activity interventions resulted in a mean reduction in infant birth weight of 31 g (95% CI −57, −4, 27 trials, 5214 women). However, individual study results were somehow heterogeneous and often no significant difference was found between the exercise and control groups, as depicted in Fig. 4.2. This could be partly explained by the differences in physical activity prescription and adherence between studies, as the type (cardiovascular, muscular, combination), volume (frequency and duration), intensity and length of the intervention varied substantially between studies. Indeed, these physical activity characteristics, in addition to maternal characteristics such as obesity and fitness, might influence fetal growth differentially, as suggested by Clapp and colleagues' early work [11].

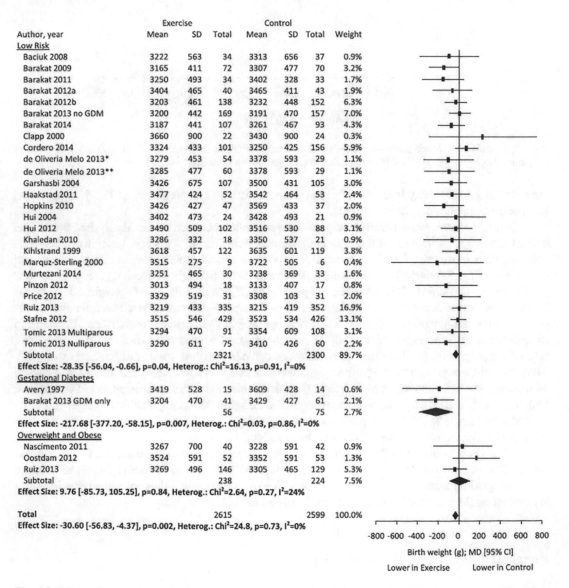

Fig. 4.2 Effect of prenatal exercise interventions on mean birth weight. Legend: Difference in mean birth weight between women randomised to prenatal exercise compared with standard care. *SD* standard deviation, *GDM* gestational diabetes mellitus, *heterog* heterogeneity, *MD* mean difference, *CI* confidence interval (Reproduced with permission from Wiebe et al. [3])

In an attempt to unravel the specific association between various physical activity exposures during pregnancy and infant birth weight, our group recently published a systematic review and meta-analysis of observational studies investigating the association between maternal physical activity and neonatal growth measures [24]. Due to important heterogeneity between studies, we were only able to evaluate the impact of physical activity volume, including intensity, on infant birth weight. High physical activity levels were defined by vigorous intensity physical activity and/or participation in at least three weekly exercise sessions lasting at least 30 min, or by the most active group in studies reporting analyses with more than two physical activity level categories. Moderate physical activity levels were below the high level criteria, but still included a minimum physical activity level above the sedentary or least active category (the lowest activity level). We then compared (1) women classified as having high levels of physical activity to women with lower physical activity volumes ("high vs low"), and (2) women with moderate levels of physical activity to women with lower physical activity volumes ("moderate vs low"). A total of 15 studies were included in both analyses, as illustrated in Figs. 4.3 and 4.4. When comparing infant birth weight of women with high and low levels of physical activity, we found that high physical activity levels were associated with a 70 g reduction in birth weight (Fig. 4.3). In contrast, infants born to women with moderate physical activity levels had a birth weight increased by 61 g compared with infants of women with low physical activity levels (Fig. 4.4).

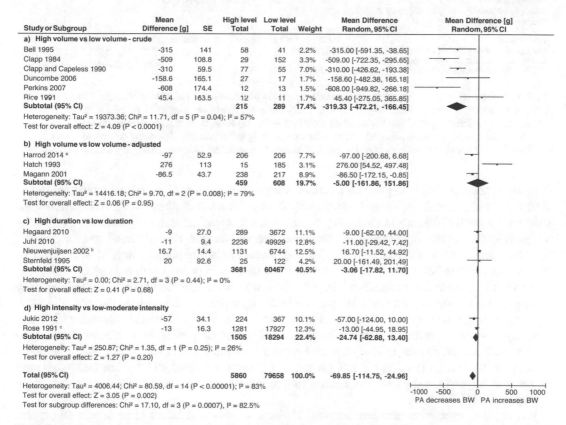

Fig. 4.3 Association between maternal physical activity during pregnancy and infant's birth weight – high levels of physical activity. Legend: (**a**) Results from studies providing crude results only, based on activity volume. (**b**) Results from studies providing adjusted results, based on activity volume. (**c**) Results from studies based on duration. (**d**) Results from studies based on intensity. (**a**) Significant difference between groups (nonsignificant here due to estimated equal sample size per quartile). (**b**) This study reported only time spent swimming. (**c**) This study compared high intensity exercise with moderate-intensity exercise. *BW* birth weight, *PA* physical activity (Reproduced with permission from Bisson et al. [24])

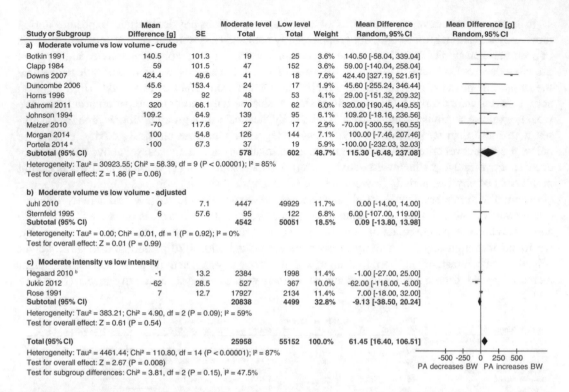

Fig. 4.4 Association between maternal physical activity during pregnancy and infant's birth weight – moderate levels of physical activity. Legend: (**a**) Results from studies providing crude results only, based on activity volume. (**b**) Results from studies providing adjusted results, based on activity volume. (**c**) Results from studies based on intensity. (**a**) This study mentioned nonsignificant adjusted results without providing estimates. (**b**) This study compared light intensity activity with no activity. *BW* birth weight, *PA* physical activity (Reproduced with permission from Bisson et al. [24])

Altogether, these findings suggest that a certain volume and intensity of exercise are required before birth weight is reduced. This could explain why the combination of results from randomized trials yield only a small difference in birth weight. Although not investigated in the previously cited meta-analyses, studies evaluating the impact of maternal exercise on infant length found no evidence of a decreased length with maternal exercise [25–29]. Accordingly, although growth in weight can be altered with maternal exercise, such stimulus does not seem to impede growth in length.

Another important issue regarding fetal growth relates to the specific moment during pregnancy when physical activity is performed. Indeed, results from previous studies suggest that physical activity in early pregnancy could decrease fetal growth and birth weight [30, 31]. Although early pregnancy appears as a sensitive period for the programming of fetal growth, other studies also suggest that physical activity in mid- or late pregnancy could also influence birth weight [32, 33]. In addition, reducing physical activity volume in mid-pregnancy has been associated with an increased infant birth weight and adiposity, compared with maintaining or increasing physical activity volume during the same period [34].

Finally, the association between maternal physical activity and infant birth weight might also depend on particular maternal characteristics. For instance, most physical activity studies found no difference in infant birth weight between overweight or obese pregnant women engaged in physical activity and those pursuing a sedentary pregnancy [3, 27, 30, 35]. In addition, a lifestyle intervention for obese women during pregnancy, including dietary guidance and exercise training, resulted in a larger infant birth weight in the intervention group despite a significant reduction in gestational weight gain [36]. Compliance issues with the exercise program were however noted in this study.

Whether the physical activity levels achieved by overweight and obese women are insufficient to positively influence birth weight or whether the beneficial effects of physical activity cannot counterbalance the deleterious effects of maternal obesity [37] remains to be established.

Physical Activity and Risk of Birth Weight Extremes

Despite a relatively small effect on birth weight, most studies investigating the impact of maternal exercise on the risk of high birth weight or large weight for gestational age found a decreased risk with maternal exercise. Indeed, Wiebe and colleagues found that women participating in a supervised exercise program during pregnancy had a 31% reduction in the risk of delivering a large infant, compared with controls (OR 0.69, 95% CI 0.55, 0.86, 18 studies, 3982 women) [3]. Importantly, the risk of low birth weight or small weight for gestational age did not seem to be increased with maternal exercise (OR 1.02, 95% CI 0.72, 1.46, 11 studies, 2183 women) [3], although some observational studies in highly active women suggested otherwise [38, 39].

Physical Activity and Infant Body Composition

Theoretically, a change in birth weight can be the consequence of a change in lean mass, fat mass, and/or bone mass in various proportions. Accordingly, changes in these tissues could imply differential long term health consequences for the child. Although neonatal body composition, and in particular neonatal adiposity, has been shown to be highly sensitive to the prenatal environment [40, 41], only a few studies have evaluated the effect of maternal exercise these specific outcomes. In previously inactive women, Clapp and colleagues found that beginning a moderate intensity exercise program in early pregnancy resulted in a proportional increase in neonatal lean and fat masses, compared with no exercise [26]. On the contrary, Hopkins and colleagues found that a moderate intensity exercise program starting in mid-pregnancy reduced proportionally neonatal fat and lean masses, compared with no exercise [25]. In previously active women, reducing exercise practice in mid-pregnancy has also been found to increase neonatal lean mass, fat mass and fat percentage, compared with maintaining or increasing exercise practice from mid-pregnancy until delivery [34].

Two observational studies also evaluated the association between maternal exercise and infant body composition, and both found that vigorous exercise and/or a high volume of physical activity was associated with a reduction in neonatal adiposity [33, 42]. Recent data from our group also suggest that maternal vigorous exercise measured by accelerometry in the first half of pregnancy is associated with an important decrease in neonatal fat mass and fat percentage (−122.6 g or −2.3% fat in newborns of women doing vigorous exercise vs not doing vigorous exercise) [43]. In contrast, time spent in moderate intensity exercise in late pregnancy was associated with an increased lean mass (2.0 g increase for each minute spent doing moderate intensity exercise). Finally, the combination of a high volume of moderate intensity physical activity with vigorous intensity physical activity was also associated with a decrease in birth weight (~ −300 g for newborns of women doing vigorous exercise and high levels of moderate exercise vs not doing vigorous exercise) and neonatal bone mineral content (BMC, −5.4 g for newborns of women doing vigorous exercise and high levels of moderate exercise vs not doing vigorous exercise), without changes in bone mineral density (BMD). However, this association was not independent from linear growth. Two previous observational studies have also found evidence for a decrease in neonatal BMC and/or BMD with maternal exercise in late pregnancy [44, 45], but the only randomised trial evaluating these outcomes found no significant differences between the exercise and control groups [25].

As for infant birth weight, the impact of maternal exercise on body composition appears to be modulated by exercise intensity, volume and timing during pregnancy. In addition, as most studies were conducted in healthy, normal weight and low-risk pregnant women, the impact of maternal physical activity on infant birth weight and body composition in other populations remains to be established.

Long-Term Impact of Maternal Physical Activity on Child Growth

An important question that needs to be addressed regards the long term impact of maternal physical activity on child growth and health, as it is not known whether the changes observed at birth in birth weight and body composition persist over time and whether other effects not obvious at birth become apparent later in life.

A few observational studies attempted to answer these questions. Clapp initially investigated whether children of women who were regularly active during pregnancy remained lighter and leaner at 5 years of age, compared with children from a group of matched sedentary women. Interestingly, offspring of active women were still lighter and leaner compared with offspring of sedentary women at this age, and also exhibited higher language skills and intellectual quotient [46]. On the contrary, the same group found neither significant difference in anthropometric measures nor neurodevelopment in 1-year old children of active women compared with those of sedentary women, although children of active women were lighter and leaner at birth [47].

In a follow-up study of a lifestyle intervention for obese pregnant women, children of the intervention and control group did not differ in terms of weight, BMI or adiposity at age 2.8 years [48]. However, as children from the intervention group were initially heavier at birth [36], this absence of difference between groups could perhaps be seen as an improvement over time. Children from both groups were also similar with respect to plasma glucose, insulin, triglyceride and HDL cholesterol levels as well as blood pressure [49].

Finally, in children aged 7–8, one large ($n = 40,280$) observational study found no association between maternal self-reported physical activity practice during pregnancy and child's BMI or obesity risk [50], while another one ($n = 5125$) found decreased odds of obesity in children form active mothers (OR 0.77, 95% CI 0.65, 0.91). Clearly, more follow-up studies are needed before definitive conclusions can be drawn regarding the long term benefits of maternal physical activity on child's growth and development.

Biological Mechanisms Proposed to Explain the Impact of Maternal Exercise on Infant Birth Weight

Numerous mechanisms have been proposed to explain the variation in infant birth weight and body composition with maternal exercise. First, exercise is thought to modulate fetal nutrients, especially glucose, and oxygen availability, which is dependent upon blood flow to the fetus and the amount of substrates in maternal blood [11]. As active muscles require more energy substrates during exercise, blood flow is redistributed to accommodate their needs, which results in a transient reduction in blood supply to the fetus [51, 52]. Glucose utilization by active muscles [53] also reduces glucose availability for the fetus, and maternal exercise can improve insulin sensitivity [54]. However, the type of dietary carbohydrates (either of low or high glycemic index) consumed by the mother also influences both glucose and insulin response to exercise [55], which can in turn modify fetal growth [11]. Maternal physical activity could also indirectly influence birth weight through an effect on gestational weight gain, as exercise has been shown to reduce this parameter [3] which highly influences birth weight [56]. Altogether, these mechanisms could explain the decreased birth weight observed with maternal physical activity in meta-analyses. However, as most of these effects appear to be intensity and time-dependent [51, 52, 57, 58], and as birth weight seems to be reduced primarily with high volumes of vigorous exercise [24], some other mechanisms must counterbalance these effects when physical activity is lower in volume and intensity. Indeed, it has been proposed that maternal cardiac output, blood volume and placental volume were increased in regularly active women [11], which could mitigate the birth weight-lowering effect of transient bouts of exercise and explain why some studies found no difference or even an increased birth weight with maternal physical activity. Indeed, placental function and volume have been shown to be enhanced by regular moderate intensity starting in early pregnancy [26], while increasing exercise volume in mid-pregnancy reduces placental growth [34].

Recent studies also suggest that maternal exercise could modulate the placental nutrient transport capacity [59, 60], which could modulate fetal growth and birth weight. Finally, epigenetic modifications resulting from maternal exercise could also be responsible for changes in birth weight. Indeed, McCullough and colleagues have shown that total energy expenditure in early pregnancy is associated with a reduced DNA methylation of the PLAGL1 gene in cord blood, a gene whose methylation level is positively associated with maternal obesity and fetal growth [31]. Since the association between maternal physical activity and birth weight association was attenuated after adjustment for the methylation levels of this gene, it is thought to be partly responsible for the effect of physical activity on birth weight.

Conclusions

In summary, maternal physical activity clearly appears to influence fetal growth, although the precise mechanisms remain to be elucidated. Physical activity parameters such as type, intensity and volume undoubtedly modulate the impact on infant birth weight and body composition, with high volume and intensity of physical activity associated with a reduced birth weight and adiposity. The moment when physical activity is performed, as well as the maternal characteristics, might also influence fetal growth adaptations to maternal exercise. Importantly, current physical activity recommendations for pregnant women appear safe for mother and child in low risk pregnancy, with no evidence of an increased risk of small weight for gestational age. More work is nevertheless required in order to assess the long term impact of maternal physical activity on child health, and to adequately counsel pregnant women with a higher risk pregnancy regarding safe physical activity levels throughout pregnancy.

References

1. Myers J, McAuley P, Lavie CJ, Despres JP, Arena R, Kokkinos P. Physical activity and cardiorespiratory fitness as major markers of cardiovascular risk: their independent and interwoven importance to health status. Prog Cardiovasc Dis. 2015;57(4):306–14.
2. Kramer MS, McDonald SW. Aerobic exercise for women during pregnancy. Cochrane Database Syst Rev. 2006;19(3):CD000180.
3. Wiebe HW, Boule NG, Chari R, Davenport MH. The effect of supervised prenatal exercise on fetal growth: a meta-analysis. Obstet Gynecol. 2015;125(5):1185–94.
4. Sanabria-Martinez G, Garcia-Hermoso A, Poyatos-Leon R, Alvarez-Bueno C, Sanchez-Lopez M, Martinez-Vizcaino V. Effectiveness of physical activity interventions on preventing gestational diabetes mellitus and excessive maternal weight gain: a meta-analysis. BJOG. 2015;122(9):1167–74.
5. Aune D, Saugstad OD, Henriksen T, Tonstad S. Physical activity and the risk of preeclampsia: a systematic review and meta-analysis. Epidemiology. 2014;25(3):331–43.

6. Singhal A, Wells J, Cole TJ, Fewtrell M, Lucas A. Programming of lean body mass: a link between birth weight, obesity, and cardiovascular disease? Am J Clin Nutr. 2003;77(3):726–30.
7. Inskip HM, Godfrey KM, Martin HJ, Simmonds SJ, Cooper C, Sayer AA. Size at birth and its relation to muscle strength in young adult women. J Intern Med. 2007;262(3):368–74.
8. Ridgway CL, Ong KK, Tammelin T, Sharp SJ, Ekelund U, Jarvelin MR. Birth size, infant weight gain, and motor development influence adult physical performance. Med Sci Sports Exerc. 2009;41(6):1212–21.
9. Stuart A, Amer-Wahlin I, Persson J, Kallen K. Long-term cardiovascular risk in relation to birth weight and exposure to maternal diabetes mellitus. Int J Cardiol. 2013;168(3):2653–7.
10. Chiavaroli V, Giannini C, D'Adamo E, de Giorgis T, Chiarelli F, Mohn A. Insulin resistance and oxidative stress in children born small and large for gestational age. Pediatrics. 2009;124(2):695–702.
11. Clapp JF. Influence of endurance exercise and diet on human placental development and fetal growth. Placenta. 2006;27(6–7):527–34.
12. Royal College of Obstetricians and Gynaecologists. Exercise in pregnancy. RCOG Statement No. 4 – January 2006 [On line]; [cited August 10th, 2016]; Available from: https://www.rcog.org.uk/globalassets/documents/guidelines/statements/statement-no-4.pdf. n.d.
13. Davies GA, Wolfe LA, Mottola MF, MacKinnon C. Joint SOGC/CSEP clinical practice guideline: exercise in pregnancy and the postpartum period. Can J Appl Physiol. 2003;28(3):330–41.
14. ACOG Committee Opinion No. 650. Physical activity and exercise during pregnancy and the postpartum period. Obstet Gynecol. 2015;126(6):e135–42.
15. PARmed-X. PARmed-X for pregacy, physical activity readiness medical examination [On line]. 2002 [cited August 10th, 2016]; Available from: http://www.csep.ca/cmfiles/publications/parq/parmed-xpreg.pdf.
16. ACSM. Benefits and risks associated with physical activity. In: Thompson WR, editor. ACSM's guidelines for exercise testing and prescription. 8th ed. Philadelphia: Lippincott Williams & Wilkins; 2009. p. 2–17.
17. Bouchard C, Rankinen T. Individual differences in response to regular physical activity. Med Sci Sports Exerc. 2001;33(6 Suppl):S446–51. discussion S52–3.
18. Bisson M, Almeras N, Plaisance J, Rheaume C, Bujold E, Tremblay A, et al. Maternal fitness at the onset of the second trimester of pregnancy: correlates and relationship with infant birth weight. Pediatr Obes. 2013;8(6):464–74.
19. Evenson KR, Wen F. Prevalence and correlates of objectively measured physical activity and sedentary behavior among US pregnant women. Prev Med. 2011;53(1–2):39–43.
20. Pomerance JJ, Gluck L, Lynch VA. Physical fitness in pregnancy: its effect on pregnancy outcome. Am J Obstet Gynecol. 1974;119(7):867–76.
21. Erkkola R. The physical work capacity of the expectant mother and its effect on pregnancy, labor and the newborn. Int J Gynaecol Obstet. 1976;14(2):153–9.
22. Erkkola R, Makela M. Heart volume and physical fitness of parturients. Ann Clin Res. 1976;8(1):15–21.
23. Laukkanen JA, Laaksonen D, Lakka TA, Savonen K, Rauramaa R, Makikallio T, et al. Determinants of cardiorespiratory fitness in men aged 42 to 60 years with and without cardiovascular disease. Am J Cardiol. 2009;103(11):1598–604.
24. Bisson M, Lavoie-Guenette J, Tremblay A, Marc I. Physical activity volumes during pregnancy: a systematic review and meta-analysis of observational studies assessing the association with infant's birth weight. AJP Rep. 2016;6(2):e170–97.
25. Hopkins SA, Baldi JC, Cutfield WS, McCowan L, Hofman PL. Exercise training in pregnancy reduces offspring size without changes in maternal insulin sensitivity. J Clin Endocrinol Metab. 2010;95(5):2080–8.
26. Clapp JF 3rd, Kim H, Burciu B, Lopez B. Beginning regular exercise in early pregnancy: effect on fetoplacental growth. Am J Obstet Gynecol. 2000;183(6):1484–8.
27. Bisson M, Almeras N, Dufresne SS, Robitaille J, Rheaume C, Bujold E, et al. A 12-week exercise program for pregnant women with obesity to improve physical activity levels: an open randomised preliminary study. PLoS One. 2015;10(9):e0137742.
28. Barakat R, Lucia A, Ruiz JR. Resistance exercise training during pregnancy and newborn's birth size: a randomised controlled trial. Int J Obes. 2009;33(9):1048–57.
29. Barakat R, Pelaez M, Cordero Y, Perales M, Lopez C, Coteron J, et al. Exercise during pregnancy protects against hypertension and macrosomia: randomized clinical trial. Am J Obstet Gynecol. 2016;214(5):649 e1–8.
30. Badon SE, Wander PL, Qiu C, Miller RS, Williams MA, Enquobahrie DA. Maternal leisure time physical activity and infant birth size. Epidemiology. 2016;27(1):74–81.
31. McCullough LE, Mendez MA, Miller EE, Murtha AP, Murphy SK, Hoyo C. Associations between prenatal physical activity, birth weight, and DNA methylation at genomically imprinted domains in a multiethnic newborn cohort. Epigenetics. 2015;10(7):597–606.
32. Fleten C, Stigum H, Magnus P, Nystad W. Exercise during pregnancy, maternal prepregnancy body mass index, and birth weight. Obstet Gynecol. 2010;115(2 Pt 1):331–7.
33. Harrod CS, Chasan-Taber L, Reynolds RM, Fingerlin TE, Glueck DH, Brinton JT, et al. Physical activity in pregnancy and neonatal body composition: the healthy start study. Obstet Gynecol. 2014;124(2 Pt 1):257–64.

34. Clapp JF 3rd, Kim H, Burciu B, Schmidt S, Petry K, Lopez B. Continuing regular exercise during pregnancy: effect of exercise volume on fetoplacental growth. Am J Obstet Gynecol. 2002;186(1):142–7.

35. Renault KM, Norgaard K, Nilas L, Carlsen EM, Cortes D, Pryds O, et al. The treatment of obese pregnant women (TOP) study: a randomized controlled trial of the effect of physical activity intervention assessed by pedometer with or without dietary intervention in obese pregnant women. Am J Obstet Gynecol. 2014;210(2):134 e1–9.

36. Vinter CA, Jensen DM, Ovesen P, Beck-Nielsen H, Jorgensen JS. The LiP (lifestyle in pregnancy) study a randomized controlled trial of lifestyle intervention in 360 obese pregnant women. Diabetes Care. 2011;34(12):2502–7.

37. Catalano P, deMouzon SH. Maternal obesity and metabolic risk to the offspring: why lifestyle interventions may have not achieved the desired outcomes. Int J Obes. 2015;39(4):642–9.

38. Clapp JF 3rd, Dickstein S. Endurance exercise and pregnancy outcome. Med Sci Sports Exerc. 1984;16(6):556–62.

39. Bell RJ, Palma SM, Lumley JM. The effect of vigorous exercise during pregnancy on birth-weight. Aust N Z J Obstet Gynaecol. 1995;35(1):46–51.

40. Catalano PM, Thomas A, Huston-Presley L, Amini SB. Increased fetal adiposity: a very sensitive marker of abnormal in utero development. Am J Obstet Gynecol. 2003;189(6):1698–704.

41. Sewell MF, Huston-Presley L, Super DM, Catalano P. Increased neonatal fat mass, not lean body mass, is associated with maternal obesity. Am J Obstet Gynecol. 2006;195(4):1100–3.

42. Clapp JF 3rd, Capeless EL. Neonatal morphometrics after endurance exercise during pregnancy. Am J Obstet Gynecol. 1990;163(6 Pt 1):1805–11.

43. Bisson M, Tremblay F, St-Onge O, Robitaille J, Pronovost E, Simonyan D, et al. Influence of maternal physical activity on infant's body composition. Pediatr Obes. 2016; doi: 10.1111/ijpo.12174.

44. Harvey NC, Javaid MK, Arden NK, Poole JR, Crozier SR, Robinson SM, et al. Maternal predictors of neonatal bone size and geometry: the Southampton Women's Survey. J Dev Orig Health Dis. 2010;1(1):35–41.

45. Godfrey K, Walker-Bone K, Robinson S, Taylor P, Shore S, Wheeler T, et al. Neonatal bone mass: influence of parental birthweight, maternal smoking, body composition, and activity during pregnancy. J Bone Miner Res. 2001;16(9):1694–703.

46. Clapp JF 3rd. Morphometric and neurodevelopmental outcome at age five years of the offspring of women who continued to exercise regularly throughout pregnancy. J Pediatr. 1996;129(6):856–63.

47. Clapp JF 3rd, Simonian S, Lopez B, Appleby-Wineberg S, Harcar-Sevcik R. The one-year morphometric and neurodevelopmental outcome of the offspring of women who continued to exercise regularly throughout pregnancy. Am J Obstet Gynecol. 1998;178(3):594–9.

48. Tanvig M, Vinter CA, Jorgensen JS, Wehberg S, Ovesen PG, Lamont RF, et al. Anthropometrics and body composition by dual energy x-ray in children of obese women: a follow-up of a randomized controlled trial (the lifestyle in pregnancy and offspring [LiPO] study). PLoS One. 2014;9(2):e89590.

49. Tanvig M, Vinter CA, Jorgensen JS, Wehberg S, Ovesen PG, Beck-Nielsen H, et al. Effects of lifestyle intervention in pregnancy and anthropometrics at birth on offspring metabolic profile at 2.8 years: results from the lifestyle in pregnancy and offspring (LiPO) study. J Clin Endocrinol Metab. 2015;100(1):175–83.

50. Schou Andersen C, Juhl M, Gamborg M, Sorensen TI, Nohr EA. Maternal recreational exercise during pregnancy in relation to children's BMI at 7 years of age. Int J Pediatr. 2012;2012:920583.

51. Erkkola RU, Pirhonen JP, Kivijarvi AK. Flow velocity waveforms in uterine and umbilical arteries during submaximal bicycle exercise in normal pregnancy. Obstet Gynecol. 1992;79(4):611–5.

52. Szymanski LM, Satin AJ. Strenuous exercise during pregnancy: is there a limit? Am J Obstet Gynecol. 2012;207(3):179 e1–6.

53. Richter EA, Hargreaves M. Exercise, GLUT4, and skeletal muscle glucose uptake. Physiol Rev. 2013;93(3):993–1017.

54. van Poppel MN, Oostdam N, Eekhoff ME, Wouters MG, van Mechelen W, Catalano PM. Longitudinal relationship of physical activity with insulin sensitivity in overweight and obese pregnant women. J Clin Endocrinol Metab. 2013;98(7):2929–35.

55. Clapp JF 3rd. Effect of dietary carbohydrate on the glucose and insulin response to mixed caloric intake and exercise in both nonpregnant and pregnant women. Diabetes Care. 1998;21(Suppl 2):B107–12.

56. Sommer C, Sletner L, Morkrid K, Jenum AK, Birkeland KI. Effects of early pregnancy BMI, mid-gestational weight gain, glucose and lipid levels in pregnancy on offspring's birth weight and subcutaneous fat: a population-based cohort study. BMC Pregnancy Childbirth. 2015;15:84.

57. Ruchat SM, Davenport MH, Giroux I, Hillier M, Batada A, Sopper MM, et al. Effect of exercise intensity and duration on capillary glucose responses in pregnant women at low and high risk for gestational diabetes. Diabetes Metab Res Rev. 2012;28(8):669–78.

58. Soultanakis HN, Artal R, Wiswell RA. Prolonged exercise in pregnancy: glucose homeostasis, ventilatory and cardiovascular responses. Semin Perinatol. 1996;20(4):315–27.

59. Day PE, Ntani G, Crozier SR, Mahon PA, Inskip HM, Cooper C, et al. Maternal factors are associated with the expression of placental genes involved in amino acid metabolism and transport. PLoS One. 2015;10(12):e0143653.

60. Brett KE, Ferraro ZM, Holcik M, Adamo KB. Prenatal physical activity and diet composition affect the expression of nutrient transporters and mTOR signaling molecules in the human placenta. Placenta. 2015;36(2):204–12.

Chapter 5
Maternal Characteristics Predisposing to Fetal Growth Restriction

Irene Cetin, Chiara Mandò, and Francesca Parisi

Key Points

- A reduction of nutrient supply and oxygenation is the final common pathway in FGR.
- Impaired placental function is mainly the final step leading to decreased nutrient and oxygen transfer to the fetus.
- Impaired maternal nutrition and nutrient absorption and maternal state of health can represent a risk factor affecting placental function.
- Maternal characteristics such as body mass index and lifestyle, can also influence both systemic and local oxidative stress and inflammation, potentially conditioning fetal growth.
- Maternal diet and environmental factors may cause epigenetic modifications, leading to alterations of oxygenation and nutrient supply to the fetus and finally to FGR.
- Growing evidence suggests a sexual dimorphism in the placental response to maternal environment.
- A cross-talk between mother-placenta-fetus compartments, further complicates the identification of the initial origin of fetal growth deficiency.

Keywords Fetal growth restriction • Maternal risk factors • Epigenetics • Oxidative stress • Inflammation • Placental function

Abbreviations

ART   Assisted reproductive technology
FGR   Fetal growth restriction
miRNAs micro-RNAs
SGA   Small for gestational age

I. Cetin, MD, PhD (✉) • C. Mandò, PhD • F. Parisi, MD
Department of Biomedical and Clinical Sciences "L. Sacco" and Centro di Ricerche Fetali Giorgio Pardi, University of Milan, Milan, Italy
e-mail: irene.cetin@unimi.it

© Springer International Publishing AG 2017
R. Rajendram et al. (eds.), *Diet, Nutrition, and Fetal Programming*, Nutrition and Health, DOI 10.1007/978-3-319-60289-9_5

Introduction

Fetal growth restriction (FGR) affects up to 10% of live-born infants representing a major cause of neonatal morbidity and mortality worldwide. Using global norms, approximately 10% of term infants in developed countries are small for gestational age (SGA) compared to 23% of term infants in developing countries [1]. Normal fetal growth is a multifactorial process, strictly dependent on genetic background, endocrine milieu and appropriate placental function [2]. Despite the clinical heterogeneity of definitions and causes, FGR is defined as the failure of a fetus to reach its growth potential according to gestational age and fetal gender [3]. The American College of Obstetricians and Gynecologists quantified the growth restriction as an estimated fetal weight below the 10th percentile for gestational age [4], warning to take into account the individualized growth potential of each fetus and avoiding to fail in this way the identification of larger fetuses that may be at risk of adverse outcome.

Constitutionally small infants (SGA babies) show by definition a birth weight below 10th percentile due to constitutional factors including maternal height, weight, ethnicity, and parity, without an increased risk for perinatal mortality or morbidity. Conversely, in FGR the nutrient supply to the fetus is compromised and the fetus, as an adaptive mechanism, responds by reducing its overall size and fat mass, preserving brain growth, accelerating lung maturation, and increasing red blood cell production [5]. Therefore, the risk of mortality and morbidity is increased in infants with FGR because of the compromised growth and reduced energy reserves that increase the vulnerability of these infants during the stressful perinatal period with the transition from intrauterine to extrauterine life.

Moreover, a new concept developed in the last decades: optimal intrauterine fetal growth represents the necessary starting point not only for good pregnancy outcome and neonatal wellbeing, but also for favorable health outcomes in childhood and adult life of the offspring. Developmental trajectories in early life have been associated with the response of the individual to later exposures, through mechanisms involving one-carbon metabolism and molecular biological processes, such as epigenetic programming, that can permanently modify the subsequent development of an individual [6]. In this scenario, FGR appears to be a significant risk factor for hypertension, hyperlipidemia, coronary heart disease, and diabetes mellitus in the adult (Barker hypothesis). This gives a new central role to intrauterine early life also in order to implement global health and wellbeing.

Assessment and Determinants of Fetal Growth

Fetal growth is currently assessed with reasonable accuracy by comparing the ultrasound measurements of fetal size parameters with reference population-based growth charts derived from populations of fetuses with assumed normal growth. When a small fetus is detected, it can be challenging to distinguish between a fetus that is constitutionally small versus growth restricted. Making the correct diagnosis is prognostically important for estimating perinatal morbidity and mortality and the risk for recurrence. In order to improve the sensitivity of in utero diagnosis and to reduce dangerous misclassification, the development of customized growth curves based on individual maternal characteristics (i.e. race, age, parity, height, weight) [7] and the use of ultrasound markers, including feto-placental Doppler velocimetry, growth velocity and fetal body composition, have been proposed (Table 5.1) [8]. In particular, reduced subcutaneous fat mass has been shown in FGR and the reduction is more significant when fat is normalized for body size [9]. Customized growth curves account for non-pathologic maternal factors including mother's height, pregestational weight, parity, and ethnicity, representing all strong contributors to birth weight. This allows the interpretation of estimated fetal weight in the context of the individual fetus' growth potential, rather than against a population-based birth weight distribution. Despite a higher reliability of this approach, routine clinical use of customized growth curves

Table 5.1 Ultrasound evaluation of FGR

Diagnosis	Reference population-based growth charts
	Estimated fetal weight below the 10th percentile for gestational age
Customized growth curves	Use of individual maternal characteristics impacting birth weight (anthropometric measures, ethnicity)
Feto-placental Doppler velocimetry	Evaluation of feto-placental perfusion and compensatory mechanisms (i.e. brain sparing)
	Evaluation of blood flow in major vessels mainly including the uterine arteries, umbilical artery, ductus venosus, and middle cerebral artery
Growth trajectories assessment	Serial ultrasound scan assessing growth velocity
Fetal body composition	Evaluation of fetal subcutaneous tissue thickness (mid-thigh, mid-arm, abdominal fat mass, subscapular fat mass), eventually normalized for body size

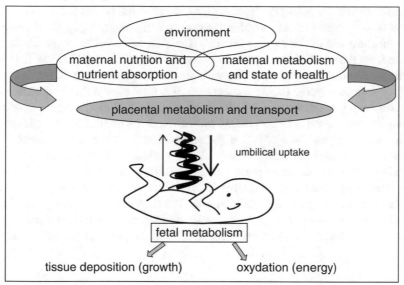

Fig. 5.1 Major determinants of fetal nutrition. Determinants of fetal growth involve a strict cross-talk between the three compartments of mother, placenta and fetus

remains controversial since clear evidence of benefit has not been demonstrated and its use has implications on resource allocation [10]. On the other hand, the assessment of the feto-placental circulation by Doppler ultrasound is employed to assist the prediction of hypoxemia and acidemia representing the most important surveillance test able to improve fetal outcome in this high-risk population [11]. Since a specific placental phenotype with increased uterine impedance leading to reduced nutrient transfer, placental respiratory failure and fetal hypoxemia, represents the most frequent pathophysiology of FGR, a temporal sequence of hemodynamic alterations has been described, involving changes in flow velocity waveforms suggesting organ-sparing effects at various levels of fetal compromise [12].

Determinants of fetal growth involve a strict cross-talk between the three compartments of mother, placenta and fetus (Fig. 5.1). Normal fetal growth reflects the interaction of the fetal genetically predetermined growth potential and its modulation by the health of fetus, placenta and mother. Firstly, an optimal maternal nutrient and oxygen supply has a critical role in feto-placental growth and development. The placenta represents the interface between maternal and fetal circulations and has a critical and active role on nutrients and oxygen delivery, depending on its size, morphology, blood supply, transporter expression and metabolic and endocrine function. Finally, fetal genetic and metabolic factors and uptake are constantly involved in the response to environmental factors and in energy production. The process of fetal growth comprises three consecutive and overlapping phases. The first phase consists of cellular hyperplasia and encompasses the first 16 weeks of gestation. Derangements in this phase are more likely to lead to symmetric FGR where fetal organs and size parameters are all decreased proportionally. The second phase, with concomitant hyperplasia and hypertrophy, occurs between 16 and 32 weeks and involves increases in cell size and number. The third and final phase, called the phase of cellular hypertrophy, occurs after the 32nd week and is characterized by a rapid increase in cell size. Quantitatively, normal singleton fetal growth increases from approximately 5 g/day at 14–15 weeks of gestation to 10 g/day at 20 weeks and 30–35 g/day at 32–34 weeks, after which the growth rate decreases.

Intrauterine growth trajectories have always been thought to be modifiable from the second trimester onwards, when maternal metabolism switches to a catabolic state, fetal growth starts to be exponential and fetal fat tissue deposition strongly depends on the endocrine, maternal and placental milieu. All these events are strongly dependent on external intervention and maternal exposures. Conversely, prior to the widespread use of ultrasound in early pregnancy, first trimester growth was thought to be uniform and under genetic control. However, these beliefs were challenged after the analysis of data from thousands of first trimester ultrasound examinations [13, 14]. Early delay in fetal growth has been documented in pregnancies with precise gestational age dating, and appears to be predictive of subsequent adverse perinatal outcomes. It is now known that maternal factors, such as age, alcohol consumption, smoking, diastolic blood pressure and diet, strongly modify embryonic growth trajectories even so early in pregnancy. Moreover, first trimester embryonic growth has been strongly related to subsequent fetal growth in the second and third trimester of pregnancy, as well as to adverse pregnancy outcome including preterm delivery and SGA babies [13, 14]. Since prospective studies showed that parental periconceptional characteristics, nutrition and lifestyle, strongly modify the developmental competence of gametes, pre-implantation embryo and fetus, with long-term health consequences in the offspring and a germline-dependent transmission across generations (transgenerational effect), the adequate planning of pregnancy and the modification of wrong exposures need to be part of a positive and necessary intervention as early as the preconceptional period (Fig. 5.2) [6].

Maternal Determinants of FGR

Although the etiology of FGR can be various and broadly categorized into maternal, fetal, and placental causes, a suboptimal nutrient supply and oxygenation of the feto-placental unit represents the final common pathway in FGR pathogenesis. The mechanisms leading to this can be heterogeneous and overlapping, depending on both external (maternal diet, lifestyle, environment and exposures) and internal (maternal/placental/fetal altered metabolism, molecular mechanisms) factors (Fig. 5.1). Impaired placental function is mainly the final step leading to decreased nutrient and oxygen transfer to the fetus. Indeed, the placenta operates as a nutrient sensor matching fetal growth rate to the ability of the mother to deliver nutrients by modifying placental transport functions.

Maternal risk factors for FGR comprise: socio-demographic factors, including race, extreme maternal age (less than 16 years and more than 35 years) and low socioeconomic status; chronic comorbidities, particularly if associated with vascular and endothelial dysfunction (i.e. hypertensive, renal and autoimmune disorders); nutritional status, including inadequate energy, micro- and macronutrients intake, inadequate gestational weight gain and extreme pregestational body mass index (BMI); assisted reproductive technology (ART) conception; lifestyle habits, including smoking, alcohol consumption and substance abuse [15]. Table 5.2 summarizes maternal risk factors for FGR.

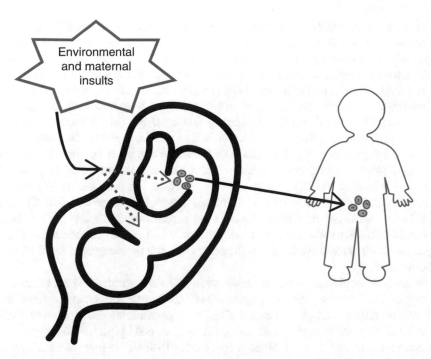

Fig. 5.2 In utero and transgenerational effect of periconceptional maternal environment. Periconceptional maternal nutrition and lifestyle may affect the development of gametes, embryo and fetus with long-term implications for health and non-communicable diseases of the offspring. A transgenerational effect could be explained by the epigenetic programming of fetal gametes

Table 5.2 Maternal risk factors for fetal growth restriction (FGR)

Maternal determinants of FGR	
Socio-economic factors	Socio-economic status
	Age
	Ethnicity
Exposures	Environmental (i.e. pollutants)
	Substance abuse
	Alcohol consumption
	Tobacco use
	Altitude
Comorbidities	Medication use
	Pre-existing medical conditions
	Associated pregnancy complications (i.e. preeclampsia)
	Maternal infections
Obstetric history	Previous FGR
	Parity
	Inter-pregnancy interval
	ART conception
Nutritional status	Pregestational BMI
	Gestational weight gain
	Diet

Maternal metabolism and health status may represent a risk factor affecting placental function and utero-placental blood flow. For example, vascular and endothelial dysfunction associated with systemic pathologies including diabetes, renal and autoimmune diseases and preexisting hypertensive disorders, may compromise placental vascular development, oxygenation and transport systems leading to reduced placental perfusion and FGR [16]. Furthermore, the delivery of a very SGA newborn has been associated with an increased risk of maternal hospitalization and death (odds ratio (OR) 1.6) in a multi-adjusted model, suggesting that maternal cardiovascular factors can affect utero-placental perfusion and fetal growth even before maternal disease becomes clinically overt [17]. Even hematological disorders (i.e. sickle cell disease) and some autoimmune diseases such as antiphospholipid syndrome may cause chronic villitis, placental vasculopathy and thrombosis, leading to fetal undernutrition and hypoxia as possible sequelae. On the contrary, the role of maternal inherited thrombophilia is controversial and not consistent as a cause of FGR. Chronic maternal hypoxemia due to pulmonary or cardiac disease or to severe anemia can lead to a reduction in oxygen supply and FGR. Even residing at high altitude results in maternal chronic hypoxemia and lower birth weight, reporting an average birth weight decline of 65 g for every additional 500 m in altitude above 2000 mt [18].

Impaired maternal nutrition and nutrient absorption represent worldwide one of the most important factor leading to FGR altering nutrient placental availability and supply to the fetus. In particular, maternal nutrition affects fetal growth either directly by determining the amount of nutrients available, and indirectly by affecting the fetal endocrine system, and epigenetically by modulating gene activity. In particular, maternal birth weight, prepregnancy BMI and weight gain during pregnancy are responsible for about 10% of the variance in fetal weight.

During the Dutch famine, severe maternal starvation has been strongly associated with FGR when it occurred in the second half of pregnancy. Maternal undernutrition, in fact, may alter fetal growth trajectory by modulating hormone production in the maternal, placental, or fetal compartments and by modifying placental weight, surface and nutrient transfer capacity. The resulting changes in placental and fetal growth depend both on the severity of the nutritional challenge and on the timing of deprivation, leading to a compensatory increase in placental mass, surface and transport when undernutrition realizes in the first part of gestation and to a decrease of the same parameters, resulting in FGR, if it realizes in the last part [19]. Modest degrees of nutritional deficiency and maternal malabsorption of nutrients (i.e. celiac disease) also have an effect on birth weight. Conversely, maternal overnutrition (i.e. obesity) may lead to FGR probably through mechanisms involving malnutrition and consequent micronutrients imbalance, vascular alteration, metabolic derangements and altered oocytes quality, but results are controversial [20, 21]. Conversely, recent studies underline the positive and strong association between dietary-caused inflammation and infant birth weight [22].

Maternal use of alcohol, cigarettes and illicit drugs may cause FGR by a direct cytotoxic effect or indirectly from related variables such as malnutrition and vascular dysfunction. Smoking during pregnancy has been independently associated with a twofold increased risk of adverse outcomes, including FGR. It has been estimated that about 3% of women smokes tobacco during the 3 months before conception, and about 54% quit during pregnancy [23]. The strongest association between smoking and FGR occurs in the third trimester of pregnancy showing a dose-response association. As expected, for women who quit smoking in pregnancy, the adjusted OR for FGR is strongly related to the trimester, reporting the highest OR when the woman quit in the third trimester compared to the first trimester [23].

In conclusion, a cross-talk between mother-placenta-fetus compartments further complicates the identification of the possible origin of fetal growth deficiency. Any insult deriving from the environment or from one of these three compartments, may also affect the entire system, possibly leading to FGR. These insults mainly result in both systemic and local status of oxidative stress and inflammation, and in epigenetic modifications, leading to alterations of placental gene expression, thus modifying placental function.

Molecular Mechanisms Undergoing Alterations of Oxygenation and Nutrients Supply

Oxidative Stress and Inflammation

Oxidative stress and inflammation have been reported in maternal, placental and fetal tissues of FGR pregnancies over the past years, both in humans and in animal models [24–26].

Maternal characteristics such as BMI and lifestyle, including oral care and maternal exercise, can influence both systemic and local oxidative stress and inflammation, potentially conditioning fetal growth (Fig. 5.3) [15, 27, 28].

Oxidative stress results from the imbalance between the generation of oxidant species and antioxidant defenses in the cell, mainly resulting in over-production of reactive oxygen species in mitochondria. Altered mitochondrial content, a marker of oxidative stress, has been reported both in FGR maternal blood and in the placenta [24, 29]. In mouse embryo, impaired mitochondrial function affects subsequent fetal and placental growth [30], and conversely, maternal undernutrition in rats induces impaired placental mitochondrial function in fetal and placental growth restriction [31]. In humans, altered mitochondrial function in the placenta has also been shown, with increased placental oxygen consumption, possibly representing a limiting step in FGR, preventing adequate oxygen delivery to the fetus [24]. Moreover, cord blood oxidative stress biomarkers have been shown to vary with the severity of FGR and of vascular disease in the twin pregnancy model in which both fetuses share the same maternal environment [25]. Oxidative stress was also recently reported as a common trait of endothelial dysfunction in chorionic arteries from fetuses with FGR [32].

Oxidative stress can stimulate an inflammatory response and, conversely an inflammatory response induces oxidative stress, generating a positive feedback system. One or more pro-inflammatory factors released from the syncytial surface of the placenta into the maternal circulation may be involved in this scenario. Several markers of systemic inflammation have been demonstrated to increase in FGR mother-child couple compared to normal pregnancies, as well as in FGR placentas and in the kidney of piglets [33, 34]. This might also be due to uneven adipose deposition in FGR, which is often accompanied by the release of pro-inflammatory signaling molecules, as recently reported in male rats [35].

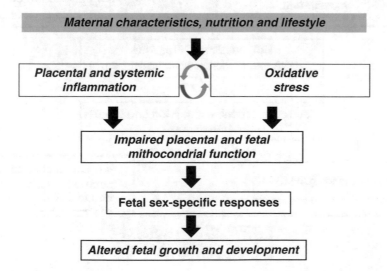

Fig. 5.3 Associations among maternal environment, oxidative stress and inflammation, potentially conditioning fetal growth. Maternal characteristics and exposures can influence both systemic and placental oxidative stress and inflammation, potentially conditioning fetal growth by modifying oxygen and nutrient delivery to the fetus

Interestingly, growing evidence suggests that fetal sex also affects fetal growth responses to the intrauterine and maternal environment [20, 36]. Sexually dimorphic differences in growth and survival of the fetus are likely mediated by the sex specific function of the human placenta, with male and female fetuses establishing different strategies to cope with the same adverse maternal environment [36]. In a rat model, adult females from undernourished mothers during perinatal life were lately reported to develop a better global antioxidant status, possibly contributing to their protection against hypertension programming. Moreover, a proteomic analysis of adipose tissue in rats showed that although FGR affected pathways of substrate and energy metabolism in both males and females, important gender differences were evident, with FGR males predisposing to later development of obesity, while females showing established obesity [37].

There is emerging knowledge on the relationship between the effect of maternal nutrition or metabolic status on placental function and the risk of non-communicable diseases later in life, with a specific impact of sexual dimorphism and epigenetic mechanisms [38].

Epigenetic Modifications

Maternal diet and environmental factors, such as pollution, smoking or psychosocial stress, are very important causes of epigenetic modifications in FGR, with sexual dimorphism in the placental response to the maternal environment (Fig. 5.4) [20, 38–40]. Indeed, epigenetic variation in the placenta is now emerging as a candidate mediator of the environmental influence on placental functioning and a key regulator of pregnancy outcome. A growing body of evidence based on epigenome-wide

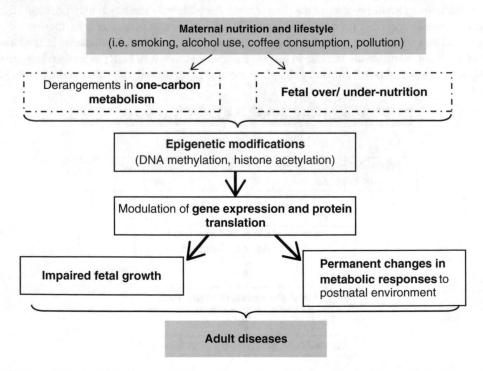

Fig. 5.4 Epigenetic changes linking maternal diet and environmental factors to fetal growth restriction (FGR) and adult diseases. Maternal exposures during critical stages of intrauterine development can influence the adult phenotype of the offspring by permanently modify gene expression and protein translation through epigenetic perturbations

association studies suggests that early life adverse environmental events may trigger widespread and persistent alterations in transcriptional profiling, which lead to the risk of development and progression of a variety of human chronic diseases [39]. Over the past years, epigenetic modifications have been extensively associated with FGR. DNA methylation is the most intensively studied epigenetic feature. Several studies associate altered DNA methylation profiles of key gene regulation and transcription pathways in umbilical cord blood [41] and placenta of FGR pregnancies. Evidence for an involvement of imprinted genes in FGR and placenta-associated complications has been extensively shown [42]. Loss of imprinting and aberrant methylation of insulin-like growth factor 2 (IGF), as well as decreased methylation in the H19 gene promoter, with a consequent increased H19 transcription, have been reported in FGR placentas [43]. The genome-wide differential DNA methylation of all known imprinted genes in normal and FGR placentas has been analyzed, suggesting that differential methylation changes occur in FGR throughout the genomic regions, including genes actively expressed in the placenta [44]. Analyses of genome-wide methylation patterns in normal, SGA and FGR human placentas shows that methylation patterns are associated with infant growth, suggesting that methylation status in the human term placenta may be a marker for the intrauterine environment, potentially playing a critical functional role in fetal development. Recently, placental DNA methylation gene levels of IGF2, AHRR, HSD11B2 and WNT2 were confirmed to associate with FGR [45]. Moreover, a correlation has been established between disrupted DNA methylation of a few genes previously shown altered in the term placenta and altered maternal serum levels of the corresponding protein, indicating that DNA methylation might be a useful tool to identify novel biomarkers for adverse pregnancy outcomes [46].

The timing of insult likely influences the degree of epigenetic alterations. Early gestation has recently been identified as a critical time-period for adult DNA methylation changes in whole blood after prenatal exposure to Dutch famine [19].

Histone modifications have also been reported in animal models. In a rat model of FGR, low-protein diet-derived offspring presented permanent repressive posttranslational histone modifications at the promoter of Cyp7a1, leading to increased blood cholesterol [47]. Prenatal caffeine ingestion induced aberrant DNA methylation and histone acetylation of the SF-1 promoter in the rat fetal adrenal, leading to the production of corticosterone during fetal development [48].

Finally, maternal circulating microRNAs (miRNAs) expression has been investigated over the past years in FGR, gaining increasing interest for their potential role as pathology biomarkers and potential therapeutic tools [49]. miRNAs are short non-coding RNAs that regulate gene expression at the post-transcriptional level. Pregnancy is associated with increased maternal plasma levels of several placenta-specific miRNAs compared to non-pregnant controls, which possibly mediate crosstalk between the feto-placental unit and the mother during pregnancy. FGR has been associated with increased circulating miRNAs regulated by hypoxia. Indeed, circulating miRNAs might also serve as biomarkers for placental function during pregnancy. Moreover, a significant increase of extracellular placental miRNAs levels in the first trimester maternal serum has been observed in pregnancies with later onset of preeclampsia and/or FGR [50].

Conclusions

Fetal growth is dependent from appropriate oxygen and nutrient supply and utilization. There are many maternal factors that may decrease fetal growth mainly affecting placental function and transfer capabilities. The interplay between mother, placenta and fetus is always involved, as fetal growth is likely matched to nutrient and oxygen availability. Any insult deriving from the environment or from one of these three compartments, seems to act at the placental level, altering mitochondrial function and oxygen consumption, possibly leading to FGR.

Epigenetic mechanisms are found to be likely involved in linking environmental exposures, such as lifestyle and nutritional inadequacies, to alterations in placental function and fetal growth. Different epigenetic responses have been described depending on fetal sex, thus leading to interesting hypothesis about sexual dimorphism occurring during intrauterine life.

These new findings may lead to interventions during preconception as well as pregnancy, with the potential to reduce the negative effects of environmental, nutritional and lifestyle exposures on fetal growth and on future health outcomes.

References

1. Bergmann RL, Bergmann KE, Dudenhausen JW. Undernutrition and growth restriction in pregnancy. Nestle Nutr Workshop Ser Pediatr Program. 2008;61:103–21.
2. Cetin I, Sparks JW. Determinants of intrauterine growth. In: Hay Jr WW, Thureen PJ, editors. Neonatal nutrition and metabolism. ed 2 ed. Cambridge: Cambridge University Press; 2006. p. 23–31.
3. Sharma D, Shastri S, Sharma P. Intrauterine growth restriction- part 1. J Matern Fetal Neonatal Med. 2016;9:1–39.
4. American College of Obstetricians and Gynecologists. ACOG practice bulletin no. 134: fetal growth restriction. Obstet Gynecol. 2013;121(5):1122–33.
5. Tudehope D, Vento M, Bhutta Z, Pachi P. Nutritional requirements and feeding recommendations for small for gestational age infants. J Pediatr. 2013;162:S81.
6. Steegers-Theunissen RP, Twigt J, Pestinger V, Sinclair KD. The periconceptional period, reproduction and long-term health of offspring: the importance of one-carbon metabolism. Hum Reprod Update. 2013;19:640–55.
7. Zhang X, Platt RW, Cnattingius S, et al. The use of customized versus population-based birthweight standards in predicting perinatal mortality. Br J Obstet Gynaecol. 2007;114:474–7.
8. Cetin I, Boito S, Radaelli T. Evaluation of fetal growth and fetal well-being. Semin Ultrasound CT MR. 2008;29(2):136–46.
9. Padoan A, Rigano S, Ferrazzi E, et al. Differences in fat and lean mass proportions in normal and growth-restricted fetuses. Am J Obstet Gynecol. 2004;191:1459–64.
10. Gardosi J, Figueras F, Clausson B, Francis A. The customised growth potential: an international research tool to study the epidemiology of fetal growth. Paediatr Perinat Epidemiol. 2011;25:2.
11. Alfirevic Z, Stampalija T, Gyte GM. Fetal and umbilical Doppler ultrasound in high-risk pregnancies. Cochrane Database Syst Rev. 2013;12(11):CD007529.
12. Unterscheider J, Daly S, Geary MP, Kennelly MM, McAuliffe FM, O'Donoghue K, Hunter A, Morrison JJ, Burke G, Dicker P, Tully EC, Malone FD. Predictable progressive Doppler deterioration in IUGR: does it really exist? Am J Obstet Gynecol. 2013;209(6):539.e1–7.
13. Mook-Kanamori DO, Steegers EA, Eilers PH, Raat H, Hofman A, Jaddoe VW. Risk factors and outcomes associated with first-trimester fetal growth restriction. JAMA. 2010;303(6):527–34.
14. Van Uitert EM, Exalto N, Burton GJ, Willemsen SP, Koning AH, Eilers PH, Laven JS, Steegers EA, Steegers-Theunissen RP. Human embryonic growth trajectories and associations with fetal growth and birthweight. Hum Reprod. 2013;28(7):1753–61.
15. Cetin I, Mando C, Calabrese S. Maternal predictors of intrauterine growth restriction. Curr Opin Clin Nutr Metab Care. 2013;16(3):310e319.
16. Maloney KF, Heller D, Baergen RN. Types of maternal hypertensive disease and their association with pathologic lesions and clinical factors. Fetal Pediatr Pathol. 2012;31(5):319–23.
17. Almasi O, Pariente G, Kessous R, Sergienko R, Sheiner E. Association between delivery of small-for-gestational-age neonate and long-term maternal chronic kidney disease. J Matern Fetal Neonatal Med. 2015;23:1–4.
18. Julian CG, Yang IV, Browne VA, Vargas E, Rodriguez C, Pedersen BS, Moore LG, Schwartz DA. Inhibition of peroxisome proliferator-activated receptor γ: a potential link between chronic maternal hypoxia and impaired fetal growth. FASEB J. 2014;28(3):1268–79.
19. Tobi EW, Slieker RC, Stein AD, Suchiman HE, Slagboom PE, van Zwet EW, Heijmans BT, Lumey LH. Early gestation as the critical time-window for changes in the prenatal environment to affect the adult human blood methylome. Int J Epidemiol. 2015;44(4):1211–23.
20. Mandò C, Calabrese S, Mazzocco MI, Novielli C, Anelli GM, Antonazzo P, Cetin I. Sex specific adaptations in placental biometry of overweight and obese women. Placenta. 2016;38:1–7.
21. Pantham P, Aye IL, Powell TL. Inflammation in maternal obesity and gestational diabetes mellitus. Placenta. 2015;36(7):709e715.

22. Sen S, Rifas-Shiman SL, Shivappa N, Wirth MD, Hébert JR, Gold DR, Gillman MW, Oken E. Dietary inflammatory potential during pregnancy is associated with lower fetal growth and breastfeeding failure: results from project viva. J Nutr. 2016;146:728–36. pii: jn225581. [Epub ahead of print].
23. Blatt K, Moore E, Chen A, Van Hook J, DeFranco EA. Association of reported trimester-specific smoking cessation with fetal growth restriction. Obstet Gynecol. 2015;125(6):1452–9.
24. Mandò C, De Palma C, Stampalija T, Anelli GM, Figus M, Novielli C, Parisi F, Clementi E, Ferrazzi E, Cetin I. Placental mitochondrial content and function in intrauterine growth restriction and preeclampsia. Am J Physiol Endocrinol Metab. 2014;306(4):E404–13.
25. Maisonneuve E, Delvin E, Edgard A, Morin L, Dubé J, Boucoiran I, Moutquin JM, Fouron JC, Klam S, Levy E, Leduc L. Oxidative conditions prevail in severe IUGR with vascular disease and Doppler anomalies. J Matern Fetal Neonatal Med. 2015;28(12):1471–5.
26. Chen F, Wang T, Feng C, Lin G, Zhu Y, Wu G, Johnson G, Wang J. Proteome differences in placenta and endometrium between normal and intrauterine growth restricted pig fetuses. PLoS One. 2015;10(11):e0142396.
27. Wiebe HW, Boulé NG, Chari R, Davenport MH. The effect of supervised prenatal exercise on fetal growth: a meta-analysis. Obstet Gynecol. 2015;125(5):1185–94.
28. Madianos PN, Lieff S, Murtha AP, et al. Maternal periodontitis and prematurity. Part II: maternal infection and fetal exposure. Ann Periodontol. 2001;6:175–82.
29. Colleoni F, Lattuada D, Garretto A, Massari M, Mandò C, Somigliana E, Cetin I. Maternal blood mitochondrial DNA content during normal and intrauterine growth restricted (IUGR) pregnancy. Am J Obstet Gynecol. 2010;203(4):365–e6.
30. Wakefield SL, Lane M, Mitchell M. Impaired mitochondrial function in the preimplantation embryo perturbs fetal and placental development in the mouse. Biol Reprod. 2011;84:572–80.
31. Mayeur S, Lancel S, Theys N, Lukaszewski MA, Duban-Deweer S, Bastide B, Hachani J, Cecchelli R, Breton C, Gabory A, Storme L, Reusens B, Junien C, Vieau D, Lesage J. Maternal calorie restriction modulates placental mitochondrial biogenesis and bioenergetic efficiency: putative involvement in fetoplacental growth defects in rats. Am J Physiol Endocrinol Metab. 2013;304:E14–22.
32. Schneider D, Hernández C, Farías M, Uauy R, Krause BJ, Casanello P. Oxidative stress as common trait of endothelial dysfunction in chorionic arteries from fetuses with IUGR and LGA. Placenta. 2015;36(5):552–8.
33. Visentin S, Lapolla A, Londero AP, Cosma C, Dalfrà M, Camerin M, Faggian D, Plebani M, Cosmi E. Adiponectin levels are reduced while markers of systemic inflammation and aortic remodelling are increased in intrauterine growth restricted mother-child couple. Biomed Res Int. 2014;2014:401595.
34. Elmhiri G, Mahmood DF, Niquet-Leridon C, Jacolot P, Firmin S, Guigand L, Tessier FJ, Larcher T, Abdennebi-Najar L. Formula-derived advanced glycation end products are involved in the development of long-term inflammation and oxidative stress in kidney of IUGR piglets. Mol Nutr Food Res. 2015;59(5):939–47.
35. Riddle ES, Campbell MS, Lang BY, Bierer R, Wang Y, Bagley HN, Joss-Moore LA. Intrauterine growth restriction increases TNF α and activates the unfolded protein response in male rat pups. J Obes. 2014;2014:829862.
36. Clifton VL. Review: sex and the human placenta: mediating differential strategies of fetal growth and survival. Placenta. 2010;31(Suppl):S33eS39.
37. de Souza AP, Pedroso AP, Watanabe RL, Dornellas AP, Boldarine VT, Laure HJ, do Nascimento CM, Oyama LM, Rosa JC, Ribeiro EB. Gender-specific effects of intrauterine growth restriction on the adipose tissue of adult rats: a proteomic approach. Proteome Sci. 2015;13:32.
38. Tarrade A, Panchenko P, Junien C, Gabory A. Placental contribution to nutritional programming of health and diseases: epigenetics and sexual dimorphism. J Exp Biol. 2015;218(Pt 1):50–8. Review.
39. Vaiserman A. Epidemiologic evidence for association between adverse environmental exposures in early life and epigenetic variation: a potential link to disease susceptibility? Clin Epigenetics. 2015;7(1):96.
40. Casas-Agustench P, Iglesias-Gutiérrez E, Dávalos A. Mother's nutritional miRNA legacy: nutrition during pregnancy and its possible implications to develop cardiometabolic disease in later life. Pharmacol Res. 2015;100:322–34.
41. Hillman SL, Finer S, Smart MC, Mathews C, Lowe R, Rakyan VK, Hitman GA, Williams DJ. Novel DNA methylation profiles associated with key gene regulation and transcription pathways in blood and placenta of growth-restricted neonates. Epigenetics. 2015;10(1):50–61.
42. Monk D. Genomic imprinting in the human placenta. Am J Obstet Gynecol. 2015;213(4 Suppl):S152–62.
43. Koukoura O, Sifakis S, Soufla G, et al. Loss of imprinting and aberrant methylation of IGF2 in placentas from pregnancies complicated with fetal growth restriction. Int J Mol Med. 2011;28:481–7.
44. Lambertini L, Lee TL, Chan WY, et al. Differential methylation of imprinted & genes in growth-restricted placentas. Reprod Sci. 2011;18:1111–7.
45. Xiao X, Zhao Y, Jin R, Chen J, Wang X, Baccarelli A, Zhang Y. Fetal growth restriction and methylation of growth-related genes in the placenta. Epigenomics. 2016;8(1):33–42.
46. Wilson SL, Blair JD, Hogg K, Langlois S, von Dadelszen P, Robinson WP. Placental DNA methylation at term reflects maternal serum levels of INHA and FN1, but not PAPPA, early in pregnancy. BMC Med Genet. 2015;16(1):111.

47. Sohi G, Marchand K, Revesz A, et al. Maternal protein restriction elevates cholesterol in adult rat offspring due to repressive changes in histone modifications at the cholesterol 7alpha-hydroxylase promoter. Mol Endocrinol. 2011;25:785–98.

48. Ping J, Wang JF, Liu L, Yan YE, Liu F, Lei YY, Wang H. Prenatal caffeine ingestion induces aberrant DNA methylation and histone acetylation of steroidogenic factor 1 and inhibits fetal adrenal steroidogenesis. Toxicology. 2014;3(321):53–61.

49. Mouillet JF, Ouyang Y, Coyne CB, Sadovsky Y. MicroRNAs in placental health and disease. Am J Obstet Gynecol. 2015;213(4 Suppl):S163–72.

50. Hromadnikova I, Kotlabova K, Doucha J, et al. Absolute and relative quanti-& fication of placenta-specific micrornas in maternal circulation with placental insufficiency-related complications. J Mol Diagn. 2012;14:160–7.

Chapter 6
Maternal Insulin Sensitivity and Fetal Brain Activity

Franziska Schleger, Katarzyna Linder, Andreas Fritsche, and Hubert Preissl

Key Points

- The adult human brain is an insulin-sensitive organ
- Central nervous insulin resistance affects peripheral glucose metabolism in adults
- Maternal metabolism influences different aspects of fetal development
- Maternal insulin sensitivity influences fetal postprandial brain activity
- Central nervous insulin resistance may be programmed already in utero

Keywords Fetal magnetoencephalography • Fetal programming • Insulin sensitivity • Fetal brain • Maternal metabolism • Central nervous insulin resistance

Abbreviations

ER	Evoked response
FFA	Free fatty acids
fMEG	Fetal magnetoencephalography
GDM	Gestational diabetes mellitus
HOMA-IR	Homeostatic model assessment of insulin resistance

F. Schleger, PhD • H. Preissl, PhD (✉)
Institute for Diabetes Research and Metabolic Diseases of the Helmholtz Center Munich at the University of Tübingen, Tübingen, Germany
e-mail: hubert.preissl@helmholtz-muenchen.de

K. Linder, MD • A. Fritsche, MD
Institute for Diabetes Research and Metabolic Diseases of the Helmholtz Center Munich at the University of Tübingen, Tübingen, Germany

Department of Internal Medicine, Division of Endocrinology, Diabetology, Angiology, Nephrology and Clinical Chemistry, University of Tübingen, Tübingen, Germany

© Springer International Publishing AG 2017
R. Rajendram et al. (eds.), *Diet, Nutrition, and Fetal Programming*,
Nutrition and Health, DOI 10.1007/978-3-319-60289-9_6

IR	Insulin resistance
IS	Insulin sensitivity
NGT	Normal glucose tolerant
OGTT	Oral glucose tolerance test
SQUIDs	Superconducting quantum interference devices

While it has been shown that children of mothers with metabolic disturbances have an increased risk of becoming obese or developing diabetes in later life [1–4], little is known about the mechanisms behind this metabolic programming. Until recently it has been assumed that changes in maternal metabolism, especially insulin sensitivity (see Table 6.1), mainly influence peripheral processes in the fetus. However, several studies showed that maternal insulin resistance leads to functional and anatomical changes in the fetal brain mainly in rodents and that the human brain is insulin sensitive. These studies were the basis for the first studies investigating the influence of maternal metabolism on the fetal brain in humans.

Insulin Sensitivity in the Adult Human Brain

The human brain is an insulin sensitive organ. Several studies have shown that peripheral insulin can pass the blood brain barrier and act in a large number of different brain areas like hypothalamus, fusiform gyrus, prefrontal areas and hippocampus [5], thereby affecting many behavioral, metabolic or cognitive processes [6, 7]. However, similarly to the periphery, brain insulin sensitivity is altered by metabolic changes and it is possible that the normal insulin is attenuated or even absent, this is called brain insulin resistance. It has been suggested that brain insulin resistance does not solely result from metabolic changes in the periphery, but could actively contribute to the development of metabolic diseases [8].

An early magnetoencephalographic study on the effects of insulin on spontaneous and evoked human brain activity showed diminished insulin action in the brain of obese as compared to lean adults. They used a stepwise euglycaemic–hyperinsulinaemic clamp, during which insulin was infused continuously and simultaneously glucose was infused to prevent hypoglycemia [9, 10]. As the peripheral insulin infusion can not exclude interactions between other insulin sensitive organs and the brain, in later studies, insulin was administered intranasally as a spray. After intranasal application, insulin is transported directly along olfactory nerves into the central nervous system, thereby almost completely avoiding the blood transport [8, 11]. Using a combination of both stepwise clamp and nasal insulin, a strong relationship between peripheral insulin resistance and insulin resistance of the human brain was found [12, 13]. Many studies delivered evidence that insulin action in the human brain may affect the peripheral metabolism. During a lifestyle intervention, obese subjects with higher brain insulin sensitivity lost more weight than obese subjects with brain insulin resistance [9]. Intranasal insulin administration could not improve insulin sensitivity in obese men, but it did in lean men [14]. The underlying mechanisms of central insulin action and insulin resistance of the human brain are not completely resolved. Better knowledge on brain insulin action seems to be essential in order to understand the pathogenesis of obesity and type 2 diabetes mellitus.

Table 6.1 What is insulin sensitivity?

Insulin sensitivity describes the degree to which cells respond to normal insulin action, as opposed to insulin resistance, which describes a state in which the cells cease to respond to insulin. In insulin sensitive subjects, a small amount of insulin is necessary for glucose metabolism in cells, in insulin resistant subjects large amounts of insulin are necessary to allow for glucose metabolism

Insulin sensitivity can be assessed via blood samples, either in a fasting state (HOMA-IR, [15]) or during a glucose challenge (oral glucose tolerance test, OGTT, see Box 6.1, [16]

Developmental Programming of Brain Insulin Sensitivity in Animals

Animal studies have repeatedly shown that maternal diet and metabolism can not only have disruptive effects on weight and metabolic diseases in offspring [17–19], but excessive nutrient supply during gestation or in early postnatal periods can directly influence fetal brain development [20–22].

In mice, maternal high-fat diet feeding during lactation (a period in rodent development which has been described as analogous to the human last fetal trimester) can predispose the offspring for obesity and impaired glucose homeostasis. The effect on the neonatal mouse brain development showed itself in abnormal insulin signaling and was associated with an impairment in circuit formation in insulin-sensitive hypothalamic areas [20]. Early postnatal overfeeding by decreasing litter size can have similar effects: Overfed rats gained more weight during the lactation period and were overweight later in life. They also showed differences in neurochemical plasticity compared to rats that grew up in normal-sized litters: Answers to anorexigenic and orexigenic neuropetides in hypothalamic neurons were altered [21].

Gupta et al. [22] investigated fetal brain development in rats (analogous to the first two trimesters of human gestation). Term fetuses of mothers that had been fed on high-fat diets before and during pregnancy showed altered leptin and insulin signaling and upregulation of orexigenic neuropeptides in the hypothalamus.

Sanguinetti et al. [23] showed an effect on fetal brain insulin sensitivity in minipigs: At birth, offspring of mothers that had been fed high-fat diets during gestation, as opposed to offspring of mothers on low-fat diets, showed higher brain glucose metabolism and more brain insulin receptors. The overexposure to glucose during the fetal phase led to a subsequent attenuated brain glucose metabolism during further development under normal feeding conditions. This indicates a change in fetal brain insulin sensitivity in response to differences in maternal diets during gestation.

This research in animals shows that changes in maternal metabolism can program a variety of changes in the fetus, and most interestingly, in the fetal brain. Studied developmental periods have been discussed as models for the second trimester (fetal period in rodents) and the third trimester (lactation period in rodents) of human gestation. The effects of human maternal metabolism on the fetal brain can be studied with specific brain imaging methods.

Fetal Magnetoencephalography: Accessing Fetal Brain Activity Noninvasively

Fetal Magnetoencephalography (fMEG) is a non-invasive technique which enables a direct measurement of fetal neuronal activity in utero (see Table 6.2 and Fig. 6.1).

FMEG allows the investigation of fetal heart dynamics [35, 36], spontaneous fetal brain activity [37, 38], fetal evoked brain activity to visual stimuli [26, 32] and auditory stimuli [28, 29, 39], mainly in the last trimester of pregnancy. Fetal evoked responses (ER) usually consist of one component, which can be described by its amplitude and latency. Amplitudes depend on fetal position and distance to the sensors, but latencies can be directly compared between different subjects. For a data example of a fetal ER, see Fig. 6.2.

Fetuses not only show evoked brain activity to a variety of tones, like different frequencies of pure tones and white noise [40], but also show discriminative responses to changes in stimulation, in so-called oddball paradigms. In this paradigm, one stimulus (or stimulation sequence, the standard) is frequently presented, interspersed with one or more infrequent stimuli (the deviant or oddball stimuli). In addition to responses evoked by the stimuli themselves, mismatch responses are elicited by the change from the standard to the deviant stimulation, if the change is perceived and the memory trace of the original

Table 6.2 Method: fetal magnetoencephalography (fMEG)

FMEG allows the direct non-invasive measurement of fetal neuronal activity. As opposed to electrical activity recorded in electroencephalographic measurements, magnetic signals recorded in magnetoencephalographic measurements are not distorted by passing through layers of biological tissue. Due to its high temporal resolution, fMEG is especially suitable to evaluate the time course of fetal neuronal activity [24]

While adult brain activity has been measured and studied with magnetoencephalography (MEG) extensively, fetal brain activity has been more elusive. Human fetal research was limited to behavioral and physiological measures based on ultrasound and electrocardiographic recordings. In the 1980s first fetal magnetoencephalography measurements have been conducted by Blum et al. [25] with a single-channel MEG system. In the following years, detection methods of fMEG signals have advanced [26–29], as have data acquisition methods, with the development of dedicated fMEG systems shaped to fit the maternal abdomen

In dedicated fMEG systems, as in MEG systems used in adults, highly sensitive sensors, so-called superconducting Quantum Interference Devices (SQUIDs), are installed. They can measure even weak magnetic fields in the femto Tesla (fT, 10^{-15} T) to pico Tesla (pT, 10^{-12} T) range, which includes the field strength of fetal brain activity. To reach superconductivity the sensors are cooled down with liquid helium to about 4°K in a temperature-isolated container [30]. Systems are operated in magnetically shielded rooms to shield from environmental noise (10^{-7} T)

FMEG systems do not directly provide fetal anatomical information. To determine fetal position, ultrasound measurements are conducted before and after fMEG measurements [24]

Activity recorded besides fetal brain activity include maternal heart activity (up to 100pT), fetal heart activity (up to 10pT), uterine muscle activity, and muscle activity due to maternal movement [31]. To analyze fetal brain data, environmental noise is cancelled, and maternal and fetal heart activity is removed [32–34]. After stimulus-locked averaging, visual analysis of evoked responses is possible [27, 28]

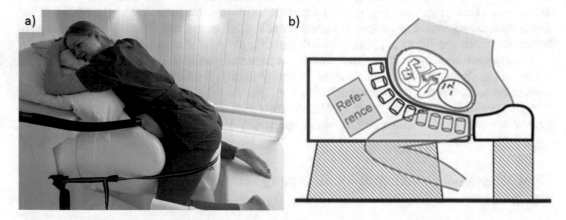

Fig. 6.1 The fMEG system installed in Tübingen. (**a**) Woman seated on the fMEG system during auditory stimulation. (**b**) Schematic of the fMEG system (The pictures were reproduced with permission of the University Hospital Tübingen, Germany (**a**, **b**) University of Arkansas for Medical Sciences, Little Rock, Arkansas, USA)

pattern persists [41]. Mismatch responses in fetuses have been shown to changes in pure tone frequencies [42, 43] and changes in the number of tones in a sequence [44]. Since there is evidence that fetal ERs habituate with repeated stimulation, with decreasing amplitudes of ERs [45, 46], oddball paradigms are also employed to avoid habituation to the stimulation of interest by interrupting the repeated presentation of a frequent standard stimulus with an infrequent deviant stimulus, to ensure that the amplitude of the ER doesn't decrease with repeated stimulation. The outcome measure of interest is the fetal response latency. It has been shown to decrease during the course of gestation and is assumed to be an indicator of cortex maturation [24, 39, 47]. In this context, delayed brain maturation has also been studied: Visual ERs have been shown to be delayed in growth-restricted fetuses with placental insufficiency but not in fetuses that were merely small for their gestational age [48, 49]. ER latency appears to be an indicator

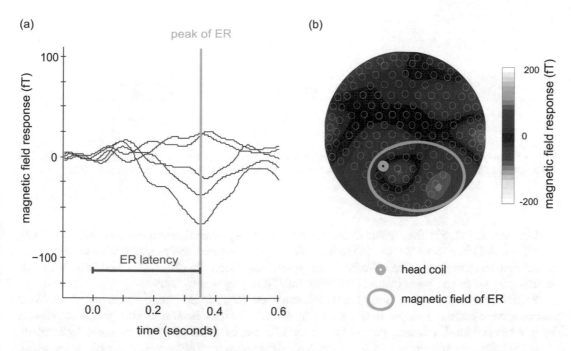

Fig. 6.2 Fetal evoked response (*ER*) to an auditory stimulus. (**a**) Magnetic field response in five channels over time. Auditory stimulation starts at 0.0 s. The time from beginning of stimulation to the peak of the ER is called ER latency. (**b**) Distribution of magnetic field activity over maternal abdomen

---

Box 6.1 Oral Glucose Tolerance Test (OGTT)

During an OGTT, blood samples are taken during fasting state and after a glucose challenge. Oral glucose tolerance tests are routinely performed in German pregnancy care between 24 and 28 weeks of gestation, to check for gestational diabetes mellitus. Maternal blood glucose levels are measured in the fasting state, then women drink a 75 mg glucose drink and maternal blood glucose levels are again measured 1 and 2 h, respectively, after ingesting the glucose drink. Gestational diabetes is diagnosed if one of the three blood glucose measures exceeds a threshold value (92, 180, 153 mg/dl, Deutsche Praxisleitlinie Gestationsdiabetes Stand 2015 [50]). Gestational diabetes is a state of hyperglycaemia and hyperinsulinaemia during gestation, in which pregnant woman are insulin resistant. Based on the blood glucose and insulin values obtained during the OGTT, maternal insulin sensitivity index can be determined [51]

---

of brain maturation over gestational age and perturbed brain development on a group level, but recent studies have also shown it to be respondent to short-term changes in fetal environment, namely changes in maternal metabolism.

Studies Showing Effects of Maternal Insulin Sensitivity and Maternal Metabolism on Fetal Brain Activity in Humans

To investigate whether maternal metabolic changes influence fetal brain activity, fMEG measurements were conducted during the course of a maternal oral glucose tolerance test (OGTT, see Box 6.1).

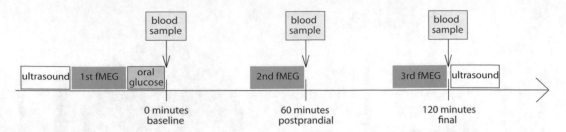

Fig. 6.3 Study protocol. Three fetal magnetoencephalographic recordings (*fMEG*) were performed. The first just before the ingestion of the glucose and two additional respectively 60 and 120 min after the ingestion [52, 53]

Linder et al. [52, 53] investigated fetal evoked brain activity in relation to maternal insulin sensitivity (see Table 6.1) in normal glucose tolerant (NGT) pregnant woman and pregnant woman with gestational diabetes mellitus (GDM). Women with gestational diabetes have elevated blood glucose levels during pregnancy and lower insulin sensitivity than NGT pregnant women.

Participants underwent an oral glucose tolerance test (OGTT, see Box 6.1), during which blood samples were taken at three main timepoints: 0, 60 and 120 min. Insulin sensitivity was determined by glucose and insulin measurements at 0, 60 and 120 min, based on a formula proposed by Stumvoll et al. [51]. Before each taking of a blood sample, fMEG measurements were performed, during which auditory stimulation was presented to the fetuses in an oddball paradigm, containing frequent 500 Hz tone bursts, interspersed with infrequent 750 Hz tone bursts to avoid habituation. Response latencies of fetal auditory evoked fields were determined [52, 53]. The timing of procedures during the studies is depicted in Fig. 6.3.

Maternal blood values of NGT and GDM subjects over the course of an OGTT are depicted in Fig. 6.4. Maternal insulin and glucose levels increased from fasting level to 60 min and decreased again at 120 min. Maternal free fatty acid (FFA) levels decreased at 60 min and further decreased at 120 min [53].

Over the same time period, fetal auditory ER latencies in the NGT group decreased from baseline to the postprandial measurement at 60 min and did not change significantly again after 120 min [53].

The timepoint of interest was the postprandial state: In fetuses in the NGT group, ER latencies were faster after 60 min than at baseline, at a timepoint where maternal blood values showed large changes relative to baseline: Increased insulin and glucose levels and decreased FFA levels. While no effect of maternal blood FFA on ER latencies was found, both maternal blood glucose and insulin levels showed a significant influence on fetal postprandial ER latency. This indicates a short-term effect of maternal metabolism on fetal brain activity. However, this postprandial effect disappeared in the GDM sample, in which fetuses did not show a change in ER latency in the postprandial state [53], see Fig. 6.4, panel D.

Maternal insulin sensitivity correlated negatively with fetal ER latencies: NGT mothers were separated into two groups based on the median of the insulin sensitivity value. Fetuses of NGT mothers with higher insulin sensitivity showed shorter postprandial ER latencies than fetuses of NGT mothers with lower insulin sensitivity and fetuses of GDM mothers showed longer ER latencies than fetuses of mother with NGT. Postprandial ER latency in the fetuses decreased with increasing insulin sensitivity [53], see Fig. 6.5.

These findings indicate that there might be a direct effect of maternal metabolism on fetal brain activity. It is not a general effect of maternal metabolic status on fetal brain activity per se, but rather a dynamic effect that only appears in the postprandial state.

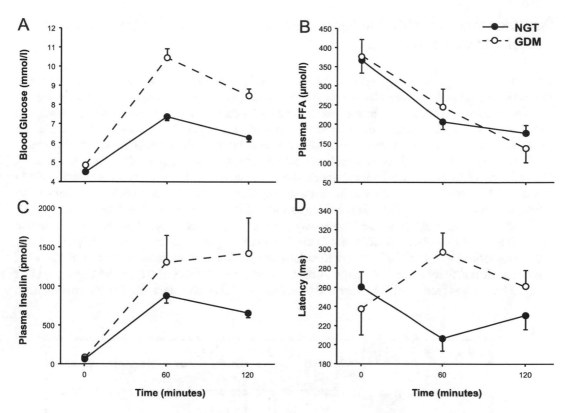

Fig. 6.4 Maternal metabolism and fetal brain. Results of the Linder [53] study during the course of the three timepoints of an OGTT in normal glucose tolerant (*NGT*) pregnant woman and woman with gestational diabetes mellitus (*GDM*). (**a**) Maternal blood glucose, (**b**) maternal free fatty acids (*FFA*), (**c**) maternal plasma insulin, (**d**) fetal auditory evoked response latencies. Values shown are mean ± SEM (Reproduced with permission from Linder [53])

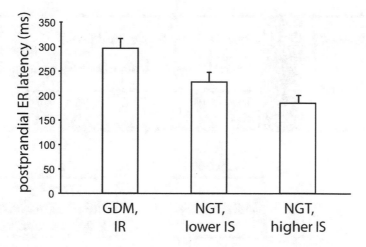

Fig. 6.5 Comparison of fetal postprandial evoked response (*ER*) latency between three maternal groups with different insulin sensitivity (*IS*). Mothers in the gestational diabetes mellitus (GDM, $n = 12$) group, with at least one blood glucose value above the diagnostic threshold (see Box 6.1) have the lowest IS; normal glucose tolerant (*NGT*) mothers were split into two groups based on the median of the IS value, into a group with lower IS and a group with higher IS (each $n = 14$). Postprandial ER latency in the fetuses decreased with increasing IS (Adapted from Linder [53])

Possible Underlying Mechanisms: How Could Maternal Insulin Sensitivity Actually Influence the Fetus?

There are several possible mechanisms that could explain the association between the amount of change in postprandial response latency in the fetal brain and the insulin sensitivity of the mother.

One speculation concerning the mechanism can be based on the Pedersen Hypothesis. Pederson postulated back in 1952, that, as glucose passes the placenta (and insulin does not), increased glucose levels in the mother lead to increased glucose levels in the fetus, and thereby induce hyperinsulinaemia in the fetus [54]. In mothers, insulin levels are higher in the postprandial state. These temporarily higher levels of insulin in mothers are assumed to correspond with temporary hyperinsulinemia in fetuses. It is possible that variations in insulin levels are important for an appropriate fetal brain maturation, but chronic hyperinsulinemia may lead to onset of fetal brain insulin resistance (see Fig. 6.6).

Alternatively maternal insulin resistance may cause a variety of other metabolic changes, which in turn might lead to the observed difference in the fetal brain response. Tschritter et al. [55] could show that elevated levels of saturated nonesterified fatty acids (FFA) reduce insulin action at the level of cerebrocortical activity in the adult brain. Already in the early 1970s, Szabo et al. [56], proposed that FFA are transferred from mother to fetus and contribute to fetal macrosomia in a diabetic environment.

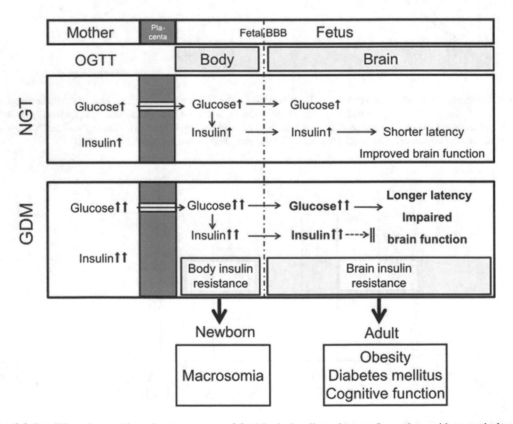

Fig. 6.6 Possible pathogenesis and consequences of fetal brain insulin resistance. In mothers with normal glucose tolerance (*NGT*), postprandially increased insulin improves brain function of the fetus. In mothers with GDM, hyperglycemia-induced insulin resistance evolves in the mother and, in parallel, in the fetal brain, which leads to impairment of fetal postprandial brain reaction because of brain insulin resistance and increases risk for obesity and type 2 diabetes in their later life (Reproduced with permission from Linder [53])

And although these first fetal brain activity studies [52, 53] didn't find any association between maternal FFA and fetal brain responses to auditory stimulation, it is still possible that specific FFA patterns play a role in this process.

In addition to FFAs, other factors have also been considered as potentially affecting brain insulin sensitivity. One of the best examined is the "satiety hormone" leptin. Leptin concentrations are higher in obese humans and a molecular crosstalk could be demonstrated between leptin and insulin signaling in some brain regions in rodents [57, 58]. Cetin et al. [59] investigated the relationship between intrauterine growth and fetal leptin levels in fetuses of healthy mothers and mothers with GDM. Significantly higher leptin levels were found in fetuses of GDM mothers and this correlated with abdominal fat mass as estimated via ultrasound. The impact of leptin (which was measurable as early as 19 weeks of gestation [59]) on the development of the human brain remains still undiscovered.

Also, reduced insulin transport into the fetal brain induced by maternal insulin resistance can be discussed as a possible mechanism [53].

As it is not possible to non-invasively measure fetal metabolic changes directly, speculation on detailed mechanisms is largely based on results from adult and animal studies. Of course, a wide range of further maternal hormonal metabolic changes may affect the fetal brain action and fetal brain development.

Conclusion

Insulin resistance of human brain is associated with obesity, age, visceral fat and FFA and can impair the peripheral metabolism in adults. As understanding the mechanism of the development of human brain insulin resistance may be crucial in the prevention and therapy of obesity and type 2 diabetes mellitus, further studies substantiating this phenomenon and providing the underlying mechanism are still needed. Research on the developmental trajectory of insulin sensitivity in the brain is still in a very early stage. Initial studies in human fetuses indicate that there might be fetal programming of central nervous insulin sensitivity. Brain insulin resistance might already be developed in utero, and might contribute to later metabolic diseases. This could mean that it is necessary to start preventive steps very early or even preconceptional. However, this remains speculation at present. There are no data on whether the postprandial differences in fetal brain activity that have been shown actually have long-term effects – longitudinal data in relation to this question are still missing. If the effects persist, it would be of interest whether they are reversible, at which stage, and how.

References

1. Dabelea D, Hanson RL, Lindsay RS, et al. Intrauterine exposure to diabetes conveys risks for type 2 diabetes and obesity: a study of discordant sibships. Diabetes. 2000;49:2208–11.
2. Kim C, Newton KM, Knopp RH. Gestational diabetes and the incidence of type 2 diabetes: a systematic review. Diabetes Care. 2002;25:1862–8.
3. HAPO Study Cooperative Research Group, Metzger BE, Lowe LP, et al. Hyperglycemia and adverse pregnancy outcomes. N Engl J Med. 2008;358:1991–2002.
4. Sobngwi E, Boudou P, Mauvais-Jarvis F, et al. Effect of a diabetic environment in utero on predisposition to type 2 diabetes. Lancet. 2003;361:1861–5.
5. Heni M, Kullmann S, Preissl H, Fritsche A, Häring HU. Impaired insulin action in the human brain: causes and metabolic consequences. Nat Rev Endocrinol. 2015;11(12):701–11.
6. Baura GD, Foster DM, Porte D Jr, Kahn SE, Bergman RN, Cobelli C, Schwartz MW. Saturable transport of insulin from plasma into the central nervous system of dogs in vivo. A mechanism for regulated insulin delivery to the brain. J Clin Invest. 1993;92(4):1824–30.

7. Brüning JC, Gautam D, Burks DJ, Gillette J, Schubert M, Orban PC, Klein R, Krone W, Müller-Wieland D, Kahn CR. Role of brain insulin receptor in control of body weight and reproduction. Science. 2000;289(5487):2122–5.

8. Heni M, Kullmann S, Ketterer C, Guthoff M, Linder K, Wagner R, Stingl KT, Veit R, Staiger H, Häring HU, Preissl H, Fritsche A. Nasal insulin changes peripheral insulin sensitivity simultaneously with altered activity in homeostatic and reward-related human brain regions. Diabetologia. 2012;55(6):1773–82.

9. Tschritter O, Preissl H, Hennige AM, Sartorius T, Stingl KT, Heni M, Ketterer C, Stefan N, Machann J, Schleicher E, Fritsche A, Häring HU. High cerebral insulin sensitivity is associated with loss of body fat during lifestyle intervention. Diabetologia. 2012;55(1):175–82.

10. Tschritter O, Preissl H, Hennige AM, Stumvoll M, Porubska K, Frost R, Marx H, Klösel B, Lutzenberger W, Birbaumer N, Häring HU, Fritsche A. The cerebrocortical response to hyperinsulinemia is reduced in overweight humans: a magnetoencephalographic study. Proc Natl Acad Sci U S A. 2006;103:12103–8.

11. Renner DB, Svitak AL, Gallus NJ, Ericson ME, Frey WH 2nd, Hanson LR. Intranasal delivery of insulin via the olfactory nerve pathway. J Pharm Pharmacol. 2012;64(12):1709–14.

12. Kullmann S, Frank S, Heni M, Ketterer C, Veit R, Häring HU, Fritsche A, Preissl H. Intranasal insulin modulates intrinsic reward and prefrontal circuitry of the human brain in lean women. Neuroendocrinology. 2013;97(2):176–82.

13. Kullmann S, Heni M, Veit R, Scheffler K, Machann J, Häring HU, Fritsche A, Preissl H. Elective insulin resistance in homeostatic and cognitive control brain areas in overweight and obese adults. Diabetes Care. 2015;38(6):1044–50.

14. Heni M, Wagner R, Kullmann S, Veit R, Mat Husin H, Linder K, Benkendorff C, Peter A, Stefan N, Häring HU, Preissl H, Fritsche A. Central insulin administration improves whole-body insulin sensitivity via hypothalamus and parasympathetic outputs in men. Diabetes. 2014;63(12):4083–8.

15. Matthews DR, Hosker JP, Rudenski AS, Naylor BA, Treacher DF, Turner RC. Homeostasis model assessment: insulin resistance and beta-cell function from fasting plasma glucose and insulin concentrations in man. Diabetologia. 1985;28(7):412–9.

16. Matsuda M, DeFronzo RA. Insulin sensitivity indices obtained from oral glucose tolerance testing: comparison with the euglycemic insulin clamp. Diabetes Care. 1999;22(9):1462–70.

17. Piotrowska I, Zgódka P, Milewska M, Błaszczyk M, Grzelkowska-Kowalczyk K. Developmental programming of metabolic diseases – a review of studies on experimental animal models [article in polish]. Postepy Hig Med Dosw (Online). 2014;68:899–911.

18. Srinivasan M, Katewa SD, Palaniyappan A, Pandya JD, Patel MS. Maternal high-fat diet consumption results in fetal malprogramming predisposing to the onset of metabolic syndrome-like phenotype in adulthood. Am J Physiol Endocrinol Metab. 2006;291(4):E792–9.

19. Taylor PD, McConnell J, Khan IY, Holemans K, Lawrence KM, Asare-Anane H, Persaud SJ, Petrie L, Hanson MA, Poston L. Impaired glucose homeostasis and mitochondrial abnormalities in offspring of rats fed a fat-rich diet in pregnancy. Am J Phys Regul Integr Comp Phys. 2005;288:R134–9.

20. Vogt MC, Paeger L, Hess S, et al. Neonatal insulin action impairs hypothalamic neurocircuit formation in response to maternal high-fat feeding. Cell. 2014;156:495–509.

21. Davidowa H, Li Y, Plagemann A. Altered responses to orexigenic (AGRP, MCH) and anorexigenic (α-MSH, CART) neuropeptides of paraventricular hypothalamic neurons in early postnatally overfed rats. Eur J Neurosci. 2003;18:613–21.

22. Gupta A, Srinivasan M, Thamadilok S, Patel MS. Hypothalamic alterations in fetuses of high fat diet-fed obese female rats. J Endocrinol. 2009;200:293–300.

23. Sanguinetti E, Liistro T, Mainardi M, Pardini S, Salvadori PA, Vannucci A, Burchielli S, Iozzo P. Maternal high-fat feeding leads to alterations of brain glucose metabolism in the offspring: positron emission tomography study in a porcine model. Diabetologia. 2016;59(4):813–21.

24. Preissl H, Lowery CL, Eswaran H. Fetal magnetoencephalography: current progress and trends. Exp Neurol. 2004;190(Suppl 1):S28–36.

25. Blum T, Saling E, Bauer R. First magnetoencephalographic recordings of the brain activity of a human fetus. Br J Obstet Gynaecol. 1985;92(12):1224–9.

26. Eswaran H, Preissl H, Wilson JD, Murphy P, Robinson SE, Rose D, Vrba J, Lowery CL. Short-term serial magnetoencephalography recordings of fetal auditory evoked responses. Neurosci Lett. 2002;331(2):128–32.

27. Eswaran H, Wilson JD, Preissl H, Robinson SE, Vrba J, Murphy D, Rose D, Lowery CL. Magnetoencephalographic recordings of visual evoked brain activity in the human fetus. Lancet. 2002;360(9335):779–80.

28. Lengle JM, Chen M, Wakai RT. Improved neuromagnetic detection of fetal and neonatal auditory evoked responses. Clin Neurophysiol. 2001;112(5):785–92.

29. Schneider U, Schleussner E, Haueisen J, Nowak H, Seewald HJ. Signal analysis of auditory evoked cortical fields in fetal magnetoencephalography. Brain Topogr. 2001;14(1):69–80.

30. Lowery CL, Eswaran H, Murphy P, Preissl H. Fetal magnetoencephalography. Semin Fetal Neonatal Med. 2006;11(6):430–6.

31. Preissl H, Lowery CL, Eswaran H. Fetal magnetoencephalography: viewing the developing brain in utero. Int Rev Neurobiol. 2005;68:1–23.

32. McCubbin J, Robinson SE, Cropp R, Moiseev A, Vrba J, Murphy P, Preissl H, Eswaran H. Optimal reduction of MCG in fetal MEG recordings. IEEE Trans Biomed Eng. 2006;53(8):1720–4.
33. Vrba J, Robinson SE, Mccubbin J, Lowery CL, Eswaran H, Wilson JD, Murphy P, Preissl H. Fetal MEG redistribution by projection operators. IEEE Trans Biomed Eng. 2004;51(7):1207–18.
34. Wilson JD, Govindan RB, Hatton JO, Lowery CL, Preissl H. Integrated approach for fetal QRS detection. IEEE Trans Biomed Eng. 2008;55(9):2190–7.
35. Brändle J, Preissl H, Draganova R, Ortiz E, Kagan KO, Abele H, Brucker SY, Kiefer-Schmidt I. Heart rate variability parameters and fetal movement complement fetal behavioral states detection via magnetography to monitor neurovegetative development. Front Hum Neurosci. 2015;9:147.
36. Stingl K, Paulsen H, Weiss M, Preissl H, Abele H, Goelz R, Wacker-Gussmann A. Development and application of an automated extraction algorithm for fetal magnetocardiography – normal data and arrhythmia detection. J Perinat Med. 2013;41(6):725–34.
37. Eswaran H, Govindan RB, Haddad NI, Siegel ER, Preissl HT, Murphy P, Lowery CL. Spectral power differences in the brain activity of growth-restricted and normal fetuses. Early Hum Dev. 2012;88(6):451–4.
38. Vairavan S, Govindan RB, Haddad N, Preissl H, Lowery CL, Siegel E, Eswaran H. Quantification of fetal magnetoencephalographic activity in low-risk fetuses using burst duration and interburst interval. Clin Neurophysiol. 2014;125(7):1353–9.
39. Holst M, Eswaran H, Lowery C, Murphy P, Norton J, Preissl H. Development of auditory evoked fields in human fetuses and newborns: a longitudinal MEG study. Clin Neurophysiol. 2005;116(8):1949–55.
40. Muenssinger J, Matuz T, Schleger F, Draganova R, Weiss M, Kiefer-Schmidt I, Wacker-Gussmann A, Govindan RB, Lowery CL, Eswaran H, Preissl H. Sensitivity to auditory spectral width in the fetus and infant – an fMEG study. Front Hum Neurosci. 2013;7:917.
41. Näätänen R. Mismatch negativity: clinical research and possible applications. Int J Psychophysiol. 2003;48(2): 179–88.
42. Huotilainen M, Kujala A, Hotakainen M, Parkkonen L, Taulu S, Simola J, Nenonen J, Karjalainen M, Näätänen R. Short-term memory functions of the human fetus recorded with magnetoencephalography. Neuroreport. 2005;16(1):81–4.
43. Draganova R, Eswaran H, Murphy P, Lowery C, Preissl H. Serial magnetoencephalographic study of fetal and newborn auditory discriminative evoked responses. Early Hum Dev. 2007;83(3):199–207. Epub 2006 Jul 24.
44. Schleger F, Landerl K, Muenssinger J, Draganova R, Reinl M, Kiefer-Schmidt I, Weiss M, Wacker-Gußmann A, Huotilainen M, Preissl H. Magnetoencephalographic signatures of numerosity discrimination in fetuses and neonates. Dev Neuropsychol. 2014;39(4):316–29.
45. Matuz T, Govindan RB, Preissl H, Siegel ER, Muenssinger J, Murphy P, Ware M, Lowery CL, Eswaran H. Habituation of visual evoked responses in neonates and fetuses: a MEG study. Dev Cogn Neurosci. 2012;2(3):303–16.
46. Muenssinger J, Matuz T, Schleger F, Kiefer-Schmidt I, Goelz R, Wacker-Gussmann A, Birbaumer N, Preissl H. Auditory habituation in the fetus and neonate: an fMEG study. Dev Sci. 2013;16(2):287–95.
47. Schleussner E, Schneider U. Developmental changes of auditory-evoked fields in fetuses. Exp Neurol. 2004; 190(Suppl 1):S59–64.
48. Kiefer I, Siegel E, Preissl H, Ware M, Schauf B, Lowery C, Eswaran H. Delayed maturation of auditory-evoked responses in growth-restricted fetuses revealed by magnetoencephalographic recordings. Am J Obstet Gynecol. 2008;199(5):503.e1–7.
49. Morin EC, Schleger F, Preissl H, Braendle J, Eswaran H, Abele H, Brucker S, Kiefer-Schmidt I. Functional brain development in growth-restricted and constitutionally small fetuses: a fetal magnetoencephalography case-control study. BJOG. 2015;122(9):1184–90.
50. Kleinwechter H, Schäfer-Graf U, Bührer C, Hoesli I, Kainer F, Kautzky-Willer A, Pawlowski B, Schunck K, Somville T, Sorger M. Gestational diabetes mellitus (GDM) diagnosis, therapy and follow-up care. Practice guideline of the German diabetes association (DDG) and the German Association for Gynaecology and Obstetrics (DGGG). Exp Clin Endocrinol Diabetes. 2014;122:395–405.
51. Stumvoll M, van Haeften T, Fritsche A, Gerich J. Oral glucose tolerance test indexes for insulin sensitivity and secretion based on various availabilities of sampling times. Diabetes Care. 2001;24:796–7.
52. Linder K, Schleger F, Ketterer C, Fritsche L, Kiefer-Schmidt I, Hennige A, Häring HU, Preissl H, Fritsche A. Maternal insulin sensitivity is associated with oral glucose-induced changes in fetal brain activity. Diabetologia. 2014;57(6):1192–8. doi:10.1007/s00125-014-3217-9. Epub 2014 Mar 28.
53. Linder K, Schleger F, Kiefer-Schmidt I, Fritsche L, Kümmel S, Heni M, Weiss M, Häring HU, Preissl H, Fritsche A. Gestational diabetes impairs human fetal postprandial brain activity. J Clin Endocrinol Metab. 2015;100(11):4029–36.
54. Pedersen J. The pregnant diabetic and her newborn: problems and management. In: Pathogenesis of the characteristic features of newborn infants of diabetic women. Baltimore: William & Wilkins; 1967. p. 128–37.
55. Tschritter O, Preissl H, Hennige AM, et al. The insulin effect on cerebrocortical theta activity is associated with serum concentrations of saturated nonesterified fatty acids. J Clin Endocrinol Metab. 2009;94:4600–7.

56. Szabo AJ, Szabo O. Placental free-fatty-acid transfer and fetal adipose-tissue development: an explantation of fetal adiposity in infants of diabetic mothers. Lancet. 1974;2(7879):498–9.

57. Scherer T, Buettner C. Yin and Yang of hypothalamic insulin and leptin signaling in regulating white adipose tissue metabolism. Rev Endocr Metab Disord. 2011;12(3):235–43.

58. Sartorius T, Heni M, Tschritter O, Preissl H, Hopp S, Fritsche A, Lievertz PS, Gertler A, Berthou F, Taouis M, Staiger H, Häring HU, Hennige AM. Leptin affects insulin action in astrocytes and impairs insulin-mediated physical activity. Cell Physiol Biochem. 2012;30(1):238–46.

59. Cetin I, Morpurgo PS, Radaelli T, Taricco E, Cortelazzi D, Bellotti M, Pardi G, Beck-Peccoz P. Fetal plasma leptin concentrations: relationship with different intrauterine growth patterns from 19 weeks to term. Pediatr Res. 2000;48(5):646–51.

Part II
Maternal Undernutrition and Protein Restriction: Effects on Fetus

Chapter 7
Dietary Restriction and the Endocrine Profiles in Offspring and Adults

Young Ju Kim

Key Points

- Undernutrition in utero and the nutritional status during postnatal life have irreversible health consequences in later life.
- Fetal growth depends on its transplacental supply of nutrient and oxygen and on its hormonal environments.
- Hormones act as maturational and nutritional signals in utero and control tissue accretion and differentiation under the environmental conditions in the fetus. Especially, glucocorticoids have a key role in intrauterine programming and induce permanent changes in system.
- Glucocorticoids can regulate intrauterine development through a wide range of different mechanism, and their actions may be mediated directly or indirectly via placental function or production of other hormones.
- During adverse conditions in pregnancy, the glucocorticoid-induced endocrine changes have immediate benefits to fetal survival by keeping pregnancy and modifying fetal growth.
- Glucocorticoids act as environmental signals that change the fetal epigenome and optimize the phenotype in utero. If the postnatal environment differs from those signals in utero, the glucocorticoid-induced changes in offspring may be maladaptive and lead to have cardiometabolic diseases and detrimental health in adults.
- Reduction in the availability of nutrients during fetal development programs, the endocrine pancreas and insulin-sensitive tissues and malnourished offsprings are born with a defect in their β-cell, and insulin-sensitive tissues will be definitely altered.

Keywords Undernutrition • Insulin • Insulin-like growth factors • Thyroid hormones • Leptin • Cortisol • Glucocorticoids • Intrauterine programming

Y.J. Kim, MD, PhD (✉)
Department of Obstetrics and Gynecology, College of Medicine, Ewha Womans University, Seoul, South Korea
e-mail: kkyj@ewha.ac.kr

© Springer International Publishing AG 2017
R. Rajendram et al. (eds.), *Diet, Nutrition, and Fetal Programming*,
Nutrition and Health, DOI 10.1007/978-3-319-60289-9_7

Abbreviations

11β-HSD 2	11β-hydroxysteroid dehydrogenase type 2
GR	Glucocorticoid receptor
HPA	Hypothalamic-pituitary-adrenal
IGFs	Insulin-like growth factors
IUGR	Intrauterine growth restriction
MR	Mineralocorticoid receptor
POMC	Proopiomelanocortin

Introduction

Recent studies have shown that in addition to genetic factors and environmental factors, undernutrition in utero and the nutritional status during postnatal life have irreversible health consequences in later life. It has been suggested that a stimulus during a critical period of development may have a permanent effect on body system, and these programmed effects may have an influence during fetal development and predispose to diseases including obesity, diabetes, metabolic syndrome, and cardiovascular disease in future life [1–3].

Because endocrine hormones including insulin, insulin-like growth factors (IGFs), thyroid hormones, leptin, cortisol, and glucocorticoid regulate fetal growth and development, they have an important role in intrauterine programming. Hormones act as maturational and nutritional signals in utero and control tissue accretion and differentiation under the environmental conditions in the fetus [4]. Especially, glucocorticoids have a key role in intrauterine programming and induce permanent changes in system. In the mechanism of action, glucocorticoids can regulate intrauterine development through a wide range of different mechanism, and their actions may be mediated directly or indirectly via placental function or production of other hormones [4].

It has been suggested that resetting of endocrine axes controlling growth and development would be one pathway for the developmental programming of later health [5]. The fetal hypothalamic-pituitary-adrenal (HPA) axis is vulnerable to changes in the intrauterine environment, and even subtle changes in the environment can disrupt the balance of fetal HPA development with glucocorticoid production, and finally alter long-term HPA activity and function [5].

In this chapter, we will review the mechanisms programming HPA axis function, hormonal profiles, endocrine pancreas, and how HPA axis and these hormones including glucocorticoids contribute to later diseases.

Premature Fetal HPA Axis Activation by Prenatal Undernutrition

HPA regulation can be programmed by undernutrition. According to Sebaai et al. (2004), rats exposed to prenatal nutrient restriction showed reduced body weight, increased hippocampal mineralocorticoid receptor (MR):glucocorticoid receptor (GR) mRNA ratio, increased proopiomelanocortin (POMC), GR mRNA in the pituitary, and an increase of corticosterone levels [6]. Maternal nutrient restriction in the sheep resulted in reductions in pituitary and adrenal responsiveness to stimulation and in significant alterations in fetal adrenal enzymes [7, 8].

In the guinea pig, after maternal nutrient restriction, maternal and fetal cortisol levels were significantly increased and also associated with elevated ACTH levels in maternal circulation [9]. This result means that nutrient restriction increased maternal HPA activity and resulted in an increase in placental transfer of maternal glucocorticoids to fetal circulation [9].

Although maternal glucocorticoid levels are much higher than fetal levels, the presence of the enzyme 11β-hydroxysteroid dehydrogenase type 2 (11β-HSD 2) in the placenta protects the fetus from maternal-derived glucocorticoids [10]. Maternal protein restriction in rats is associated with elevations of blood pressure in offspring and decreased placental 11 β-HSD 2 activity [11], and it is suggested that a deficiency in placental 11β-HSD 2 results an increased glucocorticoid levels in fetus and can program the HPA axis and postnatal endocrine dysfunction [5].

Elevated HPA axis activity in the fetus gives important implications for long-term endocrine regulation and also can be influential for preterm birth and parturition [12]. Bloomfield et al. (2003) demonstrated that periconceptional undernutrition in pregnant sheep showed high fetal cortisol levels and preterm birth [12]. These data suggested that the HPA axis programming may contribute to preterm birth and metabolic dysfunction in adulthood [5].

Endocrine Programming

Hormones have an important role in regulating normal growth and development in utero, and their concentrations and bioactivity can change in response to environmental factors including undernutrition known to cause intrauterine programming [4]. Undernutrition can alter both maternal and fetal concentrations of many hormones including insulin, IGFs, thyroid hormones, leptin, cortisol, and glucocorticoid. Because some hormones cross the placenta, the fetal endocrine response to undernutrition reflects the activity of both maternal and fetal endocrine glands [13].

The hormones present in the fetal circulation have four main sources including the fetal endocrine glands, uteroplacental tissues, transplacental diffusion from mother (steroids, thyroid hormones), and finally circulating precursor molecules by metabolism in the fetal or placental tissues [4]. In general, if fetal nutrient supply is increasing, anabolic hormones (e.g., insulin, IGF-1, thyroxine) would be increased and catabolic hormones (e.g., cortisol, catecholamines, growth hormones) would be decreased [4].

Insulin derived from the fetal pancreas is one of the anabolic hormones and increases the uptake of glucose and amino acid as well as the rates of glucose oxidation and protein synthesis by fetal tissues. Fetal insulin is positively related to the fetal glucose levels and body weight at birth [14], and its deficiency may induce a symmetrical type of intrauterine growth restriction (IUGR) [15]. In sheep, this increases the transplacental glucose concentration gradient and marterno-fetal glucose transfer without altering the transport of the placenta [16]. However, insulin stimulates placental uptake of glucose and amino acids [17]. Conversely, pancreatic agenesis and mutations in the insulin-promoting factor-1 gene in infants are associated with hypoinsulinemia and severe IUGR [18]. Fetal insulin is a growth-promoting hormone and acts as a signal of nutrient plenty [4].

IGFs including IGF-I and IGF-II are anabolic hormone of fetal growth and are derived from feto-placental tissues. These hormones are involved in the control of fetal growth. In mice, deletion of IGF gene reduces fetal growth whereas overexpression of IGF2 gene results in fetal overgrowth [19]. In human, birth weight and placental weight are positively correlated with cord blood IGF levels and related to variations in the methylation status of the IGF2-H19 gene locus [20]. The IGFs stimulate fetal growth by metabolic and non-metabolic mechanisms. They act as progression factors in cell cycle, prevent apoptosis, and increase DNA and protein synthesis in fetal tissues [21]. IGF-I has anabolic effects similar to insulin in utero and appears to be the signal of nutrient sufficiency, which regulates tissue accretion [4]. However, fetal IGF-II may provide a more general stimulus to cell growth and regulate tissue-specific changes in cell differentiation during gestation [4].

Thyroid hormones are important for the growth, metabolism, and differentiation of fetal tissues. Despite the placental transfer of maternal thyroid hormones, impaired function of the fetal thyroid gland is associated with severe IUGR, and the concentration of free thyroxine (T_4) in cord blood is related to birth weight [22]. Although short-term T_4 infusion does not alter the body weight of fetal sheep, it increases fetal oxygen consumption, glucose oxidation, bone growth, cardiomyocyte differentiation, and hepatic glycogen deposition [23]. Thyroid hormones control fetal adiposity by regulating leptin gene expression in fat [24]. It is required that thyroid hormones influence fetal growth indirectly via changes in IGFs and leptin bioavailability or by actions on placental nutrient transfer [23].

Leptin as a primary satiety factor is the obesity gene product, a 16-KDa protein synthesized by adipocytes, and this hormone suppresses food intake and increase energy expenditure [25]. In rat offspring from 50% food-restricted mother, Lee et al. (2013) found that the offsprings which showed rapid catch-up growth had significantly increased serum leptin levels and severe obesity at 6 months of age with gender differences [26] (Figs. 7.1 and 7.2). Although its role in intrauterine development

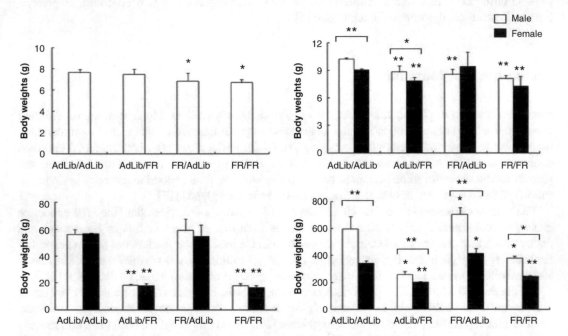

Fig. 7.1 Body weights of 1-day-old, 3-day-old, 3-week-old, 6-month-old offspring. **$p < 0.01$ versus control offspring. *$p < 0.05$ versus control offspring. (1) AdLib/AdLib, given normal diet during pregnancy, lactation, and adulthood; (2) AdLib/FR, given normal diet during pregnancy and 50% FR during lactation and adulthood; (3) FR/AdLib, given 50% FR during pregnancy and normal diet during lactation and adulthood; (4) FR/FR, given 50% FR during pregnancy and during lactation and adulthood

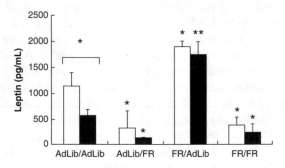

Fig. 7.2 Plasma leptin levels in the 6-month-old offspring. (1) AdLib/AdLib, given normal diet during pregnancy, lactation, and adulthood; (2) AdLib/FR, given normal diet during pregnancy and 50% FR during lactation and adulthood; (3) FR/AdLib, given 50% FR during pregnancy and normal diet during lactation and adulthood; (4) FR/FR, given 50% FR during pregnancy and during lactation and adulthood

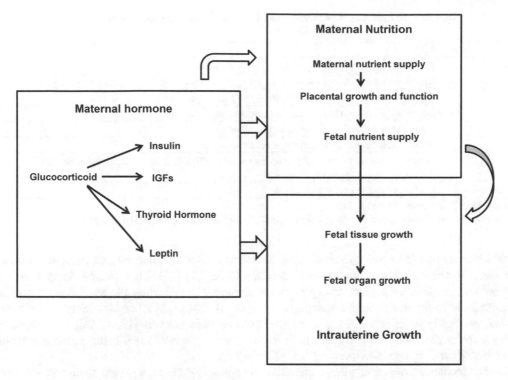

Fig. 7.3 A schematic diagram showing the interaction between maternal hormone and maternal nutrition in the control of intrauterine growth. *IGFs* Insulin-like growth factors

remains unclear, umbilical cord concentrations of leptin are correlated with placental weight and with the weight, length, and adiposity of human neonates [27]. Leptin also reduces hepatic glycogen stores and gluconeogenic enzyme activities and stimulates the growth, amino acid transport, and lipid metabolism of human trophoblast in vitro [27, 28].

Fetal growth depends on its transplacental supply of nutrient and oxygen and on its hormonal environments [23]. The nutrients provide the carbon and nitrogen required for tissue accretion, whereas the fetal hormones regulate their distribution between oxidative metabolism and mass accumulation. Fetal hormones can change the transplacental nutrient supply by modifying fetal metabolism and placental phenotype [23]. In signaling nutrient availability, fetal hormones act to optimize fetal growth (Fig. 7.3). However, disruption of normal balance between tissue accretion and differentiation in utero can lead to permanent changes in tissue structure and function with consequences for the later health of the infant and the adult [23].

Glucocorticoids as Regulatory Signals During Intrauterine Development

Glucocorticoids are important regulatory signals during intrauterine development, and they act as maturational, environmental, and programming signals that modify the developing phenotype to optimize offspring viability [29]. Changes in fetal growth in adverse environments are not due only to downregulation of growth stimulatory hormones, and fetal concentrations of growth inhibitory hormones (e.g., glucocorticoids) also increase in this environment [23]. Increasing cortisol levels switch fetal tissues from accretion to differentiation and slow fetal growth while maturing organ essential for neonatal survival (the lung, liver, gut, and kidneys) [30].

Table 7.1 Summary of the developmental effects of the glucocorticoid on visceral tissues
of fetal sheep during late gestation

Visceral tissue	Effects
Lung	Surfactant production, alveolar density, and wall thickness
	Elastin and collagen expression, β-adrenergic receptors, angiotensin-converting enzyme activity
Liver	Glycogen and gluconeogenic enzymes, *IgF* gene expression,
	β-adrenergic, growth hormones, and angiotensin II receptors
	Corticosteroid-binding globulin, angiotensinogen
Gut	Acid secretion, digestive enzyme, mucosal turnover
Kidney	Glomerular filtration rate, tubular sodium reabsorption, deiodinase activity, GR and MR receptors, renin-angiotensin II system
Adipose tissue	Leptin production, UCP expression

Data are from Fowden and Forhead [29]
Abbreviations: *GR* glucocorticoid receptor, *MR* mineralocorticoid receptor, *UCP* uncoupling protein

Glucocorticoids have a wide range of developmental effects in normal and adverse conditions, especially in tissues essential for survival at birth (Table 7.1) [29]. They induce changes in tissue expression of proteins, receptors, transporters, ion channels, and enzymes [4], and these changes lead to alterations in the morphology, metabolism, hormonal change, biochemical composition in fetal tissues, and lastly functional consequences in organ and system levels [13, 31, 32]. Therefore, they activate many physiological processes such as pulmonary gas exchange, hepatic gluconeogenesis, gastrointestinal digestion, and thermogenesis (Table 7.1).

In the mechanism of action, glucocorticoids can regulate intrauterine development through a wide range of different mechanism, and their actions may be mediated directly or indirectly via placental function or production of other hormones [4]. In placental effects, glucocorticoids can induce alterations in placental morphology, transport, and metabolism that contribute to fetal growth [29]. In effects on other endocrine systems, they affect production of sex steroids, eicosanoids, adipokines, HPA axis, renin-angiotensin system, catecholamines, somatotrophic axis, and thyroid hormone axis [29]. The glucocorticoid-induced changes in fetal endocrine function lead to prepartum increases in the fetal concentrations of other hormones including triiodothyronine, IGF-I, leptin, and adrenaline, which have independent effects on fetal tissue growth and function [27].

During adverse conditions in pregnancy, the glucocorticoid-induced endocrine changes have immediate benefits to fetal survival by keeping pregnancy and modifying fetal growth. If the endocrine changes continue after recovery of normal conditions, they may become more detrimental to intrauterine development and compromise the ability of the fetus to respond to subsequent environmental challenges [29]. Changes in endocrine function induced by early glucocorticoid exposure in utero are known to persist after birth to alter the adult endocrine environment [32]. For example, prenatal glucocorticoid exposure alters adult HPA function at every level of the axis from the brain to tissue glucocorticoid bioavailability [33]. These programmed changes in HPA function may contribute to metabolic disorders in adults. Therefore, the regulatory effects of glucocorticoids on intrauterine development involve multiple interactions between other endocrine systems, when glucocorticoids are acting as both maturational and environmental signals [29].

In epigenetic effects, glucocorticoids act via several different mechanisms to alter gene expression. They are known to alter gene expression more indirectly via epigenetic modifications of the genome and chromatin structure postnatally [34]. These include DNA methylation, histone modifications, and changes in noncoding long and microRNA [34]. However, little is known about the epigenetic effects of glucocorticoids in utero. Glucocorticoids may act by changing the imprint status of growth-regulatory imprinted genes, such as IGF2, which are expressed from only one allele in a parent-of-origin manner [29]. Whether these changes in IGF2 expression are due to altered expression of the H19-derived noncoding RNA or to changes in methylation at the differentially methylated region and imprinted control region of the IGF2-H19 locus remains unknown [29]. Glucocorticoid exposure in early life, therefore, affects the developing epigenome through many different ways, with dynamic results for epigenetic marks through the life of the offspring.

Programming of the Endocrine Pancreas

Animal models have demonstrated that reduction in availability of nutrients during fetal development programs the endocrine pancreas and insulin-sensitive tissues [35]. Whatever the type of fetal malnutrition, malnourished offsprings are born with a defect in their β-cell, and insulin-sensitive tissues will be definitely altered [35]. Hormones during fetal life like insulin, IGFs and glucocorticoids were implicated as possible factors amplifying the defect. The poor development of the endocrine pancreas after early malnutrition gives the offspring with deficient functional unit of pancreas [35]. Normal glucose tolerance with low insulin secretion has been explained by an adaptation of the peripheral tissue through an increased number of insulin receptors in the liver, adipose tissue, and muscle [36–38]. These adaptations declined with age, and insulin resistance appeared in the adult low-protein offspring [35].

During pregnancy, the endocrine pancreas of the mother has to adapt in response to the higher demand of insulin required for fetal growth. Whenever the pregnant mother was the offspring of a protein or calorie-restricted dam, it became glucose intolerant and hyperglycemic [39, 40]. In consequence, the pups whose grandmothers were protein or calorie restricted during pregnancy showed lower plasma insulin levels and pancreatic insulin content, as a consequence of their reduced β-cell mass development [41].

Conclusion

Undernutrition in utero and the nutritional status during postnatal life have irreversible health consequences in later life. Resetting of endocrine axes controlling growth and development would be one pathway for the developmental programming of later health. The fetal HPA axis is vulnerable to changes in the intrauterine environment, and even subtle changes in the environment can disrupt the balance of fetal HPA development with glucocorticoid production, and finally alter long-term HPA activity and function. Elevated HPA axis activity in the fetus gives important implications for long-term endocrine regulation and also can be influential for preterm birth and parturition. Therefore, the HPA axis programming may contribute to preterm birth and metabolic dysfunction in adulthood.

Reduction in the availability of nutrients during fetal development programs, the endocrine pancreas and insulin-sensitive tissues and malnourished offsprings are born with a defect in their β-cell, and insulin-sensitive tissues will be definitely altered. Hormones during fetal life like insulin, IGFs, and glucocorticoids were implicated as possible factors amplifying the defect. The poor development of the endocrine pancreas after early malnutrition gives the offspring with deficient functional unit of pancreas.

Because endocrine hormones including insulin, IGFs, thyroid hormones, leptin, cortisol, and glucocorticoid regulate fetal growth and development, these hormones have an important role in intrauterine programming. Hormones act as maturational and nutritional signals in utero and control tissue accretion and differentiation under the environmental conditions in the fetus. Glucocorticoids are important regulatory signals during intrauterine development, and they act as maturational, environmental, and programming signals that modify the developing phenotype to optimize offspring viability. Earlier in gestation, glucocorticoids act as environmental signals that change the fetal epigenome and optimize the phenotype in utero. If the postnatal environment differs from those signals in utero, the glucocorticoid-induced changes in offspring may be maladaptive and lead to have cardiometabolic diseases and detrimental health in adults.

References

1. Barker DJ, Osmond C, Simmonds SJ, Wield GA. The relation of small head circumference and thinness at birth to death from cardiovascular disease in adult life. BMJ. 1993;306:422–6.
2. Huxley RR, Shiell AW, Law CM. The role of size at birth and postnatal catch-up growth in determining systolic blood pressure: a systemic review of literature. J Hypertens. 2000;18:815–31.
3. Newsome CA, Shiell AW, Fall CH, Phillips DI, Shier R, Law CM. Is birth weight related to later glucose and insulin metabolism? A systemic review. Diabet Med. 2003;20:339–48.
4. Fowden AL, Forhead AJ. Endocrine mechanisms of intrauterine programming. Reproduction. 2004;127:515–26.
5. Sloboda DM, Newnham JP, Moss TJ, Challis JR. The fetal hypothalamic-pituitary-adrenal axis: relevance to developmental origins of health and disease. In: Gluckman P, Hanson M, editors. Developmental origins of health and disease. 1st ed. New York: Cambridge University Press; 2006. p. 191–205.
6. Sebaai N, Lesage J, Breton C, Vieau D, Deloof S. Perinatal food deprivation induces marked alterations of the hypothalamic-pituitary-adrenal axis in 8-month-old male rats both under basal conditions and after a dehydration period. Neuroendocrinology. 2004;79:163–73.
7. Hawkins P, Steyn C, McGarridge HH, Saito T, Ozaki T, Stratford LL, et al. Effect of maternal nutrient restriction in early gestation on development of the hypothalamic pituitary adrenal axis in fetal sheep at 0.8–0.9 of gestation. J Endocrinol. 1999;163:553–61.
8. Fraser M, Oliver MH, Harding JE, Gluckman PD, Challis JRG. Alterations in ovine fetal adrenal corticotropin receptor and steroidogenic enzyme mRNA expression following maternal undernutrition in late pregnancy. J Soc Gynecol Investig. 2001;6:116A.
9. Lingas R, Dean F, Matthews SG. Maternal nutrient restriction (48h) modifies brain corticosteroid receptor expression and endocrine function in the fetal guinea pig. Brain Res. 1999;846:236–42.
10. Edwards CRW, Benediktsson R, Lindsay RS, Seckl JR. Dysfunction of placental glucocorticoids barrier: link between fetal environment and adult hypertension? Lancet. 1993;341:355–7.
11. Langley-Evans SC, Phillips GJ, Benediktsson R, Gardner DS, Edwards CR, Jackson AA, et al. Protein intake in pregnancy, placental glucocorticoid metabolism and the programming of hypertension in the rat. Placenta. 1996;17:169–72.
12. Bloomfield FH, Oliver MH, Hawkins P, et al. A periconceptional nutritional origin for noninfectious preterm birth. Science. 2003;300:606.
13. Fowden AL, Giussani DA, Forhead AJ. Intrauterine programming of physiological systems: causes and consequences. Physiology. 2006;21:29–37.
14. Fowden AL. Endocrine regulation of fetal growth. Reprod Fertil Dev. 1995;7:351–63.
15. Fowden AL, Hill DJ. Intrauterine programming of the endocrine pancreas. Br Med Bull. 2001;60:123–42.
16. Fowden AL, Forhead AJ. Insulin deficiency alters the metabolic and endocrine responses to undernutrition in fetal sheep near term. Endocrinology. 2012;153:4008–18.
17. Jones HN, Powell TL, Jasson T. Regulation of placental nutrient transport – a review. Placenta. 2007;28:763–74.
18. Thomas IH, Saini NK, Adhikari A, Lee JM, Kasa-Vubu JZ, Vazquez DM, et al. Neonatal diabetes mellitus with pancreatic agenesis in an infant with homozygous IPF-1 Pro63fsX60 mutation. Pediatr Diabetes. 2009;10:492–6.
19. Efstratiadis A. Genetics of mouse growth. Int J Dev Biol. 1998;42:955–76.
20. Fowden AL, Coan PM, Angiolini E, et al. Imprinted genes and the epigenetic regulation of placental phenotype. Prog Biophys Mol Biol. 2010;106:281–8.
21. Hill DJ, Petrik J, Arany E. Growth factors and the regulation of fetal growth. Diabetes Care. 1998;21(Suppl 2): B60–9.
22. Shields BM, Knight BA, Hill A, Hattersley AT, Vaidya B. Fetal thyroid hormones level at birth is associated with fetal growth. J Clin Endocrinol Metab. 2012;96:E934–8.
23. Sferruzzi-Perri AN, Vaughan OR, Forhead AJ, Fowden AL. Hormonal and nutritional drivers of intrauterine growth. Curr Opin Clin Nutr Metab Care. 2013;16:298–309.
24. O'Connor DM, Blache D, Hoggard N, Brookes E, Wooding FB, Fowden AL, et al. Developmental control of plasma leptin and adipose leptin messenger ribonucleic acid in the ovine fetus during late gestation: role of glucocorticoids and thyroid hormones. Endocrinology. 2007;148:3750–7.
25. Yuen BS, McMilen IC, Symonds ME, Owens PC. Abundance of leptin mRNA in fetal adipose tissue is related to fetal body weight. J Endocrinol. 1999;163:R11–4.
26. Lee S, Lee KA, Choi GY, Desai M, Lee SH, Pang MG, et al. Feed restriction during pregnancy/lactation induces programmed changes in lipid, adiponectin and leptin levels with gender differences in rat offspring. J Matern Fetal Neonatal Med. 2013;26(9):908–14.
27. Forhead AJ, Fowden AL. The hungry fetus? Role of leptin as a nutritional signal before birth. J Physiol. 2009;587:1145–52.

28. White V, Gonzalez E, Capobianco E, Pustovrh C, Martinez N, Higa R, et al. Leptin modulates nitric oxide production and lipid metabolism in human placenta. Reprod Fertil Dev. 2006;18:425–32.
29. Fowden AL, Forhead AJ. Glucocorticoids as regulatory signals during intrauterine development. Exp Physiol. 2015;100(12):1477–87.
30. Vaughan OR, Forhead AJ, Fowden AL. Glucocorticoids and placental programming. In: Burton GJ, DJP B, Moffett A, editors. The placenta and human developmental programming. Cambridge: Cambridge University Press; 2011. p. 175–87.
31. Harris A, Seckl J. Glucocorticoids, prenatal stress and the programming of disease. Horm Behav. 2011;59:279–89.
32. Moisiadis VG, Matthews SG. Glucorcorticoids and fetal programming part 1: outcomes. Nat Rev Endocrinol. 2014;10:391–402.
33. Jellyman JK, Valenzuela OA, Fowden AL. Glucocorticoid programming of the hypothalamic-pituitary-adrenal axis and metabolic function: animal studies from mouse to horse. J Anim Sci. n.d. doi: 10.2527/jas2014-6812.
34. Weaver IC. Epigenetic effects of glucocorticoids. Semin Fetal Neonatal Med. 2009;14:143–50.
35. Remacle C, Dumortier O, Bol V, Goosse K, Romanus P, Theys N, et al. Intrauterine programming of the endocrine pancreas. Diabetes Obes Metab. 2007;9(Suppl 2):196–209.
36. Holness MJ, Fryer LG, Sugden MG. Protein restriction during early development enhances insulin responsiveness but selectively impairs sensitivity to insulin at low concentrations in white adipose tissue during a later pregnancy. Br J Nutr. 1999;81:481–9.
37. Ozanne SE, Nave BT, Wang CL, Shepherd PR, Prins J, Smith GD, et al. Poor fetal nutrition causes long- term changes in expression of insulin signaling components in adipocytes. Am J Phys. 1997;273(Pt 1):E46–51.
38. Shepherd PR, Nave BT, Rincon J, Nolte LA, Bevan AP, Siddle K, et al. Differential regulation of phosphoinositide 3-kinase adapter subunit variants by insulin in human skeletal muscle. J Biol Chem. 1997;272:19000–7.
39. Mericq V, Ong KK, Bazaes R, Pena V, Avila A, Salazar T, et al. Longitudinal changes in insulin sensitivity and secretion from birth to age three years in small-and appropriate-for-gestational-age children. Diabetologia. 2005;48:2609–14.
40. Blondeau B, Garofano A, Czernichow P, Breant B. Age-dependent inability of the endocrine pancreas to adapt to pregnancy: a long-term consequence of perinatal malnutrition in the rat. Endocrinology. 1999;140:4208–13.
41. Boloker J, Gertz SJ, Simmons RA. Gestational diabetes leads to the development of the diabetes in adulthood in the rat. Diabetes. 2002;51:1499–506.

Chapter 8
Maternal Undernutrition and Visceral Adiposity

Prabhat Khanal and Mette Olaf Nielsen

Key Points

- Increased prevalence of visceral obesity and associated metabolic disorders appear to be associated not only with intake of an unhealthy postnatal diet and lack of physical activity but also with prenatal malnutrition exposures during critical periods of foetal development.
- Maternal undernutrition during pregnancy leads to an increased prevalence of central obesity in offspring, both in childhood and in adult life.
- Prenatal undernutrition, particularly during the later stages of gestation, interferes in a differential manner with adipose tissues to expand by hyperplasia as compared to hypertrophy, resulting in reduced expandability of subcutaneous adipose tissue, which in a sheep model led to extreme hypertrophic expansion of visceral adipose tissues.
- Prenatally induced changes in intrinsic and obesity induced cellularity of adipose tissues can then lead to adipose tissue-derived elevated pro-inflammatory response and associated systematic metabolic dysregulation.
- It is not clear how maternal nutritional status during pregnancy affects recruitment of mesenchymal stem cells into adipose lineages, differentiation of preadipocytes into mature adipocytes or extracellular matrix remodelling.

Keywords Adipocyte development • Fat distribution • Maternal undernutrition • Subcutaneous expandability • Visceral adiposity

P. Khanal, PhD
Department of Veterinary and Animal Sciences, Faculty of Health and Medical Sciences,
University of Copenhagen, Frederiksberg, Denmark

Institute of Basic Medical Sciences, Department of Nutrition, Faculty of Medicine,
Norwegian Transgenic Centre, University of Oslo, Oslo, Norway
e-mail: pbt@sund.ku.dk

M.O. Nielsen, PhD (✉)
Department of Veterinary and Animal Sciences, Faculty of Health and Medical Sciences,
University of Copenhagen, Frederiksberg, Denmark
e-mail: mette.olaf.nielsen@sund.ku.dk

© Springer International Publishing AG 2017
R. Rajendram et al. (eds.), *Diet, Nutrition, and Fetal Programming*,
Nutrition and Health, DOI 10.1007/978-3-319-60289-9_8

- Maternal undernutrition is associated with permanent epigenetic regulation of key genes which are potentially involved in development of visceral obesity later in life, but detailed mechanisms as well as identification of early (epigenetic) markers to identify susceptible individuals remain a key challenge.
- Proper maternal nutrition during critical periods of foetal development is an important issue to counteract the increasing trend of visceral obesity and associated metabolic disorders in humans.

Abbreviations

ATM   Adipose tissue macrophages
BMI   Body mass index
CD-68   Cluster of differentiation-68
HIF   Hypoxia inducible factor
IL-6   Interleukin-6
PPARγ   Peroxisome proliferator-activated receptor γ
SGA   Small for gestational age
SREBP-1   Sterol regulatory binding protein-1
TLR-4   Toll-like receptor-4
TNF-α   Tumour necrosis factor-α
VEGF   Vascular endothelial growth factor

Introduction

The global epidemic of obesity and associated disorders in on the increase in the world today seriously affecting the quality of human life [1]. In 2005, 33% of the world's adult population were reported to be overweight or obese, and it is predicted that if the recent trend continues, 57.8% of the total world's population (3.3 billion people) could be either overweight or obese by 2030 [2]. Thus, presently obesity is considered a serious public health issue worldwide affecting people of all ages, gender, ethnicities and nationalities [3].

Obesity is defined as 'a condition of abnormal or excessive fat accumulation in adipose tissue, to the extent that health may be impaired' [4], and it is well known that development of obesity and metabolic disorders generally is associated with high intakes of energy-rich foods [5] or sedentary lifestyles [6]. However, it is still not very clear why some individuals appear to be more vulnerable to development of obesity-associated metabolic disorders such as diabetes and cardiovascular diseases than others. It appears that the site of excessive fat deposition in the body rather than absolute fat deposition per se is a key factor for the development of obesity-induced alterations in metabolic traits [7]. Visceral obesity is considered to be a particular risk factor and a marker of 'dysfunctional adipose tissue' and associated with other disorders such as the metabolic syndrome, cardiovascular diseases and some types of cancers [8, 9]. Thus, it is crucial to understand underlying mechanisms behind the development of central or visceral obesity and associated disorders to limit or even inhibit a further escalation of the obesity epidemic.

Previous epidemiological and animal studies have convincingly demonstrated that obesity and associated metabolic disorders are not only related to genotype and/or postnatal environmental factors such as an unhealthy diet or lack of adequate physical activity, but it is also influenced by circumstances taking place during foetal life [10, 11] due to a phenomenon termed 'foetal metabolic programming' [12, 13]. The foetal nutritional history appears to have a much greater role in the current epidemic of obesity and associated diseases than hitherto anticipated [14]. Thus, a better understanding of how the early life nutrition can programme for adiposity and health outcomes later in life is essential to be able to design proper nutritional or other interventions to contribute to reverse the obesity epidemic [15]. This review aims to evaluate the impacts of intrauterine growth restriction

(IUGR) caused by prenatal undernutrition on the development of visceral obesity after birth (*Part I*) and to discuss the potential mechanisms underlying a foetal predisposition for visceral adiposity (*Part II*). In the first part, impact of prenatal undernutrition on the manifestation of visceral obesity in young and adult offspring and its association with an early postnatal obesogenic diet will be discussed. Secondly, mechanistic insights will be provided into the relationship between foetal undernutrition and later visceral obesity and programming impacts based on timing of undernutrition exposure in utero, adipose tissue development and distribution, changes in inflammatory responses, etc.

Part I: Association Between Prenatal Undernutrition and Later Fat Deposition and Distribution

Prenatal Undernutrition and Fat Deposition Patterns in Young Offspring

Previous human epidemiological studies provided evidence that deposition of visceral fat is affected by foetal nutrition and consequently foetal growth. It was shown that individuals born small for gestational age (SGA) have a higher percentage of body fat in infancy and childhood [16]. Furthermore, adolescent girls with smaller birth weight tended to store their fat in the trunk rather than limbs [17]. Moreover central fat deposition was found to be higher in children, who were stunted in early childhood and born small for gestational age [18]. We have shown that undernutrition (50% of daily energy and protein requirements) of twin pregnant ewes during the last trimester (last 6 weeks of gestation) predisposed for visceral obesity in the offspring by altering fat distribution patterns related to a reduced propensity for subcutaneous fat deposition [19, 20]. Early-to mid-gestation nutrient restriction in sheep has also been shown to increase fat deposition in adolescent male offspring along with poor glucose uptake [21]. Similar findings were also revealed in a swine model, where offspring underfed in utero increased visceral fatness from early postnatal stages [22]. Thus, these studies clearly indicate across many animal models that it is possible to observe early signs of upregulated visceral obesity in fetally nutritionally programmed individuals.

Prenatal Undernutrition and Fat Distribution Patterns in Adult Offspring

Several human epidemiological and experimental animal studies have demonstrated an inverse relationship between birth weight and central obesity persisting into adulthood. Interestingly this appears to be specifically related to abdominal visceral fat deposition but not with subcutaneous abdominal fat in adulthood [23]. Reduced growth during foetal life and infancy and associated increased abdominal obesity in adult men is evidenced by a higher waist to hip ratio [24]. During the Second World War in the Western Netherlands, these populations were exposed to a limited and well-defined period of extreme nutritional scarcity, and women who were pregnant during that time and their offspring have given rise to a Dutch birth cohort, in which the association between foetal nutrition and subsequent health outcomes later in life has been examined [25]. Women, who were exposed to famine during early gestation, were shown to have higher incidence of abdominal obesity at the age of 50 with higher body mass index (BMI) and waist circumference [26]. On the other hand, prenatal exposure to famine during late gestation was associated with decreased glucose tolerance and increased plasma insulin levels, thus influencing the glucose-insulin homeostasis and increasing type 2 diabetes risk [27]. Impacts of timing of prenatal nutrition exposure on later development of visceral adiposity will be discussed in a separate section below. In a study involving a Chinese adult population, it was demonstrated that birth weight had a U-shaped association with waist circumference and systolic blood pressure, but individuals with the lowest birth weight had higher fasting glucose levels and those having a combination of lowest birth weight and higher abdominal obesity had highest prevalence of type 2 diabetes [28].

These epidemiological studies suggest that sub optimal nutrition during pregnancy favours more fat deposition in visceral regions, potentially contributing to several obesity-induced metabolic disorders. Such associations of poor nutrition level during pregnancy and later development of visceral obesity have been confirmed in several animal models. Maternal low-protein diet during the last third of pregnancy resulted in increased visceral fat deposition along with higher low-density lipoprotein cholesterol, glucose, insulin and leptin levels in adult male rat offspring [29]. A low-protein diet during pregnancy, particularly during late or throughout pregnancy, increased more visceral and reduced subcutaneous fat deposition in adult male rat offspring [30]. Moreover, rat offspring exposed to a low-protein diet throughout pregnancy and lactation developed visceral adiposity in young adulthood along with upregulation of adipocyte differentiation, angiogenesis and extracellular matrix remodelling [31]. Thus, epidemiological evidences in humans as well as studies in different animal species have shown a clear association between poor maternal nutrition during pregnancy and increased visceral adiposity in offspring in adulthood.

Interactive Impacts of Prenatal Undernutrition with Postnatal Diet on Visceral Adiposity

Obesity, especially central obesity, is associated with development of a range of metabolic disorders [8, 32]. Human as well as animal studies have shown that foetal undernutrition will not only predispose for permanent and irreversible changes in body composition, metabolism and endocrine function in itself but also provide an additional risk of development of metabolic disorders upon exposure to an obesogenic diet postnatally [13, 26, 33]. Several studies in both humans and experimental animal models have confirmed such an unfortunate additive or even synergistic impact of mismatching pre- and postnatal nutrition exposures.

Young adult Ethiopians who migrated in Israel for up to 4 years had increased prevalence of diabetes associated with increased intake of refined carbohydrates as compared to the Ethiopian diet [34]. In rats, deposition of epididymal white adipose tissue was increased in high-fat fed offspring born to dams that were protein restricted during pregnancy and lactation [35] and undernutrition in the third trimester of gestation in sheep increased preference for visceral rather than subcutaneous fat deposition, when they were exposed to an obesogenic diet in early postnatal life [19, 20]. Even chickens have been found to have higher abdominal fat deposition when ad libitum fed if their mothers had been feed restricted compared to offspring from normally fed hens [36]. Reduced subcutaneous adipose expandability in prenatally undernourished sheep has in our Copenhagen sheep model been shown to be associated with occurrence of a special subpopulation of very small adipocytes (<40 μm in diameter) and increased collagen infiltration in subcutaneous adipose tissue (Fig. 8.1) [37]. We have furthermore observed that prenatal undernutrition reduces intrinsic and obesity-induced hyperplasia in subcutaneous and perirenal fat depots, thus predisposing for visceral obesity and massive perirenal adipocyte hypertrophy during obesity development (Khanal et al. Unpublished results; Fig. 8.2).

Increased abdominal fat accumulation has been proposed as an important risk factor for various renal disorders as well as cardiovascular and metabolic diseases associated with obesity-induced metabolic syndrome [38, 39]. Thus, implications of a mismatching pre- and postnatal nutrition exposure for fat deposition patterns have been suggested to explain why incidence of, e.g. cardiovascular diseases, is increasing more in developing than in developed countries considering that a significant proportion of overweight people in the developed world are capable of maintaining an apparently healthy metabolic phenotype [40]. So although adaptive responses induced by undernutrition in utero may be important for short-term survival, this can lead to increased risk of obesity and associated disorders in offspring later in life if the predicted postnatal environment is not matched [41]. Therefore, obesity development is of particular concern in prenatally undernourished individuals, where postnatal dietary interventions are less likely to be effective in reversing associated adverse outcomes [42].

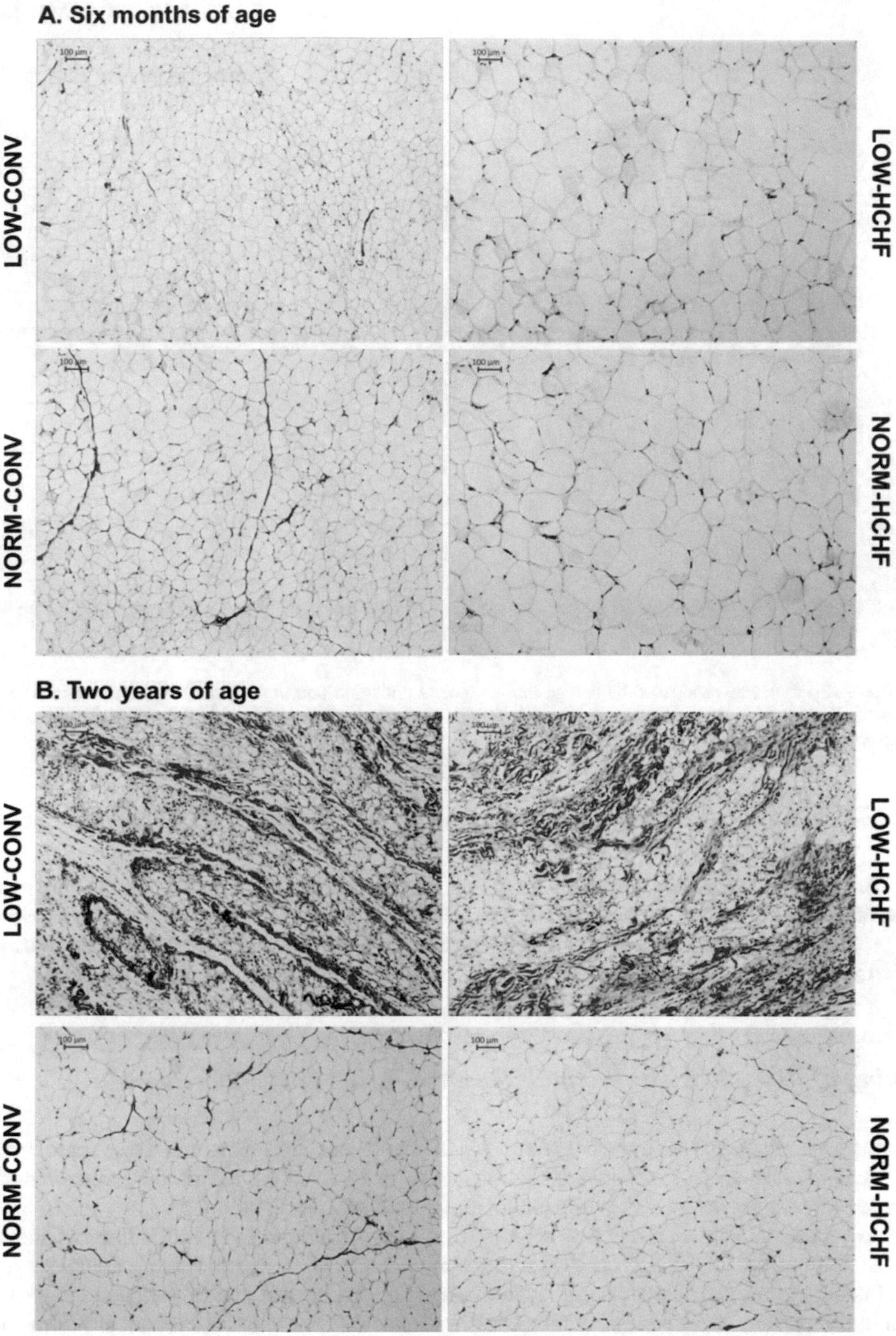

Fig. 8.1 Morphology of Van Gieson stained subcutaneous adipose tissue from 6-month-old adolescent lambs and 2-year-old adult sheep. Panel (**a**): larger population of very small cells in the individuals exposed to prenatal undernutrition during late gestation followed by normal nutrition during postnatal life (LOW-CONV) and extensive hypertrophy in adipocytes from lambs fed HCHF diet postnatally. Panel (**b**): extensive collagen infiltration in animals exposed to prenatal undernutrition during late gestation (LOW). NORM, 100% of daily energy and protein requirements during the last 6 weeks of gestation; LOW 50% of NORM; CONV, moderate postnatal diet, HCHF postnatal obesogenic, high-carbohydrate-high-fat diets (until 6 months after birth) (Adapted from Nielsen et al. [37])

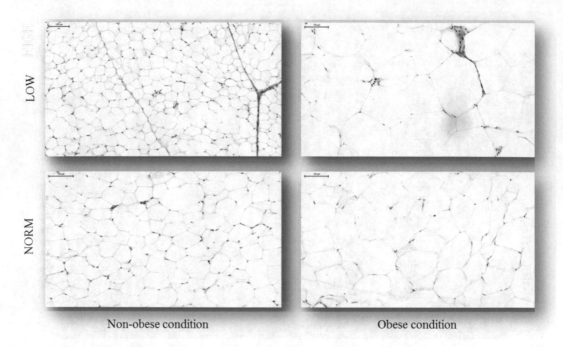

Fig. 8.2 Adipocyte size as affected by late gestation prenatal undernutrition in perirenal adipose tissue in adolescent lambs. NORM, provided normal energy and protein requirements during late gestation; LOW, provided 50% of NORM (Adapted from Khanal et al. Unpublished data)

Part II: Mechanisms Underlying Foetal Predisposition for Visceral Adiposity

The mechanisms underlying foetal programming are still incompletely understood. In this section, some of the important mechanisms known or suggested to be implicated in foetal programming leading to a predisposition for visceral obesity will be discussed with the main focus on timing of undernutrition exposure in utero and subsequent adipose tissue development, distribution and function.

Timing of Abnormal Nutritional Exposure During Foetal Development

The maternal nutritional environment affects foetal growth and development in a distinct manner, as brain and cardiovascular function are most sensitive to malnutrition during the embryonic stage, whereas adipose tissues are more susceptible during the foetal phase [43], where they are formed. In humans, the foetal adipose tissue first appears from second trimester [44], and in humans and other animals born precocial (such as sheep with a gestation length of around 145 days), the major part of foetal adipogenesis and adipose differentiation occurs during the last part of gestation [45, 46]. The quantitative growth of perirenal-abdominal adipose tissue thus commences at about day 70 of gestation in sheep, and fat mass increases rapidly along with a parallel increase in lipid content until 110–120 days of gestation [47], and a marked increase in proliferation of mitochondria and development of nerves become visible in the perirenal fat depot during late gestation [48]. In humans, perirenal fat develops at the beginning of the second trimester, and complete differentiation of perirenal fat has been observed after 21st week of pregnancy [44]. In sheep, the growth of subcutaneous fat commences 2–3 weeks later than perirenal-abdominal fat depots, but a significant regression of subcutaneous fat occurs about day 115, resulting in a virtual disappearance by term [47]. Also in humans, the

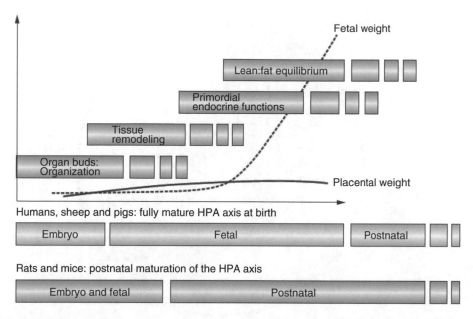

Fig. 8.3 Critical windows for foetal organogenesis and changes in placental and body weight between conception and early postnatal life, in a range of species; *HPA axis* hypothalamic–pituitary–adrenal axis (Adapted from Symonds et al. [14])

subcutaneous fat is visually absent during the first and second trimesters [49]. Thus nutritional insults during pregnancy may potentially have differential impacts on development of adipose tissues and fat deposition patterns depending upon the timing of nutritional exposure in utero, since different organs have their distinct pattern of organogenesis and maturation and hence developmental stages during foetal life, as shown in Fig. 8.3 [14]. In precocial species, foetal development of abdominal and peri-renal adipose tissues may be most sensitive to foetal malnutrition during mid- to late gestation and subcutaneous adipose tissue in late gestation, since the major growth and development of these respective tissues occur during those periods.

In rodents, it is not possible to detect white adipose tissue macroscopically during the embryonic stage or at birth [50]. Timing of adipose development relative to birth and implications of foetal nutrition insults may thus be widely different from those of humans and other precocial species.

Changes in Adipocyte Development and Growth

It is known that maternal malnutrition in utero can programme the growth and development of adipocytes and hence predisposition for later obesity development [51]. However, the detailed mechanisms whereby adipocyte structure and function are programmed and have implications for visceral obesity development are still subjects of investigation. As described earlier, white adipose tissue cannot be detected in any substantial amounts prior to birth in rodents, in humans and in other higher mammals; differentiation of mesenchymal cells, adjacent formation of blood vessels and subsequent adipogenesis appear to initiate during the second trimester of gestation [44, 52]. During late gestation, maturation of already existing adipocytes occurs, and the gradual increment in body fat after birth is mainly due to increased adipocyte size [52]. How maternal undernutrition regulates the commitment of mesenchymal stem cells to develop into different lineages, myocytes or fibrocytes, and hence subsequent foetal adipose and other tissues development is not yet known. Involvement of microRNA and epigenetic changes has been proposed as a possible mechanism [53].

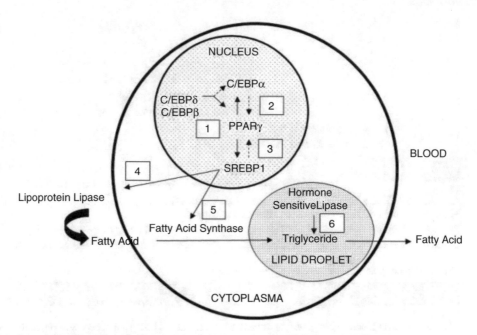

Fig. 8.4 Sequential regulation of adipogenesis and lipogenesis (*1*) C/EBPδ and C/EBPβ upregulate PPARγ and C/EBPα; (*2*) PPARγ₂ upregulates C/EBPα and vice versa, resulting in adipocyte differentiation; (*3*) PPARγ₂ upregulates lipogenic transcription factor, SREBP1c; (*4*) SREBP1c upregulates extracellular lipolytic enzyme, lipoprotein lipase facilitating fatty acid uptake by adipocytes; (*5*) SREBP1c upregulates lipogenic enzyme, fatty acid synthase facilitating lipogenesis within adipocytes; (*6*) intracellular lipolytic enzyme, hormone sensitive lipase acts on triglyceride to release fatty acid from adipocyte (Adapted from Desai and Ross [51])

Adipose tissue development involves the two processes: adipogenesis and lipogenesis (Fig. 8.4). Adipogenesis involves recruitment and proliferation of preadipocytes or adipocyte precursor cells and their subsequent differentiation into lipid filled mature fat cells [54]. Adipogenic transcription factors mainly peroxisome proliferator-activated receptor-γ (PPAR-γ) and CCAAT/enhancer binding protein-α (C/EBP-α) regulate the expression of genes necessary for the development of mature adipocytes [55]. Adipose tissue adipogenesis is also coupled to angiogenesis, and regulatory factors involved in angiogenesis can therefore potentially affect adipose development. Vascular endothelial growth factor (VEGF) is one of the most critical angiogenic factors initiating the formation of immature blood vessels [56]. The growth and expansion of adipose tissue, e.g. during obesity development, are governed by hyperplasia (increase in cell number) and hypertrophy (increase in cell size) [57]. In the obese situation, the increase in fat mass can lead to a hypoxic situation in adipose tissue, which can activate hypoxia-inducible factor-1 (HIF-1), which in turn inhibits preadipocyte differentiation and initiates adipose tissue fibrosis [58]. It is not clear whether and to what extent such developmental events in adipose tissue are programmed by poor nutrition in foetal life and to what extent this can account for the associated greater risk of obesity development in foetal programmed individuals. However, adult rats born by dams subjected to protein restriction throughout gestation and lactation had increased visceral fat (combination of mesenteric, omental and retroperitoneal fat) mass due to hyperplasia, and expression of a number of genes involved in adipogenesis, angiogenesis and extracellular matrix remodelling was upregulated in the visceral adipose tissue [31]. More specifically, mRNA expression of genes involved in cell proliferation and differentiation, lipogenesis, uptake of free fatty acids from circulation, cholesterol synthesis and angiogenesis was increased in the visceral adipose tissue studied. In pigs, young adult males born with a low birth weight as a result of uteroplacental insufficiency had increased relative weight of epididymal white adipose tissue with increased lipid content, cellular hypertrophy and elevated mRNA expression of genes associated with lipid synthesis and storage [59].

Moreover, intrauterine growth restricted male adolescent rat offspring had an increased relative amount of visceral (retroperitoneal) adipose tissue with increased mRNA expression of genes associated with lipid and energy metabolism, whereas such changes were interestingly not evident in subcutaneous adipose tissue [60]. Recently, we have as previously mentioned shown that late gestation undernutrition in sheep led to occurrence of very small adipocytes and increased collagen infiltration in subcutaneous, but not in perirenal adipose tissue [37]. This was associated not only with a reduced ability for obesity-induced subcutaneous fat deposition, but it has been revealed that occurrences of such a population of very small adipocytes is associated with upregulated adipose inflammatory responses and impaired whole-body insulin sensitivity in overweight and obese humans [61, 62]. Thus, through interference with the normal process of adipocyte proliferation and differentiation, foetal malnutrition can lead to differential functional changes in adipose tissues, which will (1) reduce subcutaneous expandability, thereby (2) increasing fat deposition in intra-abdominal adipose tissues and (3) relying more on unhealthy hypertrophic rather than hyperplasic growth in this respect. Hence, prenatal events can determine fat distribution patterns in the body and associated risk of visceral obesity, since adipogenesis basically takes place before birth in larger mammals [63]. Future studies should clarify, whether abnormal features related to adipose development can be detected already at birth and hence potentially be used as a much needed reliable biomarker for adverse foetal programming.

Changes in Fat Deposition Patterns

Any disturbance in the distinct cellular events leading to adipocyte development may alter the tissue expandability and fat distribution patterns and increase the risk of deposition of fat in non-adipose tissues, also called ectopic fat accumulation. Fat deposition pattern is an important factor linking obesity to development of metabolic disturbances. Thus, visceral and ectopic fat deposition is associated with insulin resistance and type 2 diabetes [64]. Subcutaneous adipose tissue, however, appears to have unique beneficial properties related to improvement of insulin sensitivity [65], and subcutaneous fat accumulation is therefore considered to be a relatively healthy form of adiposity. Expandability of subcutaneous adipose tissue therefore becomes important to allow it to act as a 'sink' and prevent unhealthy lipid overflow for deposition in visceral adipose and non-adipose tissues [66, 67].

As already discussed, it has been acknowledged for some time that fat deposition patterns depend upon the nutrition supplied in utero [68], although the underlying mechanisms are not well understood. Thus, old English men born with a high birth weight (average: 4.23 kg) had higher body fat percentage and trunk-to-limb fat mass ratio and lower muscle mass than those born with a low birth weight (average: 2.76 kg) [69]. Moreover, in growth-restricted infants, subcutaneous adipose tissue, but not other fat depots, mass was reduced as compared to appropriate-for-gestational-age infants [70]. In adolescent sheep subjected to late gestation undernutrition, the reduced subcutaneous expandability resulted in relative preference for fat deposition in mesenteric and perirenal tissues during obesity development [19, 20]. A more unhealthy pattern of fat deposition in visceral and/or ectopic regions of the body will thereby be predisposed for, when expandability of subcutaneous adipose tissue becomes limited due to unfavourable nutrition exposure in utero, particularly during mid- to late gestation. Recently, we have found evidence in sheep to suggest that such a foetal-derived shift in fat deposition patterns is associated with intrinsic adipose cellularity and capacity to undergo hyperplasic rather than hypertrophic growth – not only in subcutaneous but also in perirenal and mesenteric adipose tissues. Thus in adolescent sheep with a history of late gestation undernutrition, intrinsic cellularity was reduced in subcutaneous and mesenteric adipose tissues in the non-obese state (Khanal et al., Unpublished data; Table 8.1). Even more important, the ability to expand cell numbers during obesity development was also reduced in these two tissues and even more pronounced in perirenal adipose tissue. Thus, during obesity development, the visceral adipocyte underwent extreme hypertrophy to store the additional flow of lipids

Table 8.1 Effects of prenatal nutrition combined with postnatal obesity on adipocyte cross-sectional area and cell number index in different adipose tissues

Item	LOW-HCHF	LOW-CONV	NORM-HCHF	NORM-CONV
Subcutaneous fat				
Adipocyte CSA (μm^2)	6088 ± 94^a	2426 ± 90^b	6088 ± 139^a	2107 ± 111^c
CNI	51.5 ± 1.2^b	27.6 ± 0.8^c	62.5 ± 1.8^a	48.5 ± 1.4^b
Mesenteric fat				
Adipocyte CSA (μm^2)	8567 ± 146^a	4233 ± 111^c	7949 ± 207^b	4251 ± 137^c
CNI	53.2 ± 1.3^b	34.8 ± 0.7^e	84.5 ± 2.7^a	46.3 ± 1.2^c
Perirenal fat				
Adipocyte CSA (μm^2)	$11{,}980 \pm 149^a$	2991 ± 131^d	7354 ± 214^b	5338 ± 176^c
CNI	57.9 ± 1.3^b	32.4 ± 0.7^{cd}	112.6 ± 3.2^a	31.5 ± 0.9^d

Data are presented as least square means±SEM. Effects of prenatal (LOW vs NORM) nutrition in obese or non-obese situation (HCHF vs CONV) were significant ($P < 0.05$) if the data within a row and within the respective columns are marked by different superscripts

CSA cross-sectional area, *CNI* cell number index calculated as adipocyte mass (total fat mass (kg) multiplied by the %'age of adipocytes in the tissue) divided by the volume of a spherical adipocyte with a radius derived from the measured mean cross-sectional area, *LOW* ($N = 10$; five males, five females; diet fed to twin-pregnant dams during the last trimester and fulfilling 50% of their daily energy and protein requirements), *NORM* ($N = 6$; six males, 0 female; diet fed to twin-pregnant dams during the last trimester and fulfilling 100% of their daily energy and protein requirements), *HCHF* ($N = 13$; eight males, five females; high-carbohydrate-high-fat postnatal diet fed to lambs and consisting of cream-milk replacer mix in a 1:1 ratio supplemented with rolled maize), and *CONV* ($N = 13$; seven males, six females; conventional postnatal diet fed to lambs and consisting of milk replacer and hay until 8 weeks of age and hay only thereafter and adjusted to achieve moderate and constant growth rates of approx. 225 g/day) (Adapted from Khanal et al. Unpublished data)

(Khanal et al., Unpublished data; Table 8.1) due to limited hyperplasic ability in general and hypertrophic ability of subcutaneous adipocytes. Studies in pigs have also indicated that the perirenal adipose tissue development can be affected by foetal nutrition, since undernutrition during pregnancy in sows increased perirenal adiposity in their foetuses and increased lipid locules size in the perirenal adipocytes [71, 72].

Thus, not only subcutaneous but also perirenal and potentially other visceral fats are targets of foetal programing. Increased preference for fat distribution in the visceral region in individuals exposed to prenatal undernutrition is likely linked to coexistence of not only poor expandability of subcutaneous fat but a general interference with ability of adipose tissues to undergo hyperplasic growth, resulting in an extreme hypertrophic expansion in visceral depots during obesity development. Very little knowledge is available from humans about distinct metabolic and development features of individual visceral adipose tissues, including the perirenal. The validity of findings from animal studies therefore needs to be confirmed in humans.

Upregulated Inflammatory Responses and Epigenetic Regulation

Adipose tissue is not only a passive responder to nutrient provision and signals from different hormonal systems but also acts as an important endocrine organ secreting and expressing different factors (adipokines), which have important endocrine functions [73]. It has been hypothesized that increased free fatty acids and pro-inflammatory factors released from visceral fat into the portal vein towards the liver play an important role for insulin resistance in obese individuals [74, 75]. Visceral adipose tissues and adipose-tissue resident macrophages produce more proinflammatory cytokines like tumour necrosis factor-alpha (TNF-α) and interleukin-6 (IL-6) and less adiponectin than other adipose tissues [76]. Overexpansion of visceral adipocytes interferes with the normal sequestration and storage of lipid resulting in increased release of lipids and pro-inflammatory signals, thereby promoting systemic insulin resistance [77]. Various studies have provided evidence to suggest that the processes of inflammation in adipose tissues could also be targets of foetal programming.

In sheep, gestational nutrient restriction resulted in overexpression in perirenal adipose tissue of inflammatory markers such as cluster of differentiation 68 (CD 68) and toll-like receptor (TLR4) [78]. Intrauterine growth restriction increased inflammation also in subcutaneous adipose tissue prior to onset of obesity and along with impaired glucose tolerance in male rats [79]. In insulin insensitive foetally undernourished adult rats, adipose explants and stromal vascular fraction cultures had enhanced secretion of TNFα and IL-1β, and adipose expression of several key proinflammatory genes and markers of macrophage infiltration were increased [80]. Adipose tissue macrophages (ATM) are the source of inflammatory adipokines such as TNF-α (tumour necrosis factor) and IL-6 (interleukin-6), and rodent studies showed that ATMs may significantly contribute to development of systemic insulin resistance [81]. A macrophage marker (F4/80) in perigonadal, perirenal, mesenteric and subcutaneous adipose tissues of mice was positively correlated with adipocyte size and body mass [82]. Undernutrition in utero can therefore be expected to predispose for increased macrophage infiltration, pro-inflammatory adipose responses and associated metabolic disorders. This is due to the abovementioned changes in adipose expandability traits leading to overexpansion (hypertrophic growth) of particularly visceral adipocytes during obesity development.

It is now widely believed that a relatively brief environmental malnutrition challenge during embryonic or foetal development can induce permanent imprinting of the genome, which may not manifest their metabolic impacts until much later in life. Prenatal exposures can induce epigenetic modifications such as gene promoter region methylation (i.e., the CpG sites), chromatin histone acetylation/methylation and changes expression of miRNA [83]. However, studies on how early life nutrition influence epigenetic regulation of key genes associated with obesity development are limited. Suggested targets for epigenetic modifications induced by foetal malnutrition include cell lineage determinants (transformation of stem cells to pre-adipocytes) and determinants of pre-adipocyte differentiation (during adipogenesis) and adipose inflammation. The cellular mechanisms linking foetal malnutrition to epigenetic modifications are as yet unknown, and how epigenetic marks and the transcriptional regulation interact also remains to be established [84–87]. In mice, maternal undernutrition during pregnancy and lactation was shown to result in permanent removal of methyl groups at CpG sites in the promoter region of the leptin gene in adult offspring, which was associated with reduced leptin mRNA expression [87]. Although, perinatal epigenetic analysis may become a useful tool in the future for early identification of individuals susceptible to obesity development and associated adverse metabolic traits [88], identification of reliable epigenetic biomarkers is still a major challenge.

Conclusion

Proper nutrition during critical periods of foetal development is important to counteract the increased trend of visceral obesity and associated disorders in humans, and a healthy diet postnatally appears particular important for individuals exposed to undernutrition prenatally. The impact of foetal nutrition on adipose tissue development and function later in life depends upon timing of the exposures in relation to formation, differentiation and growth of the different adipose tissues. For the quantitatively most important adipose tissues, mid- to late gestation is the most important periods in humans and other precocial animal species, inducing some limitations in the use of rodent models in this respect. Maternal undernutrition during periods of adipose formation and development can induce alterations in development of stem cells into preadipocytes and differentiation of preadipocytes into mature lipid filled adipocytes cells. This can permanently alter the mechanisms, whereby different adipose tissues expand later in life. Detailed studies in sheep have shown that undernutrition during late foetal life reduces the intrinsic cellularity (cell formation) in subcutaneous, perirenal and mesenteric adipose tissues. This will reduce expandability of subcutaneous adipose tissue and its ability to act as a 'nutrient overflow sink', since hypertrophic ability in this tissue appears to be limited. In turn, visceral and ectopic fat deposition is predisposed for. However, foetal undernutrition also interferes with the ability of visceral adipose tissues to form new adipocytes during obesity development in postnatal life, resulting in increased reliance on hypertrophic expansion with formation of very large adipocytes, rather than expansion by formation of a greater number of adipocytes of a more normal size. Hypertrophic adipose expansion with formation of very large adipocytes is associated with elevated adipose tissue-derived pro-inflammatory responses, which are linked to development of metabolic disorders such as type 2 diabetes, which are known to be associated with obesity. Much remains to be understood about the specific role of epigenetic changes in foetal programming of adipose tissue development and postnatal function.

References

1. Kopelman PG. Obesity as a medical problem. Nature. 2000;404:635–43.
2. Kelly T, Yang W, Chen CS, Reynolds K, He J. Global burden of obesity in 2005 and projections to 2030. Int J Obes. 2008;32:1431–7.
3. Prentice AM. The emerging epidemic of obesity in developing countries. Int J Epidemiol. 2006;35:93–9.
4. WHO, Obesity: preventing and managing the global epidemic. Working group on obesity. Geneva: World Health Organization; 1998.
5. Putnam J, Allshouse J, Kantor LS. U.S. per capita food supply trends: more calories, refined carbohydrates, and fats. Food Rev. 2002;25:1–15.
6. Sturm R. The economics of physical activity: societal trends and rationales for interventions. Am J Prev Med. 2004;27:126–35.
7. Björntorp P. Metabolic implications of body fat distribution. Diabetes Care. 1991;14:1132–43.
8. Despres JP, Lemieux I. Abdominal obesity and metabolic syndrome. Nature. 2006;444:881–7.
9. Shuster A, Patlas M, Pinthus JH, Mourtzakis M. The clinical importance of visceral adiposity: a critical review of methods for visceral adipose tissue analysis. Br J Radiol. 2012;85:1–10.
10. Taylor PD, Poston L. Developmental programming of obesity in mammals. Exp Physiol. 2007;92:287–98.
11. Dyer JS, Rosenfeld CR. Metabolic imprinting by prenatal, perinatal, and postnatal overnutrition: a review. Semin Reprod Med. 2011;29:266–76.
12. Lucas A. Programming by early nutrition in man. Ciba Found Symp. 1991;156:38–50.
13. Godfrey KM, Barker DJ. Fetal nutrition and adult disease. Am J Clin Nutr. 2000;71:1344S–52S.
14. Symonds ME, Sebert SP, Hyatt MA, Budge H. Nutritional programming of the metabolic syndrome. Nat Rev Endocrinol. 2009;5:604–10.
15. Fall CHD. Evidence for the intra-uterine programming of adiposity in later life. Ann Hum Biol. 2011;38:410–28.
16. Hediger ML, Overpeck MD, Kuczmarski RJ, McGlynn A, Maurer KR, Davis WW. Muscularity and fatness of infants and young children born small- or large-for-gestational-age. Pediatrics. 1998;102:E60.
17. Barker M, Robinson S, Osmond C, Barker DJ. Birth weight and body fat distribution in adolescent girls. Arch Dis Child. 1997;77:381–3.
18. Walker SP, Gaskin PS, Powell CA, Bennett FI. The effects of birth weight and postnatal linear growth retardation on body mass index, fatness and fat distribution in mid and late childhood. Public Health Nutr. 2002;5:391–6.
19. Khanal P, Husted SV, Axel AM, Johnsen L, Pedersen KL, Mortensen MS, Kongsted AH, Nielsen MO. Late gestation over- and undernutrition predispose for visceral adiposity in response to a post-natal obesogenic diet, but with differential impacts on glucose–insulin adaptations during fasting in lambs. Acta Physiol. 2014;210:110–26.
20. Nielsen MO, Kongsted AH, Thygesen MP, Strathe AB, Caddy S, Quistorff B, Jørgensen W, Christensen VG, Husted S, Chwalibog A, Sejrsen K, Purup S, Svalastoga E, McEvoy FJ, Johnsen L. Late gestation undernutrition can predispose for visceral adiposity by altering fat distribution patterns and increasing the preference for a high-fat diet in early postnatal life. Br J Nutr. 2013;109:2098–110.
21. Ford SP, Hess BW, Schwope MM, Nijland MJ, Gilbert JS, Vonnahme KA, Means WJ, Han H, Nathanielsz PW. Maternal undernutrition during early to mid-gestation in the ewe results in altered growth, adiposity, and glucose tolerance in male offspring. J Anim Sci. 2007;85:1285–94.

22. Barbero A, Astiz S, Lopez-Bote CJ, Perez-Solana ML, Ayuso M, Garcia-Real I, Gonzalez-Bulnes A. Maternal malnutrition and offspring sex determine juvenile obesity and metabolic disorders in a swine model of leptin resistance. PLoS One. 2013;8:e78424.
23. Rolfe Ede L, Loos RJ, Druet C, Stolk RP, Ekelund U, Griffin SJ, Forouhi NG, Wareham NJ, Ong KK. Association between birth weight and visceral fat in adults. Am J Clin Nutr. 2010;92:347–52.
24. Law CM, Barker DJ, Osmond C, Fall CH, Simmonds SJ. Early growth and abdominal fatness in adult life. J Epidemiol Community Health. 1992;46:184–6.
25. Lumey LH, Ravelli AC, Wiessing LG, Koppe JG, Treffers PE, Stein ZA. The Dutch famine birth cohort study: design, validation of exposure, and selected characteristics of subjects after 43 years follow-up. Paediatr Perinat Epidemiol. 1993;7:354–67.
26. Ravelli AC, van Der Meulen JH, Osmond C, Barker DJ, Bleker OP. Obesity at the age of 50 y in men and women exposed to famine prenatally. Am J Clin Nutr. 1999;70:811–6.
27. Ravelli AC, van der Meulen JH, Michels RP, Osmond C, Barker DJ, Hales CN, Bleker OP. Glucose tolerance in adults after prenatal exposure to famine. Lancet. 1998;351:173–7.
28. Tian JY, Cheng Q, Song XM, Li G, Jiang GX, Gu YY, Luo M. Birth weight and risk of type 2 diabetes, abdominal obesity and hypertension among Chinese adults. Eur J Endocrinol. 2006;155:601–7.
29. de Oliveira JC, Gomes RM, Miranda RA, Barella LF, Malta A, Martins IP, Franco CC, Pavanello A, Torrezan R, Natali MR, Lisboa PC, Mathias PC, de Moura EG. Protein restriction during the last third of pregnancy malprograms the neuroendocrine axes to induce metabolic syndrome in adult male rat offspring. Endocrinology. 2016;157:1799–812.
30. Bellinger L, Sculley DV, Langley-Evans SC. Exposure to undernutrition in fetal life determines fat distribution, locomotor activity and food intake in ageing rats. Int J Obes. 2006;30:729–38.
31. Guan H, Arany E, van Beek JP, Chamson-Reig A, Thyssen S, Hill DJ, Yang K. Adipose tissue gene expression profiling reveals distinct molecular pathways that define visceral adiposity in offspring of maternal protein-restricted rats. Am J Physiol Endocrinol Metab. 2005;288:E663–73.
32. Fox CS, Massaro JM, Hoffmann U, Pou KM, Maurovich-Horvat P, Liu CY, Vasan RS, Murabito JM, Meigs JB, Cupples LA, D'Agostino RB Sr, O'Donnell CJ. Abdominal visceral and subcutaneous adipose tissue compartments: association with metabolic risk factors in the Framingham Heart Study. Circulation. 2007;116:39–48.
33. Jones RH, Ozanne SE. Fetal programming of glucose-insulin metabolism. Mol Cell Endocrinol. 2009;297:4–9.
34. Cohen MP, Stern E, Rusecki Y, Zeidler A. High prevalence of diabetes in young adult Ethiopian immigrants to Israel. Diabetes. 1988;37:824–8.
35. Gosby AK, Maloney CA, Caterson ID. Elevated insulin sensitivity in low-protein offspring rats is prevented by a high-fat diet and is associated with visceral fat. Obesity. 2010;18:1593–600.
36. van der Waaij EH, van den Brand H, van Arendonk JA, Kemp B. Effect of match or mismatch of maternal–offspring nutritional environment on the development of offspring in broiler chickens. Animal. 2011;5:741–8.
37. Nielsen MO, Hou L, Johnsen L, Khanal P, Bechshøft CL, Kongsted AH, Vaag A, Hellgren LI. Do very small adipocytes in subcutaneous adipose tissue (a proposed risk factor for insulin insensitivity) have a fetal origin? Clin Nutr Exp. 2016;8:9–24.
38. Matsuzawa Y, Funahashi T, Nakamura T. The concept of metabolic syndrome: contribution of visceral fat accumulation and its molecular mechanism. J Atheroscler Thromb. 2011;18:629–39.
39. Chen J, Muntner P, Hamm LL, Jones DW, Batuman V, Fonseca V, Whelton PK, He J. The metabolic syndrome and chronic kidney disease in U.S. adults. Ann Intern Med. 2004;140:167–74.
40. López-Jaramillo P1, Silva SY, Rodríguez-Salamanca N, Duràn A, Mosquera W, Castillo V. Are nutrition-induced epigenetic changes the link between socioeconomic pathology and cardiovascular diseases? Am J Ther. 2008;15:362–72.
41. Gluckman PD, Hanson MA, Spencer HG. Predictive adaptive responses and human evolution. Trends Ecol Evol. 2005;20:527–33.
42. Khanal P, Johnsen L, Axel AM, Hansen PW, Kongsted AH, Lyckegaard NB, Nielsen MO. Long-term impacts of foetal malnutrition followed by early postnatal obesity on fat distribution pattern and metabolic adaptability in adult sheep. PLoS One. 2016;11:e0156700.
43. Symonds ME, Stephenson T, Gardner DS, Budge H. Long-term effects of nutritional programming of the embryo and fetus: mechanisms and critical windows. Reprod Fertil Dev. 2006;19:53–63.
44. Poissonnet CM, Burdi AR, Garn SM. The chronology of adipose tissue appearance and distribution in the human fetus. Early Hum Dev. 1984;10:1–11.
45. Symonds ME, Lomax MA. Maternal and environmental influences on thermoregulation in the neonate. Proc Nutr Soc. 1992;51:165–72.
46. Symonds ME, Stephenson T. Maternal nutrition and endocrine programming of fetal adipose tissue development. Biochem Soc Trans. 1999;27:97–104.
47. Alexander G. Quantitative development of adipose tissue in foetal sheep. Aust J Biol Sci. 1978;31:489–503.

48. Gemmell RT, Alexander G. Ultrastructural development of adipose tissue in foetal sheep. Aust J Biol Sci. 1978;31:505–15.
49. Weinreb JC, Lowe T, Cohen JM, Kutler M. Human fetal anatomy: MR imaging. Radiology. 1985;157:715–20.
50. Ailhaud G1, Grimaldi P, Négrel R. Cellular and molecular aspects of adipose tissue development. Annu Rev Nutr. 1992;12:207–33.
51. Desai M, Ross MG. Fetal programming of adipose tissue: effects of intrauterine growth restriction and maternal obesity/high-fat diet. Semin Reprod Med. 2011;29:237–45.
52. Kiess W, Petzold S, Töpfer M, Garten A, Blüher S, Kapellen T, Körner A, Kratzsch J. Adipocytes and adipose tissue. Best Pract Res Clin Endocrinol Metab. 2008;22:135–53.
53. Yan X, Zhu MJ, Dodson MV, Du M. Developmental programming of fetal skeletal muscle and adipose tissue development. J Genomics. 2013;8:29–38.
54. Avram MM, Avram AS, James WD. Subcutaneous fat in normal and diseased states 3. Adipogenesis: from stem cell to fat cell. J Am Acad Dermatol. 2007;56:472–92.
55. Morrison RF, Farmer SR. Hormonal signaling and transcriptional control of adipocyte differentiation. J Nutr. 2000;130:3116s–21s.
56. Hausman GJ, Richardson RL. Adipose tissue angiogenesis. J Anim Sci. 2004;82:925–34.
57. Hausman DB, DiGirolamo M, Bartness TJ, Hausman GJ, Martin RJ. The biology of white adipocyte proliferation. Obes Rev. 2001;2:239–54.
58. Buechler C, Krautbauer S, Eisinger K. Adipose tissue fibrosis. World J Diabetes. 2015;6:548–53.
59. Sarr O, Thompson JA, Zhao L, Lee TY, Regnault TR. Low birth weight male guinea pig offspring display increased visceral adiposity in early adulthood. PLoS One. 2014;9:e98433.
60. Joss-Moore LA, Wang Y, Campbell MS, Moore B, Yu X, Callaway CW, McKnight RA, Desai M, Moyer-Mileur LJ, Lane RH. Uteroplacental insufficiency increases visceral adiposity and visceral adipose PPARγ2 expression in male rat offspring prior to the onset of obesity. Early Hum Dev. 2010;86:179–85.
61. McLaughlin T, Deng A, Yee G, Lamendola C, Reaven G, Tsao PS, Cushman SW, Sherman A. Inflammation in subcutaneous adipose tissue: relationship to adipose cell size. Diabetologia. 2009;53:369–77.
62. McLaughlin T, Lamendola C, Coghlan N, Liu TC, Lerner K, Sherman A, Cushman SW. Subcutaneous adipose cell size and distribution: relationship to insulin resistance and body fat. Obesity. 2014;22(3):673–80.
63. Muhlhausler B, Smith SR. Early-life origins of metabolic dysfunction: role of the adipocyte. Trends Endocrinol Metab. 2009;20:51–7.
64. Gastaldelli A. Role of beta-cell dysfunction, ectopic fat accumulation and insulin resistance in the pathogenesis of type 2 diabetes mellitus. Diabetes Res Clin Pract. 2011;93:S60–5.
65. Tran TT, Yamamoto Y, Gesta S, Kahn CR. Beneficial effects of subcutaneous fat transplantation on metabolism. Cell Metab. 2008;7:410–20.
66. Lemieux I. Energy partitioning in gluteal-femoral fat: does the metabolic fate of triglycerides affect coronary heart disease risk? Arterioscler Thromb Vasc Biol. 2004;24:795–7.
67. Miranda PJ, DeFronzo RA, Califf RM, Guyton JR. Metabolic syndrome: definition, pathophysiology, and mechanisms. Am Heart J. 2005;149:33–45.
68. Symonds ME, Pearce S, Bispham J, Gardner DS, Stephenson T. Timing of nutrient restriction and programming of fetal adipose tissue development. Proc Nutr Soc. 2004;63:397–403.
69. Kensara OA, Wootton SA, Phillips DI, Patel M, Jackson AA, Elia M. Fetal programming of body composition: relation between birth weight and body composition measured with dual-energy X-ray absorptiometry and anthropometric methods in older Englishmen. Am J Clin Nutr. 2005;82:980–7.
70. Harrington TA, Thomas EL, Frost G, Modi N, Bell JD. Distribution of adipose tissue in the newborn. Pediatr Res. 2004;55:437–41.
71. Nguyen LT, Muhlhausler BS, Botting KJ, Morrison JL. Maternal undernutrition alters fat cell size distribution, but not lipogenic gene expression, in the visceral fat of the late gestation guinea pig fetus. Placenta. 2010;31:902–9.
72. Kind KL, Roberts CT, Sohlstrom AI, Katsman A, Clifton PM, Robinson JS, Owens JA. Chronic maternal feed restriction impairs growth but increases adiposity of the fetal guinea pig. Am J Physiol Regul Integr Comp Physiol. 2005;288:R119–26.
73. Kershaw EE, Flier JS. Adipose tissue as an endocrine organ. J Clin Endocrinol Metab. 2004;89:2548–56.
74. Després JP, Moorjani S, Lupien PJ, Tremblay A, Nadeau A, Bouchard C. Regional distribution of body fat, plasma lipoproteins, and cardiovascular disease. Arteriosclerosis. 1990;10:497–511.
75. Item F, Konrad D. Visceral fat and metabolic inflammation: the portal theory revisited. Obes Rev. 2012;13:30–9.
76. Hamdy O, Porramatikul S, Al-Ozairi E. Metabolic obesity: the paradox between visceral and subcutaneous fat. Curr Diabetes Rev. 2006;2:367–73.
77. Hajer GR, van Haeften TW, Visseren FL. Adipose tissue dysfunction in obesity, diabetes, and vascular diseases. Eur Heart J. 2008;29:2959–71.
78. Sharkey D, Symonds ME, Budge H. Adipose tissue inflammation: developmental ontogeny and consequences of gestational nutrient restriction in offspring. Endocrinology. 2009;150:3913–20.

79. Riddle ES, Campbell MS, Lang BY, Bierer R, Wang Y, Bagley HN, Joss-Moore LA. Intrauterine growth restriction increases TNF alpha and activates the unfolded protein response in male rat pups. J Obes. 2014;2014:829862.
80. Reynolds CM, Li M, Gray C, Vickers MH. Preweaning growth hormone treatment ameliorates adipose tissue insulin resistance and inflammation in adult male offspring following maternal undernutrition. Endocrinology. 2013;154:2676–86.
81. Zeyda M, Stulnig TM. Obesity, inflammation, and insulin resistance-a mini-review. Gerontology. 2009;55:379–86.
82. Weisberg SP, McCann D, Desai M, Rosenbaum M, Leibel RL, Ferrante AW Jr. Obesity is associated with macrophage accumulation in adipose tissue. J Clin Invest. 2003;112:1796–808.
83. Lillycrop KA, Burdge GC. Epigenetic mechanisms linking early nutrition to long term health. Best Pract Res Clin Endocrinol Metab. 2012;26:667–76.
84. Musri MM, Parrizas M. Epigenetic regulation of adipogenesis. Curr Opin Clin Nutr Metab Care. 2012;15:342–9.
85. Li HX, Xiao L, Wang C, Gao JL, Zhai YG. Epigenetic regulation of adipocyte differentiation and adipogenesis. J Zhejiang Univ Sci B. 2010;11:784–91.
86. Toubal A, Treuter E, Clément K, Venteclef N. Genomic and epigenomic regulation of adipose tissue inflammation in obesity. Trends Endocrinol Metab. 2013;24:625–34.
87. Jousse C, Parry L, Lambert-Langlais S, Maurin AC, Averous J, Bruhat A, Carraro V, Tost J, Letteron P, Chen P, Jockers R, Launay JM, Mallet J, Fafournoux P. Perinatal undernutrition affects the methylation and expression of the leptin gene in adults: implication for the understanding of metabolic syndrome. FASEB J. 2011;25:3271–8.
88. Godfrey KM, Sheppard A, Gluckman PD, Lillycrop KA, Burdge GC, McLean C, Rodford J, Slater-Jefferies JL, Garratt E, Crozier SR, Emerald BS, Gale CR, Inskip HM, Cooper C, Hanson MA. Epigenetic gene promoter methylation at birth is associated with child's later adiposity. Diabetes. 2011;60:1528–34.

Chapter 9
Maternal Undernutrition and Long-Term Effects on Hepatic Function

Daniel B. Hardy

Key Points

- This chapter focuses on human and animal data linking undernutrition in utero (i.e., placental insufficiency, nutrient restriction, maternal low protein) with long-term hepatic dysfunction in postnatal life.
- Undernutrition in utero influences lipid homeostasis, gluconeogenesis, insulin sensitivity, drug metabolism, and overall growth leading to liver fibrosis and long-term symptoms of the metabolic syndrome.
- Some of the direct mechanisms linking undernutrition in perinatal life to hepatic dysfunction include hypoxia and epigenetic influences (i.e., DNA methylation, posttranslational histone modifications, and microRNAs).
- Rapid postnatal catch-up growth can indirectly augment hepatic ER stress leading to impaired insulin signaling and alterations in microRNAs in the liver.
- Animal studies have indicated that intervention in perinatal life with essential nutrients, hormones, or modulators of nuclear receptors can rescue hepatic gene expression and may prevent the long-term metabolic deficits associated with the undernourished liver.

Keywords DOHaD • Epigenetics • Maternal low-protein diet • Hypoxia • Uterine ligation • Nuclear receptors • Posttranslational histone modifications • DNA methylation • Endoplasmic reticulum stress • MicroRNAs

Abbreviations

11β-HSD1	11β-hydroxysteroid dehydrogenase type 1
ADP	Adenine diphosphate
Akt1	Protein kinase B

Supported by: CIHR Operating Grant and Natural Sciences and Engineering Research Council of Canada.

D.B. Hardy, PhD (✉)
The Departments of Obstetrics & Gynecology and Physiology & Pharmacology, The Children's Health Research Institute and the Lawson Health Research Institute, The University of Western Ontario, London, ON, Canada
e-mail: Daniel.Hardy@schulich.uwo.ca

CpG	Cysteine-phosphate-guanine
CVD	Cardiovascular disease
Cyp2c11	Cytochrome P450 2c11
Cyp3a1	Cytochrome P450 3a1
Cyp7a1	Cytochrome P450 7a1
EPO	Erythropoietin
ER stress	Endoplasmic reticulum stress
Ex-4	Exendin-4
G6Pase	Glucose-6 phosphatase
GLP-1	Glucagon-like peptide-1
GR	Glucocorticoid receptor
HDL	High-density lipoproteins
IGF-1	Insulin growth factor 1
IUGR	Intrauterine growth restriction
JMJD	Jmj domain-containing histone demethylation protein
LDL	Low-density lipoproteins
LP	Low protein
LXR	Liver X receptor
miRs	MicroRNAs
MMP2	Matrix metalloproteinase 2
MNR	Maternal nutrition restriction
MPR	Maternal protein restriction
pAkt1 (Ser473)	Phospho Akt1 (serine 473)
Pck1	Phosphoenolpyruvate carboxykinase 1 (soluble)
pEIF2α	Phospho-eukaryotic translation initiation factor 2
PND	Postnatal day
PPAR	Peroxisome proliferator-activated receptor
SGA	Small for gestational age
SMAD4	SMAD family member 4
TGFB1	Transforming growth factor β1
TUDCA	Tauroursodeoxycholic acid
UPR	Unfolded protein response
VEGF	Vascular endothelial growth factor

Introduction

The liver plays a critical role in mammals for metabolism, digestion, detoxification, storage, protein production, and immunity. Given the role of the liver in cholesterol, fatty acid, and glucose homeostasis, it is not surprising hepatic dysfunction underlies several of the symptoms (i.e., hypercholesterolemia, obesity, glucose intolerance) characterizing the metabolic syndrome [1, 2]. The surge in the incidence of the metabolic syndrome worldwide is of great concern considering that it raises the risk of developing cardiovascular disease (CVD) by ~20-fold, and CVD is responsible for 1 out 2.9 deaths in the United States [3–6]. In addition to the metabolic syndrome, impaired liver health and function also can lead to liver fibrosis (and the end-stage cirrhosis), which is estimated to contribute up to 45% of deaths in the developed world [7, 8]. Liver fibrosis is a major predictor for diabetes, overall liver failure, portal hypertension, and liver cancer [9–11]. Since diet (i.e., "Western diet") is a major contributor to defects in liver function and ultimately liver fibrosis or CVD, current therapeutic strategies are aimed at lifestyle modifications (i.e., physical activity and healthy eating) and/or pharmaceutical interventions to treat the disease once manifested [12–15]. While pharmaceuticals may be effective reducing the risk of CVD, the long-term dependency on them can be dangerous for the liver. For example, statins can reduce the risk of ischemic heart disease by up to 60%; however, the existence of statin-induced rhabdomyolysis and hepatitis-associated liver failure emerges in some patients [16]. Clearly additional studies are warranted for hepatic disease prevention versus treatment. A major preventative strategy is in recognizing the early origins of adult disease so that efficacious interventions can be targeted to prevent long-term defects in liver function.

Maternal Undernutrition and Impaired Hepatic Function: Clinical Evidence

Over 25 years ago, Professor David Barker revealed that adverse in utero events can permanently alter physiological processes leading to the metabolic syndrome [17]. The early evidence that an impairment of liver size and/or function was involved came from the fact that there was a strong correlation between reduced abdominal circumference at birth with elevated total and LDL cholesterol in adulthood [18]. Secondly, intrauterine growth restriction (IUGR), caused by either placental insufficiency or maternal malnutrition, often results in asymmetric organ development whereby there is a reduction in the growth of less essential organs such as the liver, lungs, and kidneys [19, 20]. Thirdly, there is a strong inverse relationship between birth weight and obesity or glucose intolerance; both under the regulation of the liver [21–24]. It is noteworthy that the majority of these links to metabolic disease arose from large population-based studies whereby under nutrition in utero (i.e., due to famine) was the major factor leading to impaired fetal growth [21, 25–28].

Postpartum, the major factor influencing this inverse relationship between low birth weight and metabolic disease is nutrition-induced accelerated growth in neonatal life, which leads to an earlier onset of the symptoms of the metabolic syndrome [25, 29–31]. Barker explained this phenomenon with the "predictive adaptive response" hypothesis, which suggests that "adverse events during development induce adaptations suited for survival in a similar predictive environment but can become maladaptive if a mismatch to the predictive environment occurs, leading to a thrifty phenotype" [32, 33]. Since IUGR leads to major decreases in fetal liver development, it seems conceivable that the liver has the most to gain in growth during postnatal life [19, 20]. Animal models of IUGR support that the undernourished liver undergoes rapid postnatal catch-up growth leading to further metabolic dysfunction, but there is evidence from human studies as well [34–36]. For example, infants born small for gestational age (SGA) undergo hypersomatotropism as early as 4 days as a result of increased circulating insulin growth factor 1 (IGF-1) produced by the liver [37]. Elegant studies by Singhal et al. have also demonstrated that low birth weight infants with rapid postnatal growth (due to growth-promoting formula diets) exhibited a higher LDL/HDL ratio, likely derived from impaired cholesterol homeostasis in the liver [38]. While future noninvasive imaging studies are warranted to tract liver development (i.e., liver growth, lipid composition) in IUGR infants long-term, animal models of maternal undernutrition have shed great light into the mechanisms underlying the fetal programming of the liver. More importantly, by elucidating some of the underlying mechanisms involved, new pharmaceutical and dietary intervention strategies can be employed to prevent these defects in liver function.

Uterine Ligation or Ablation Model of Undernutrition and Long-Term Hepatic Function

As previously mentioned, IUGR can occur due to placental insufficiency which occurs in about 8% of pregnancies [39, 40]. Animal studies have demonstrated that placental insufficiency-induced IUGR leads to decreases in oxygenation and substrate availability for the fetus [41–43]. Therefore, the uterine ligation or uterine ablation serves as excellent models for examining idiopathic IUGR and the short- and long-term effects on liver function. Both models lead to decreased birth weight and lower liver to body weight ratios [35, 44]. In the guinea pig, uterine ablation led to a greater incidence of hepatic perisinusoidal or periportal fibrosis in 5-month offspring with increased expression of profibrogenic markers including TGFβ1, MMP2, and SMAD4 [44]. In rats, uterine ligation leads to development of the metabolic syndrome in the offspring including type 2 diabetes, dyslipidemia, and hypertriglyceridemia [45–47]. Interestingly, many of these symptoms were reciprocated into the F2 generation [48]. These metabolic deficits exist, in part, due to altered glucose transporter expression, impairment of fatty acid metabolism, increased glucocorticoid activity, augmented glucose production, and blunted insulin suppression all within the liver [45, 47, 49–51]. These offspring also exhibited decreased hepatic and circulating insulin growth factor 1 (Igf-1) which is critical for insulin function, glucose metabolism, and growth [52]. While other models of maternal dietary-induced IUGR led to hypercholesterolemia in postnatal life, uterine ligation appears to have no effect on cholesterol homeostasis unless the offspring were challenged with a high-fat diet in postnatal life [34, 53, 54]. Although this animal model is physiologically relevant to idiopathic IUGR, it is distinct from dietary-induced undernutrition as it leads to direct decreases in both oxygen and nutrients to the fetus. Other exclusive dietary models are essential in understanding the contribution of maternal malnutrition alone on long-term hepatic function and disease.

Maternal Nutrient Restriction (MNR) Model of Undernutrition

Human and animal studies of food restriction during pregnancy confirm that maternal undernourishment leads to IUGR depending upon the timing (pre- vs postconception) and severity of the insult [28, 29, 55–57]. Moreover, like models of uterine ligation, fetal liver growth from MNR dams is compromised at birth followed by rapid postnatal catch-up growth [36, 55, 58]. However, with models of MNR, the impact of a decrease in maternal and placental weight during pregnancy must also be taken into consideration [55, 59]. Sheep and rat studies have demonstrated that MNR leads to glucose intolerance and insulin insensitivity, along with greater hepatic lipid and glycogen content in the offspring [58, 60]. The impaired glucose tolerance in MNR sheep offspring is attributed, in part, to increased circulating cortisol and augmented hepatic PEPCK expression in MNR offspring [60]. In contrast to offspring of uterine ligation, MNR offspring with catch-up growth exhibited increases in Igf-1 which the authors attribute is associated with decreased longevity, but not necessarily metabolic disease [58].

Maternal Protein Restriction (MPR) Model of Undernutrition

Placental insufficiency in humans often leads to protein (and amino acid) deficiencies in the fetus, which are critical for fetal growth [61, 62]. Therefore, the MPR model is a relevant model to study placental insufficiency-IUGR as it leads to asymmetric IUGR, without any effects on maternal weight gain or food intake [22, 63]. Moreover, MPR offspring have decreases in fetal liver weight at birth and, depending on the timing of protein restoration, display liver and whole body catch-up growth despite no differences in food intake [34, 64]. Remarkably, MPR offspring, more predominantly in males, exhibit several symptoms of the metabolic syndrome including glucose intolerance, visceral obesity, hypercholesterolemia, and hypertension [34, 63, 65–69]. The glucose intolerance is attributed to augmented gluconeogenesis (e.g., G6Pase, 11β-HSD1), diminished glucokinase expression, decreased pAkt1 (Ser473), and decreased glucagon receptor in the livers of MPR offspring [64, 67, 70, 71]. With respect to lipids, MPR male offspring with catch-up growth show increases in circulating hepatic cholesterol due to decreases in the expression of Cyp7a1, the critical enzyme in cholesterol metabolism [34]. Aside from alterations in glucose and cholesterol homeostasis, MPR male offspring with catch-up also exhibit increases in hepatic Cyp3a and Cyp2c11 expression and activity influencing long-term drug metabolism (i.e., statins) in these offspring [72]. As testosterone is a major substrate for these Cyp enzymes, it may explain why MPR male offspring have lower circulating testosterone levels, and consequentially, the long-term sexual dimorphism which exists in this model [68]. Similar to uterine-ligated offspring, MPR offspring with catch-up growth have decreases in hepatic Igf-1; however, the decrease in Igf-1 is mainly attributed to the effects of protein restriction during lactation [63]. All in all, the MPR model truly reinforces the main principle of Barker's "predictive adaptive response" given that when there is no nutritional mismatch in postnatal life, MPR offspring do not exhibit any decreases in cholesterol catabolism, insulin sensitivity, or drug metabolism in the liver [34, 64, 72].

Direct Mechanisms Linking Maternal Undernutrition and Adverse Metabolic Outcomes

While human and animal studies have certainly established the strong links between an undernourished in utero environment and metabolic deficits in the offspring, we are only just beginning to unravel the direct and indirect molecular events involved. Interestingly, one of the major direct drivers of altered hepatic gene expression and function short- and long-term is hypoxia. While it is not surprising that uterine ligation directly leads to hypoxia in the liver, maternal undernutrition alone in guinea pigs also led to increases in the expression of markers for hypoxia (EPO, EPO receptor, VEGF) in the fetal liver and kidney [35, 73]. In uterine ligation studies, decreases in oxygenation reduced hepatic mitochondrial oxidative phosphorylation further led to oxidative stress in young rat offspring [35, 47]. Collectively, this explains the increased hepatic gluconeogenesis and impaired insulin signaling exhibited in this young offspring.

Epigenetic forces have also been implicated to play a direct and sustaining role in the fetal programming of the liver. Epigenetic mechanisms, which include direct DNA methylation, posttranslational histone modifications, and microRNAs (miRs), influence the long-term expression of a gene by altering the ability of the transcriptional machinery to interact with the chromatin environment. Elegant studies in the baboon fetus have demonstrated that 70% undernutrition during pregnancy led to augmented hepatic gluconeogenesis associated with both increased Pck1 mRNA and decreases in the methylation of CpG dinucleotides of the *Pck1* promoter [59]. Moreover, uterine ligation has been shown to directly increase DNA methylation in the promoter of hepatic *Igf-1* at birth and that this persists into the F2 generation even when F1 IUGR offspring are adequately nourished [48, 74]. Interestingly, in this study, supplementation of the diet in the F1 IUGR offspring with folic acid, choline, betaine, vitamin B_{12}, and other essential nutrients prevented the methylation of the *Igf-1* promoter in the F2 generation along with symptoms of the metabolic syndrome [48]. However, caution is necessary in the overall interpretation of these studies given undernutrition-induced alterations in DNA methylation can vary between sexes and within different CpG islands of the same promoter [74].

Posttranslational histone modifications, which include methylation, acetylation, phosphorylation, ubiquitination, and ADP-ribosylation of histones, serve as another epigenetic mechanism to influence long-term gene expression by perinatal undernutrition. This is evident when maternal dietary protein is restricted during pregnancy and lactation leading to long-term hypercholesterolemia as a result of decreased expression of hepatic Cyp7a1, the critical enzyme involved in cholesterol catabolism [34]. Remarkably, the histone modifications involved in MPR-induced silencing the expression of *Cyp7a1* promoter, namely, increased trimethylation and decreased acetylation of histone H3 [lysine 9, 14], are sustained from 3 weeks to 4 months in postnatal life [34]. The origin of these histone modifications is due, in part, to MPR-mediated decreased in Jmjd2a and Jmjd2c, demethylases involved in removing trimethyl groups of histone H3 [lysine 9]. It is noteworthy that while both male and female MPR offspring exhibited decreased Cyp7a1 expression at 3 weeks, female MPR offspring at 4 months are protected from the posttranslational histone modifications silencing the *Cyp7a1* promoter. MPR has also been demonstrated to lead to long-term posttranslational histone modifications (e.g., decreased histone H3 acetylation [lysine 9, 14] silencing the expression of the hepatic liver X receptor (LXRα) at 4 months (Fig. 9.1) [67]. The decrease in the expression of this repressive glucose sensor permitted

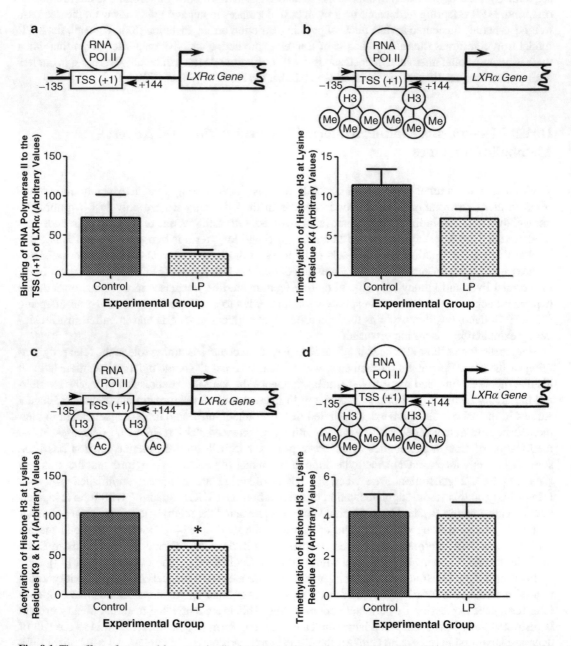

Fig. 9.1 The effect of maternal low-protein diet in utero on the in vivo transcriptional and epigenetic regulation of the *LXRα* transcriptional start site (−135 to +144 bp) at 4 months of age. (**a**) Binding of RNA polymerase II to the LXRα TSS, (**b**) trimethylation of histone H3 lysine 4, (**c**) acetylation of histone H3 lysine 9 and 14, and (**d**) trimethylation of histone H3 lysine 9. Primers were designed based on sequencing from *Ensembl*. Livers were immunoprecipitated with antibodies specific to RNA polymerase II, trimethylated histone H3 [K4], acetylated histone H3 [K9, 14], and trimethylated histone H3 [K9]. Quantification was performed using qRT-PCR (*Sso-Fast EvaGreen*) with primers specific to the proposed LXR element sites. The relative amount of immunoprecipitated genomic DNA was normalized to total genomic DNA. Data are represented as arbitrary values using the ΔΔCt method. Results are expressed as the mean ± standard error (SEM). * = Statistically significant. $n = 4$–6 (Reprinted from Vo et al. [67], with permission from BioScientifica Ltd.)

augmented expression of hepatic gluconeogenic enzymes (e.g., G6Pase and 11β-HSD1) contributing to glucose intolerance [67].

MiRs, which consist of short, noncoding RNA molecules of 20–25 nucleotides in length, can also act in an epigenetic manner to regulate gene expression by repressing the translation of proteins or decreasing messenger RNA (mRNA) stability. MPR during pregnancy and lactation has been demonstrated to increase the expression of miR-29a, miR-29b, and miR-29c in the liver by 3 weeks and 4 months of age which silences the expression of Igf-1 and decreases body weight [63]. Interestingly, protein restriction during lactation alone had a greater effect to augment the miR-29 family and suppress Igf-1, while restoration of maternal dietary proteins in MPR offspring at birth prevented miR-29 repression of Igf-1 [63]. In the guinea pig, uterine ligation in pregnancy led to decreases in hepatic miR-146a expression in the 5-month offspring, concomitant with an increase in its target profibrotic gene, SMAD4 [44]. Further studies are warranted to investigate how the expression of miRs in the liver is altered by perinatal undernutrition via direct (i.e., regulation of 5′-UTR of miR promoters) and indirect (i.e., ER stress) mechanisms [75].

Indirect Mechanisms Linking Maternal Undernutrition and Adverse Metabolic Outcomes: The Contribution of Catch-Up Growth

In several animal models of maternal undernutrition leading to metabolic disease, often the changes in hepatic gene expression do not occur directly at the time of the perinatal insult but manifests later in life [58, 64, 72]. This may be attributed to long-term global changes (e.g., epigenetic mechanisms), initiated by the perinatal environment, which precedes the eventual alterations in gene function. For example, in MPR offspring whereby increases in trimethylation of histone H3 [lysine 9] silencing the promoter of *Cyp7a1* was present in 3 week and 4 month offspring, alterations in histone methylation were not yet occurring in embryonic life [34]. However, the stage was beginning to be set as MPR-mediated decreases in the fetal expression of histone demethylases in the liver were apparent [34].

The more probable reason for indirect effects of a perinatal undernutrition and long-term alterations in hepatic gene expression is rapid postnatal catch-up growth. As previously mentioned, in humans postnatal catch-up growth can accelerate the onset and exacerbate the symptoms of metabolic disease in low birth weight children [25, 29–31]. Given the undernourished neonatal liver undergoes major catch-up growth postpartum, it is quite conceivable that the "stress" of active hepatocyte growth and replication during this period of time may confer detrimental metabolic deficits which only arise after this window of recovery. The major mechanism likely involved in this rapid growth-triggered process is endoplasmic reticulum (ER) stress.

ER stress occurs when perturbation in the function or homeostasis of the ER leads to luminal accumulation of misfolded or unfolded proteins. Many known triggers of ER stress include impaired disulfide bond formation, compromised Ca^{2+} homeostasis, low amino acids, hypoxia, decreased N-linked glycosylation, increased lipid load, and greater oxidative stress. In response to ER stress, the unfolded protein response (UPR) tries to restore ER homeostasis by attenuating protein translation (i.e., increased pEIF2α) while at the same time increasing the expression of chaperone proteins involved in refolding proteins to alleviate the ER. However, if ER stress persists, apoptosis is initiated leading to alterations in gene expression and cell function. In MPR offspring with postnatal catch-up growth (due to restoration of proteins at weaning), the livers at 4 months exhibit ER stress (i.e., increased pEIF2α) attributed to impaired insulin sensitivity (e.g., decreased pAkt1[Ser473]) despite the fact that the food intake is similar (Fig. 9.2, *LP2*) [63, 64]. Conversely, if there is no catch-up growth, protein translation is enhanced with higher hepatic insulin sensitivity (Fig. 9.2, *LP1*) [64]. The low-protein diet itself does not appear to be playing a direct role given alterations in the ER stress pathway were not detected in the fetal liver. Given oxidative stress is present in the undernourished liver, and that the "mismatch" in the nutritional environment likely leads to lipid overload and/or

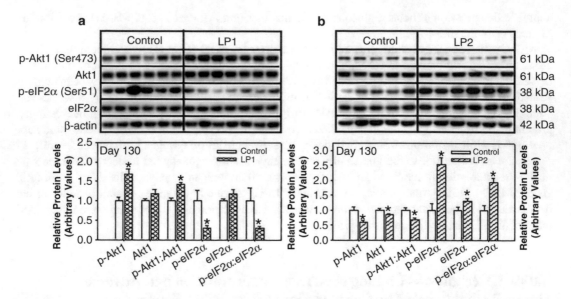

Fig. 9.2 The effect of maternal low-protein dietary regimes on hepatic phosphorylated eIF2α (Ser51) protein levels at 4 months of age. The effect of (**a**) LP1 (low protein all life) and (**b**) LP2 (low-protein pregnancy and lactation) dietary regimes on phosphorylated protein kinase B (Akt1) at serine 473, Akt1, phosphorylated eukaryotic initiation factor 2 α (eIF2α) at serine 51, and eIF2α protein levels in the livers of male offspring at postnatal day 130. Relative p-Akt1 (S473), Akt1, p-eIF2α (S51), and eIF2α protein levels were determined using Western blot analysis. Total protein was isolated and p-Akt1 (S473), Akt1, p-eIF2α (S51), and eIF2α protein were detected on a Western blot using p-Akt1 (S473), Akt1, p-eIF2α (S51), and eIF2α primary antibody. Their protein levels were quantified using densitometry and normalized to that of β-actin protein levels. Results were expressed as the mean ± SEM. *, significant difference ($P < 0.05$); $n = 5$–6 for control and $n = 6$–7 for LP1 and LP2 group, where each n represents a single offspring derived from a different mother (Reprinted from Sohi et al. [64], with permission from Elsevier Ltd.)

impaired disulfide bond formation, it is apparent that these triggers during perinatal life, coupled with postnatal catch-up growth, may initiate the cascade leading to chronic ER stress [35, 47]. It is noteworthy that in a perinatal rat model of nicotine exposure leading to postnatal catch-up growth and dyslipidemia, ER stress was also evident in the adipose tissue of 6-month offspring [76]. Aside from directly influencing hepatic gene expression and function, augmented ER stress in the liver may also alter epigenetic mechanisms such as miRs. For example, activation of ER stress has been demonstrated to induce miR-29a which is known to silence Igf-1 and pAkt-1 (Ser473) [75]. It is noteworthy that miR-29a is increased in 4-month MPR offspring with catch-up growth and ER stress, coupled with decreased Igf-1 an pAkt-1 (Ser473) [63, 64]. An overview of the direct and indirect mechanism involved in the nutritional programming of the perinatal liver is illustrated in Fig. 9.3.

The "Plastic Liver": Intervening in Early Life to Prevent Long-Term Metabolic Dysfunction

From fetal to neonatal life, the liver undergoes extensive growth, differentiation, and remodeling creating an ideal window for intervention given its plasticity. During fetal life, the liver is considered mainly hematopoietic, while in postnatal life is considered more hepatocyte-like [77]. This may explain why certain perinatal nutritional insults altering postnatal gene expression are differentially altered in fetal life [67, 72]. By mid-gestation in rodents, the liver bud is formed containing progenitor cells that differentiate into either hepatocytes or ductal cells; however, in the last 3 days of gestation,

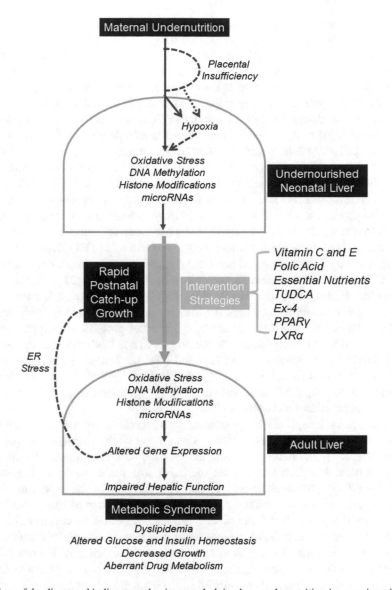

Fig. 9.3 Overview of the direct and indirect mechanisms underlying how undernutrition in utero impairs liver function from neonatal to adult life. Direct pathways altered by maternal undernutrition are indicated by *red solid arrows*, while indirect pathways affected by placental insufficiency and postnatal catch-up growth are indicated by *red dashed arrows*. Neonatal intervention strategies are illustrated in *cyan arrows*

the liver mass triples due to extensive proliferation [78, 79]. After birth in rodents, there is a greater transition from fetal to adult hepatocytes accompanied by high rates of replication, neogenesis, and apoptosis [79]. The human liver develops in a similar pattern, although the majority of liver differentiation occurs in prenatal life [80]. It is estimated that the postnatal rodent liver at 3 weeks is equivalent to the human liver at the third trimester. Regardless of the species, the perinatal liver is undergoing extensive remodeling and is subject to alterations by environmental cues during this period. These cues can consist of alterations in nutrition, hormones/cell signaling, epigenetic forces, and/or by the actions of pharmaceuticals.

From a nutrition standpoint, several studies have investigated the role of vitamins, folic acid, and proteins to reverse the effects of undernutrition on hepatic health. In a rodent model of maternal diabetes leading to IUGR and decreased liver weight, supplementation of vitamins C and E in pregnancy prevented decreases in fetal liver weight, but not total bodyweight [81]. The IUGR-associated lipid peroxidation in these fetal livers was also significantly reduced due to maternal vitamin supplementation attributed to increases in superoxide dismutase antioxidant activity [81]. Given its role a methyl donor for DNA methylation, intervention studies with folic acid show promise in reversing some of the epigenetic mechanisms associated with the undernourished liver. Elegant studies by Lillycrop demonstrated that administration of folic acid during MPR pregnancy reversed the decreases in DNA methylation to the promoters of *PPARα* and *GR* and subsequently diminished the MPR increases in their fetal gene expression [82, 83]. But with respect to DNA methylation, the benefits of folic acid appear to be promoter specific given periconceptional intake of folic acid (400 μg/day) led to an increase in DNA methylation of hepatic insulin growth-like factor 2 and, subsequently, low birth weight [84]. As mentioned previously, introduction of a combination of nutrients (i.e., folic acid, vitamin B_{12}) to the diet of IUGR offspring has multigenerational effects given the F2 generation did not exhibit impairments in hepatic and lipid homeostasis [48]. The use of the bile acid tauroursodeoxycholic acid (TUDCA) could be considered as a promising safe therapeutic agent in neonatal life given its ability to reduce ER stress (e.g., promote protein refolding) and consequentially improve liver insulin sensitivity [85]. With regard to protein supplementation, the beneficial effects of restoring maternal proteins also appear to be very promoter specific in the liver. In rats, restoring maternal proteins at birth prevents long-term decreases in hepatic cholesterol metabolism (e.g., Cyp7a1) and Igf-1 but leads to greater expression of genes involved in gluconeogenesis (e.g., G6Pase and 11β-HSD1) [34, 63, 67]. These studies illustrate the complexity between the length of the nutritional insult, epigenetics, and catch-up growth on long-term hepatic gene expression and function.

Hormones and nuclear receptors have promise in reversing the adverse effects of undernutrition on hepatic dysfunction. One of the best examples is with the use of the glucagon-like peptide-1 (Glp-1) analog, exendin-4 (Ex-4). Neonatal administration of Ex-4 to uterine-ligated IUGR offspring prevented the long-term development of hepatic oxidative stress and insulin resistance [47]. It also exerted beneficial effects on the pancreatic β cells via increases in the expression of Pdx-1 [86]. Another hormone and antioxidant, melatonin, has been demonstrated to increase umbilical blood flow during gestation in sheep, but it did not rescue growth restriction in undernourished ewes [87]. Targeting nuclear receptors may have a more sustained impact given their widespread roles in influencing endocrine function along with glucose and lipid homeostasis. Female IUGR offspring treated with agonists to the lipid-sensing nuclear receptor PPARγ have long-term insulin-sensitizing effects, although hypoglycemia was also exhibited [88]. Given the role of the liver X receptor (LXRα) in regulating cholesterol, glucose, and fatty acid homeostasis, altering LXR activity in early life could impair several symptoms of the metabolic syndrome. A pilot study using the LXR agonist (GW3695) during neonatal life (PND5-15) in MPR offspring led to ameliorated total cholesterol levels concomitant with increased LXRα and Cyp7a1 by 3 weeks of age [89]. An overview of the known neonatal interventions is summarized in Fig. 9.3.

Regardless of the success of particular intervention strategies in animal models, caution must be approached in assessing its overall efficacy. The intervention must be examined in the context of the species examined and how the timing of intervention relates to liver development (e.g., plasticity) between species. The impact of the intervention on epigenetic mechanisms must also be considered to determine its sustainability long-term but, more importantly, on the specificity (or lack thereof) to particular target promoters. For the time being, the safer approach may be in general dietary implementation to reduce catch-up growth and the indirect burden it exerts on hepatic development and function.

Conclusion

In response to maternal undernutrition and placental insufficiency, the fetal liver takes a huge hit with respect to development and growth. Consequentially, the undernourished neonatal liver has the most to gain in postnatal life leading to accelerated catch-up growth. However, both developmental events end up being detrimental to long-term liver function. The present review illustrates the direct epigenetic mechanisms underlying the aberrant expression of hepatic genes in malnourished offspring which persists into adulthood. Hypoxia in the neonatal liver also plays a role in driving some of these epigenetic mechanisms along with increased oxidative stress. With ensuing rapid catch-up growth in postnatal life, this places a burden on the normal growth trajectory of the liver leading to onset of ER stress. This culminates in further metabolic dysfunction such as ER-mediated insulin insensitivity in the liver. In this chapter, nutritional, hormonal, and pharmaceutical interventions early in life are cited which mitigate the effects of undernutrition on hepatic gene expression and function short- and long-term. However, further studies are warranted to address the safety, specificity, and sustainability of these interventions to the whole organism. Until that time, more conventional nutritional steps are necessary to reduce postnatal catch-up growth of IUGR offspring in the hope to reduce global effects (e.g., ER stress) on the recovering liver.

References

1. Wilson PW, D'Agostino RB, Levy D, Belanger AM, Silbershatz H, Kannel WB. Prediction of coronary heart disease using risk factor categories. Circulation. 1998;97(18):1837–47.
2. Mathieu P, Pibarot P, Despres JP. Metabolic syndrome: the danger signal in atherosclerosis. Vasc Health Risk Manag. 2006;2(3):285–302.
3. Writing Group Members, Lloyd-Jones D, Adams RJ, Brown TM, Carnethon M, Dai S, et al. Heart disease and stroke statistics – 2010 update: a report from the American Heart Association. Circulation. 2010;121(7):e46–215.
4. Lamarche B, Lemieux S, Dagenais GR, Despres JP. Visceral obesity and the risk of ischaemic heart disease: insights from the Quebec Cardiovascular Study. Growth Hormon IGF Res Off J Growth Horm Res Soc Int Res Soc. 1998;8(Suppl B(Journal Article)):1–8.
5. Schocken DD, Benjamin EJ, Fonarow GC, Krumholz HM, Levy D, Mensah GA, et al. Prevention of heart failure: a scientific statement from the American Heart Association Councils on Epidemiology and Prevention, Clinical Cardiology, Cardiovascular Nursing, and High Blood Pressure Research; Quality of Care and Outcomes Research Interdisciplinary Working Group; and Functional Genomics and Translational Biology Interdisciplinary Working Group. Circulation. 2008;117(19):2544–65.
6. Lloyd-Jones D, Adams RJ, Brown TM, Carnethon M, Dai S, De Simone G, et al. Executive summary: heart disease and stroke statistics – 2010 update: a report from the American Heart Association. Circulation. 2010;121(7):948–54.
7. Mehal WZ, Iredale J, Friedman SL. Scraping fibrosis: expressway to the core of fibrosis. Nat Med. 2011;17(5):552–3.
8. Henderson NC, Iredale JP. Liver fibrosis: cellular mechanisms of progression and resolution. Clin Sci Lond Engl 1979. 2007;112(5):265–80.
9. McCullough AJ. The clinical features, diagnosis and natural history of nonalcoholic fatty liver disease. Clin Liver Dis. 2004;8(3):521–33. viii.
10. Ekstedt M, Franzén LE, Mathiesen UL, Thorelius L, Holmqvist M, Bodemar G, et al. Long-term follow-up of patients with NAFLD and elevated liver enzymes. Hepatol Baltim Md. 2006;44(4):865–73.
11. Bhaskar ME. Management of cirrhosis and ascites. N Engl J Med. 2004;351(3):300–1. author reply 300–1.
12. Kohli R, Kirby M, Xanthakos SA, Softic S, Feldstein AE, Saxena V, et al. High-fructose, medium chain trans fat diet induces liver fibrosis and elevates plasma coenzyme Q9 in a novel murine model of obesity and nonalcoholic steatohepatitis. Hepatol Baltim Md. 2010;52(3):934–44.
13. Ishimoto T, Lanaspa MA, Rivard CJ, Roncal-Jimenez CA, Orlicky DJ, Cicerchi C, et al. High-fat and high-sucrose (western) diet induces steatohepatitis that is dependent on fructokinase. Hepatol Baltim Md. 2013;58(5):1632–43.
14. Nordestgaard BG, Benn M, Schnohr P, Tybjaerg-Hansen A. Nonfasting triglycerides and risk of myocardial infarction, ischemic heart disease, and death in men and women. JAMA J Am Med Assoc. 2007;298(3):299–308.
15. Bansal S, Buring JE, Rifai N, Mora S, Sacks FM, Ridker PM. Fasting compared with nonfasting triglycerides and risk of cardiovascular events in women. JAMA J Am Med Assoc. 2007;298(3):309–16.

16. Law MR, Wald NJ, Rudnicka AR. Quantifying effect of statins on low density lipoprotein cholesterol, ischaemic heart disease, and stroke: systematic review and meta-analysis. BMJ. 2003;326(7404):1423.
17. Barker DJ. The fetal and infant origins of adult disease. BMJ. 1990;301(6761):1111.
18. Barker DJ, Martyn CN, Osmond C, Hales CN, Fall CH. Growth in utero and serum cholesterol concentrations in adult life. BMJ. 1993;307(6918):1524–7.
19. Valsamakis G, Kanaka-Gantenbein C, Malamitsi-Puchner A, Mastorakos G. Causes of intrauterine growth restriction and the postnatal development of the metabolic syndrome. Ann N Y Acad Sci. 2006;1092:138–47.
20. Neerhof MG. Causes of intrauterine growth restriction. Clin Perinatol. 1995;22(2):375–85.
21. Ravelli GP, Stein ZA, Susser MW. Obesity in young men after famine exposure in utero and early infancy. N Engl J Med. 1976;295(7):349–53.
22. Desai M, Hales CN. Role of fetal and infant growth in programming metabolism in later life. Biol Rev Camb Philos Soc. 1997;72(2):329–48.
23. Hales CN, Barker DJ, Clark PM, Cox LJ, Fall C, Osmond C, et al. Fetal and infant growth and impaired glucose tolerance at age 64. BMJ. 1991;303(6809):1019–22.
24. McCance DR, Pettitt DJ, Hanson RL, Jacobsson LT, Knowler WC, Bennett PH. Birth weight and non-insulin dependent diabetes: thrifty genotype, thrifty phenotype, or surviving small baby genotype? BMJ. 1994;308(6934):942–5.
25. Finken MJ, Inderson A, Van Montfoort N, Keijzer-Veen MG, van Weert AW, Carfil N, et al. Lipid profile and carotid intima-media thickness in a prospective cohort of very preterm subjects at age 19 years: effects of early growth and current body composition. Pediatr Res. 2006;59(4 Pt 1):604–9.
26. Ravelli AC, van der Meulen JH, Michels RP, Osmond C, Barker DJ, Hales CN, et al. Glucose tolerance in adults after prenatal exposure to famine. Lancet. 1998;351(9097):173–7.
27. Forsdahl A. Living conditions in childhood and subsequent development of risk factors for arteriosclerotic heart disease. The cardiovascular survey in Finnmark 1974-75. J Epidemiol Community Health. 1978;32(1):34–7.
28. Yudkin JS, Stanner S. Prenatal exposure to famine and health in later life. Lancet. 1998;351(9112):1361–2.
29. Yajnik C. Interactions of perturbations in intrauterine growth and growth during childhood on the risk of adult-onset disease. Proc Nutr Soc. 2000;59(2):257–65.
30. Eriksson JG. Early growth, and coronary heart disease and type 2 diabetes: experiences from the Helsinki Birth Cohort studies. Int J Obes 2005. 2006;30(Suppl 4(Journal Article)):S18–22.
31. Martin RM, McCarthy A, Smith GD, Davies DP, Ben-Shlomo Y. Infant nutrition and blood pressure in early adulthood: the Barry Caerphilly growth study. Am J Clin Nutr. 2003;77(6):1489–97.
32. Hales CN, Barker DJ. Type 2 (non-insulin-dependent) diabetes mellitus: the thrifty phenotype hypothesis. Diabetologia. 1992;35(7):595–601.
33. Hales CN, Barker DJ. The thrifty phenotype hypothesis. Br Med Bull. 2001;60(Journal Article):5–20.
34. Sohi G, Marchand K, Revesz A, Arany E, Hardy DB. Maternal protein restriction elevates cholesterol in adult rat offspring due to repressive changes in histone modifications at the cholesterol 7alpha-hydroxylase promoter. Mol Endocrinol Baltim Md. 2011;25(5):785–98.
35. Peterside IE, Selak MA, Simmons RA. Impaired oxidative phosphorylation in hepatic mitochondria in growth-retarded rats. Am J Physiol Endocrinol Metab. 2003;285(6):E1258–66.
36. Nevin CMY, Matushewski B, Regnault TRH, Richardson BS. Maternal nutrient restriction (MNR) in guinea pigs leads to fetal growth restricted (FGR) offspring with differential rates of organ catch-up growth. Reprod Sci. 2016;23:149A.
37. Deiber M, Chatelain P, Naville D, Putet G, Salle B. Functional hypersomatotropism in small for gestational age (SGA) newborn infants. J Clin Endocrinol Metab. 1989;68(1):232–4.
38. Singhal A, Cole TJ, Fewtrell M, Lucas A. Breastmilk feeding and lipoprotein profile in adolescents born preterm: follow-up of a prospective randomised study. Lancet. 2004;363(9421):1571–8.
39. Jaquet D, Gaboriau A, Czernichow P, Levy-Marchal C. Insulin resistance early in adulthood in subjects born with intrauterine growth retardation. J Clin Endocrinol Metab. 2000;85(4):1401–6.
40. Ross MG, Beall MH. Prediction of preterm birth: nonsonographic cervical methods. Semin Perinatol. 2009;33(5):312–6.
41. Murotsuki J, Challis JR, Han VK, Fraher LJ, Gagnon R. Chronic fetal placental embolization and hypoxemia cause hypertension and myocardial hypertrophy in fetal sheep. Am J Phys. 1997;272(1 Pt 2):R201–7.
42. Ogata ES, Bussey ME, Finley S. Altered gas exchange, limited glucose and branched chain amino acids, and hypo-insulinism retard fetal growth in the rat. Metabolism. 1986;35(10):970–7.
43. Simmons RA, Gounis AS, Bangalore SA, Ogata ES. Intrauterine growth retardation: fetal glucose transport is diminished in lung but spared in brain. Pediatr Res. 1992;31(1):59–63.
44. Sarr O, Blake A, Thompson JA, Zhao L, Rabicki K, Walsh JC, et al. The differential effects of low birth weight and western diet consumption upon early life hepatic fibrosis development in guinea pig. J Physiol. 2015;594(6):1753–72.
45. Lane RH, Kelley DE, Gruetzmacher EM, Devaskar SU. Uteroplacental insufficiency alters hepatic fatty acid-metabolizing enzymes in juvenile and adult rats. Am J Phys Regul Integr Comp Phys. 2001;280(1):R183–90.

46. Simmons RA, Templeton LJ, Gertz SJ. Intrauterine growth retardation leads to the development of type 2 diabetes in the rat. Diabetes. 2001;50(10):2279–86.
47. Raab EL, Vuguin PM, Stoffers DA, Simmons RA. Neonatal exendin-4 treatment reduces oxidative stress and prevents hepatic insulin resistance in intrauterine growth-retarded rats. Am J Phys Regul Integr Comp Phys. 2009;297(6):R1785–94.
48. Goodspeed D, Seferovic MD, Holland W, Mcknight RA, Summers SA, Branch DW, et al. Essential nutrient supplementation prevents heritable metabolic disease in multigenerational intrauterine growth-restricted rats. FASEB J Off Publ Fed Am Soc Exp Biol. 2015;29(3):807–19.
49. Baserga M, Hale MA, McKnight RA, Yu X, Callaway CW, Lane RH. Uteroplacental insufficiency alters hepatic expression, phosphorylation, and activity of the glucocorticoid receptor in fetal IUGR rats. Am J Phys Regul Integr Comp Phys. 2005;289(5):R1348–53.
50. Lane RH, Crawford SE, Flozak AS, Simmons RA. Localization and quantification of glucose transporters in liver of growth-retarded fetal and neonatal rats. Am J Phys. 1999;276(1 Pt 1):E135–42.
51. Lane RH, MacLennan NK, Hsu JL, Janke SM, Pham TD. Increased hepatic peroxisome proliferator-activated receptor-gamma coactivator-1 gene expression in a rat model of intrauterine growth retardation and subsequent insulin resistance. Endocrinology. 2002;143(7):2486–90.
52. Fu Q, Yu X, Callaway CW, Lane RH, McKnight RA. Epigenetics: intrauterine growth retardation (IUGR) modifies the histone code along the rat hepatic IGF-1 gene. FASEB J Off Publ Fed Am Soc Exp Biol. 2009;23(8):2438–49.
53. Zinkhan EK, Chin JR, Zalla JM, Yu B, Numpang B, Yu X, et al. Combination of intrauterine growth restriction and a high-fat diet impairs cholesterol elimination in rats. Pediatr Res. 2014;76(5):432–40.
54. Zhang J, Lewis RM, Wang C, Hales N, Byrne CD. Maternal dietary iron restriction modulates hepatic lipid metabolism in the fetuses. Am J Physiol Integr Comp Physiol. 2005;288(1):R104–11.
55. Elias AA, Ghaly A, Matushewski B, Regnault TRH, Richardson BS. Maternal nutrient restriction in guinea pigs as an animal model for inducing fetal growth restriction. Reprod Sci. 2016;23(2):219–27.
56. Lumey LH. Compensatory placental growth after restricted maternal nutrition in early pregnancy. Placenta. 1998;19(1):105–11.
57. Sohlström A, Katsman A, Kind KL, Roberts CT, Owens PC, Robinson JS, et al. Food restriction alters pregnancy-associated changes in IGF and IGFBP in the guinea pig. Am J Phys. 1998;274(3 Pt 1):E410–6.
58. Tosh DN, Fu Q, Callaway CW, McKnight RA, McMillen IC, Ross MG, et al. Epigenetics of programmed obesity: alteration in IUGR rat hepatic IGF1 mRNA expression and histone structure in rapid vs. delayed postnatal catch-up growth. Am J Physiol Gastrointest Liver Physiol. 2010;299(5):G1023–9.
59. Nijland MJ, Mitsuya K, Li C, Ford S, McDonald TJ, Nathanielsz PW, et al. Epigenetic modification of fetal baboon hepatic phosphoenolpyruvate carboxykinase following exposure to moderately reduced nutrient availability. J Physiol. 2010;588(Pt 8):1349–59.
60. George LA, Zhang L, Tuersunjiang N, Ma Y, Long NM, Uthlaut AB, et al. Early maternal undernutrition programs increased feed intake, altered glucose metabolism and insulin secretion, and liver function in aged female offspring. Am J Phys Regul Integr Comp Phys. 2012;302(7):R795–804.
61. Petry CJ, Ozanne SE, Hales CN. Programming of intermediary metabolism. Mol Cell Endocrinol. 2001;185(1–2):81–91.
62. Crosby WM. Studies in fetal malnutrition. Am J Dis Child 1960. 1991;145(8):871–6.
63. Sohi G, Revesz A, Ramkumar J, Hardy DB. Higher hepatic miR-29 expression in undernourished male rats during the postnatal period targets the long-term repression of IGF-1. Endocrinology. 2015;156(9):3069–76.
64. Sohi G, Revesz A, Hardy DB. Nutritional mismatch in postnatal life of low birth weight rat offspring leads to increased phosphorylation of hepatic eukaryotic initiation factor 2 α in adulthood. Metabolism. 2013;62(10):1367–74.
65. Guan H, Arany E, van Beek JP, Chamson-Reig A, Thyssen S, Hill DJ, et al. Adipose tissue gene expression profiling reveals distinct molecular pathways that define visceral adiposity in offspring of maternal protein-restricted rats. Am J Physiol Metab. 2005;288(4):E663–73.
66. Petrik J, Reusens B, Arany E, Remacle C, Coelho C, Hoet JJ, et al. A low protein diet alters the balance of islet cell replication and apoptosis in the fetal and neonatal rat and is associated with a reduced pancreatic expression of insulin-like growth factor-II. Endocrinology. 1999;140(10):4861–73.
67. Vo T, Revesz A, Ma N, Hardy DB. Maternal protein restriction leads to enhanced hepatic gluconeogenic gene expression in adult male rat offspring due to impaired expression of the liver x receptor. J Endocrinol. 2013;218(Journal Article):85–97.
68. Chamson-Reig A, Thyssen SM, Hill DJ, Arany E. Exposure of the pregnant rat to low protein diet causes impaired glucose homeostasis in the young adult offspring by different mechanisms in males and females. Exp Biol Med Maywood NJ. 2009;234(12):1425–36.
69. Petry CJ, Ozanne SE, Wang CL, Hales CN. Early protein restriction and obesity independently induce hypertension in 1-year-old rats. Clin Sci Lond Engl 1979. 1997;93(2):147–52.
70. Burns SP, Desai M, Cohen RD, Hales CN, Iles RA, Germain JP, et al. Gluconeogenesis, glucose handling, and structural changes in livers of the adult offspring of rats partially deprived of protein during pregnancy and lactation. J Clin Invest. 1997;100(7):1768–74.

71. Ozanne SE, Smith GD, Tikerpae J, Hales CN. Altered regulation of hepatic glucose output in the male offspring of protein-malnourished rat dams. Am J Phys. 1996;270(4 Pt 1):E559–64.
72. Sohi G, Barry EJ, Velenosi TJ, Urquhart BL, Hardy DB. Protein restoration in low-birth-weight rat offspring derived from maternal low-protein diet leads to elevated hepatic CYP3A and CYP2C11 activity in adulthood. Drug Metab Dispos Biol Fate Chem. 2014;42(2):221–8.
73. Elias AA, Maki B, Matushewski B, Nygard K, Regnault TRH, Richardson BS. Maternal nutrient restriction in guinea pigs leads to fetal growth restriction with evidence for chronic hypoxia. Pediatric Res. 2017; in press; doi:10.1038/pr.2017.92.
74. Fu Q, McKnight RA, Callaway CW, Yu X, Lane RH, Majnik AV. Intrauterine growth restriction disrupts developmental epigenetics around distal growth hormone response elements on the rat hepatic IGF-1 gene. FASEB J Off Publ Fed Am Soc Exp Biol. 2015;29(4):1176–84.
75. Nolan K, Walter F, Tuffy LP, Poeschel S, Gallager R, Haunsberger S, Bray I, Stallings RL, Concannon CG, Prehn HM. Endoplasmic reticulum stress-mediated upregulation of miR-29a enhances sensitivity to neuronal apoptosis. Eur J Neurosci. 2016;43:640–52.
76. Barra NG, VanDuzer T, Holloway AC, Hardy DB. Maternal nicotine exposure (MNE) leads to decreased visceral adipocyte size associated with endoplasmic reticulum (ER) stress in 26 week old rat offspring. Reprod Sci. 2016; 23:314A.
77. Gualdi R, Bossard P, Zheng M, Hamada Y, Coleman JR, Zaret KS. Hepatic specification of the gut endoderm in vitro: cell signaling and transcriptional control. Genes Dev. 1996;10(13):1670–82.
78. Cascio S, Zaret KS. Hepatocyte differentiation initiates during endodermal-mesenchymal interactions prior to liver formation. Dev Camb Engl. 1991;113(1):217–25.
79. Greengard O, Federman M, Knox WE. Cytomorphometry of developing rat liver and its application to enzymic differentiation. J Cell Biol. 1972;52(2):261–72.
80. Kung JWC, Currie IS, Forbes SJ, Ross JA. Liver development, regeneration, and carcinogenesis. J Biomed Biotechnol. 2010;2010:984248.
81. Ornoy A, Tsadok MA, Yaffe P, Zangen SW. The Cohen diabetic rat as a model for fetal growth restriction: vitamins C and E reduce fetal oxidative stress but do not restore normal growth. Reprod Toxicol Elmsford N. 2009;28(4):521–9.
82. Lillycrop KA, Phillips ES, Jackson AA, Hanson MA, Burdge GC. Dietary protein restriction of pregnant rats induces and folic acid supplementation prevents epigenetic modification of hepatic gene expression in the offspring. J Nutr. 2005;135(6):1382–6.
83. Lillycrop KA, Rodford J, Garratt ES, Slater-Jefferies JL, Godfrey KM, Gluckman PD, et al. Maternal protein restriction with or without folic acid supplementation during pregnancy alters the hepatic transcriptome in adult male rats. Br J Nutr. 2010;103(12):1711–9.
84. Steegers-Theunissen RP, Obermann-Borst SA, Kremer D, Lindemans J, Siebel C, Steegers EA, et al. Periconceptional maternal folic acid use of 400 microg per day is related to increased methylation of the IGF2 gene in the very young child. PLoS One. 2009;4(11):e7845.
85. Kars M, Yang L, Gregor MF, Mohammed BS, Pietka TA, Finck BN, et al. Tauroursodeoxycholic acid may improve liver and muscle but not adipose tissue insulin sensitivity in obese men and women. Diabetes. 2010;59(8):1899–905.
86. Pinney SE, Jaeckle Santos LJ, Han Y, Stoffers DA, Simmons RA. Exendin-4 increases histone acetylase activity and reverses epigenetic modifications that silence Pdx1 in the intrauterine growth retarded rat. Diabetologia. 2011;54(10):2606–14.
87. Lemley CO, Meyer AM, Camacho LE, Neville TL, Newman DJ, Caton JS, et al. Melatonin supplementation alters uteroplacental hemodynamics and fetal development in an ovine model of intrauterine growth restriction. Am J Physiol Integr Comp Physiol. 2012;302(4):R454–67.
88. Garg M, Thamotharan M, Pan G, Lee PW, Devaskar SU. Early exposure of the pregestational intrauterine and postnatal growth-restricted female offspring to a peroxisome proliferator-activated receptor-{gamma} agonist. Am J Physiol Metab. 2010;298(3):E489–98.
89. Sohi G, Revesz A, Arany E, Hardy DB. The liver X receptor mediates the impaired cholesterol metabolism exhibited in the offspring of maternal protein restricted rats. Reprod Sci. 2011;18(4):F163.

Chapter 10
Maternal Protein Restriction and Its Effects on Heart

Heloisa Balan Assalin, José Antonio Rocha Gontijo, and Patrícia Aline Boer

Key Points

- Intrauterine environment, mainly maternal nutritional status, represents a predictive factor for adult hypertension and cardiovascular disease.
- Protein restriction in pregnancy is associated with intrauterine growth restriction, which implies in low birth weight, hypertension development, and higher cardiovascular risk in adulthood.
- Cardiovascular disease might be secondary to several alterations that occur due to gestational protein restriction such as progressive increase in blood pressure, altered hypothalamic-pituitary-adrenal axis, insulin resistance, and enhanced baseline sympathetic activity;
- Gestational protein restriction induces morphological primary changes in the heart, which might predispose to cardiovascular dysfunction later in life.
- Impaired cardiomyocyte proliferation and differentiation, with reduced cardiomyocyte number, altered expression of structural proteins and increased interstitial fibrosis could progressively result in cardiovascular dysfunction in adulthood.

Keywords Fetal programming • Maternal protein restriction • Intrauterine growth restriction • Heart development • Cardiovascular disease

Abbreviations

CVD   Cardiovascular disease
HPA   Hypothalamic-pituitary-adrenal axis
IUGR   Intrauterine growth restriction
LP   Low protein
LPD   Low-protein diet
LVMI   Left ventricular mass index
NP   Normal protein
TIMP-2   Tissue inhibitor of metalloprotease 2
US   United States

H.B. Assalin, BSc, PhD • J.A.R. Gontijo, MD, PhD • P.A. Boer, BSc, PhD (✉)
Department of Internal Medicine, Faculty of Medical Sciences at University of Campinas, Campinas, SP, Brazil
e-mail: alineboer@yahoo.com.br; boer@fcm.unicamp.br

© Springer International Publishing AG 2017
R. Rajendram et al. (eds.), *Diet, Nutrition, and Fetal Programming*,
Nutrition and Health, DOI 10.1007/978-3-319-60289-9_10

Introduction

Cardiovascular diseases (CVD) are the first cause of death in the world, and over three quarters of CVD deaths take place in low- and middle-income countries. In 2012, an estimated 17.5 million people died from CVDs, representing 31% of all global deaths [1].

It is well known that the etiology of CVD is related to genetic factors; postnatal environmental and behavioral risk factors such as unhealthy diet, physical inactivity, tobacco use; and harmful use of alcohol. However, more recently, attention has also focused on environment experienced in utero as a factor predictive of later hypertension and CVD [2].

It has been widely accepted that the major programming influence upon the fetus is maternal nutritional status [3]. Protein restriction in pregnancy is related to low birth weight or disproportion of the fetus (thinness or shortness to head circumference) at birth, a marker of intrauterine growth restriction (IUGR) [4]. As gestational malnutrition (caloric and protein) causes IUGR, we could expect that poor countries were the hardest hit by the effects of fetal programming; however, the US population is subject to "high calorie malnutrition" by choosing more palatable food to the detriment of those with higher amounts of nutrients [5]. Thus, the prevalence of chronic diseases that represent risk factors for cardiovascular diseases such as obesity, diabetes, and hypertension is growing (Fig. 10.1). IUGR affects up to 7–10% of pregnancies and is the major cause of perinatal mortality and long-term morbidity, being a high relevant condition [6, 7].

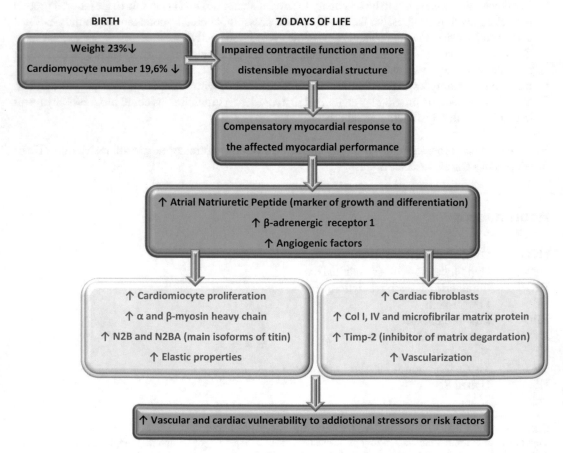

Fig. 10.1 Structural and functional cardiovascular changes that might reflect primary programmed events during organogenesis. Gestational low-protein programmed offspring were termed LP, and offspring from normal protein dams were termed NP. At birth, cardiomyocytes number reduction was observed [30], and after 70 days (no hypertension, no hypercholesterolemia, and no atherosclerosis), compensatory hyperplasia and enhanced content of stromal structures were observed [25, 34]

Epidemiological Evidences

Several epidemiological studies have demonstrated the association between small size at birth and CVD and its biological risk factors in Europe [8], North America [9], and India [10].

Reduced growth in fetal life and small birth weight, along with accelerated growth in childhood, result in greater risk of coronary heart disease in adult life [10, 11]. Furthermore, it is associated with an increased risk of hypertension and noninsulin-dependent diabetes, two disorders closely linked to CVD [10–12].

The Dutch famine (1944–1945) allowed the study of gestation undernutrition effects on humans. People who had been exposed to famine in any stage of gestation had reduced glucose tolerance [13]. Conversely, people exposed to famine in early gestation had a more atherogenic lipid profile, disturbed blood coagulation, increased stress responsiveness, obesity [13], and a higher risk of CVD [14].

Mechanisms of Programed Risk to CVD

Epidemiological studies are strongly supported by animal models, which attempt to investigate the possible change-related mechanisms in cardiac physiology of protein-restricted animals. Langley-Evans et al. were among the first to show that prenatal nutritional environment could have a powerful impact on cardiovascular function in the offspring in an animal model [12]. These authors have used synthetic diets containing 18% or 9% of casein during rat gestation, and systolic blood pressures of male and female pups were significantly enhanced at the age of 4 weeks [12]. Thus, these and other animal models have been used to understand the possible mechanisms involved in programming.

Several possible mechanisms by which nutritional restriction during gestation might lead to CVD are related to reduced fetal growth followed by accelerated weight gain in childhood if exists incompatibility between intra- and extra-uterine supply of nutrients.

Small babies and low-protein restricted rat offspring have reduced nephron number [15, 16]. It has been suggested that this leads to hyperperfusion of each nephron due to the increased blood flow through each glomerulus, which may lead to early development of glomerulosclerosis in adult life. Rapid childhood growth is thought to increase hyperperfusion. Normal aging brings glomeruli loss and results in accelerated age-related glomeruli loss and a self-perpetuating cycle of rising blood pressure and glomerular loss [17].

However, the mechanisms underlying the programming of hypertension by maternal undernutrition are likely to be multifactorial and complex. In addition to the influences of intrauterine undernutrition on nephrogenesis, which may underlie the programming of hypertension, fetal exposure to an excess of glucocorticoid appears to be a critical step in programming of hypertension [18]. Furthermore, low birth weight and nutrient availability have been associated with numerous endocrine changes later in life [19, 20] and programming of the hypothalamic-pituitary-adrenal axis (HPA) [21], which themselves may influence cardiovascular risk.

In fact, a number of studies support that the relationship between cardiovascular risk and low birth weight might be explained in part by fetal metabolic programming leading to diseases associated with cardiovascular disease. Babies with low birth weight have reduced muscle tissue due to lower cell replication during intrauterine development. In case of excessive and rapid weight gain in childhood, these children are liable to put on fat rather than muscle, leading to a disproportionately high fat mass in later life. This might be associated with the development of insulin resistance [22].

Barker et al. suggest that another mechanism linking poor weight gain in gestation and infancy with CVD is altered liver function, which reflects on raised plasma fibrinogen and factor VII concentration [23].

Furthermore, Alves et al. suggested that juvenile offspring from protein restricted dams exhibit enhanced baseline sympathetic activity [24]. β-adrenergic pathways are often activated to maintain an appropriate cardiac output which could explain the augmented myocardial expression of β_1-adrenergic receptor in IUGR animals [25]. Another important factor to regulate myocardial inotropy is Na/K-ATPase, which was also overexpressed in IUGR animals [25].

However, several studies have demonstrated that gestational protein restriction induces primary changes in heart, which might predispose to cardiovascular dysfunction later in life. It has been proposed that a suboptimal intrauterine environment results in fetal adaptations, which act to maintain heart growth, but which result in permanent changes to cardiac structure and function [26]. Cardiac myocytes rapidly proliferate during fetal life, but in the perinatal period and shortly after birth, proliferation ceases and myocytes undergo an additional cycle of DNA synthesis and nuclear mitosis without cytokinesis that leaves most adult cardiomyocytes binucleated [27]. Fetal growth restriction retarded cardiomyocyte maturation and is associated with lower binucleation and enlarged cardiomyocytes relative to heart size [28].

However, the impact of heart growth and development on heart weight is still controversial (Table 10.1). In IUGR rats that were exposed to maternal protein restriction, a reduced heart weight is often found [29, 30]. Alternatively, an increased heart weight has also been documented [31, 32]. Otherwise, no changes on heart weight have also been reported [33, 34]. In human studies, these discrepancies of results can be from diverse etiologies and differences in severity of IUGR fetuses recruited. Similarly, in animal models, the differences in results may arise from several factors: differences in the strain of rats studied, levels of maternal dietary protein restriction, timing of dietary administration to dams, and postnatal differences in body growth and levels of blood pressure of the offspring [35].

Low-protein diet (LPD) influences on cardiomyocyte number are more consistent. Several authors have shown the reduction in cardiomyocyte number, both in humans and animals [30, 36]. Because cardiomyocytes in general cease proliferating soon after birth, postnatal growth of heart is predominantly due to cardiomyocyte hypertrophy [27]. This may lead to impaired cardiac function later in life, especially if the heart is stimulated to hypertrophy, such as after the induction of hypertension [30].

Table 10.1 Studies investigating the effects of administration of a maternal low-protein diet (LPD) in rats on cardiac weight of offspring – highlighting differences in rat strains studied, severity of dietary protein restriction, and timing of diet administration

Author and year of study	Rat strain and age of offspring at investigation	Diets	Diet timing	Major findings in LPD group
Muaku et al. (1997) [29]	Wistar 23-days old	NP: 20% casein	During pregnancy	↓ Body weight
		LP: 5% casein		↓ Heart weight
Cortius et al. (2005) [30]	Wistar Kyoto at birth	NP: 20% casein	2 weeks prior to and during pregnancy and 2 weeks postnatally	↓ Birth weight
		LP: 8.7% casein		↓ Heart weight
				↓ Cardiomyocytes number
				↓ Binucleated cardiomyocytes
Jackson et al. (2002) [31]	Wistar 4-weeks old	NP: 18% casein		↑ Relative heart weight
		LP: 9% casein		
Lim et al. (2012) [32]	Wistar Kyoto 32-weeks old	NP: 20% casein	2 weeks prior to and during pregnancy and 2 weeks postnatally	↓ Body weight at 32 weeks
		LP: 8.7% casein		↑ Relative heart weight
Desai et al. (1996) [33]	Wistar	NP: 200 g protein/kg diet	During pregnancy	↓ Birth weight
				↔ Heart weight
	21 days old and 11 months old	LP: 80 g protein/kg diet		
Menendez-Castro et al. (2011) [34]	Wistar	NP: 17.2% casein	During pregnancy	↓ Body weight
	10-weeks old	LP: 8.4% casein		↔ Relative heart weight

Modified from Zohdi et al. [35]

NP normal protein diet, *LP* low-protein diet, ↑ increased, ↓ decreased, ↔ unchanged

The analysis of cardiac tissue showed that left ventricular expression of structural proteins, associated with pathological cardiac remodeling, was increased by maternal protein restriction. In 7-month-old rats exposed to undernutrition during pregnancy – the ratio of β- to α-myosin heavy chain protein and the expression of collagen I and III – were all increased [36]. Consistent with these observed changes in structural protein expression, the expression of matrix metalloproteinase 2 was lower in 7-month-old IUGR rats [36] and the expression of tissue inhibitor of metalloprotease 2 (TIMP-2) was higher in 70-day-old rats exposed to gestational protein restriction [34]. Therefore, in adult rats, restricting maternal protein intakes during gestation increases the number of cardiac fibroblasts in IUGR rats [25] and the amount of interstitial fibrosis in left ventricle [32].

Accumulation of extracellular matrix structural proteins in heart adversely affects myocardial viscoelasticity with accumulation of fibrillary collagen, leading to cardiac dysfunction [37]. Furthermore, the isolation of cardiomyocyte groups by collagens can cause a reduction in gap junctions in cardiac muscle and lead to electrical load variations, thus triggering arrhythmias [38].

The sarcomere is a key element of heart contractility and shorter sarcomeres have less actin and myosin cross bridges and less contractile force and reduced range of shortening [39]. Iruretagoyena et al. recently showed changes in sarcomere length in human fetuses with IUGR [40]. Furthermore, the expression of both N2B and N2BA titin isoforms, another important component of myocardial sarcomeres, is increased in 70-day-old rats from LPD dams [25].

Furthermore, endothelial dysfunction, with loss of modulatory role of endothelium, may be a critical factor in the development of hypertension. Newborns with fetal growth restriction have an increase in aortic intima-media thickness [41], which supports the existence of vascular remodeling. Increased coronary flow perfusion in severely growth-restricted fetuses and abnormal results on Doppler velocimetry in peripheral vessels were described [42]. Thus, alterations in the composition of the vascular extracellular matrix could possibly reduce vascular compliance, which is known to be a marker of CVD [34].

Children with fetal growth restriction have an altered cardiac geometry and shape, with less elongated and more globular ventricles, which also could be seen in animal models of IUGR. Morphometric measurements confirmed quantitatively an overall increase in transverse cardiac diameters, which lead to apparent ventricular cavity dilatation [43, 44]. This different architecture is not as efficient in generating the normal stroke volume, which results in the need for an increased heart rate to maintain cardiac output [43]. Furthermore, IUGR fetuses had echocardiographic signs of cardiac dysfunction from early stages [45]. Cardiac dysfunction deteriorates further with the progression of fetal compromise, along with the appearance of biochemical signs of cell damage, such as increased levels of b-type natriuretic peptide [45].

Myocardial hypertrophy (i.e., higher LVMI) was observed in IUGR patients [46]. Although remodeled ventricles could compensate for their lower efficiency in childhood, any additional changes in their working conditions (e.g., hypertension) at a later age would result in an abnormally high increase in local wall stress and dilatation [43].

Echocardiographic analysis of IUGR fetuses showed a significant decline in cardiac systolic function [43]. Crispi et al. showed that fetal growth restriction was associated with systolic and diastolic dysfunction, with preserved ejection fraction [44]. Echocardiography in gestational protein restricted rats at the 70th day of life revealed significantly higher values of left ventricular end-systolic diameter and left ventricular end-diastolic diameter with consecutively reduced fractional shortening [25]. Furthermore, these animals showed decreased ejection fraction and a reduction in left ventricular anterolateral wall thickness, which suggested an impaired contractile function and indicated a more distensible myocardial structure [25].

Apart from these structural and functional cardiovascular changes in offspring born from protein-restricted dams, the British research group of Dr. Fleming has shown the impact of maternal periconceptional protein restriction on long-term health outcomes in rodents.

To investigate the importance of periconceptional period, this research group established a rat model to which a maternal low-protein diet (9% casein; Emb-LPD) was administered exclusively during the 4 days of preimplantation development, followed by a control diet (18% casein) postnatally and thereafter [47]. Emb-LPD rat and mouse presented altered blastocyst cell number and more rapid growth during either fetal or postnatal period and led to long-term changes in perinatal and postnatal growth rate [47, 48]. Although Emb-LPD both in rat and mouse models had no effect on gestational length and litter size, the offspring had increased mean systolic blood pressure at 4 and 11 weeks [47], accompanied by attenuated arterial responsiveness in vitro to acetylcholine- and isoprenaline-induced vasodilatation [49] and increased cardiovascular disease risk in adult offspring.

Thus, both the periconceptional and the gestational period are windows during which environmental factors may cause permanent changes in the pattern and characteristics of development, leading to risk of adult-onset disease. Epigenetics consists in an advanced explanation for long-term or later-onset outcomes of early life experiences. Therefore, these environmental factors, by adaptive or maladaptive responses, result in a permanent resetting of gene expression programs that is mediated by altered epigenetic marking (DNA methylation, posttranslational modifications of histones, and microRNAs action), which can persist long after the duration of the initiating factor [50]. In our laboratory, we are currently investigating the microRNA expression profile on the left ventricle of protein-restricted offspring rats in both 12 days and 16 weeks old. And, not surprising, we could detect two downregulated microRNAs and seven upregulated microRNAs in 12-day-old offspring and ten downregulated microRNAs and seven upregulated microRNAs in 16-week-old offspring (unpublished data).

Catch-Up Growth

Helsinki cohort studies showed that both women and men with accelerated IUGR or "catch-up" growth during childhood presented increased risk of coronary heart disease [11].

Programming of metabolic disease by faster early growth is a finding seen across populations, and when nutrient-enriched formula is used for infants born small for gestational age at term, weight gain and higher diastolic blood pressure at ages 6–8 years were observed [51]. Studies suggest that there exist a "dose-response" association between early growth and later CVD risk [51].

In addition, experimental results have shown that catch-up growth is detrimental. Recently, Zohdi et al. reviewed the works in which IUGR was induced by protein restriction, and we can observe that, when the restriction was made only during pregnancy, the programed offspring present hypertension and when the restriction is during pregnancy and 2–3 weeks postnatally, the offspring is normotensive [35]. In our lab we observed, in the same rat model, that when protein restriction occurs only during pregnancy, the systolic blood pressure is enhanced from 8 to 16 weeks of age, and when protein restriction is maintained during lactation period, the rise occurs in the 16th week (Fig. 10.2). Thus, we suggest that cardiovascular function may be early adversely affected when there is a mismatch in prenatal and postnatal growth.

Some possible mechanisms have been proposed and a possibility is that catch-up growth is achieved by overgrowth of a limited cell mass reduced by fetal growth restriction that can disrupt cell function [52]. In addition, a large body size imposes an excessive metabolic demand on a reduced cell mass. Another possible link between catch-up growth and coronary heart disease is that hormonal changes during development can persist after birth, affecting heart disease development [53].

Conclusions

Evidences from epidemiology and animal studies demonstrate that IUGR is a factor predictive of later hypertension and CVD in adulthood. The mechanisms underlying the programming of hypertension by maternal undernutrition are likely to be multifactorial and complex (Fig. 10.3). The incompatibility between intrauterine restricted diet and normal diet nutrient content after birth can be excessive for

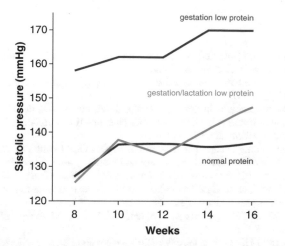

Fig. 10.2 Systolic blood pressure of male offspring whose mothers received normal (17% casein) or low-protein (6% casein) diet at gestational period or during gestation and lactation

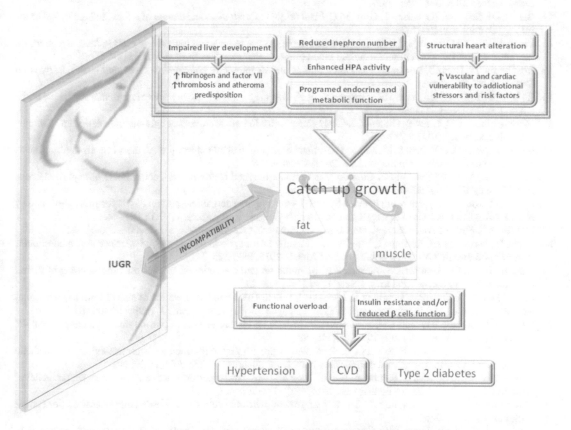

Fig. 10.3 Schematic summarization of mechanisms and consequences of IUGR and catch-up growth. *IUGR* intrauterine growth restriction, *HPA* hypothalamic-pituitary-adrenal axis, *CVD* cardiovascular disease

economic phenotype molded for a restrict environment. This mismatch results in accelerated or "catch-up" growth during childhood represent an overload for systems and organs with detrimental metabolic and physiological consequences. The end-stage consequences are diseases as hypertension, diabetes, and CVD.

References

1. Cardiovascular diseases (CVDs) [Internet]. World Health Organization. 2015 [cited 3 Jan 2016]. Available from: http://www.who.int/mediacentre/factsheets/fs317/en/.
2. Langley-Evans S, Gardner D, Welham S. Intrauterine programming of cardiovascular disease by maternal nutritional status. Nutrition. 1998;14(1):39–47.
3. Godfrey K, Barker D. Maternal nutrition in relation to fetal and placental growth. Eur J Obs Gynae. 1995;61(1):15–22.
4. Langley-Evans SC, Langley-Evans AJ, Marchand MC. Nutritional programming of blood pressure and renal morphology. Arch Physiol Biochem. 2003;111(1):8–16.
5. Thornburg KL. The programming of cardiovascular disease. J Dev Orig Health Dis. 2015;6(5):366–76.
6. Bernstein IM, Horbar JD, Badger GJ, et al. Morbidity and mortality among very low-birthweight neonates with intrauterine growth restriction: the Vermont Oxford Network. Am J Obstet Gynecol. 2000;182:198–206.
7. Turan S, Turan OM, Salim M, et al. Cardiovascular transition to extrauterine life in growth-restricted neonates: relationship with prenatal Doppler findings. Fetal Diagn Ther. 2013;33:103–9.
8. Barker DJP, Osmond C, Winter PD, Margetts B, Simmonds SJ. Weight in infancy and death from ischaemic heart disease. Lancet. 1989;ii:577–80.
9. Rich-Edwards JW, Stampfer MJ, Manson JE, et al. Birth weight and risk of cardiovascular disease in a cohort of women followed up since 1976. BMJ. 1997;315:396–400.
10. Stein CE, Fall CHD, Kumaran K, Osmond C, Cox V, Barker DJP. Fetal growth and coronary heart disease in South India. Lancet. 1996;348:1269–73.
11. Barker DJ, Eriksson JG, Forsen T, Osmond C. Fetal origins of adult disease: strength of effects and biological basis. Int J Epidemiol. 2002;31:1235–9.
12. Langley-Evans SC, Phillips GJ, Jackson AA. In utero exposure to maternal low protein diets induces hypertension in weanling rats, independently of maternal blood pressure changes. Clin Nutr. 1994;13:319–24.
13. Roseboom TJ, Rooij S, Painter R. The Dutch famine and its long-term consequences for adult health. Early Hum Dev. 2006;82(8):485–91.
14. Roseboom TJ, van der Meulen JHP, Osmond C, et al. Coronary heart disease in adults after prenatal exposure to the Dutch famine. Heart. 2000;84:595–8.
15. Merlet-Bénichou C, Leroy B, Gilbert T, Lelièvre-Pégorier M. Retard de croissance intra-utérin et déficit en néphrons. Médecine/Sciences. 1993;9:777–80.
16. Langley-Evans SC, Welham SJM, Jackson AA. Fetal exposure to maternal low protein diets impairs nephrogenesis and promotes hypertension in the rat. Life Sci. 1999;64:965–74.
17. Lucas SRR, Miraglia SM, Gil FZ, Coimbra TM. Intrauterine food restriction as a determinant of nephrosclerosis. Am J Kidney Dis. 2001;37:467–76.
18. Langley-Evans SC. Hypertension induced by foetal exposure to maternal low-protein diet in the rat is prevented by pharmacological blockade of maternal glucocorticoid synthesis. J Hypertens. 1997;15:537–44.
19. Fowden AL, Forhead AJ. Endocrine mechanisms of intrauterine programming. Reproduction. 2004;127(5):515–26.
20. Briffa JF, McAinch AJ, Romano T, Wlodek ME, Hryciw DH. Leptin in pregnancy and development: a contributor to adulthood disease? Am J Physiol Endocrinol Metab. 2015;308:E335–50.
21. Langley-Evans SC, Gardner DS, Jackson AA. Maternal protein restriction influences the programming of the rat hypothalamic-pituitary-adrenal axis. J Nutr. 1996;126:1578–85.
22. Lithell HO, McKeique PM, Berglund L, Mohsen R, Lithell UB, Leon DA. Relation of size at birth to non-insulin dependent diabetes and insulin concentrations in men aged 50–60 years. Br Med J. 1996;312:406–10.
23. Barker DJP, Meade TW, Fall CH, et al. Relation to fetal and infant growth to plasma fibrinogen and factor VII concentrations in adult life. BMJ. 1992;304:148–52.
24. Alves JLB, Nogueira VO, Neto MPC, et al. Maternal protein restriction increases respiratory and sympathetic activities and sensitizes peripheral chemoreflex in male rat offspring. J Nutr. 2015;145:907–14.
25. Menendez-Castro C, Toka O, Fahlbusch F, et al. Impaired myocardial performance in a normotensive rat model of intrauterine growth restriction. Pediatr Res. 2014;25(6):697–706.
26. Thornburg KL, Louey S, Giraud GD. The role of growth in heart development. Nestle Nutr Workshop Ser Pediatr Program. 2008;61:39–51.
27. Ahuja P, Sdek P, MacLellan WR. Cardiac myocyte cell cycle control in development, disease, and regeneration. Physiol Rev. 2007;87:521–44.
28. Morrison JL, Botting KJ, Dyer JL, Williams SJ, Thornburg KL, McMilen IC. Restriction of placental function alters heart development in the sheep fetus. Am J Phys Regul Integr Comp Phys. 2007;293:R306–13.
29. Muaku SM, Thissen JP, Gerard G, Ketelslegers JM, Maiter D. Postnatal catch-up growth induced by growth hormone and insulin-like growth factor-I in rats with intrauterine growth retardation caused by maternal protein malnutrition. Pediatr Res. 1997;42:370–7.

30. Cortius HB, Zimanyi MA, Maka N, et al. Effect of intrauterine growth restriction on the number of cardiomyocytes in rat hearts. Pediatr Res. 2005;57:796–800.
31. Jackson AA, Dunn RL, Marchand MC, Langley-Evans SC. Increased systolic blood pressure in rats induced by a maternal low-protein diet is reversed by dietary supplementation with glycine. Clin Sci (Lond). 2002;103:633–9.
32. Lim K, Lombardo P, Schneider-Kolsky M, Black MJ. Intrauterine growth restriction coupled with hyperglycemia: effects on cardiac structure in adult rats. Pediatr Res. 2012;72:344–51.
33. Desai M, Crowther NJ, Lucas A, Hales CN. Organ-selective growth in the offspring of protein-restricted mothers. Br J Nutr. 1996;76:591–603.
34. Menendez-Castro C, Fahlbusch F, Cordasic N, et al. Early and late postnatal myocardial and vascular changes in a protein restriction rat model of intrauterine growth restriction. PLoS One. 2011;6(5):1–10.
35. Zohdi V, Lim K, Pearson JT, Black MJ. Development programming of cardiovascular disease following intrauterine growth restriction: findings utilizing a rat model of maternal protein restriction. Forum Nutr. 2015;7:119–52.
36. Xu Y, Williams SJ, O'Brien D, Davidge ST. Hypoxia or nutrient restriction during pregnancy in rats leads to progressive cardiac remodeling and impairs post-ischemic recovery in adult male offspring. FASEB J. 2006;20:1251–3.
37. Weber KT, Brilla CG, Janicki JS. Myocardial fibrosis: functional significance and regulatory factors. Cardiovasc Res. 1993;27:341–8.
38. Spach MS, Boineau JP. Microfibrosis produces electrical load variations due to loss of side-to-side cell connections: a major mechanism of structural heart disease arrhythmias. Pacing Clin Electrophysiol. 1997;20:397–413.
39. Sela G, Yadid M, Landesberg A. Theory of cardiac sarcomere contraction and the adaptive control of demands. Ann N Y Acad Sci. 2010;1188:222–30.
40. Iruretagoyena JI, Gonzalez-Tendero A, Garcia-Canadilla P, et al. Cardiac dysfunction is associated with altered sarcomere ultrastructure in intrauterine growth restriction. Am J Obstet Gynecol. 2014;210:550. e1–50.e7.
41. Skilton MK, Evans N, Griffiths KA, Harmer JA, Celermajer D. Aortic wall thickness in newborns with intrauterine restriction. Lancet. 2005;23:1484–6.
42. Chaoui R. Coronary arteries in fetal life: physiology, malformations and the "heart-sparing effect". Acta Paediatr Suppl. 2004;93:6–12.
43. Crispi F, Bijnens B, Figueras F, et al. Fetal growth restriction results in remodeled and less efficient hearts in children. Circulation. 2010;121:2427–36.
44. Crispi F, Bijnens B, Sepulveda-Swatson E, et al. Postsystolic shortening by myocardial deformation imaging as a sign of cardiac adaptation to pressure overload in fetal growth restriction. Circ Cardiovasc Imaging. 2014;7:781–7.
45. Crispi F, Hernandez-Andrade E, Pelsers M, et al. Cardiac dysfunction and cell damage across clinical stages of severity in growth-restricted fetuses. Am J Obstet Gynecol. 2008;199:254e1–4.
46. Leipälä JA, Boldt T, Turpeinen U, Vuolteenaho O, Fellman V. Cardiac hypertrophy and altered hemodynamic adaptation in growth-restricted preterm infants. Pediatr Res. 2003;53:989–93.
47. Kwong WY, Wild AE, Roberts P, Willis AC, Fleming TP. Maternal undernutrition during the preimplantation period of rat development causes blastocyst abnormalities and programming of postnatal hypertension. Development. 2000;127:4195–202.
48. Watkins AJ, Ursel E, Panton R, et al. Adaptive responses by mouse early embryos to maternal diet protect fetal growth but predispose to adult onset disease. Biol Reprod. 2008;78:299–306.
49. Watkins AJ, Lucas ES, Torrens C, et al. Maternal low-protein diet during pre-implantation development induces vascular dysfunction and altered renin-angiotensin-system homeostasis in the offspring. Br J Nutr. 2010;103:1762–70.
50. Hochberg Z, Feil R, Constancia M, et al. Child health, developmental plasticity, and epigenetic programming. Endocr Rev. 2011;32:159–224.
51. Singhal A. The global epidemic of noncommunicable disease: the role of early life factors. In: Black RE, Singhal A, Uauy R, editors. International nutrition: achieving millennium goals and beyond, vol. 78. Vevey: Nestlé Nutr Inst Workshop Ser; 2014. p. 123–32.
52. Pitts GC. Cellular aspects of growth and catch-up growth in the rat: a reevaluation. Growth. 1986;50:419–36.
53. Barker DJP, Gluckman PD, Godfrey KM, Harding JE, Owens JA, Robinson JS. Fetal nutrition and cardiovascular disease in adult life. Lancet. 1993;341:938–41.

Chapter 11
Effects of Maternal Protein Restriction on Nephrogenesis and Adult and Aging Kidney

Patrícia Aline Boer, Ana Tereza Barufi Franco, and José Antonio Rocha Gontijo

Key Points

- Intrauterine environment, mainly maternal nutritional status, represents a predictive factor for kidney dysfunction and arterial hypertension in adulthood.
- Protein restriction in pregnancy is associated with intrauterine growth restriction resulting in low birth weight and subsequent arterial hypertension, development, decreased renal sodium excretion and glomerulosclerosis.
- Decreased urinary sodium fractional excretion (FE_{Na}) was accompanied by a fall in fractional proximal sodium excretion and occurred despite unchanged creatinine clearance.
- In animal models of gestational programming animal by protein restriction, the reduction in glomerular filtrated area and hyperflow promoted increased ultrafiltration pressure with progressive lesion of the nephron.
- Studies demonstrate that dipsogenic and natriuretic effects of intracerebroventricular (i.c.v.) angiotensin II (AngII) was significantly lower in low-protein (LP) offspring than in normoprotein (NP) rats. These results may be related to the decreased type 1 and type 2 angiotensin II receptors ($AT1_R/AT2_R$) ratio appearing in LP offspring in neuronal areas related to water and salt balance.
- Low-protein (LP) offspring is associated with that pronounced reduction in cellularity and type 1 angiotensin II receptor (AT_1R) density in the solitary tract nucleus (nTS). Conversely, the reduced cellularity and AT_1R density are reverted by diet taurine supplementation, normalizing arterial pressure and urinary sodium excretion in adult offspring.

Keywords Angiotensin receptors • Arterial hypertension • CNS • Foetal programming • Intrauterine growth restriction • Maternal protein restriction • RAS • Renal function

Abbreviations

ADH   Antidiuretic hormone
AngII   Angiotensin II
AVP   Arginine vasopressin

P.A. Boer, BSc, PhD (✉) • A.T.B. Franco, BSc, MSc • J.A.R. Gontijo, MD, PhD
Department of Internal Medicine, Faculty of Medical Sciences, University of Campinas, Campinas, SP, Brazil
e-mail: alineboer@yahoo.com.br; boer@fcm.unicamp.br

© Springer International Publishing AG 2017   131
R. Rajendram et al. (eds.), *Diet, Nutrition, and Fetal Programming*,
Nutrition and Health, DOI 10.1007/978-3-319-60289-9_11

AT1$_R$/AT2$_R$	Type 1 and type 2 angiotensin receptors
CKD	Chronic kidney disease
CNS	Central nervous system
CVD	Cardiovascular disease
CVO	Circumventricular organs
DOHaD	Developmental origins of health and disease
FE$_{Na}$	Fractional urinary sodium excretion
GD	Gestational day
HPA	Hypothalamic-pituitary-adrenal axis
i.c.v.	Intracerebroventricular
L	Lactation
LP	Low protein
LPD	Low-protein diet
LVMI	Left ventricular mass index
MM	Mesenchymal metanephron
MRI	Magnetic resonance imaging
nTS	Medial solitary tract nucleus
NP	Normal protein
PVN	Paraventricular nucleus
RAS	Renin-angiotensin system
SD	Sprague-Dawley rats
Ub	Ureteral bud
US	United States
W	Wistar rats
WKY	Wistar Kyoto rats

Introduction

Chronic kidney disease (CKD) is a major problem of public health worldwide, affecting more than 50 million individuals [1, 2]. In 2006, more than one million people received renal replacement therapy, and even with the availability of this therapy, the absolute number of deaths was greater than that caused by cervical, prostate, breast and colon/rectum cancers [3]. In recent years, CKD has been regarded as a global epidemic and high mortality disorder, in which diagnosis and stabilization of disease progression are unpredictable and occur late [2, 3]. For this reason, there is a need to identify the beginning and risk factors for CKD progression to allow innovative and early therapy interventions [1, 2].

In low-income countries, underweight birth children are often associated with arterial hypertension and cardiovascular and renal diseases in adulthood. Conversely, in developed countries, malnutrition is well characterized by high calorie and more-palatable processed food consumption [4, 5], which is associated with low birthweight and higher blood pressure in adulthood. In addition, it has been demonstrated that arterial hypertension is associated with an early decreased nephron numbers. The Developmental Origins of Health and Disease (DOHaD) concept defines those gestational conditions that determinate changes to optimize phenotype for adaptation to postnatal environment. However, in many situations, the incompatibility between programmed phenotype and postnatal exposure environments may result in adult health disorders.

Studies have been shown that maternal, emotional and nutritional stresses are related to programming process, and the kidney is among the structures most affected in offspring [4, 5]. Ontogeny is a process finely orchestrated by a number of biochemical factors whose concentration and time of appearance affect the final result. Thus, small changes can have an important effect on this process.

The conditions, to which the mother and consequently the foetus and/or embryo are exposed, such as psychological and/or nutritional stresses, will have predominant role during organogenesis and particularly during nephrogenesis. Although not fully elucidated, various mechanisms have been identified as directly or indirectly involved in the genesis or maintenance of renal disorders. This chapter aimed to present evidences of the association among maternal low-protein ingestion, low nephron number, arterial hypertension and kidney dysfunction in adulthood and aging.

Gestational Protein Restriction and Reduced Nephron Number

In 1967 [6], Zeman showed that in the rat, at the first time, gestational protein restriction (LP, 6% casein) results in smaller kidneys when compared with control offspring, whose mothers were fed normal protein diet (NP, 24% casein). In gestational low-protein intake model, Zeman also found kidneys from pups with predominantly fewer and undifferentiated glomeruli 8 h after birth [6, 7] compared with control offspring. In humans, nephrogenesis is complete prior to birth, but in rats it occurs from approximately midgestation to 10 days after birth [8]. Though reduction of 17.5% in the number of glomeruli has been verified, these animals had 50% more immature glomeruli, which led him to suggest that a major effect of intrauterine protein malnutrition on the kidneys could be retardation in development [2]. At the same year, Hall and Zeman [9] published the results from kidney functional study of these animals from birth until 6 days after birth, and LP offspring presented reduced excretion of water and glomerular filtration rate one-quarter less than NP. Allen and Zeman [10] also demonstrated that an increased postnatal nutrient intake during the suckling period had no influence on nephron number in low-protein intake (LP) offspring. Additional study from these authors showed that renal response to antidiuretic hormone (ADH) was impaired in 6-day-old LP but not in 13-day and 22-day-old pups, and the glomerular filtration rate and tubular function were significantly reduced [11]. For two decades, scarce studies were performed establishing the number of nephrons in maternal protein-restricted model. From 1994 to here, a lot of findings demonstrating the nephron number reduction, from 15% to 43%, were presented (Table 11.1).

This apparent reduced nephron number discrepancy may be explained by different factors such as decrease in rodent casein chow concentrations (from 5% to 9%), period of time to diet consumption, rodent lineage and animal age of glomeruli count. Thus, in studies by Langley-Evans et al. [13, 22] and Sahajpal

Table 11.1 Works investigating kidney programming by protein restriction

Author (year)	Animal and time of diet exposition	NP/LP casein%	Age of counting	Nephron reduction%
Zeman (1968) [6, 7]	SD, all GDs	24/6	8 h	♂17.5
Merlet-Benichou et al. (1994) [12]	SD, 8–22°GD	22/5	2 weeks	♂30
Langley-Evans et al. (1999) [13]	W, all GDs	18/9	4 weeks	♂15
Woods et al. (2001) [14]	SD, all GDs	21/8.5	15 h	♂25.4
Vehascari et al. (2001) [15]	SD, 12–22°GD	24/6	8 weeks	♂28/♀29
Welham et al. (2002) [16]	W, all GDs	18/9/6	2 weeks	♂30/♂41
Sahajpal and Ashton (2005) [17]	W, all GDs	18/9	4 weeks	♂34
Woods et al. (2004) [18]	SD, all GDs	19/5	22 weeks	♂43
Makrakis et al. (2007) [19]	WKY 2 weeks before, all GDs, L	20/8.7	4 weeks	♂29
Hoppe et al. (2007) [20]	C57, 2 weeks before, all GDs, L	20/9	3 weeks	♂22/♀16
Hoppe et al. (2007) [21]	SD, 2 weeks before, all GDs, L	20/8	19.3 weeks	♂31
Harrison and Langley-Evans (2009) [22]	W, all GDs	18/9	10 weeks	♂33/♀35
Mesquita et al. (2010) [23]	SD, all GDs	17/6	1.7/16 weeks	♂28/♂27

SD Sprague-Dawley, *W* Wistar, *GD* gestational day, *L* lactation

and Ashton [17], in which all of these parameters are similar, the reduction of nephron number (~19%) was also the same. Technically, they accessed three to five sections from the full range of sections for each kidney, in which the glomeruli number is counted and the total number of sections multiplied the averaged nephron number from each section [13]. Conversely, Sahajpal and Ashton [17] performed mechanic maceration and digestion of kidney tissue and counted the number of glomeruli in the suspension. Thus, in many studies, it raises the possibility that reduced nephron count is, at least in part, related to the method used for quantification of glomerular number. Bertram et al. [24] have described an unbiased stereological method by physical dissector-fractionator combination for glomerular quantification, also used in our lab, with very similar results. Welham et al. [16] findings showed 13% fewer glomeruli using tissue homogenate, such as Harrison and Langley-Evans [22], both showing similar results. Recently, Chacon-Caldera et al. [25] presented a new method for glomerular unit quantification by magnetic resonance imaging in kidney labelled with cationized ferritin. These authors have acquired the glomeruli number by using a scanning time of 33 min and 20 s, with reproducible results described above, however, with easier and faster access compared with stereological technique.

Mechanisms for Cessation of Nephrogenesis

Ontogenesis is a process finely orchestrated by a number of chemical factors whose concentration and time of appearance affect the final result. Thus, small changes can have an important effect on this process. The conditions, to which the mother and consequently the embryo/foetus are exposed, such as psychological and/or nutrient stress, will have predominant role during organogenesis and particularly during nephrogenesis. In humans, nephrogenesis initiates at week 5 (it is complete between weeks 32 and 36) [26] and at day 9, in rats (being finalized at postnatal, between days 8 and 11) [27], by dual induction, when signals from the mesenchymal metanephron (MM) induce sprouting of ureteral bud (UB). In parallel, signals from UB lead to MM cell condensation on its top forming a hood called CAP. Stem cells present in this CAP lead to UB branches and in their points will be formed new CAPs. While at one end UB continues to grow and branching in the others, the CAP nephrogenic stem cells differentiate into nephrons. The developing MM is particularly vulnerable to gestational protein restriction, and, although not fully elucidated, various mechanisms have been suggested as directly or indirectly involved in the genesis or maintenance of disorders in the renal development. Also, the exact period in which protein restriction may induce changes is not known.

Observations by Kwong et al. [28] identified the relationship between preimplantation period and early changes that propagate into postnatal life. In this study, pregnant rats have been exposed to 9% casein intake (LP group) from 0 to 4.25 days after mating followed by analysis of 16-cell morulae, early and expanding blastocyst stages. Here, cell numbers at the morulae stage were not affected by low-protein diet; however, the blastocyst cell number in the internal cell mass and also the trophectoderm cell number were 15% comparatively reduced to control group (females supplied with 18% casein diet). Additionally, isoleucine, leucine, methionine, proline, threonine and valine amino acids were depleted from the LP dam's serum. These authors concluded that serum amino acid depletion and/or hyperglycaemic maternal environment were important mechanisms involved in reduced blastocyst cell proliferation. Thus, the early-reduced stem cell number may exert long-term effects on maternal LP models [28].

Welham et al. [16], using gestational low-protein diet in rats, observed that, on embryonic day 13, the number of cells in the metanephron was not modified comparatively to control, but the number of apoptotic cells was 122% (using 9% casein diet) and 87% (using 6% casein diet) enhanced. At embryonic day 15, the number of metanephric cells was 54% and 72% reduced in embryo exposed to 9% and 6% casein content diet, respectively. Thus, the authors concluded that early-enhanced apoptotic deletion of metanephric progenitor cells is associated with reduced number of glomeruli. In cultural

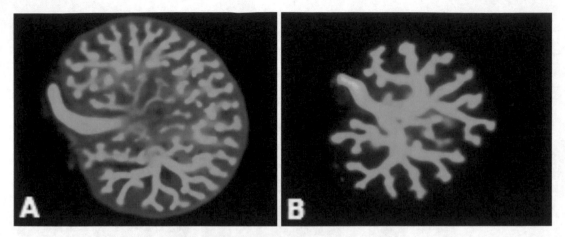

Fig. 11.1 Ureteral branches reduction by gestational protein restriction. Ureteral branches extracted from embryo metanephroi of mothers that received normal protein (**a**) or low-protein (**b**) diet during gestation. Immunofluorescence using pan-cytokeratin

study, we had demonstrated that embryo metanephroi extracted from LP mothers at 14.5 gestational days and grown for 48 h presented 28% reduced ureteral branches when compared with control (NP, normal protein diet) (Mesquita FF, Arena D, Ewen-McCullen L, Gontijo JA, Bertram J, Boer PA, Armitage J, unpublished data, Fig. 11.1).

Recently, studies in our laboratory have demonstrated that nephrogenic stem cells in the CAPs are 27% reduced in LP metanephroi (6% casein) embryos at 17 gestational days (unpublished observations) when compared with NP group. At 12-day-old and 16 week-old rats submitted to the same diets, we observed, respectively, a reduction of 28% and 27% in nephron number [23]. Different mechanisms can contribute to foetal programming phenotype: exposure to foetal glucocorticoid, alterations in RAS components, apoptosis and DNA methylation. During gestational development, glucocorticoids may induce early cell differentiation in detriment of proliferation, which may be related to reduction in kidney stem cells. An LP diet during gestation decreases the activity of placental 11ß-hydroxysteroid dehydrogenase, exposing the foetus to glucocorticoids and resetting the hypothalamic-pituitary-adrenal axis in the offspring [29].

Hypertension Development as an Interaction Between Neurohumoral and Kidney Dysfunction

Maternal dietary protein restriction during pregnancy is associated with renal morphological and physiological changes. Brenner et al. [30] have postulated: "…a renal abnormality that contributes to essential hypertension in the general population is a reduced number of nephrons". These authors have correlated this abnormality with reduced nephron number and/or decreased glomerular filtration area in animals with a higher propensity to glomerulosclerosis and chronic renal failure. Thus, in gestational programming animal models, the effective reduction of glomerular filtrated area and hyperflow promote increased ultrafiltration pressure with progressive lesion of nephron. Hence, premature glomerular senescence associated with low renal reserve to compensate injury can be, at least in part, the mechanism that contributes to developing arterial hypertension (Fig. 11.2). Otherwise, a number of studies suggest that reduced nephron number alone is not enough to lead to arterial hypertension and renal disease [31]. It is necessary to consider that reduced nephron number is only a part

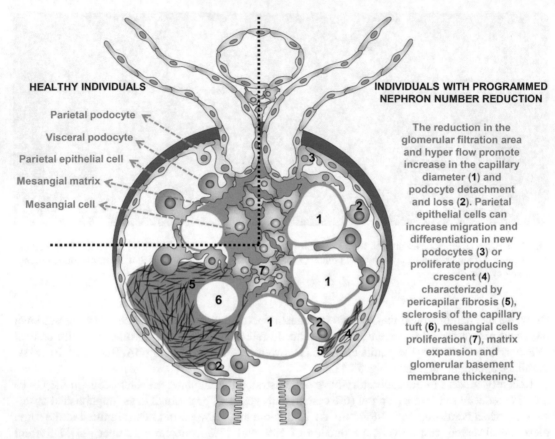

HEALTHY INDIVIDUALS

Parietal podocyte
Visceral podocyte
Parietal epithelial cell
Mesangial matrix
Mesangial cell

INDIVIDUALS WITH PROGRAMMED NEPHRON NUMBER REDUCTION

The reduction in the glomerular filtration area and hyper flow promote increase in the capillary diameter (**1**) and podocyte detachment and loss (**2**). Parietal epithelial cells can increase migration and differentiation in new podocytes (**3**) or proliferate producing crescent (**4**) characterized by pericapilar fibrosis (**5**), sclerosis of the capillary tuft (**6**), mesangial cells proliferation (**7**), matrix expansion and glomerular basement membrane thickening.

Fig. 11.2 The reduction on nephron number promotes glomerular injury by overload. Premature glomerular loss in low renal reserve individuals can contribute to development of arterial hypertension in adulthood (Modified from Shankland et al. Nat Rev Nephrol. 2014;10:158–173)

in this multifactorial process. Thus, Brawley et al. [32] have shown that maternal protein deprivation in rat results in blunted vasorelaxation of small resistance arteries in male offspring, causing the development of cardiovascular disease in adulthood. Recently, studies have demonstrated that, in later life, offspring programmed by maternal low-protein diet presents exaggerated proliferative response to vascular injury induced by enhancement [34] of oxidative stress, inflammatory response and hypoxia, resulting in exaggerated vascular remodelling through the reactions to vascular injury.

The abnormal function/expression of AngII receptors during any period of life may be a cause or consequence of renal adaptation. Compared with controls, AT_1R is upregulated on the first day after LP offspring birth, but this receptor appears to be downregulated by 12 days of age and thereafter. Otherwise, in this offspring, AT_2R expression differs from controls at 1 day of age, but it is also downregulated thereafter, with low nephron numbers at all ages: from the foetal period, at the end of nephron formation and during adulthood [23, 33]. Modulations in renal, vascular and neural renin-angiotensin system (RAS) have been also implicated in the genesis of gestational low-protein programmed hypertension. In LP offspring, ACE inhibition and AT1 receptor antagonists significantly reduced the systolic blood pressure. Otherwise, foetal malnutrition model is associated with decreased kidney expression of angiotensin receptors, resulting in the inability of renal tubules to handle the hydroelectrolyte balance, consequently implying in hypertension development. Supporting this hypothesis recently, it has been demonstrated that experimentally induced maternal protein restriction reduces renal tissue renin and angiotensin II levels and the expression of AT1 and AT2 receptors in newborn

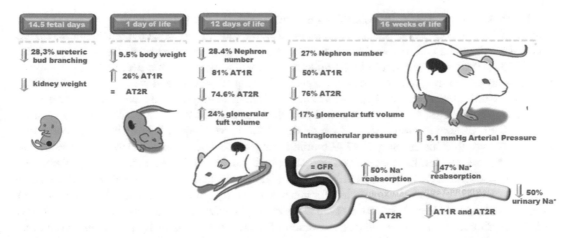

Fig. 11.3 Time-course effects of experimental kidney programming. We used male rats from mothers submitted to gestational low protein (6% casein) comparatively to normal protein (17% casein) diet [23, 33]

rats [23, 33]. These investigations also show an early and pronounced decrease in fractional urinary sodium excretion (FE_{Na}) in maternal LP offspring, in addition to 8 weeks of age when compared with age-matched NP. Decreased FE_{Na} was accompanied by a fall in fractional proximal sodium excretion, which occurred despite unchanged creatinine clearance, used to estimate glomerular filtration rate and enhanced fractional post-proximal sodium excretion (Fig. 11.3). In this case, fluid is reabsorbed to the same degree, resulting in the concentration in the end of the proximal tubule, being the same as in the beginning. In other words, the reabsorption in the proximal tubule is isosmotic without a change in plasma osmolality. These effects were associated with a significant extracellular isotonic expansion and supposedly enhanced arterial blood pressure in the LP group; however, the precise mechanism of these phenomena remains unknown.

Although the precise mechanism by which blood pressure rises in the programmed offspring kept being elucidated, renal control of the fluid and electrolyte balance are thought to play a dominant role in the long-term control of arterial blood pressure. As described above, intrauterine growth restriction has been associated with maternal low-protein intake (LP), and although the specific nature of this condition is unclear, a number of mechanisms have been proposed. Since these initial discoveries, most intrinsic components of RAS, including angiotensinogen, angiotensin and converting enzymes, have been well described and demonstrated in different areas of the central nervous system (CNS) [35]. However, notably most previous studies in this field have focused on peripheral angiotensin receptors and their roles in prenatal imprinting. The role of the CNS in the control of blood pressure and hydrosaline homeostasis has been demonstrated by several studies [36, 37]. The existence of an isolated brain RAS was proposed by the discovery of renin-like activity in the brain [38].

Conversely, the central role of RAS in the control of blood pressure and hydroelectrolytic homeostasis has been demonstrated by prior studies [39]. It acts specifically by activating at least two well-characterized transmembrane G protein-coupled receptors belonging to the seven-transmembrane-spanning receptor family, type 1 ($AT1_R$) and type 2-angiotensin receptor ($AT2_R$). Recent studies have shown that the CNS, during development, can be influenced by alterations in the intrauterine environment. Utero programming of arterial hypertension, via alteration of RAS before birth, has attracted great attention. Data from our laboratory, confirming prior reports, indicate that LP kidneys, even after higher blood pressure development, excrete a lesser amount of salt under basal conditions than kidneys of NP rats [23, 33]. Additionally, for the first time, our studies demonstrate that the dipsogenic effect of i.c.v. 4 nmol AngII was significantly lower in the LP offspring than in NP rats. These results may be related to the decreased $AT1_R/AT2_R$ ratio appearing in LP offspring, in neuronal areas, related to water and salt balance [40, 41].

The physiological regulatory role of brain-derived arginine vasopressin (AVP) and AngII in the control of water intake awaits further examination. Dysfunction of the foetal hypothalamus areas rich in AngII receptors can affect foetal tissue maturation, leading to profound consequences in postnatal life [23, 33]. Previous immunoblotting studies have shown a hypothalamic decreased AT_1R expression in 1-day-old LP rats [42], but there is a significant enhance in AT_1R at 4 weeks of age, when these animals are still normotensive [42]. Lima et al. [40], using 12-day-old rats, partially confirm these studies and demonstrate an early hypothalamic decreased AT_1R expression, by western blotting (minus 20%), without recovery of AT_1R expression in the 16-week-old LP offspring when compared with the NP group. This unchanged AT_1R blotting in the whole hypothalamic extract of 16-week-old LP rats may indicate results of uneven AT_1R diencephalic nuclei expression as revealed by qualitative immunohistochemistry of different analysed hypothalamic structures. AT_1R located on circumventricular organ (CVO) neurons may project for many other brain regions behind the blood-brain barrier [43]. The reduced AT_1R expression observed in the choroid plexus and paraventricular nucleus (PVN) of LP offspring may indicate a reduced activation of neural receptor ends by inborn and circulating AngII [40], and the reduction of dipsogenic response to AngII i.c.v. administration in LP is possibly explained by lower hypothalamic AVP expression than observed in NP rats. In addition, it is plausible to consider that the association of decreasing AT_1R/AT_2R ratio attenuated AngII dipsogenic and natriuretic responses mediated by neural pathways with origin in CVO.

While circulating, AngII tends to retain sodium by a direct renal action [44] as well as through aldosterone release from the adrenal gland; stimulation of brain AngII receptors has been reported to induce natriuresis [45]. The mechanism by which central AngII induces its natriuretic effects remains to be elucidated. There is considerable evidence to support a role for the sympathetic nervous system in the control of urinary sodium excretion [36, 37]. Thus, we may state that a reduced hypothalamic AVP and AT_1R/AT_2R ratio expression could promote an attenuated urinary excretion of salt and water in LP offspring compared with the NP group.

Additionally, the medial solitary tract nucleus (nTS) – the central site of termination of baroreceptor afferents – is intimately involved in the arterial pressure control. This nucleus contains a high density of AngII AT_1 receptors located both presynaptically, on vagal and carotid sinus afferents and on interneurons [46]. AngII reduces blood pressure and heart rate after injection of low doses in the nTS, as previously reported in several strains of rats [47]. Study from our lab evaluates changes of postnatal nTS angiotensin receptors by maternal protein restriction and its impact on in utero programming of hypertension in adult life [41]. This study shows that maternal LP restriction during prenatal life decreases the mass and neuronal proliferation (about 21%) in this encephalic area. These disorders of the foetal brain areas, including the brainstem, may affect foetal neural cell maturation and hence have profound consequences in functional neural postnatal life. The nTS – the central site of termination of baroreceptor afferents – is intimately involved in the arterial pressure control. Our study also has shown a striking reduction of AT_1 receptors in the nTS of the maternal LP offspring when compared with unchanged AT_1R density in NP and taurine-treated LPT rats [41]. Thus, at least in part, the AngII-mediated hypotensive effect may result from inhibition of the sympathetic nervous system activity by direct connections of vagal sensory afferent fibbers with cells in the A_2-catecholamine cell group in the ventral nTS. Study has also shown previously that the level of taurine is markedly reduced in the plasma of foetuses of dams fed an LP diet [48]. Additionally, taurine supplementation of the maternal LP intake restored to normal the foetal plasma taurine concentration [49]. The physiologic function of this amino acid remains elusive. In animal experiments, including primate models, taurine deficiency during pregnancy and lactation is associated with growth failure, abnormal cerebellar development, neurologic deficits, retinal degeneration and cardiac damage [50]. Taking into account the above findings, we may suppose that progressive enhanced blood pressure in addition to 8 weeks of age in LP offspring may be associated with that pronounced reduction in cellularity and AT_1R density in the nTS. Conversely, this finding reverted by diet taurine supplementation, normalizing the arterial pressure and urinary sodium excretion in adult offspring.

Maternal Protein Restriction Effects on the Aging Kidney

So far, studies about the effects of gestational nutrition and aging are scarce. The aging process occurs on a global level, which is demanding and increasing public health costs. A natural and peculiar process in which overriding results include increased rates of chronic diseases, morbidity and consequently mortality. Aging is an expected event regulated by an interaction among genetic profile and environmental circumstances that affect, in different proportions, the functionality of the neural, urinary, gastrointestinal, cardiovascular, endocrine and immune systems. Together, such modulatory and effector systems maintain the homeodynamics of the *milieu intérieur* and its fast response to environmental imbalance [51].

Take into account the kidney considerations, the expected changes on aging kidneys include enhanced renal vascular resistance, low plasma flow, increased filtration fraction, decreased cortical mass and consequently gradual function decay and increased glomerulosclerosis, interstitial fibrosis and tubular atrophy [52]. Such natural changes are known as "senescence", attributed to age-dependent factor, corresponding to gradual deterioration of function characteristic of most complex organs and biological system, which refer either to cellular senescence or to senescence of the whole organism [53]. Numerous mechanisms contribute to advance this natural aging process, in which include mitochondrial injury and oxidative stress, alteration of cell signalling, defects in membrane permeability and disorder of calcium homeostasis, promoting imbalances among cell repair, apoptosis and cell death [54] and culminating with early senescence. Within this scenario, the influences of critical events that may occur during ontogenical period in maternal protein-restricted model could lead to later life-course consequences and aging health. Thus, the exposure to gestational protein restriction in the key developmental period of nephrogenesis may be associated with alterations in longtime health and to emanate crucial influences on aging frailty and on prevalent age-related chronic diseases [55] (Fig. 11.4). Such alterations include anatomic, physiologic and histological changes of the kidney.

Anatomic changes from aging programmed kidney include early alterations in renal mass characterized by progressive ischemic injury with loss of the remaining nephrons, which contribute to declining cortical volume with an increased medullar thickness. These changes are accompanied by tubular atrophy and interstitial fibrosis associated with renal tubular progressive dysfunction [55]. Such anatomical replacements are also found at the glomerular level, characterized by pericapsular fibrosis, sclerosis of capillary tuft, mesangial matrix expansion and glomerular basement membrane thickening. Furthermore, hyaline nodules emerge early within Bowman, promoting collapse of glomeruli; increased podocyte effacement and glomerulosclerosis are prevalent with aging [14, 18] (Fig. 11.2). Normally, glomerular structure changes in regular aging process. However, in programmed individual aging, this occurs quickly, including reduction of lobular areas, decrease in glomerular number, tubular atrophy and changes in glomerular basement membrane structure and function [14, 18]. Additionally, tubulointerstitial fibrosis is frequently observed in aging process, since it is linked to fibroblast, an activation factor that alters the kidney diluting capacity and urine osmolality [56]. In fact, many glomerular alterations are observed in premature aging linked to features of renal pathological conditions [55].

Vascular changes are observed during aging, including hypertrophy and arteriosclerosis, which are associated with sclerotic glomeruli and arterial hypertension [57]. In addition, increased activity of renal ACE and renal AT_2R expression as deregulations of renin-angiotensin system is observed. It is well known that high blood pressure is an age-dependent abnormality. However, gestational malnutrition causes a striking reduction in nephron number and increased tubular reabsorption of water and salt [23, 33], which probably accentuated and turned early the occurrence of hypertension during the aging process. This blood pressure elevation also occurs by resetting cardiovascular baroreflex effects as peculiar aggravating component in aging [58].

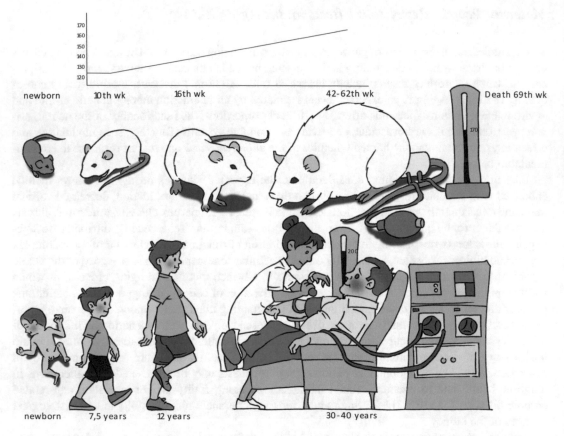

Fig. 11.4 Results obtained in rat comparatively with human. We have observed that the male rat from mothers submitted to gestational protein restriction present low birthweight and enhanced arterial pressure beyond tenth week of life. In 62-week-old rats, the functional kidney dysfunctions may be compatible with renal failure development in man (unpublished dates)

Nephron loss naturally befalls; however, this decay behaviour significantly enhanced is associated with foetal programming [13, 23, 33]. Therefore, the remaining nephron filtration is compensated by kidney overload characterized by hyperflow/hyperfiltration associated with increased glomerular capillary pressure, glomerular enlargement, increased mesangial matrix that promotes premature podocyte senescence, accelerated proteinuria and development of glomerulosclerosis in later life, accompanied by decline in the glomerular filtration rate [59].

Changes in the glomerular level are widespread, as, for example, the functional lifespan of the metanephric kidneys depends on a big amount of nephron supply [60]. Prior researches suggest that low-protein intake during all gestational period may affect foetal growth and cause alterations in the function and morphological structure of body system and its homeostasis, programming the individual for adjustment, due to permanent changes, and it contributes to the progression of chronic kidney disease and severity of hypertension [61], an increased prevalence of nephrosclerosis and end-stage renal disease in later life [55].

Perspectives

Current techniques for counting nephron number are applicable only in autopsy studies. Non-invasive methods for obtaining direct measurements of nephron number in vivo have not yet been established and must be developed to monitor nephron number in patients at risk of arterial hypertension and cardiovascular and chronic kidney diseases. Recent studies have attempted to estimate nephron unit number taking in account non-invasive procedures, evaluating the detailed structure of the kidneys by magnetic resonance imaging (MRI) [62]. This approach is based on the marked glomeruli with cationic ferritin, in vivo, allowing for whole-kidney detection of each labelled glomerulus. Although the total MRI-based count is lower than the stereological count, the error is near to 10%. Beeman et al. [63] assess glomerular number and volume in intact human kidneys using this technique. They further demonstrated MRI-detectable changes in glomerular and vascular morphology in the setting of renal vascular disease and hypertension. Thus, MRI techniques have a potential to enable direct measurements of the actual nephron number in living (human and animal) subjects as well as in experimental and pathological situations.

The question of the potential adaptive significance of foetal programming is an important one, both theoretically and practically. It affects the way in which the phenomena clustered under the DOHaD aegis are integrated in a broader context of evolutionary biology and the practical responses and interventions that might be made to affect health outcomes. However, it is a question that is still keenly debated.

Conclusion

In conclusion, maternal dietary protein restriction during pregnancy is associated with low foetal birth weight and leads to renal morphological and physiological changes. Different mechanisms can contribute to this phenotype: exposure to foetal glucocorticoid, alterations in the components of the renin-angiotensin system, apoptosis and DNA methylation. A low-protein diet during gestation decreases the activity of placental 11ß-hydroxysteroid dehydrogenase, exposing the foetus to glucocorticoids and resetting the hypothalamic-pituitary-adrenal axis in the offspring. The abnormal function/expression of type 1 (AT_1R) or type 2 (AT_2R) AngII receptors during any period of life may be the consequence or cause of renal adaptation. AT_1R is upregulated, compared with control, on the first day after birth of offspring born to low-protein diet mothers, but this protein appears to be downregulated by 12 days of age and thereafter. In these offspring, AT_2R expression differs from control at 1 day of age but is also downregulated thereafter, with low nephron numbers at all ages: from the foetal period, at the end of nephron formation and during adulthood. However, during adulthood, the glomerular filtration rate is not altered, due to glomerulus and podocyte hypertrophy. Kidney tubule transporters are regulated by physiological mechanisms; Na^+/K^+-ATPase is inhibited by AngII, and, in this model, the downregulated AngII receptors fail to inhibit Na^+/K^+-ATPase, leading to increased Na^+ reabsorption, contributing to the hypertensive status. We also considered the modulation of pro-apoptotic and anti-apoptotic factors during nephrogenesis, since organogenesis depends upon a tight balance between proliferation, differentiation and cell death.

Studies also showed changes in the postnatal hypothalamic angiotensin receptors by maternal protein restriction and its impact on in uteri programming of hypertension in adult life. In data shown in LP male pup by immunoblotting analysis, a significant decrease in the expression of AT_1R in the entire hypothalamic tissue extract of LP rats at 12 days of age compared to age-matched NP offspring. Conversely, the expression of the AT_2R in 12-day- and 16-week-old LP hypothalamus was significantly increased. The current data show the influence of central AngII administration on water consumption in a concentration-dependent fashion but also demonstrate that the water intake response to AngII was strikingly attenuated in 16-week-old LP. These results may be related to decreased brain arginine vaso-pressin (AVP) expression appearing in maternal protein-restricted offspring. Recent studies suggest that maternal low taurine ingestion may lead to changes in nTS cardiovascular and sympathetic nerve activity that are conducive to excess hydroelectrolytic tubule reabsorption and that this might potentiate the programming of adult hypertension. The present investigation shows an early decrease in fractional urinary sodium excretion in maternal protein-restricted offspring. The decreased fractional sodium excretion was accompanied by a fall in proximal sodium excretion and occurred despite unchanged creatinine clearance. These effects were associated with a significant enhancement in arterial blood pressure in the LP group, but the precise mechanism of these phenomena remains unknown.

References

1. Boucquemont J, Heinze G, Jager KJ, Oberbauer R, Leffondre K. Regression methods for investigating risk factors of chronic kidney disease outcomes: the state of the art. BMC Nephrol. 2014;15:45.
2. Van Pottelbergh G, Bartholomeeusen S, Buntinx F, Degryse J. The evolution of renal function and the incidence of end-stage renal disease in patients aged $50 years. Nephrol Dial Transplant. 2012;27:2297–303.
3. Wijewickrama ES, Weerasinghe D, Sumathipala PS, Horadagoda C, Lanarolle RD, Sheriff RM. Epidemiology of chronic kidney disease in a Sri Lankan population: experience of a tertiary care center. Saudi J Kidney Dis Transpl. 2011;22(6):1289–93.
4. Wallack L, Thornburg K. Developmental origins, epigenetics, and equity: moving upstream. Matern Child Health J. 2016;20(5):935–40.
5. Thornburg KL, Marshall N. The placenta is the center of the chronic disease universe. Am J Obstet Gynecol. 2015;213(4 Suppl):S14–20.
6. Zeman FJ. Effect of the young rat of maternal protein restriction. J Nutr. 1967;93(2):167–73.
7. Zeman FJ. Effects of maternal protein restriction on the kidney of the newborn young of rats. J Nutr. 1968;94(2):111–6.
8. Larsson L, Aperia A, Wilton P. Effect of normal development on compensatory renal growth. Kidney Int. 1980;18:29–35.
9. Hall SM, Zeman FJ. Kidney function of the progeny of rats fed a low protein diet. J Nutr. 1968;95:111–6.
10. Allen LH, Zeman FJ. Influence of increased postnatal food intake on body composition of protein-deficient rats. J Nutr. 1971;101:1311–8.
11. Allen LH, Zeman FJ. Kidney function in the progeny of protein-deficient rats. J Nutr. 1973;103(10):1467–78.
12. Merlet-Benichou C, Gilbert T, Muffat-Joly M, Lelievre-Pegorier M, Leroy B. Intrauterine growth retardation leads to a permanent nephron deficit in the rat. Pediatr Nephrol. 1994;8:175–80.
13. Langley-Evans SC, Welham SJM, Jackson AA. Fetal exposure to a maternal low protein diet impairs nephrogenesis and promotes hypertension in the rat. Life Sci. 1999;64:965–74.
14. Woods LL, Ingelfinger JR, Nyengaard JR, Rasch R. Maternal protein restriction suppresses the newborn renin-angiotensin system and programs adult hypertension in rats. Pediatr Res. 2001;49(4):460–7.
15. Vehaskari VM, Aviles DH, Manning J. Prenatal programming of adult hypertension in the rat. Kidney Int. 2001;59(1):238–45.
16. Welham SJ, Wade A, Woolf AS. Protein restriction in pregnancy is associated with increased apoptosis of mesen-chymal cells at the start of rat metanephrogenesis. Kidney Int. 2002;61(4):1231–42.
17. Sahajpal V, Ashton N. Increased glomerular angiotensin II binding in rats exposed to a maternal low protein diet in utero. J Physiol. 2005;563(Part1):193–201.
18. Woods LL, Weeks DA, Rasch R. Programming of adult blood pressure by maternal protein restriction: role of nephrogenesis. Kidney Int. 2004;65(4):1339–48.
19. Makrakis J, Zimanyi MA, Black MJ. Retinoic acid enhances nephron endowment in rats exposed to maternal protein restriction. Pediatr Nephrol. 2007;22:1861–7.
20. Hoppe CC, Evans RG, Bertram JF, Moritz KM. Effects of dietary protein restriction on nephron number in the mouse. Am J Phys Regul Integr Comp Phys. 2007;292(5):R1768–74.
21. Hoppe CC, Evans RG, Moritz KM, Cullen-McEwen LA, Fitzgerald SM, Dowling J, Bertram JF. Combined prenatal and postnatal protein restriction influences adult kidney structure, function, and arterial pressure. Am J Phys Regul Integr Comp Phys. 2007;292(1):R462–9.
22. Harrison M, Langley-Evans SC. Intergenerational programming of impaired nephrogenesis and hypertension in rats following maternal protein restriction during pregnancy. Br J Nutr. 2009;101(7):1020–30.

23. Mesquita FF, Gontijo JA, Boer PA. Maternal undernutrition and the offspring kidney: from fetal to adult life. Braz J Med Biol Res. 2010;43(11):1010–8.
24. Bertram JF. Combined prenatal and postnatal protein restriction influences adult kidney structure, function, and arterial pressure. Am J Phys Regul Integr Comp Phys. 2007;292(1):R462–9.
25. Chacon-Caldera J, Geraci S, Krämer P, Cullen-McEwen L, Bertram JF, Gretz N, Schad LR. Fast glomerular quantification of whole ex vivo mouse kidneys using Magnetic Resonance Imaging at 9.4 Tesla. Z Med Phys. 2016;S0939-3889(15):158–60.
26. Hinchliffe SA, Sargent PH, Howard CV, Chan YF, van Velzen D. Human intrauterine renal growth expressed in absolute number of glomeruli assessed by the disector method and Cavalieri principle. Lab Investig. 1991;64(6):777–84.
27. Barasch J, Pressler L, Connor J, Malik A. A ureteric bud cell line induces nephrogenesis in two steps by two distinct signals. Am J Phys. 1996;271(1 Pt 2):F50–61.
28. Kwong WY, Wild AE, Roberts P, Willis AC, Fleming TP. Maternal undernutrition during the preimplantation period of rat development causes blastocyst abnormalities and programming of postnatal hypertension. Development. 2000;127:4195–202.
29. McCalla CO, Nacharaju VL, Muneyyirci-Delale O, Glasgow S, Feldman JG. Placental 11 beta-hydroxysteroid dehydrogenase activity in normotensive and pre-eclamptic pregnancies. Steroids. 1998;63(10):511–5.
30. Brenner BM, Garcia DL, Anderson S. Glomeruli and blood pressure. Less of one, more the other? Am J Hypertens. 1988;1:335–47.
31. Kanzaki G, Tsuboi N, Haruhara K, Koike K, Ogura M, Shimizu A, Yokoo T. Factors associated with a vicious cycle involving a low nephron number, hypertension and chronic kidney disease. Hypertens Res. 2015;38(10):633–41.
32. Brawley L, Itoh S, Torrens C, Barker A, Bertram C, Poston L, Hanson M. Dietary protein restriction in pregnancy induces hypertension and vascular defects in rat male offspring. Pediatr Res. 2003;54:83–90.
33. Mesquita FF, Gontijo JA, Boer PA. Expression of renin angiotensin system signaling compounds in maternal protein restricted rats: effect on renal sodium excretion and blood pressure. Nephrol Dial Transplant. 2010;25:380–8.
34. Sherman RC, Langley-Evans SC. Antihypertensive treatment in early postnatal life modulates prenatal dietary influences upon blood pressure in the rat. Clin Sci (Lond). 2000;98:269–75.
35. Saavedra JM. Brain angiotensin II: new developments, unanswered questions and therapeutic opportunities. Cell Mol Neurobiol. 2005;25:485–512.
36. Gontijo JAR, Garcia WE, Figueiredo JF, et al. Renal sodium handling after noradrenergic stimulation of the lateral hypothalamus area in rats. Braz J Med Biol Res. 1992;25:937–42.
37. DiBona GF. Nervous kidney. Interaction between renal sympathetic nerves and renin-angiotensin system in the control of renal function. Hypertension. 2000;36:1083–8.
38. Ganten D, Marquez-Julio A, Granger P, et al. Renin in the dog brain. Am J Phys. 1971;221:1733–7.
39. Ferguson AV, Washburn DL, Latchford KJ. Hormonal and neurotransmitter roles for angiotensin in the regulation of central autonomic function. Exp Biol Med. 2001;226:85–96.
40. Lima MC, Scabora JE, Lopes A, et al. Early changes of hypothalamic angiotensin II receptors expression in gestational protein-restricted offspring: effect on water intake, blood pressure and renal sodium handling. J Renin-Angiotensin-Aldosterone Syst. 2013;14(3):271–82.
41. Scabora JE, de Lima MC, Lopes A, de Lima IP, Mesquita FF, Torres DB, Boer PA, Gontijo JA. Impact of taurine supplementation on blood pressure in gestational protein-restricted offspring: effect on the medial solitary tract nucleus cell numbers, angiotensin receptors, and renal sodium handling. J Renin-Angiotensin-Aldosterone Syst. 2015;16(1):47–58.
42. Vehaskari VM, Stewart T, Lafont D. Kidney angiotensin and angiotensin receptor expression in prenatally programmed hypertension. Am J Physiol Ren Physiol. 2004;287:F262–7.
43. McKinley MJ, McAllen RM, Davern P, et al. The sensory circumventricular organs of the mammalian brain. Berlin: Springer; n.d.
44. Hall JE, Brands MW. The renin-angiotensin-aldosterone systems. In: Seldin DW, Giebisch G, editors. The kidney: physiology and pathophysiology. New York: Lippincott Williams & Wilkins; 2000. p. 1009–46. Chapter 40.
45. Mathai ML, Evered MD, McKinley M. Central losartan blocks natriuretic, vasopressin, and pressor responses to central hypertonic NaCl in sheep. Am J Physiol Ren Physiol. 1998;275:R548–54.
46. Healy DP, Rettig R, Nguyen T, et al. Quantitative autoradiography of angiotensin II receptors in the rat solitary-vagal area: effects of nodose ganglioectomy or sinoaortic denervation. Brain Res. 1989;484:1–12.
47. Diz DI, Fantz DL, Benter IF, et al. Acute depressor actions of angiotensin II in the nucleus of the solitary tract are mediated by substance P. Am J Phys. 1997;273:R28–34.
48. Boujendar S, Remacle C, Hill D, et al. Taurine supplementation to the low protein maternal diet restores a normal development of the endocrine pancreas in the offspring. Diabetologia. 2000;43(Suppl 1):A128.
49. Cherif H, Reusens B, Ahn MT, et al. Effects of taurine on the insulin secretion of rat fetal islets from dams fed a low-protein diet. J Endocrinol. 1998;159:341–8.
50. Gaull G, Sturman JA, Raiha NCR. Development of mammalian sulfur metabolism: absence of cystathionase in human fetal tissue. Pediatr Res. 1972;6:538–47.

51. Esposito C, Plati A, Mazzullo T, et al. Renal function and functional reserve in healthy elderly individuals. J Nephrol. 2007;20:617–25.
52. Poggio ED, Rule AD. A critical evaluation of chronic kidney disease – should isolated reduced estimated glomerular filtration rate be considered a 'disease'? Nephrol Dial Transplant. 2009;24:698–700.
53. Martin JE, Sheaff MT. The pathology of ageing: concepts and mechanisms. J Pathol. 2007;211:111–3.
54. Joaquin AM, Gollapudi S. Functional decline in aging and disease: a role for apoptosis. J Am Geriatr Soc. 2001;49:1234–40.
55. Black JM, Lim K, Zimanyi MA, et al. Accelerated age-related decline in renal and vascular function in female rats following early-life growth restriction. Am J Phys Regul Integr Comp Phys. 2015;309:R1153–61.
56. Musso CG, Oreopoulos DG. Aging and physiological changes of the kidneys including changes in glomerular filtration rate. Nephron Physiol. 2011;119:p1–5.
57. Karam Z, Tuazon J. Anatomic and physiologic changes of the aging kidney. Clin Geriatr Med. 2013;29:555–64.
58. Kaur M, Chandran DS, Jaryal AK, Bhowmik D, Agarwal SK, Deepak KK. Baroreflex dysfunction in chronic kidney disease. World J Nephrol. 2016;5:53–65.
59. Gilbert JS, Lang AL, Grant AR, Nijland MJ. Maternal nutrient restriction in sheep: hypertension and decreased nephron number in offspring at 9 months of age. J Physiol. 2005;15:137–47.
60. Chen S, Brunskill EW, Potter SS, Dexheimer PJ, Salomonis N, Aronow BJ, Hong CI, Zhang T, Kopan R. Intrinsic age-dependent changes and cell-cell contacts regulate nephron progenitor lifespan. Dev Cell. 2015;35:49–62.
61. Yuasa K, Kondo T, Nagai H, Mino M, Takeshita A, Okada T. Maternal protein restriction that does not have an influence on the birth weight of the offspring induces morphological changes in kidneys reminiscent of phenotypes exhibited by intrauterine growth retardation rats. Congenit Anom (Kyoto). 2015;56:79.
62. Heilmann M, Neudecker S, Wolf I, Gubhaju L, Sticht C, Schock-Kusch D, Kriz W, Bertram JF, Schad LR, Gretz N. Quantification of glomerular number and size distribution in normal rat kidneys using magnetic resonance imaging. Nephrol Dial Transplant. 2012;27:100–7.
63. Beeman SC, Cullen-McEwen LA, Puelles VG, et al. MRI-based glomerular morphology and pathology in whole human kidneys. Am J Physiol Ren Physiol. 2014;306(11):F1381–90.

Chapter 12
Maternal Protein Restriction and Effects on Behavior and Memory in Offspring

Agnes da Silva Lopes Oliveira, José Antonio Rocha Gontijo, and Patrícia Aline Boer

Key Points

- Exposure to an adverse intrauterine environment promotes intrauterine growth restriction.
- Nutritional changes during the fetal period result in adaptations that can permanently change the structure and physiology of several organs.
- Early postnatal dietary restrictions influence cognitive performance and can lead to behavioral abnormalities and disorders in memory and learning.
- High stimulation results in changes of glucocorticoid receptors expression in the hippocampus.
- Chronic exposure to glucocorticoid caused by maternal protein restriction alters the morphological structure of the hippocampus, and these changes have been linked to impaired learning and memory ability and with altered long-term behavior.

Keywords Fetal programming • Behavior and memory • Maternal protein restriction • Hippocampal formation • Hippocampus and memory

Abbreviations

$5HT_1A$	Serotonin-specific receptors
$5HT_2A$	Serotonin-specific receptors
ACTH	Adrenocorticotrophic hormone
AT_1	Type 1 angiotensin II receptor
CNS	Central nervous system
CRH	Corticotrophin-releasing hormone

A. da Silva Lopes Oliveira, BSc, PhD
Department of Internal Medicine, School of Medicine at State University of Campinas, Campinas, SP, Brazil

J.A.R. Gontijo, MD, PhD • P.A. Boer, BSc, PhD (✉)
Department of Internal Medicine, Faculty of Medical Sciences at University of Campinas, Campinas, SP, Brazil
e-mail: alineboer@yahoo.com.br; boer@fcm.unicamp.br

© Springer International Publishing AG 2017
R. Rajendram et al. (eds.), *Diet, Nutrition, and Fetal Programming*,
Nutrition and Health, DOI 10.1007/978-3-319-60289-9_12

DEX   Dexamethasone
DOHaD   Developmental origins of health and disease
GR   Glucocorticoid receptor
HHPA   Hippocampus-hypothalamic-pituitary-adrenal axis
HPA   Hypothalamic-pituitary-adrenal axis
IUGR   Intrauterine growth restriction
LP   Low protein
MRs   Mineralocorticoid receptors
MWM   Morris water maze
NP   Normal protein

Introduction

The implications of events that occurred in early periods of life and its relationship to health in the long term are of great interest for public health in both developed and underdeveloped countries and have resulted in a number of studies to elucidate underlying biological mechanisms. It is well established that the disturbances at critical periods of fetal development may cause permanent changes in the physiology and morphology of organs [1]. Epidemiological evidence suggests that exposure to an adverse intrauterine environment promotes intrauterine growth restriction (IUGR) which has been associated with decreased supply of substrates for the fetus affecting their growth and development [2–4].

Maternal Protein Restriction and Brain

The central nervous system (CNS) is very sensitive to modifications in the environment. Its development is dependent on internal and external factors to the system itself. However external factors have been receiving increasing attention due to their influence on neuroplasticity. There is a strong association between IUGR, low birth weight and maternal low-protein intake. Maternal low nutritional levels decrease the supply of nutrients to the fetus. Thus, maternal nutrition plays a critical role in the growth and development of offspring. Nutritional changes during the fetal period result in adaptations that can permanently change the structure and physiology of organs, predisposing the individual to metabolic and endocrine diseases in adulthood and several cognitive disorders.

Considering the fact that the structural brain development begins in the early days of the embryonic period and extends to the first years of life, changes in prenatal and early postnatal development can be highly detrimental to the neurodevelopment [5]. The brain maturation happens through a series of temporally overlapping phases (Fig. 12.1). The final structure of the brain arises during ontogenesis phase, in which there is a migration of postmitotic cells in germinal zones, which differentiate and interact with other nonneural tissues nearby in a highly ordered sequence. However, the normal brain development is dependent not only of this exact sequence but also of many metabolic reactions that regulate these cellular events. These sequences are determined mainly by the genome, but the genetic regulation of brain development is highly influenced by environmental factors such as stress, smoking, infections, and nutritional changes. Thus, protein-restricted intake during the prenatal period followed by the low birth weight of the offspring acts as a risk factor for the development of neurological and psychiatric diseases. Substantial evidence from studies in animals and in humans shows that gestational as well as early postnatal dietary restrictions influence cognitive performance and can lead to behavioral abnormalities and disorders in memory and learning [6–8].

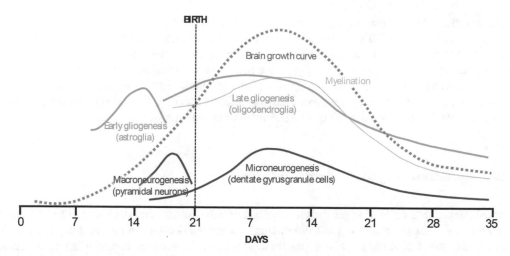

Fig. 12.1 Rat brain growth curve showing the time of cell types differentiation. The rat brain at birth has approximately 12% of adult brain weight, while that found in humans is about 27% of the adult brain weight (Adapted from Morgane et al. [5])

Critical Period of the Brain Development

The life evolution is integrated, cumulative, and continuous and not episodic, static, or discrete. Behavioral researchers rarely forget this, but medicine doctors and biologists often do. Developmental biology is the one domain of the life sciences where the organism as a progressively unfolding phenomenon is a central concept. The reemergence of developmental biology as a vigorous discipline, intersecting in important ways with genetics [9], evolution [10], and epidemiology [11–13], has injected new ideas into all those fields. Within epidemiology a seminal impact of this new attention to developmental biology has been in the formulation of the "fetal programming hypothesis," also known as the *fetal origins hypothesis* or, more generally, as the *developmental origins of health and disease* (DOHaD). Simply put, this hypothesis suggests that conditions very early in development, even in utero, can leave lasting imprints of an organism's physiology, imprints that may affect susceptibility to diseases with onsets that may occur many decades later [14, 15].

The concept of fetal programming is, of course, not new. Behavioral endocrinologists and neuroscientists, for example, have long recognized organizational effects of prenatal androgen hormones in *programming* certain aspects of reproductive axis function and reproductive behavior that emerges later in an animal's life [16]. The ontogenetic critical periods, including fetal development, are familiar concepts in psychology even as they are in biology. So, rather than being a radically new concept, the ascendancy of the fetal programming hypothesis should be seen as representing a new appreciation for these kinds of effects together with a deeper understanding of the mechanisms that produce them and the significance they may play for individuals and species. The question of the potential adaptive significance of fetal programming is an important one, both theoretically and practically. It affects the way in which the phenomena clustered under the DOHaD aegis are integrated in a broader context of evolutionary biology and the practical responses and interventions that might be made to affect health outcomes. It is a question that is still keenly debated, however.

As stated above, there are periods during the development in which the organism is highly vulnerable. Such periods are known as critical period, which represents a stage of development that cannot be reversed or repeated later, and in which organizational processes are more easily modified. If the progression of morphological, physiological, and biochemical development does not occur at the correct time, there will be a permanent functional deficits being determined by severity of the insult and the duration of the development period and which is imposed. In animals and human beings, the period of greatest vulnerability of the CNS occurs from the second third of pregnancy to early week or year of life (in humans); however, the peak of the curve brain growth occurs during pregnancy. At this stage occurs the genesis of glial and pyramidal neurons cells, resulting in the birth in 27% of brain weight. Already in rodents, this phase comprises from birth until about third week of life, when there is a development of the hippocampus and cerebellum. Thus, the impact on brain development of the fetus by maternal nutritional deficiency can be irreversible (Fig. 12.1).

Fetal Programming of Behavioral Outcomes

The most elegant example of epigenetic modification of behavior by early environments is not strictly an example of fetal programming but offers clear documentation of the epigenetic processes that determine the effect. Meaney and his colleagues have focused on maternal behavior in rats, describing individual variation in the pattern of arch-backed nursing intense licking and grooming of pups [17, 18]. Pups who receive greater degrees of maternal stimulation show less anxiety in open field tests and other indices as adults. Females who receive greater stimulation as pups give greater amounts of stimulation to their own pups, inducing the same low-anxiety behavioral phenotype in their own offspring. The entire effect appears to be mediated by epigenetic alterations in histone acetylation and methylation of the promoter region of the glucocorticoid receptor (GR) gene in the hippocampus of the rat pups depending on the type of maternal behavior they receive [19, 20]. High stimulation results in changes of glucocorticoid receptors expression in the hippocampus, which is in turn associated with modification in sensitivity to corticosteroid feedback, a pattern that persists into adulthood [21]. In hippocampus, the effect of standard glucocorticoid signaling is to suppress hypothalamic release of corticotrophin-releasing hormone (CRH), leading to lower pituitary release of adrenocorticotrophic hormone (ACTH) and lower secretion of glucocorticoid from the adrenal cortex. Adults who receive high levels of maternal stimulation as pups thus show relatively low HHPA axis reactivity to stress, while the reverse is true in those who receive less stimulation as pups. This appears to correlate with their behavior in open field and other tests and with the maternal style that females may display toward their own pups. In this way a stable difference in HPA axis sensitivity is transferred across generations through females based on an *inherited* epigenetic pattern. Interestingly, the epigenetic pattern is passed through first being translated into a behavioral pattern in the mothers and then back into an epigenetic pattern in the offspring. Prior studies have documented the effect of maternal behavior to similarly program reproductive axis activity through epigenetic effects on steroid receptor expression [22]. Although this example of rat maternal behavior is not an example of "fetal" programming, it is an elegant demonstration of the potential for programming of the HHPA axis to have behavioral consequences [23, 24]. Furthermore, one of the most impressive studies to implicate fetal programming in psychiatric outcomes is the work of Susser and colleagues on the follow-up of individuals conceived during the Nazi occupation of Holland at the end of World War II [25]. The so-called Dutch hunger winter provides a rather gruesome natural experiment in which pregnant women, along with the rest of the civilian population, were subject to extreme food deprivation during a relatively discrete period [25]. Susser's parents conducted seminal studies of the effects of this famine resulting in the recognition of the importance of folate nutrition in pregnancy in avoiding neural tube defects [26]. The younger Susser undertook to determine whether less debilitating effects on nervous system development as a consequence of famine exposure in utero might have consequences for psychiatric risk after birth. He found a significant increase of risk of schizophrenia and related disorders among those whose mothers went through the peak of the famine during their second trimester of pregnancy [25, 27]. Subsequent work with individuals born during discrete famines in China has yielded similar results [28]. Whether the mechanisms mediating these effects are epigenetic in nature remains to be determined [29].

Costello and colleagues provide a second example of prenatal influences on psychiatric outcomes [30]. They assessed a population-based sample of over 1400 boys and girls in North Carolina between at the ages of 9 and 16 for psychiatric symptoms. They found that the rates of adolescent depression were over four times higher (38.1%) in girls who were low birth weight compared to normal weight girls at birth (8.4%) and seven times higher than in boys of any birth weight (4.9%). The well-known sex difference in adolescent depression was thus almost entirely accounted for by the higher risk in low birth weight girls. However, there was an interesting interaction. Low and normal birth weight girls who experienced no subsequent adversities showed no incidence of depression. But with each additional adverse circumstance, the rate of depression in low birth weight girls, but not normal ones, increased significantly. The authors suggest that low birth weight girls are more sensitive to adverse circumstances later in life in terms of their risk of depression, a result that suggests possible alteration of physiological responses to stress, perhaps involving the HPA axis.

Mechanism of Genesis Changes

Although some nutritional effects are the result of direct change in substrate availability, part of these results is due to hormonal mediation, which can alter the development of specific fetal tissues at critical periods of development and lead to permanent changes in hormone secretion (Fig. 12.2). Animal evidences have suggested that a maternal nutritional or emotional stress during pregnancy is associated with behavioral outcomes in offspring [31, 32] . The nature of the stressing event applied may differ, but it is often assumed that the mother's HPA axis responds with higher levels of glucocorticoid hormones. It is unlikely that higher levels of maternal cortisol affect fetal physiology in humans, however, since the placenta is rich in type 2 11-ß-steroid-dehydrogenase, which converts cortisol to inactive cortisone, thus buffering the fetus from maternal cortisol levels [33]. The glucocorticoid secretion is made by the adrenal cortex and controlled by HHPA, a classic endocrine regulator of negative feedback. Glucocorticoids exert their effects by binding to GRs, a member of the family of nuclear steroid receptors. Additionally, in some tissues, glucocorticoid has higher affinity to mineralocorticoid receptors (MRs), also deeply related to the modulation of hippocampus function.

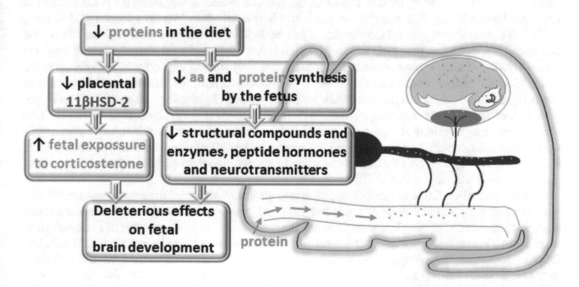

Fig. 12.2 A reduction in diet protein content lead to alterations on structural, physiological, biochemical, and psychological maturation of the brain

Although positive correlations between baseline levels of maternal and fetal cortisol have been observed [34] which in turn increases the concentration of glucocorticoids to the fetus, thereby promoting growth retardation of offspring and a possible programming of response related to cardiovascular diseases metabolic and psychiatric, evidence of changes in maternal and fetal cortisol responses to stress are independent [34]. Such buffering makes physiological sense since in late pregnancy the mother is essentially in a catabolic state, while the fetus is in an anabolic state with transient suppression of HHPA axis. In fetal programming context, cross talk between the energy metabolism of mother and fetus would be disastrous.

In addition, the exogenous administration of glucocorticoids in the mother or fetus, results in low birth weight plus several long-term diseases such as hypertension, hyperglycemia, and behavioral disorders in the offspring. Indeed, these effects are transmitted over generations without reexposure to glucocorticoids, suggesting the involvement of epigenetic mechanisms. However, dexamethasone (DEX) has been administered to mothers known to be carrying fetuses deficient in 21-hydroxylase and therefore at risk of congenital adrenal hyperplasia [35]. A secondary consequence is overproduction of adrenal androgens that can lead to varying degrees of genital androgenization [36]. Some studies have indicated potential effects on childhood and adult behavior, including sexual orientation, as well [37, 38]. DEX is often administered to head off these consequences, since it readily crosses the placenta; is not metabolized by 11-ß-steroid-dehydrogenase; and interacts with glucocorticoid receptors in the fetal hypothalamus to suppress excess production of ACTH and its corollary effects [39]. In animal studies using prenatal administration of DEX as a treatment alterations of offspring behavior and HHPA axis reactivity is observed. This suggests that the feedback sensitivity of the HHPA axis may be partially regulated through the level of activation of the axis during fetal development.

Hippocampal Formation

Given their prominent role in brain plasticity and in the regulation of cognitive processes, the hippocampal formation has been the focus of many studies designed to identify the morphological, biochemical, and physiological substrates' long-term disability of brain functions associated with dietary restrictions in the beginning of life. The hippocampus is a structure located in the medial temporal lobe. Anatomically, the hippocampus of mammals is divided into different subfields: CA1, CA2, CA3, CA4, and dentate gyrus. Functionally, it can be divided into two different regions: the ventral and dorsal hippocampus. While the ventral portion is involved primarily the *emotional processing*, the dorsal is mainly linked to *memory and learning*. It is a widely studied region for its importance in the acquisition and memory consolidation, but highly vulnerable to various environmental stresses due to plasticity of hippocampal circuits necessary for their functions in learning and memory. The hippocampal formation is a different target structure changes from the maternal environment. Studies have shown that changes during the prenatal period had influence on neurogenesis in the hippocampus immaturity and remodeling of dendrites of CA3 region, with possible cognitive changes. Furthermore, it is a preferred target region of the action of stress hormones, and through this brain area, it is part of a negative feedback mechanism in HPA axis.

Morphological studies in the hippocampus in animals that experienced maternal protein restriction showed that the pyramidal cells of CA1 and CA3 and granule cells of the dentate gyrus regions showed reduction in cell size in dendritic branching and a decrease in the number of synaptic spines in mice of various ages. However, chemical inhibitors, suggesting that hormones HHPA axis can modulate dendritic morphology in the hippocampus, can suppress these effects. Additionally, changes in the regulation of HHPA axis are consistent components in various types of affective disorders such as depression, panic disorders, and obsessive-compulsive disorder. Thus, adrenal steroids appear to be crucial factor in the structural remodeling of the hippocampus.

Fetal Programming of Psychological and Psychiatric Outcomes

Animal evidence has long suggested that maternal emotional and nutritional stress during pregnancy is associated with behavioral outcomes in offspring [31, 32]. The nature of the stresses applied may differ, but it is often assumed that the mother's HHPA axis respond releases higher levels of glucocorticoid hormones. It is unlikely that higher levels of maternal cortisol/corticosterone affect fetal physiology in humans and rodents, however, since the placenta is rich in type 2 11-β-steroid-dehydrogenase, which converts cortisol to inactive cortisone, thus buffering the fetus from maternal cortisol levels [33]. Such buffering makes physiological sense since in late pregnancy the mother is essentially in a catabolic state, while the fetus is in an anabolic state. Cross talk between the energy metabolism of mother and fetus would be disastrous.

However, dexamethasone, a synthetic glucocorticoid, has long been administered to mothers known to be carrying fetuses deficient in 21-hydroxylase and therefore at risk of congenital adrenal hyperplasia [35]. Because affected congenital adrenal hyperplasia individuals are impaired in their ability to produce cortisol, inadequate negative feedback leads to overproduction of adrenocorticotrophic hormone (ACTH) and hyperplasia of the adrenal glands. A secondary consequence is overproduction of adrenal androgens that can lead to varying degrees of genital androgenization [36]. Some studies have indicated potential effects on childhood and adult behavior, including sexual orientation, as well [37]. Dexamethasone is often administered to head off these consequences, since it readily crosses the placenta, is not metabolized by 11-β steroid-dehydrogenase, and interacts with GR receptors in the fetal hypothalamus to suppress excess production of ACTH and its corollary effects [39].

Although maternal stress may not be communicated to the fetus via maternal cortisol, there are other pathways possible, including alterations of placental blood flow [34] and changes in energy available for fetal growth. In addition, conditions that lead to fetal stress, such as restricted energy availability [34], may directly affect the level of activity of the fetal HHPA axis, as opposed to the maternal axis, with potential programming consequences. Achieving a better understanding the potential for prenatal conditions to have lasting effects on an individual's physiology, with possibly serious implications for psychiatric risk, must be considered one of the high priorities for psychological research stemming from the fetal programming hypothesis [40].

As sustained above, glucocorticoids play a role in the normal development of the brain and have been associated with neuronal maturation and survival. Thus, as mentioned above, fetal exposure to excess glucocorticoids during critical periods of brain development can lead to structural changes in neuronal dendritic morphology and the number of synapses [32]. Additionally, chronic exposure to glucocorticoid caused by maternal protein restriction alters the morphological structure of the hippocampus, and these changes in the structure of the hippocampus have been linked to learning and memory problems and long-term behavior. It is well established that children exposed to restriction of nutrients during fetal period have cognitive deficits as well as increasing the risk of psychiatric disorders development as depression and schizophrenia, changes in memory and learning, increased response to stress, and changes in drug sensitivity psychotropic. These disorders are usually studied in well-known brain regions such as the hippocampal formation where much of the internal and external connectivity and the chemical cellular architecture are well known.

Hippocampus and Memory

The different kinds of stresses affects neural regions including gestational hippocampus, amygdala, corpus callosum, neocortex, cerebellum, and hypothalamus and often results in a reduction in the volume of the tissues that make up these structures. It is known that the limbic system, particularly the hippocampus, plays a central role in the memory/cognition and control of emotions. The hippocampal

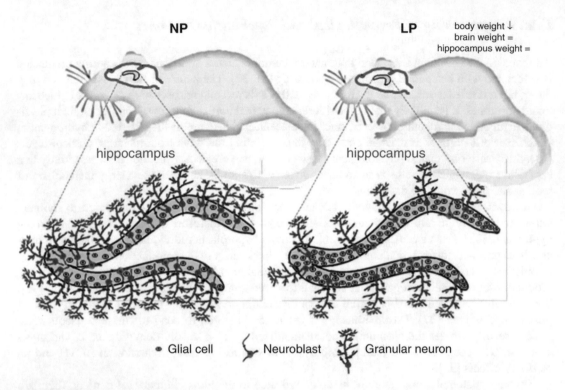

Fig. 12.3 The low-protein diet during gestation and lactation lead to marked cellular imbalances in dentate gyrus. We used male rats from mothers submitted to low protein (6% casein) comparatively to normal protein (17% casein) diet. The brain and hippocampus weight are not altered as well as cell number. However we found altered cell ratio (unpublished data)

gyrus has been the subject of several studies due to its importance in neural plasticity in neurogenesis and regulation of cognitive processes. Changes in efficiency and structural plasticity of hippocampal synaptic connections can compromise crucial neurobiological mechanisms involved in cognitive processes. As previously described, gestational protein restriction may produces, at long-term, deleterious consequences in offspring adulthood. Several animal studies have shown atrophy of hippocampal neurons and reduction in the number of neurons in this region, the result of disturbances in the maternal environment (Fig. 12.3) [41].

Prior studies have shown that changes in memory and learning from fetal exposure to glucocorticoids is the result of many cellular and molecular events which include downregulation receptors [42], reduced dendritic branching [41, 43], changes in the synapses [44], inhibiting LTP which is the best-documented neuronal substrate for memory formation [45], and impairment of energy metabolism [46]. Moreover, there may still be a reduction in BDNF, a factor involved in tropism and survival of neurons and synapses (unpublished data). There is also evidence of the interaction between fetal exposure to glucocorticoids and the serotonergic and cathecolaminergic systems by the modulation of the $5HT_1A$ and $5HT_2A$ receptors [47]. Furthermore, there is evidence that gestational protein restriction impairs the inhibitory control of the HHPA axis, leading to excessive secretion of CRF/ACTH and increased plasma levels of glucocorticoid, contributing to further damage in hippocampal and consequently higher cognitive deficits neurons, impairing the different types of declarative memory (verbal memory, social memory, and spatial memory). Chronic exposure to glucocorticoids by GRs activation induces neuronal death and mitigation of neurogenesis.

We and others have demonstrated that maternal nutritional restriction during pregnancy or in early postnatal life results in hippocampus cognitive impairment and structural abnormalities in the 16-week-old offspring. In an attempt to analyze whether gestational protein restriction might induce learning and memory impairment associated with structural changes in the hippocampus, we carried out Morris water maze (MWM) test and a detailed morphometric analysis of dendritic cytoarchitecture of the hippocampus from male adult rats [41]. In addition, we analyzed the dorsal and ventral hippocampal expression and localization of mineralocorticoid (MR) and glucocorticoid (GR), type 1 angiotensin II receptor (AT_1) and serotonin-specific receptors ($5HT_1A$ and $5HT_2A$). By MWM we did not found significant differences between LP and NP groups, in any of the parameters analyzed, suggesting that such functions of the hippocampus were not altered by gestational protein restriction. However, by applying three-dimensional analysis of dendrites from the dorsal hippocampus, this study demonstrates that gestational protein restriction leads to decreases in total basal dendritic length and in apical intersections of CA3 pyramidal neurons. The dendritic architecture of CA1 and dentate gyros was unchanged. This study revealed a clear dissociation between behavioral test response and hippocampal neuron changes as a consequence of fetal programming. We found different patterns of dorsal and ventral expression of analyzed receptors, and we suggests that reduced GR and $5HT_1A$ and enhanced $5HT_2A$ expression are involved in anxious behavior and that AT1 downregulation may have a protective effect. These neurochemical alterations may have important consequences for anxiety- and depressive-like behavior. A recent study in our lab (unpublished data) assessed the effects of maternal protein restriction, during pregnancy and breastfeeding, on the structure of the hippocampus, their duties on the memory and emotions (anxiety/fear) as well as on the cellular composition of this brain structure and influence over these morphological and behavioral parameters, and the exposure of the offspring of male rats to the enriched environment. The findings of this study represent the perinatal impact of malnutrition protein in the hippocampus, which is involved in emotional behavior as well as in memory and learning. The study revealed decoupling the behavioral test response and changes in the number of hippocampus neurons, as a consequence of fetal programming. The absence of basal changes in performance of these tests occurred in spite of reduction in the number of neurons in the dentate gyrus of the hippocampus. Several authors have suggested that the observed atrophy in the hippocampus may be a compensatory response to protect the hippocampus of additional damage. We have demonstrated, for the first time, that maternal exposure to protein restriction during neural development of offspring that cause important morphological changes in the hippocampus may make these animals vulnerable to neural disorders in adulthood. This study, at least under morphological aspect, confirmed the "selfish brain" theory, a recent paradigm that posits that in order to keep its own energy supply stable, the brain modulates the energy metabolism in the periphery by regulating both the allocation as the intake of nutrients. In this work, the unmodified brain mass do not match with the intensity of cytological composition changes, particularly of the hippocampal nucleus, in different experimental groups. Although it seems that the nutritional changes promote irreversible changes in body mass, but not in the brain and some of its fundamental structures, composition, and neuronal structure and its recovery from primordial cells, are deeply modified by the maternal dietary restriction and, surprisingly, by exposure to oxygen-enriched environment. Thus, we can affirm that the selfish brain theory explains the maintenance of brain matter; however, the proportion of the different cell types has profoundly changed what can expand our understanding of the adaptation to stress and neuron regeneration in neuron behavioral states regarded as abnormal. Moreover, we must emphasize that, while we have observed a significant reduction in the number of neurons after the period of breastfeeding, we also demonstrate, for the first time, that this parameter is reversed by stimulus in enriched environment. Ours studies are not able to answer the question whether these alterations are related to in utero underdevelopment or results from a postnatal adaptation to programmed physiology in adult life. Further time course studies should be done to answer this question.

Conclusions

Fetal gestational programming protein restriction leads to intrauterine growth restriction, which is associated with the decrease in the supply of substrates crucial to the fetus affecting growth and development. This situation has repercussions in birth weight and several changes in organs and tissues in adult life. These changes from adaptations to the maternal environment have long-term effect producing numerous structural and neurochemical deficits in key brain regions for the development of the offspring. In addition, these changes can achieve brain systems that play a key role in behavioral processes and memory and learning. Moreover, considerable attention has been focused, therefore, on the degree to which HHPA axis reactivity may be established in utero, the potential for maternal nutritional status to affect these aspects of metabolic physiology, and the cellular mechanisms by which these effects are mediated.

References

1. Martin-Gronert MS, Ozanne SE. Maternal nutrition during pregnancy and health of the offspring. Biochem Soc Trans. 2006;34:779–82.
2. Rose G. Familial patterns in ischaemic heart disease. Br J Prev Soc Med. 1964;18:75–80.
3. Forsdahl S. Are poor living conditions in childhood and adolescence an important risk factor for arteriosclerotic heart disease? Brit J Prev and Soc Medicine. 1967;31:91–5.
4. Barker DJ, Osmond C. Diet and coronary heart disease in England and Wales during and after the second world war. J Epidemiol Community Health. 1986;40:37–44.
5. Morgane PJ, Mokler DJ, Galler JR. Effects of prenatal protein malnutrition on the hippocampal formation. Neurosci Biobehav Rev. 2002;26:471–83.
6. De Oliveira LM. Malnutrition and environment: interaction effects upon animal behavior. Child Nutr Rev. 1985;13:99–108.
7. Riul TR, Carvalho AF, Almeida OS, De-Oliveira LM, Almeida SS. Ethological analysis of mother-pup interactions and other behavioral reactions in rats: effects of malnutrition and tactile stimulation of the pups. Braz J Med Biol Res. 1999;32:975–83.
8. Wainwright PE, Colombo J. Nutrition and the development of cognitive functions: interpretation of behavioral studies in animals and human infants. Am J Clin Nutr. 2006;84:961–70.
9. Badayev AV. Maternal effects as generators of evolutionary change: a reassessment. Ann N Y Acad Sci. 2008;1133:151–61.
10. West-Eberhard MJ. Developmental plasticity and evolution. Oxford: Oxford University Press; 2003.
11. Barker DJP. Mothers, babies, and disease in later life. London: BMJ Publishing; 1994.
12. Gluckman P, Hanson M, editors. Developmental origins of health and disease. Cambridge, UK: Cambridge University Press; 2006.
13. Kuh D, Ben-Shlomo Y, Lynch J, Hallqvist J, et al. Life course epidemiology. J Epidemiol Community Health. 2003;57:778–83.
14. Barker DJ, Eriksson JG, Forsen T, et al. Fetal origins of adult disease: strength of effects and biological basis. Int J Epidemiol. 2002;31(6):1235–9.
15. Gluckman P, Hanson M. The fetal matrix. Cambridge, UK: Cambridge University; 2005.
16. Nelson RJ. An introduction to behavioral endocrinology. 3rd ed. Sunderland: Sinauer; 2005.
17. Meaney MJ, Diorio J, Francis D, et al. Environmental regulation of the development of glucocorticoid receptor systems in the rat forebrain. The role of serotonin. Ann N Y Acad Sci. 1994;746:260–73. discussion 274, 289-293.
18. Meaney MJ, Mitchell JB, Aitken DH, et al. The effects of neonatal handling on the development of the adrenocortical response to stress: implications for neuropathology and cognitive deficits in later life. Psychoneuroendocrinology. 1991;16(1–3):85–103.
19. Meaney MJ, Szyf M. Environmental programming of stress responses through DNA methylation: life at the interface between a dynamic environment and a fixed genome. Dialogues Clin Neurosci. 2005;7(2):103–23.
20. Weaver IC, Cervoni N, Champagne FA, et al. Epigenetic programming by maternal behavior. Nat Neurosci. 2004;7(8):847–54.
21. Weaver IC, Meaney MJ, Szyf M. Maternal care effects on the hippocampal transcriptome and anxiety-mediated behaviors in the offspring that are reversible in adulthood. Proc Natl Acad Sci U S A. 2006;103(9):3480–5.

22. Champagne FA, Weaver IC, Diorio J, et al. Maternal care associated with methylation of the estrogen receptor-alpha1b promoter and estrogen receptor-alpha expression in the medial preoptic area of female offspring. Endocrinology. 2006;147(6):2909–15.
23. Champagne DL, Bagot RC, van Hasselt F, et al. Maternal care and hippocampal plasticity: evidence for experience-dependent structural plasticity, altered synaptic functioning, and differential responsiveness to glucocorticoids and stress. J Neurosci. 2008;28(23):6037–45.
24. Meaney MJ, Szyf M. Maternal care as a model for experience-dependent chromatin plasticity? Trends Neurosci. 2005;28(9):456–63.
25. Susser E, Brown AS, Klonowski E, et al. Schizophrenia and impaired homocysteine metabolism: a possible association. Biol Psychiatry. 1998;44(2):141–3.
26. Stein Z, Susser M, Saenger G, Marolla F. Nutrition and mental performance. Science. 1972;178(62):708–13.
27. Susser E, Neugebauer R, Hoek HW, et al. Schizophrenia after prenatal famine. Further evidence. Arch Gen Psychiatry. 1996;53(1):25–31.
28. Susser E, St Clair D, He L. Latent effects of prenatal malnutrition on adult health: the example of schizophrenia. Ann N Y Acad Sci. 2008;1136:185–92.
29. de Rooij SR, Painter RC, Phillips DI, et al. Cortisol responses to psychological stress in adults after prenatal exposure to the Dutch famine. Psychoneuroendocrinology. 2006;31(10):1257–65.
30. Costello EJ, Worthman C, Erkanli A, Angold A. Prediction from low birth weight to female adolescent depression: a test of competing hypotheses. Arch Gen Psychiatry. 2007;64(3):338–44.
31. Burton CL, Chatterjee D, Chatterjee-Chakraborty M, et al. Prenatal restraint stress and motherless rearing disrupts expression of plasticity markers and stress-induced corticosterone release in adult female Sprague-Dawley rats. Brain Res. 2007;1158:28–38.
32. Kapoor A, Matthews SG. Prenatal stress modifies behavior and hypothalamic-pituitary-adrenal function in female guinea pig offspring: effects of timing of prenatal stress and stage of reproductive cycle. Endocrinology. 2008;149(12):6406–15.
33. McCalla CO, Nacharaju VL, Muneyyirci-Delale O, et al. Placental 11 beta-hydroxysteroid dehydrogenase activity in normotensive and pre-eclamptic pregnancies. Steroids. 1998;63(10):511–5.
34. Gitau R, Fisk NM, Teixeira JM, Cameron A, Glover V. Fetal hypothalamic-pituitary-adrenal stress responses to invasive procedures are independent of maternal responses. J Clin Endocrinol Metab. 2001;86(1):104–9.
35. Speiser PW, New MI. Prenatal diagnosis and treatment of congenital adrenal hyperplasia. J Pediatr Endocrinol Metab. 1994;7(3):183–91.
36. Pang S. Congenital adrenal hyperplasia. Endocrinol Metab Clin N Am. 1997;26(4):853–91.
37. Arlt W, Krone N. Adult consequences of congenital adrenal hyperplasia. Horm Res. 2007;68(Supplement 5):158–64.
38. New MI. An update of congenital adrenal hyperplasia. Ann N Y Acad Sci. 2004;1038:14–43.
39. Hughes IA. Management of fetal endocrine disorders. Growth Hormon IGF Res. 2003;13(Supplement A):S55–61.
40. Kaplan LA, Evans L, Monk C. Effects of mothers' prenatal psychiatric status and postnatal caregiving on infant biobehavioral regulation: can prenatal programming be modified? Early Hum Dev. 2008;84(4):249–56.
41. Lopes A, Torres DB, Rodrigues AJ, et al. Gestational protein restriction induces CA3 dendritic atrophy in dorsal hippocampus neurons but does not alter learning and memory performance in adult offspring. Int J Dev Neurosci. 2013;31(3):151–6.
42. Mcewen BS. Stress and hippocampal plasticity (review). Annu Rev Neurosci. 1999;22:105–22.
43. Radley JJ, Rocher AB, Janssen WG, et al. Reversibility of apical dendritic retraction in the rat medial prefrontal cortex following repeated stress. Exp Neurol. 2005;196:199–203.
44. Antonow-Schlorke I, Schwab M, Li C, Nathanielsz PW. Glucocorticoid exposure at the dose used clinically alters cytoskeletal proteins and presynaptic terminals in the fetal baboon brain. J Physiol. 2003;547:117–23.
45. Brunson KL, Kramar E, Lin B, et al. Mechanisms of late-onset cognitive decline after early-life stress. J. Neurosci. 2005;25(41):9328–38.
46. Simerly RB. Hypothalamic substrates of metabolic imprinting. Physiol Behav. 2008;94:79–89.
47. Fontenot M, Kaplan JR, Manuck SB, Arango V, et al. Long-term effects of chronic social stress on serotonergic indices in the prefrontal cortex of adult male cynomolgus macaques. Brain Res. 1995;705:105–8.

Part III
Effects of Obesity, High Fat Diet and Junk Food on Fetal Outcomes

Chapter 13
Trends in Obesity and Implications for the Fetus

Jamie O. Lo and Antonio E. Frias

Key Points

- Obesity is a worldwide pandemic.
- Maternal obesity is associated with adverse pregnancy outcomes.
- Maternal obesity negatively impacts infant and future adult health.
- Maternal obesity affects fetal programming.
- Preconception weight loss is ideal, but not applicable to a large portion of pregnancies.
- Current interventions aimed at preventing the progression of obesity have resulted in only minimal improvement in maternal and infant outcomes.

Keywords Obesity epidemic • Fetal programming • Increased adult disease risk • Obesity • Trends

Abbreviations

ACOG   American College of Obstetricians and Gynecologists
BMI   Body mass index
HSE   Health Survey for England
IOM   Institute of Medicine
PRAMS Pregnancy Risk Assessment Monitoring System
WHO   World Health Organization

Introduction

Obesity, defined as a body mass index (BMI) ≥ 30 kg/m^2, is a worldwide pandemic (Table 13.1). The World Health Organization (WHO) estimates the prevalence of obesity to have doubled worldwide since 1980 [1]. In some countries, over 40% of women of childbearing age are overweight or obese [2].

J.O. Lo, MD • A.E. Frias, MD (✉)
Department of Obstetrics and Gynecology, Oregon Health & Science University, Portland, OR, USA
e-mail: Loj@ohsu.edu

© Springer International Publishing AG 2017
R. Rajendram et al. (eds.), *Diet, Nutrition, and Fetal Programming*,
Nutrition and Health, DOI 10.1007/978-3-319-60289-9_13

Table 13.1 Body mass index (BMI)

Classification	BMI category (kg/m^2)
Normal weight	18.5–24.9
Overweight	25.0–29.9
Obese class 1	30.0–34.9
Obese class 2	35.0–39.9
Obese class 3	≥ 40

Economic changes, technologic advances, and lifestyle alterations have produced an abundance of cheap, high-calorie food coupled with reduced physical activity contributing to the obesity crisis. The high prevalence of obesity and the projected increasing trend have adverse implications for pregnant women including thromboembolic complications, gestational diabetes, hypertension, cesarean section, maternal hemorrhage, and infection [3–5]. Offspring are at increased risk for spontaneous miscarriage, fetal malformations, fetal macrosomia, stillbirth, and preterm delivery [3–5]. Overall, the risk of any form of obstetrical complication is approximately three times higher in obese mothers [6].

Despite the revised 2009 Institute of Medicine (IOM) guidelines, 43% of pregnant women continue to exceed gestational weight gain recommendations [7]. Maternal obesity results from a combination of factors including, but not limited to, genetic predisposition, in utero determinants related to prenatal health, lack of physical activity, poor nutrition, socioeconomics, gender, lack of sleep, and medication use, in addition to underlying medical problems that promote weight gain. Current lifestyle modifications, such as diet and exercise, recommended for pre-pregnancy and pregnancy weight loss have been challenging for women to adopt. Also contributing is the lack of obesity awareness and education. Among women of reproductive age intending to become pregnant, half have low obesity risk knowledge, a third misperceive their body weight, and two thirds are unable to define a healthy diet [8].

There has been an increasing prevalence of obese reproductive-aged women, and obstetrician gynecologists are essential to preventing and treating this epidemic. This alarming trend highlights the public health significance of adverse reproductive outcomes stemming from obesity and the strong need for patient education and weight loss interventions. Efforts to increase awareness and successfully reduce pre-pregnancy and maternal obesity would have a measurable impact on infant and future adult health. The prenatal period also provides a window of opportunity for intervention to curtail the intergenerational cycle of obesity as it is a critical time of fetal growth, development, and physiological change.

Trends of Maternal Obesity

Trends in the United States

In the United States, approximately four million births occur annually, and currently approximately 60% of women of childbearing age are either overweight or obese [9, 10]. This incidence has increased by 14% nationally for women (from 44 to 58%) in the past three decades [7]. The Pregnancy Risk Assessment Monitoring System (PRAMS) is an ongoing population-based surveillance system that studies trends in pre-pregnancy obesity by maternal demographic and behavioral characteristics based on self-reported data from questionnaires in nine states. Data collected from PRAMS has demonstrated that the prevalence of pre-pregnancy obesity has increased in a decade alone from 13% in 1993–1994 to 22% in 2000–2003 regardless of maternal age, race, and education [11].

Trends in the United Kingdom

The 2014 Health Survey for England (HSE) was notable for 58.1% of women being overweight or obese. The proportion of women in England with a normal BMI decreased between 1993 and 2014 from 49.5 to 40.4%, and instead, the prevalence of obesity in pregnancy has increased from 9–10% in the early 1990s to 16–19% in the 2000s [12, 13]. Currently, the prevalence of women with a BMI ≥ 35 kg/m^2 at any point in pregnancy is 4.99%, with a BMI ≥ 40 kg/m^2 is 2.01%, and with a BMI ≥ 50 kg/m^2 it is 0.19% of all women giving birth [14].

Maternal Obesity and Disparities

Obesity disproportionately affects various ethnic populations, those of low socioeconomic status or educational level, and those living in remote or rural locations [15]. Although genetic predisposition may be a factor, ethnic groups have different norms and pressures around socially acceptable body weight, physical activity, and nutrition that may contribute to the difference.

In the United States, there is an increased incidence of obesity among Hispanic (43%), non-Hispanic black (51%), and non-Hispanic white women (33%) [16]. A prior study noted that ethnic and racial factors affected gestational weight gain. Brawarsky et al. found that African-American women were more likely to have pre-pregnancy obesity and most likely to undergo weight gain in excess of the IOM guidelines, while Caucasian and Asian females were more like to achieve target weight gain [17]. Conversely, Hispanic women were most likely to gain less weight than recommended [17]. In addition, low socioeconomic status plays a role since obesity prevalence is higher in those less educated or earning lower incomes [18].

Similarly in England, obesity in women varies by socioeconomic indicators. Women in the lowest income households or most deprived areas were most likely to be obese [19]. Approximately 31% of women in the lowest income households and 33% of women in the most deprived areas were obese, in contrast with 20% of women in the highest income households and 22% of women in the least deprived areas [19].

Pre-pregnancy Obesity

Consequences of Pre-pregnancy Obesity

Women who are obese during their childbearing years are at risk for a variety of conditions including polycystic ovary syndrome, menstrual irregularities, cardiovascular diseases, insulin resistance, type 2 diabetes, mental health issues, respiratory issues, and thromboembolic disease [20–22]. In addition, obese women are more prone to irregular cycles and infertility and thus are more likely to delay prenatal care because they may not realize they are pregnant.

Obesity is a modifiable risk factor. There are numerous approaches to obesity management in the preconception period including diet, physical activity, sleep hygiene, and surgical options. As obese women in the postpartum period have difficulty losing the weight gained during pregnancy, especially if the weight gain was excessive, preconception may be an opportune time for primary obesity prevention and intervention including slowing or stopping weight gain.

Lifestyle Modifications for Maternal Obesity

Diet and exercise are significant behavioral risk factors that influence a woman's obesity risk. Healthy eating patterns, access to healthy foods, physical activity, and daily energy expenditure are key determinants to developing obesity. The American College of Obstetricians and Gynecologists recommends regular physical activity in pregnancy for at least 20–30 min per day on most or all days of the week as it is associated with minimal risks, benefits most women, helps with weight management, and reduces obesity and its associated comorbidities [23]. There is also increasing evidence to support the role of insufficient sleep in the development of obesity and decreased effectiveness of common weight loss recommendations [24]. Thus, as women are contemplating becoming pregnant, they should undergo diet, physical activity level, and sleep hygiene assessment.

Bariatric Surgery for Maternal Obesity

Weight loss through lifestyle modification during the preconception period poses a serious challenge for most women; thus, bariatric surgery may be an option for some women. Bariatric surgery procedures have increased sixfold from 1998 to 2005 in the United States with over half performed in reproductive-aged women [25]. Overall, the data on the effect of bariatric surgery on subsequent pregnancy outcomes is limited but suggests that pregnancy after bariatric surgery appears safe and is associated with improved outcomes. The majority of studies report that following bariatric surgical procedures, obese women have improved fertility outcomes, substantial and sustained weight loss, improved fetal and neonatal outcomes, reduced risk of large for gestational age infants, and decreased rates of gestational diabetes and preeclampsia [25–28].

Other studies have demonstrated lower birthweight, stillbirth, neonatal death, shorter gestation, and up to a two to three times higher risk of small for gestational age infants born after maternal bariatric surgery [27–30]. Although most studies indicate that a history of bariatric surgery is associated with improved maternal obstetric outcomes and decreased large for gestational age infants, increased antenatal and neonatal surveillance is needed secondary to the increased risk of small for gestational age infants, shorter gestational time, and stillbirth or neonatal death.

Maternal Obesity and Maternal Outcomes

Pregnancy

As a woman's BMI increases, so does the risk of negative maternal, fetal, and neonatal outcomes. In early pregnancy, the risks associated with maternal obesity include miscarriage and fetal anomalies [31]. It is concerning that the protective effects of periconceptional folic acid supplementation do not appear to be beneficial to obese women. The benefits of an increased dose of folic acid for these women have not been well studied [32]. Thus, early ultrasounds, potentially transvaginally, should be performed to establish viability, to exclude multiple gestations, and to identify congenital anomalies. A complete ultrasound fetal anatomic survey may be limited by the poor ultrasound resolution, and thus arranging for this to be performed at 20–22 weeks should be considered [33].

In late pregnancy, there is an increased risk for thromboembolism, biliary disease, gestational diabetes, pregnancy-induced hypertension, and stillbirth with maternal obesity [34, 35]. Stratified by BMI, a prior study demonstrated that the incidence of thromboembolism was 2.5% in obese women with a BMI >29 kg/m^2 compared to 0.6% in women with a BMI of 19.8–26.0 kg/m^2 [36]. Another study noted that maternal obesity is associated with a higher risk of pulmonary embolus (adjusted OR 14.9, 95% CI, 3.0–74.8) than of deep vein thrombosis (adjusted OR 4.4, 95% CI, 1.6–11.9) [37]. As a result of this increased risk, the Royal College of Obstetricians and Gynaecologists recommend thromboprophylaxis for 10 days following delivery in women either with a pre-pregnancy or early BMI ≥40 kg/m^2 or that are greater than 35 years old with a BMI ≥30 kg/m^2 [38].

Lastly, increased peripartum risks associated with maternal obesity include postpartum hemorrhage, wound infection, anesthetic complications, shoulder dystocia, need for cesarean section, and third- or fourth-degree laceration [34, 35]. The likelihood of a successful vaginal delivery decreases as maternal BMI increases. The magnitude of this association was demonstrated by a prior meta-analysis of 33 studies noting the odds ratios of cesarean delivery were 1.46 (95% CI, 1.34–1.6), 2.06 (95% CI, 1.86–2.27), and 2.89 (95% CI, 2.28–3.79) among overweight, obese, and severely obese women, respectively, compared with normal weight pregnant women [39].

Secondary to an increased risk of anesthetic complications, an early anesthesia consultation has been demonstrated to be beneficial in this patient population as they often have difficult airways and comorbidities including sleep apnea, and an anesthesia-free pregnancy is discouraged because of the increased mortality and morbidity with general anesthesia. These patients are not ideal candidates for spinal anesthesia because the typical landmarks for placement are difficult to identify and thus epidural anesthesia is preferred because it decreases oxygen consumption in labor and increases cardiac output [40].

Pregestational and Gestational Diabetes

Maternal obesity is associated with an increased risk of diabetes, both pregestational and gestational, because insulin sensitivity is reduced by half in pregnancy and obesity is a common risk factor for insulin resistance [3, 5]. Throughout the duration of pregnancy, obese women have higher insulin resistance than women of normal weight, which increases the availability of lipids for fetal growth and development [41]. Compared to women with a normal BMI, the odds of gestational diabetes exponentially increases with increasing BMI: 1.97 for overweight, 3.01 for obese, and 5.55 for morbidly obese women [42]. In particular, obese women with increased intra-abdominal fat mass have the highest risk of insulin resistance in pregnancy. Even weight gain in the 5 years prior to conception at a rate of 1.1–2.2 kg per year will increase the risk of developing gestational diabetes, specifically in women with an initially normal BMI [43].

This is concerning because gestational diabetes is associated with increased pregnancy complications including preeclampsia, cesarean section, fetal macrosomia, shoulder dystocia, neonatal respiratory distress, and neonatal intensive care unit admission [34, 35]. Also, women who are diagnosed with gestational diabetes are at an increased risk for developing gestational diabetes in a subsequent pregnancy, and more than half develop type 2 diabetes later in life [44, 45].

Hypertensive Disorders and Preeclampsia

Maternal obesity is associated with an increased risk of pregnancy-induced hypertension and pre-eclampsia spectrum. When compared to women with a normal pregnancy BMI, those who are obese have an increased two- to threefold risk of developing gestational hypertension or preeclampsia [46, 47]. A prior study stratified women by maternal pre-pregnancy weight and contrasted women whose weight was 55–75 kg with those greater than 90 kg [34]. This study found that the odds ratio of developing pregnancy-induced hypertension was 2.38 (95% CI, 2.24–2.52) and 3 (95% CI, 2.49–3.62) in the moderately versus severely obese group, respectively [34]. It was also demonstrated that the severity of hypertensive complications correlated with the degree of obesity [34]. Moderately obese women had an odds ratio of severe pregnancy-induced hypertension, which included HELLP syndrome, of 1.56 (95% CI, 1.35–1.80), while severely obese women had an odds ratio of 2.34 (95% CI, 1.59–3.46).

The risk of preeclampsia has also been reported to double with each 5–7 kg/m² increase in BMI above normal weight [4]. These risks will decrease with weight loss but will increase with weight gain in between pregnancies. The mechanism of this increased risk is unclear, but both obesity and preeclampsia are associated with increased markers of inflammation such as interleukin-6, interleukin-8, inflammatory cytokines, and C-reactive protein [47].

Gestational Weight Gain in the Obese Population

Weight gain in overweight and obese patients can be detrimental to pregnancy outcomes. A growing evidence has demonstrated that no weight gain, and even weight loss, is associated with reduced rates of preeclampsia, fetal macrosomia, cesarean section, admissions to a neonatal intensive care unit, and low Apgar score [47]. As such, in 2009, the IOM modified the recommended weight gain in pregnant women with a BMI ≥30 kg/m² to 11–20 lbs (Table 13.2) [9]. Since then, more evidence has advocated for less weight gain and even weight loss in patients at the upper tier of obesity with an adequately growing fetus [48]. In 2013, the American College of Obstetricians and Gynecologists (ACOG) issued a committee opinion recommending that "for an obese pregnant woman who is gaining less weight than the recommended but has an appropriately growing fetus, no evidence exists that encouraging increased weight gain to conform with the updated IOM guidelines will improve maternal or fetal outcomes" [49].

Medical Management of Gestational Obesity

Ideally, weight loss should be achieved by nonsurgical means. Pregnancy is a unique time where women are motivated to adopt healthy behaviors that may potentially benefit their child. Weight management during pregnancy can be approached with nutrition and physical activity interventions during pregnancy in addition to addressing barriers to overall health. More recent studies have also evaluated the benefit of metformin on pregnancy outcomes, and while this appears promising, studies thus far have not validated this approach.

Prior studies have demonstrated that pregnancy lifestyle modification programs can reduce gestational weight gain [50–52] in addition to gestational diabetes [53]. A recent randomized controlled trial compared obese pregnant women undergoing comprehensive dietary and lifestyle intervention

Table 13.2 Recommended weight gain (2009 Institute of Medicine IOM guidelines)

Weight status	Recommended weight gain (lb)
Underweight (BMI <18.5)	28–40
Normal weight (BMI = 18.5–24.9)	25–35
Overweight (BMI = 25–29.9)	15–25
Obese (BMI ≥30)	11–20

compared with standard prenatal care and reported that the rate of ultrasound-detected adipose tissue deposition slowed among fetuses of women receiving lifestyle advice [54]. The use of a dietician and social worker to facilitate these lifestyle modifications has been shown to improve patient outcomes when a patient has access to these services [51, 52]. However, overall study conclusions are inconsistent, and knowledge gaps remain regarding the benefits and potential harms associated with nutrition and physical activity interventions for obese pregnant women.

There have been several large studies examining the effect of metformin on maternal and fetal outcomes in obese pregnant women. In 2015, a large, randomized, double-blind, placebo-controlled trial of 449 women with a BMI $\geq$30 kg/m^2 and a negative glucose tolerance test was carried out [55]. Women were randomized to receive metformin 500 mg (increasing to a maximum of 2500 mg) or matched placebo from 12 to 16 weeks gestation until delivery. This study concluded that metformin had no significant effect on miscarriage, stillbirth, neonatal death, or birthweight in obese women [55]. More recently in 2016, another large, double-blind, placebo-controlled trial examined 400 pregnant women without diabetes with a BMI $\geq$35 kg/m^2 randomized to either metformin 3000 mg or placebo from 12 to 18 weeks gestation until delivery [56]. The results of this study reported a reduction in maternal weight gain in women treated with metformin, but no significant difference between groups in the incidence of gestational diabetes, neonatal birthweight, or adverse neonatal outcomes [56]. As the results of these recent studies are incongruent and report potentially only marginal maternal benefit, this highlights the need for additional research on innovative and safe treatments for this important issue.

Long-Term Maternal Obesity Outcomes and Management

Women whose pregnancies are complicated by obesity are at increased risk for postpartum weight retention in addition to diabetes and cardiovascular disease later in life [57, 58]. Both women who are obese, and those who exceed their gestational weight gain recommendations, are less likely to return to their pre-pregnancy weight [58], which exacerbates the intergenerational cycle of obesity and increases the risk of subsequent pregnancies. Oken et al. demonstrated that 12% of women retained at least 11 lbs 1-year postpartum [59]. These women were also more likely to be younger, primiparous, of lower socioeconomic status, and unmarried and have experienced excessive gestational weight gain and heavier pre-pregnancy [59]. An increase in 3 BMI points between pregnancies, even in a women with a normal BMI, has been shown to result in a greater risk of pregnancy-induced hypertension, cesarean delivery, stillbirth, fetal macrosomia, and preeclampsia [60].

As postpartum weight retention and obesity are modifiable factors, it is important that women are counseled regarding interventions, such as diet and exercise, to achieve their pre-pregnancy weight and ultimately their ideal body weight. Postpartum television viewing of greater than 2 h daily, daily activity consisting of less than 30 min of walking, and increased trans-fat intake have all been shown to be associated with weight retention [61]. Prior studies have also demonstrated that pregnancy intervention programs can reduce postpartum weight retention, specifically those that provide supervised physical activity and diet interventions were found to be most effective [50–52, 62]. Breastfeeding is also beneficial in assisting with postpartum weight loss and is also important for infant health [63]. The American Academy of Pediatrics supports the unequivocal evidence that breastfeeding has maternal benefits including earlier return to pre-pregnancy weight, and it also protects against many diseases and conditions in the infant including childhood obesity. Unfortunately, prior studies have demonstrated that maternal obesity is associated with lower initiation of breastfeeding; although reasons for why this association exists are unknown, it has not been shown to be associated with pregnancy-related psychological factors such as depression, stress, or anxiety [64].

Effects of Maternal Obesity on Offspring

Fetal and Neonatal Period

Maternal obesity is associated with an increased risk of fetal and neonatal complications such as stillbirth, neonatal death, meconium aspiration, shoulder dystocia, low Apgar scores, fetal distress, and fetal anomalies [31, 47, 65]. Specifically, the fetal anomalies most frequently involved are neural tube defects, cardiovascular anomalies, and cranial-facial anomalies such as cleft lip and palate [31, 47, 65]. The severity of these complications increases with the degree of maternal obesity.

As the prevalence of maternal obesity increases, mean birthweight has dramatically risen to unprecedented levels during human evolution [66]. From 1985 to 1998, the mean birthweight in the United States has increased from 3423 to 3431 g and in Canada from 3391 to 3427 g [67]. Similarly, in Denmark, the mean birthweight increased between 1990 and 1999 from 3474 to 3519g [68]. Both maternal obesity at the beginning of pregnancy and maternal weight gain during pregnancy are associated with increased neonatal birthweight [3, 59] independent of a diagnosis of gestational diabetes [41]. The risk of fetal macrosomia more than doubled in obese women [47].

Impact on Adult Disease Risk

The effects of maternal obesity on offspring extend past the neonatal period. There is an accumulating evidence to suggest that maternal obesity and gestational weight gain predispose offspring to later obesity in childhood, adolescence, and early adulthood [70, 71]. A prior record linkage study demonstrated that maternal obesity was associated with a 35% increase in the hazard of all-cause offspring mortality in adulthood, even after adjustment for confounders [71].

This relationship between maternal pre-pregnancy obesity and offspring obesity may be secondary to shared genetic, behavioral, environmental, and in utero influences. Dr. David Barker previously presented evidence of fetal programming linking birthweight and the risk of disease later in life as well as the basis of adult obesity [72]. Fetal programming describes a process in which critical development is influenced by external factors, such as nutrition, and the future functionality of organs and regulatory systems is permanently set. A greater maternal-offspring BMI association has been shown compared with a paternal-offspring BMI association, supporting the hypothesis for an intrauterine effect and "malprogramming" [73]. In utero fetal programming on childhood obesity can occur as early as the first trimester [74]. The relative risk of childhood obesity associated with maternal obesity in the first trimester is 2 (95% CI 1.7–2.3) at 2 years of age, 2.3 (95% CI, 2–2.6) at 3 years of age, and 2.3 (95% CI, 2–2.6) at 4 years of age [74].

There is also evidence from animal models to support that maternal body composition and diet are major contributors to adverse childhood outcomes. A prior murine study showed that maternal high-fat diet exposure lead to increased cardiac lipid content with associated diminished cardiac function and an increase in hypertrophy, apoptosis, and fibrosis in offspring [75]. Juvenile offspring from a nonhuman primate model revealed that a high-fat/high-calorie diet in pregnancy results in damage and reprogramming of the fetal liver, brain, and pancreas [76–80]. In the postnatal period, these offspring also had accelerated weight gain and increased adiposity and glucose intolerance [76].

Several studies have investigated possible pathological processes involved in fetal programming of chronic diseases later in life. One hypothesis is the effect of nutritional stimuli on fetal programming secondary to fetal adaption to transplacental nutrition, either undernourishment or overnourishment, which may permanently alter fetal physiology and metabolism [81]. Overall, there has not been a clear consensus, but different pathways and factors have been implicated such as effects on hyperglycemia, inflammatory environment, growth hormone and insulin-like growth factor-I, beta-cell development, and fetal appetite centers. These programmed changes may then later serve as the basis for health conditions later in life such as hypertension, diabetes, and heart disease. In addition, as maternal obesity is a risk factor for insulin resistance, studies in offspring of mothers with pregestational or gestational diabetes in pregnancy are associated with an increased risk of obesity and diabetogenic disturbances in childhood through adulthood [66].

Conclusion

The obesity pandemic will continue to afflict future generations without successful prevention, intervention, and management. The times before, during, and after pregnancy are all critical periods for obesity awareness and reduction. Although preconception weight loss is ideal in obese women, this recommendation is unavailable to at least 30–50% of women whom pregnancies are unplanned [82]. Pregnancy is a unique time when women are motivated to adopt healthy behaviors that may potentially benefit their child. Knowing that a high preconception BMI is a primary determinant for gestational weight gain and a significant predictor of childhood obesity, it is critical to identify maternal obesity in pregnancy early as a primary target to prevent downstream childhood obesity and to alleviate the obesity pandemic [46, 51]. Current interventions aimed at preventing the progression of obesity in future generations by limiting gestational weight gain and reducing pre-pregnancy obesity have resulted in only minimal improvement in maternal and infant outcomes. Development of additional interventions that more successfully modify the behaviors associated with obesity may help mitigate excessive postpartum weight gain or retention. Therefore, innovative research studies are vital to mitigating the obesity pandemic. By achieving a better understanding of the mechanisms influencing fetal programming, effective treatment strategies aimed at improving maternal and fetal outcomes can be conceived.

References

1. World Health Organization. Jan 2015. Obesity and overweight fact Sheet no. 311. Available: http://www.who.int/mediacentre/factsheets/fs311/en/.
2. Tjepkema M. Measured obesity: adult obesity in Canada: measured height and weight. Statistics Canada. 2005.
3. Heslehurst N, Simpson H, Ells LJ, et al. The impact of maternal BMI status on pregnancy outcomes with intermediate short-term obstetric resource implications: a meta-analysis. Obes Rev. 2008;9(6):635–83.
4. O'Brien TE, Ray JG, Chan WS. Maternal body mass index and the risk of preeclampsia: a systematic overview. Epidemiology. 2003;14(3):368–74.
5. Johansson S, Villamor E, Altman M, Bonamy AK, Granath F, Cnattingius S. Maternal overweight and obesity in early pregnancy and risk of infant mortality: a population based cohort study in Sweden. BMJ. 2014;349:g6572.
6. Salihu HM, Weldeselasse HE, Rao K, Marty PJJ, Whiteman VE. The impact of obesity on maternal morbidity and feto-infant outcomes among macrosomic infants. J Matern Fetal Neonatal Med. 2011;24(9):1088–94.
7. Flegal KM, Carroll MD, Ogden CL, Curtin JR. Prevalence and trends in obesity among US adults, 1999–2008. JAMA. 2010;303(3):235–41.
8. Berenson AB, Pohlmeier AM, Laz TH, Rahman M, Saade G. Obesity risk knowledge, weight misperception, and diet and health attitudes among women intending to become pregnant. J Acad Nutr Diet. 2016;116(1):69–75.
9. Institute of Medicine Weight gain during pregnancy: reexamining the guidelines. Washington, DC: National Academies Press; 2009.
10. Dalenius K, Brindley P, Smith B, Reinold C, Grummer-Strawn L. Pregnancy nutrition surveillance 2010 report. Atlanta: Centers for Disease Control and Prevention; 2012. (http://www.cdc.gov/pednss/pdfs/2010-PNSS-Summary-Report-Text% 20File.pdf).
11. Kim SY, Dietz PM, England L, et al. Trends in pre-pregnancy obesity in nine states, 1993–2003. Obestiy. 2007;15(4):986–93.

12. Heslehurst N, Ells LJ, Simpson H, Batterham A, Wilkinson J, Summerbell CD. Trend in maternal obesity incidence rates, demographic predictors, and health inequalities in 36,821 women over a 15-year period. BJOG. 2007;114(2):187–94.
13. Kanagalingam MG, Forouhi NG, Greer IA, Sattar N. Changes in booking body mass index over a decade: retrospective analysis from a Glasgow Maternity Hospital. BJOG. 2005;112(10):1431–3.
14. Centre for Maternal and Child Enquiries (CMACE). Maternal obesity in the UK: findings from a national project. London: CMACE; 2010.
15. Public Health Agency of Canada and Canadian Institute for Health Information. Obesity in Canada: a joint report from the Public Health Agency of Canada and the Canadian Institute for Health Information. 2011.
16. Freedman DS. Obesity-United States, 1988–2008. Cent Dis Control Prev Morb Mortal Wkly Rep. 2011;60(1):73–7.
17. Brawarsky P, Stotland NE, Jackson RA, et al. Pre-pregnancy and pregnancy-related factors and the risk of excessive or inadequate gestational weight gain. Int J Gynaecol Obstet. 2005;91(2):125–31.
18. Ogden CL, Lamb MM, Carroll MD, Flegal KM. Obesity and socioeconomic status in adults: United States 1988–1994 and 2005–2008. NCHS data brief no 50. Hyattsville: National Center for Health Statistics; 2010.
19. Scantlebury R, Moody A. Adult obesity and overweight. Chapter 9. In: Craig R, Mindell J, editors. Health survey for England 2014: health, social care and lifestyles. Leeds: Health and Social Care Information Center; 2014.
20. Dietl J. Maternal obesity and complications during pregnancy. J Perinat Med. 2005;33(2):100–5.
21. Singh J, Huang CC, Driggers RW, et al. The impact of pre-pregnancy body mass index on the risk of gestational diabetes. J Matern Fetal Neonatal Med. 2012;25(1):5–10.
22. Bellamy L, Casas JP, Hingorani AD, Williams D. Type 2 diabetes mellitus after gestational diabetes: a systematic review and meta-analysis. Lancet. 2009;373(9688):1773–9.
23. ACOG Committee opinion no. 650: physical activity and exercise during pregnancy and the postpartum period. Obstet Gynecol. 2015:126(6):135–42.
24. Patel SR, Hu FB. Short sleep duration and weight gain: a systematic review. Obesity. 2008;16(3):643–53.
25. Shekelle PG, Newberry S, Maglione M, et al. Bariatric surgery in women of reproductive age: special concerns for pregnancy. Evid Rep Technol Assess (Full Rep). 2008;169:1–51.
26. Maggard MA, Yermilov I, Li Z, et al. Pregnancy and fertility following bariatric surgery: a systematic review. JAMA. 2008;300(19):2286–96.
27. Galazis N, Docheva N, Simillis C, Nicolaides KH. Maternal and neonatal outcomes in women undergoing bariatric surgery: a systematic review and meta-analysis. Eur J Obstet Gynecol Reprod Biol. 2014;181:45–53.
28. Johansson K, Cnattingius S, Naslund I, et al. Outcomes of pregnancy after bariatric surgery. NEJM. 2014;372(9):814–24.
29. Kjaer MM, Nilas L. Pregnancy after bariatric surgery – a review of benefits and risks. Acta Obstet Gynecol Scand. 2013;92(3):264–71.
30. Kjaer MM, Lauenborg J, Breum BM, Nilas L. The risk of adverse pregnancy outcome after bariatric surgery: a nationwide register-based matched cohort study. Am J Obstet Gynecol. 2013;208(6):464.e1-5.
31. Boots C, Stephenson MD. Does obesity increase the risk of miscarriage in spontaneous conception: a systematic review. Semin Reprod Med. 2011;29(6):507–13.
32. Werler MM, Louik C, Shapiro S, Mitchell AA. Prepregnant weight in relation to risk of neural tube defects. JAMA. 1996;275(14):1089–92.
33. Davies GA, Maxwell C, McLeod L, et al. SOGC clinical practice guidelines: obesity in pregnancy. No 239, February 2010. Int J Gynaecol Obstet. 2010;110(2):167–73.
34. Robinson HE, O'Connell CM, Joseph KS, McLeod NL. Maternal outcomes in pregnancies complicated by obesity. Obstet Gynecol. 2005;106(6):1357–64.
35. Siega-Riz AM, Siega-Riz AM, Laraia B. The implications of maternal overweight and obesity on the course of pregnancy and birth outcomes. Matern Child Health J. 2006;10(Suppl 1):153–6.
36. Edwards LE, Hellerstedt WL, Alton IR, Story M, Himes JH. Pregnancy complications and birth outcomes in obese and normal-weight women: effects of gestational weight change. Obstet Gynecol. 1996;87(3):389–94.
37. Larsen TB, Sørensen HT, Gislum M, Johnsen SP. Maternal smoking, obesity, and risk of venous thromboembolism during pregnancy and the puerperium: a population-based nested case-control study. Thromb Res. 2007;120(4):505–9.
38. RCOG 2015. Reducing the risk of venous thromboembolism during pregnancy and the puerperium (Green-top 37a). Available at: https://www.rcog.org.uk/globalassets/documents/guidelines/gtg-37a.pdf. Accessed 14 Apr 2016.
39. Chu SY, Kim SY, Schmid CH, Dietz PM, Callaghan WM, Lau J, Curtis KM. Maternal obesity and risk of cesarean delivery: a meta-analysis. Obes Rev. 2007;8(5):385–94.
40. Sarvanakumar K, Rao SG, Cooper GM. Obesity and obstetric anesthesia. Anesthesia. 2006;61(1):36–48.
41. Catalano PM, Ehrenberg HM. The short- and long-term implications of maternal obesity on the mother and her offspring. BJOG. 2006;113(10):1126–33.
42. Torloni MR, Betran AP, Horta BL, et al. Pre-pregnancy BMI and the risk of gestational diabetes: a systematic review of the literature with meta-analysis. Obes Rev. 2009;10(2):194–203.

43. Hedderson MM, Williams MA, Holt VL, et al. Body mass index and weight gain prior to pregnancy and risk of gestational diabetes mellitus. Am J Obstet Gynecol. 2008;198(4):409.e1-7.
44. Kim C, Berger DK, Chamany S. Recurrence of gestational diabetes mellitus: a systematic review. Diabetes Care. 2007;30(5):1314–9.
45. Kim C, Newton KM, Knopp RH. Gestational diabetes and the incidence of type 2 diabetes: a systematic review. Diabetes Care. 2002;25(10):1862–8.
46. Nohr EA, Vaeth M, Baker JL, Sorensen TI, Olsen J, Rasmussen KM. Combined associations of prepregnancy body mass index and gestational weight gain with the outcome of pregnancy. Am J Clin Nutr. 2008;87(6):1750–9.
47. Ovesen P, Rasmussen S, Kesmodel U. Effect of pre-pregnancy maternal overweight and obesity on pregnancy outcome. Obstet Gynecol. 2011;118(2):305–12.
48. Artal R, Lockwood CJ, Brown HL. Weight gain recommendations in pregnancy and the obesity epidemic. Obstet Gynecol. 2010;115(1):152–5.
49. ACOG Committee opinion no. 548: weight gain during pregnancy. Obstet Gynecol. 2013;121(1):210–12.
50. Bechtel-Blackwell DA. Computer-assisted self-interview and nutrition education in pregnant teens. Clin Nurs Res. 2002;11(4):450–62.
51. Wolff S, Legarth J, Vansgaard K, Toubro S, Astrup A. A randomized trial of the effects of dietary counseling on gestational weight gain and glucose metabolism in obese pregnant women. Int J Obses (Lond). 2008;32(3):495–501.
52. Asbee SM, Jenkins TR, Butler JR, White J, Elliot M, Rutledge A. Preventing excessive weight gain during pregnancy through dietary and lifestyle counseling: a randomized controlled trial. Obstet Gynecol. 2009;113(2 Pt 1):305–12.
53. Quinlivan JA, Lam LT, Fisher J. A randomised trial of four-step multidisciplinary approach to the antenatal care of obese pregnant women. Aust N Z J Obstet Gynaecol. 2011;51(2):141–6.
54. Grivell RM, Yelland LN, Deussen A, Crowther CA, Dodd JM. Antenatal dietary and lifestyle advice for women who are overweight or obese and the effect on fetal growth and adiposity: the LIMIT randomized trial. BJOG. 2016;123(2):233–43.
55. Chiswick C, Reynolds RM, Denison F, et al. Effect of metformin on maternal and fetal outcomes in obese pregnant women (EMPOWaR): a randomized, double-blind, placebo-controlled trial. Lancet. 2015;3(10):778–86.
56. Syngelaki A, Nicolaides KH, Balani J, et al. Metformin versus placebo in obese pregnant women without diabetes mellitus. NEJM. 2016;374(5):434–43.
57. Sattar N, Greer IA. Pregnancy complications and maternal cardiovascular risk: opportunities for intervention and screening? BMJ. 2002;325(7356):157–60.
58. Keppel KG, Taffel SM. Pregnancy-related weight gain and retention: implications of the 1990 Institute of Medicine guidelines. Am J Public Health. 1993;83(8):1100–3.
59. Oken E, Taveras EM, Kleinman KP, Rich-Edwards JW, Gillman MW. Gestational weight gain and child adiposity at age 3 years. AJOG. 2007;196(4):322.31–8.
60. Villamor E, Cnattingius S. Interpregnancy weight change and risk of adverse pregnancy outcomes: a population-based study. Lancet. 2006;368(9542):1164–70.
61. Oken E, Taveras EM, Popoola FA, Rich-Edwards JW, Gillman MW. Television, walking, and diet associations with postpartum weight retention. Am J Prev Med. 2007;32(4):305–11.
62. Choi J, Fukuoka Y, Lee JH. The effects of physical activity and physical activity plus diet interventions on body weight in overweight or obese women who are pregnant or in postpartum: a systematic review and met-analysis of randomized controlled trials. Prev Med. 2013;56(6):351–64.
63. Kramer MS, Kakuma R. Optimal duration of exclusive breastfeeding. Cochrane Database Syst Rev. 2012;8:CD003517.
64. Mehta UJ, Siega-Riz AM, Herring AH, Adair LS, Bentley ME. Maternal obesity, psychological factors and breast-feeding initiation. Breastfeed Med. 2011;6(6):369–76.
65. Stothard KJ, Tennant PW, Bell R, Rankin J. Maternal overweight and obesity and the risk of congenital anomalies: a systematic review and meta-analysis. JAMA. 2009;301(6):66–650.
66. Harder T, Dudenhausen JW, Plagemann A. Maternal diabesity and developmental programming in the offspring. In: Ovesen PG, Jensen DM, editors. Maternal obesity and pregnancy. Springer. 2012; p. 133–54.
67. Anath CV, Wen SW. Trends in fetal growth among singleton gestations in the United States and Canada, 1985 through 1998. Semin Perinatol. Berlin Heidelberg. 2002;26(4):260–7.
68. Orskou J, Kesmodel U, Henriksen TB, Secher NJ. An increasing proportion of infants weigh more than 4000 grams at birth. Acta Obstet Gynaecol Scand. 2001;80(10):931–6.
69. Catalano PM, McIntyre HD, Cruickshank JK, et al. The hyperglycemia and adverse pregnancy outcome study: associations of GDM and obesity with pregnancy outcomes. Diabetes Care. 2012;35(4):780–6.
70. Graversen L, Sorensen TI, Gerds TA, et al. Prediction of adolescent and adult adiposity outcomes from early life anthropometrics. Obesity. 2014;23(1):162–9.
71. Reynolds RM, Allan RM, Raja EA, et al. Maternal obesity during pregnancy and premature mortality from cardiovascular event in adult offspring: follow-up of 1,323,275 person years. BMJ. 2013;347:f4539.

72. Barker DJ. The fetal and infant origins of adult disease. BMJ. 1990;301(6761):1111.
73. Lawlor DA, Smith GD, O'Callaghan M, et al. Epidemiologic evidence for fetal overnutrition hypothesis: findings from the mater-university study of pregnancy and its outcomes. Am J Epidemiol. 2007;165(4):418–24.
74. Whitaker RC. Predicting preschooler obesity at birth: the role of maternal obesity in early pregnancy. Pediatrics. 2004;114(1):e29–36.
75. Turdi S, Ge W, Hu N, Gradley KM, Wang X, Ren J. Interaction between maternal and postnatal high fat diet leads to a greater risk of myocardial dysfunction in offspring via enhanced lipotoxicity, irs-1 serine phosphorylation and mitochondrial defects. J Mol Cell Cardiol. 2013;55:117–29.
76. McCurdy C, Bishop JM, Williams S, et al. Maternal high-fat diet triggers lipotoxicity in the fetal livers of nonhuman primates. J Clin Invest. 2009;119(2):323–35.
77. Frias A, Morgan T, Evans A, et al. Maternal high-fat diet disturbs uteroplacental hemodynamics and increases the frequency of stillbirth in a nonhuman primate model of excess nutrition. Endocrinology. 2011;152(6):2456–64.
78. Frias A, Grove K. Obesity: a transgenerational problem linked to nutrition during pregnancy. Semin Reprod Med. 2012;30(6):472–8.
79. Grayson B, Levasseur P, Williams S, Smith M, Marks D, Grove K. Changes in melanocortin expression and inflammatory pathways in fetal offspring of nonhuman primates fed a high-fat diet. Endocrinology. 2010;151(4):1622–32.
80. Sullivan E, Grayson B, Takahashi D, et al. Chronic consumption of a high-fat diet during pregnancy cause perturbations in the serotonergic system and increased anxiety-like behavior in nonhuman primate offspring. J Neurosci. 2010;30(10):3826–30.
81. de Boo HA, Harding JE. The developmental origins of adult disease (Barker) hypothesis. Aust N Z J Obstet Gynecol. 2006;45(1):4–14.
82. Finer LB, Zolna MR. Unintended pregnancy in the United States: incidence and disparities. 2006. Contraception. 2011;84(5):478–85.

Chapter 14
Maternal Obesity and Implications for Fetal Programming

Stephen P. Ford and John F. Odhiambo

Key Points

- Obesity develops as a result of the imbalance between energy intake and energy expenditure.
- Obesity among women of reproductive age ranges from 20% to 30% rendering maternal obesity a major public health concern worldwide.
- Human clinical findings demonstrate that both maternal obesity prior to conception, and excessive weight gain during pregnancy have the greatest impact on increasing childhood obesity and metabolic dysregulation in their offspring.
- Obesity is an important contributor to the global incidence of cardiovascular disease, type 2 diabetes mellitus, osteoarthritis, workforce disability and sleep apnea.
- Studies in animal models indicate that these metabolic sequelae are initiated by a proinflammatory milieu in the placenta creating an inflammatory environment for the fetus.
- This leads to alterations in fetal growth, metabolism and organ development resulting in metabolic dysregulation in the postnatal offspring.
- Our research further indicates that maternal obesity has multigenerational effects, thus intervention strategies aimed at mitigating nutritional stress in the mother not only benefit the mother and her own health, but also the health of her progenies and their progenies.

Keywords Maternal obesity • Animal models • High fat diet • Rodents • Sheep • Non-human primates

S.P. Ford, PhD (✉) • J.F. Odhiambo, PhD
Center for the Study of Fetal Programming, Department of Animal Science, University of Wyoming, Laramie, WY 82070, USA
e-mail: spford@uwyo.edu

© Springer International Publishing AG 2017
R. Rajendram et al. (eds.), *Diet, Nutrition, and Fetal Programming*,
Nutrition and Health, DOI 10.1007/978-3-319-60289-9_14

Current State of Clinical Understanding of the Impacts of Maternal Obesity on Offspring

We have been asked to summarize our current understanding of the impacts of maternal obesity, which has doubled since 1980, on programming the health of future generations. Our group has spent the past decade developing and characterizing an ovine model of diet-induced maternal obesity (MO) that has critically important developmental and physiological similarities to humans. In the analyses for the Global Burden of Disease Study, it was reported that between 1980 and 2013 the worldwide proportion of adults with a body mass index (BMI) of 25 or greater, signifying overweight/obesity, increased from 29% to 37% in men and from about 30% to 38% in women [1]. Further, it was reported that the prevalence of overweight and obesity among children and adolescents in developed countries was also very high, averaging about 24% for boys and 23% for girls [1]. This study also reported that a trend for increasing overweight/obesity was also seen in developing countries increasing from 8% in 1980 to 13% in 2013 for boys and girls. Further, the WHO (www.who.int/nut/obs.htm) has declared obesity one of the top ten adverse health risks in the world and one of the top five in developed nations where obesity among women of reproductive age ranges from 20% to 34% [2]. Thus, maternal obesity has become a major public health issue with maternal complications as well as programming of offspring metabolic disease risk. In particular, obesity is an important contributor to the global incidence of cardiovascular disease, type 2 diabetes mellitus, cancer, osteoarthritis, work disability and sleep apnea [3, 4].

A longitudinal study of 179 individuals, found that children exposed to MO, with or without gestational diabetes, exhibit an increased incidence of obesity and metabolic disease [5, 6]. This may relate to the fact that obese pregnant women exhibit an increased incidence of glucose intolerance, hypertensive disorders, hyperlipidemia and increased circulating inflammatory markers [7]. Maternal obesity is often but not always associated with the birth of large for gestational age infants [8, 9]. This increase in birth weight of infants born to obese women is a result of increased fat mass and not lean body mass [10]. Further, this increased body fat is centrally distributed [11] and there is a strong correlation between this increased fetal adiposity and insulin resistance [12].

Both maternal obesity prior to conception, and excessive weight gain during pregnancy are highly associated with increased childhood obesity [13] and metabolic dysregulation [5]. Further, newborn offspring of obese women were more obese and insulin resistant than offspring born to normal weight women [14]. These data suggest that MO has already impacted offspring prior to birth and underpins the need to study the specific mechanisms mediating the effects of MO on both the fetus and newborn [15]. Mother-child cohorts show associations between maternal BMI and/or gestational weight gain and childhood metabolism and cardiovascular function [16, 17] but although these associations are vitally important they remain only associations, due to the presence of uncontrolled confounders. This conclusion is highlighted by the results of the UPBEAT study, a large multicenter, randomized controlled trial conducted in the UK targeting diet and physical activity in obese patients to reduce the incidence of gestational diabetes and large-for-gestational-age infants [18]. These authors reported no intervention associated reductions in gestational diabetes or large-for-gestational-age fetuses, and concluded that the current focus on behavioral interventions to prevent gestational diabetes would seem to be unwarranted.

The phenotype of each unique mammalian organism is the result of the interaction of that organism's genotype with environmental influences exerted upon it. The principle of developmental programming is based on strong evidence that there are critical periods of vulnerability to suboptimal conditions during development both pre- and post-natally. Overwhelming evidence from animal studies shows that these critical vulnerable periods occur at different times for different tissues and that timing and susceptibility differ between species and sex [19]. Human epidemiological and controlled animal studies show that unwanted effects of altered in utero development may persist into later life and predispose to chronic diseases such as type 2 diabetes mellitus, obesity, and hypertension [20, 21]. Unwanted effects of changed development may remain dormant for years to reemerge and cause health problems when the internal and/or external environment (e.g. pregnancy, challenges to the immune system by infectious diseases, nutritional challenges of deficiency or excess, stress, etc.) of the individual changes. While puberty is one particularly important time of endocrine change, human epidemiological studies suggest that the chronic diseases programmed by MO now occur well before puberty. The incidence of type 2 diabetes (T2D, a condition clearly related to MO) in metropolitan Tokyo in prepubertal children between 6 and 15 years quadrupled between 1975 and 1995 [22].

Multigenerational Versus Transgenerational Impacts of Maternal Obesity

This topic is complicated by the fact that besides in utero exposure of first filial [F1] offspring during the time of maternal obesity, their developing gonads and the associated germ cells were also exposed to the same in utero insult. Thus both the F1 and F2 generations are not independent of the initial obesity exposure and the potential impact on these offspring and are referred to as multigenerational effects [23]. The mechanisms underlying the effects of multigenerational programming of obesity are largely unknown, but are likely a result of interplay between environmental, metabolic and epigenetic factors [24]. The programming impacts on offspring beginning in the F3 generation and beyond are considered independent of the initial in utero obesity exposure of the fetus or its germ cells to MO. These impacts are thought to result from meiotically-stable epigenetic inheritance, resulting from altered DNA methylation patterns, histone modifications or siRNA expression differences, and are referred to as transgenerational effects [24–26].

As one might surmise, it is much easier experimentally to discern transgenerational inheritance through the paternal lineage as the male only contributes gametes as opposed to the female who has a prolonged physiological interaction with the progeny. There is also the possibility of nongenomic transmission of F1 phenotype through altered maternal responses to the significant physiological stresses of pregnancy which may be equated to a "second hit" and unmask sub-clinical tendencies in these women such as type 2 diabetes and vascular dysfunction [27, 28]. Thus F1 females expressing a relatively normal phenotype outside of pregnancy may fail to adapt to this significant metabolic stress and thus pass on adverse effects to the F2 generation. The most obvious example would be gestational diabetes where the resulting hyperglycemia exerts significant and well characterized impacts on the fetus, as it readily crosses the placenta [29]. As evidence of this possibility, transmission of gestational diabetes via the maternal line in the rat to an F2 generation was one of the earliest transgenerational developmental programming phenotypes reported [30]. A suggested potential mechanism may be through early reprogramming of oocyte mitochondria [31] which are derived exclusively via the maternal line in mammalian species [32]. While studies have presented evidence demonstrating the impacts of multigenerational familial patterns of adult obesity on the development of childhood overweight/obesity [33, 34], they do not differentiate between behaviors, genetics or environmental impacts. Interestingly, Davis et al. [34] reported that childhood overweight was associated with grandparental obesity whether or not parents were overweight, suggesting multigenerational programming effects.

As previously discussed, human epidemiological studies investigating the transmission of maternal obesity to subsequent generations are largely observational in nature and thus poorly controlled, therefore providing little information on the mechanisms involved. It is well controlled and relevant animal models that will help elucidate whether physiological or epigenetic programming is involved. The remainder of this paper will focus on what is known about the multigenerational impacts of maternal obesity on offspring (F1 and F2 generations), as little evidence has been presented to date for transgenerational epigenetic inheritance.

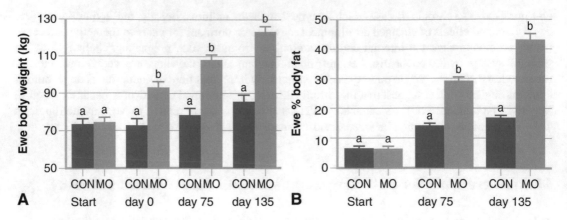

Fig. 14.1 Ewe body weight (**a**) and % body fat (**b**) for control (CON) and obese (MO) groups at different time points of gestation. (**a**, **b**) Means ± SEM between treatment groups within a time point differ ($P < 0.01$) (Adapted with permission from Ref. [46])

Animal Models of Maternal Obesity

Effects of maternal obesity in the offspring have been evaluated in several animal species, with rodents, sheep and nonhuman primates (NHP) being the most cited. Further, chronic long term MO studies have almost exclusively been conducted in rodents [35]. In rodent studies, obesogenic diets are imposed on dams either through feeding of high fat/energy diets (HFD) or allowing dams to choose among obesogenic food items often referred to as 'cafeteria' diets. High fat/energy diets have fixed ratios of nutrients hence animals can only regulate how much is consumed, whereas cafeteria diets permit active adjustment of energy intake thereby allowing animals to potentially stay closer to their nutritional optimum by balancing nutrient ratios depending on the compositional range of food components [36]. Similarly in NHP, obesity is induced nutritionally through high fat diets or by overfeeding highly palatable diets as in rodents [37–39]. In ovine studies carried out by our group at the University of Wyoming, highly palatable pelleted feed has been fed at 150% of National Research Council (NRC) requirements for adult pregnant sheep. Our feeding regimen begins 60 days prior to breeding and continues to term, resulting in the MO animals becoming overweight/obese by conception and to progressively develop to severe obesity by the end of gestation [40, 41], (Fig. 14.1).

Offspring Obesity Studies in Animal Models

Obesity develops as a result of the imbalance between energy intake and energy expenditure. In rodents, maternal cafeteria or high fat diets (HFD) during gestation induced obesity in adult offspring despite offspring being raised on standard chow during postnatal development [42, 43] and this offspring obesity was independent of maternal preconception diet [44].

Studies in sheep models provide data that parallels those in the rodent model. Further, we have reported that these metabolic sequelae are initiated by a proinflammatory milieu in the placenta creating an inflammatory environment for the fetus [45]. Our own previously published work has shown that maternal obesity at conception and throughout gestation increased adiposity of late gestation fetuses [46] and neonatal lambs [40], (Fig. 14.2). Of interest, offspring born to these obese ewes exhibited no phenotypic differences from offspring born to ewes fed only to requirements from weaning

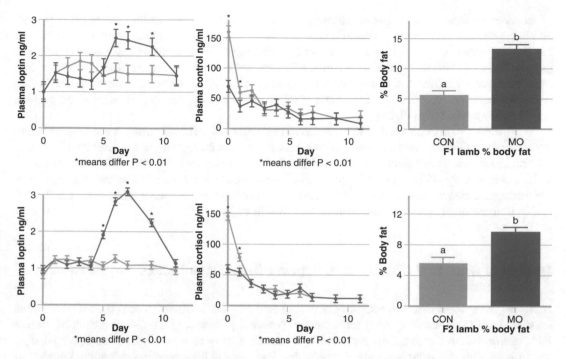

Fig. 14.2 Plasma leptin, cortisol, and % body fat in the early postnatal period in F1 (*top row*) and F2 (*bottom row*) lambs from control (CON, *open symbols*) and obese (MO, *closed symbols*) mothers and grandmothers respectively. (**a**, **b**) Means ± SEM differ ($P < 0.01$) (Adapted with permission from Refs. [55, 58])

to adulthood. When subjected to ad libitum feeding as adults, however, offspring from obese mothers exhibited macrophagia, as well as increased body weight gain and adiposity compared to offspring of control fed mothers [41, 47].

In NHP, McCurdy et al. [37] observed a twofold increase in body fat accumulation in HFD fetuses compared to fetuses gestated by control fed mothers by day 130G of gestation (gestation length = 180 days). Further, offspring of HFD mothers maintained this increased adiposity into the postnatal period and also developed early-onset obesity independent of postnatal diet [48]. This increased risk of obesity in the offspring of HFD mothers was linked to a reduction in central dopamine signaling [49]. Indeed, decreased abundance of dopamine fiber projections to the prefrontal cortex as well as decreased dopamine receptor expression have been observed in the offspring of HFD dams indicative of impairments to the development of the dopamine system [49].

Offspring Insulin Resistance

Several animal studies have demonstrated that maternal overnutrition/obesity perturbs the development of the fetal pancreas resulting in hyperinsulinemia, impaired glucose sensing and β-cell dysfunction. In rodents insulin resistance expressed as the ratio of insulin: glucose was markedly increased by a maternal HFD during gestation in neonates, weanlings and adult offspring [50, 51]. Even mild maternal overnutrition has been shown to induce glucose intolerance [52] and hyperinsulinemia independent of the level of obesity before pregnancy [44]. Further, offspring of HFD mothers exhibited reduced glucose tolerance at weaning following either an oral glucose bolus [35] or an intra-peritoneal glucose bolus [53].

In sheep studies, maternal overnutrition/obesity resulted in glucose/insulin dysregulation in mid- and late gestation fetuses and neonatal lambs [46, 54]. Further, the dysregulation of glucose control has been observed to persist into adulthood in F1 offspring of obese dams and F2 neonates of obese grand dams [55]. This dysregulation is attributed to accelerated pancreatic growth and β-cell development as observed in first half of gestation, followed by a reduction in pancreatic growth and insulin secretory capacity demonstrating the failure of the pancreas to return to normal cellular composition and function postnatally [40, 54].

Very limited data exists on diet-induced insulin resistance in NHP offspring. A recent study demonstrated that offspring born to dams fed high-fat/calorie diets during pregnancy displayed increased plasma insulin levels and glucose-stimulated insulin secretion compared to those of control-fed dams at 13 months of age [56]. An earlier study utilizing the same model observed an early activation of gluconeogenic genes in fetal liver of HFD dams and hypothesized that this might predispose the offspring to increased hepatic gluconeogenesis and insulin resistance [37].

Impact of Maternal Obesity on Offspring Blood Metabolites and Hormones

It is well recognized that maternal obesity during gestation markedly influences the metabolite and hormonal milieu in the developing fetus thereby potentially increasing the risk of metabolic disease later in life. Notable metabolites impacted by maternal obesity include glucose and lipids whereas cortisol, insulin, and leptin are some of the widely investigated hormones in most animal models of maternal obesity. In the rat model, when the maternal cafeteria diet was fed throughout lactation and gestation, there was a sexually dimorphic pattern of glucose and insulin secretion, with male offspring displaying normal glycaemia and hyperinsulinemia and female offspring exhibiting hyperglycemia, but normal insulin levels [57]. Sex differences were, however, not apparent for serum lipid levels with triglycerides and cholesterol being elevated in both males and females from the cafeteria fed dams. In the same study, leptin gene expression in perirenal fat pads of female offspring was greater compared to male offspring. In another study, Howie et al. [44] reported that offspring of high fat fed dams exhibited lower plasma insulin and leptin concentrations at postnatal day 2 compared to those from control-fed dams, however, these patterns were later reversed in adulthood (postnatal day 160). Plasma glucose was also higher in adult male offspring from HFD dams but not in female offspring [44].

In our sheep model, overfed/obese mothers exhibited hyperglycemia and hyperinsulinemia, as well as a markedly elevated insulin resistance as measured by a midgestation intravenous glucose tolerance test (Fig. 14.3). Fetuses gestated by these obese dams have elevated plasma levels of glucose, insulin, cortisol, triglycerides and cholesterol at mid-gestation and late-gestation [45, 46]. Further, neonatal offspring of obese ewes had increased plasma cortisol and insulin at birth and lacked the early postnatal leptin spike necessary for setting up hypothalamic appetite control centers and leading to hyperphagia and leptin resistance in adulthood [41, 58], (Fig. 14.2). Further, adult F1 offspring from obese ewes had higher baseline plasma glucose and insulin as well as higher concentrations of plasma leptin following a 12-week ad libitum feeding trial than F1offspring from control fed lean ewes [41]. Interestingly, adult F1 ewes from obese dams exhibited hyperglycemia, hyperinsulinemia and marked insulin resistance like their overfed/obese mothers during their subsequent pregnancies despite being fed only to requirements during gestation [55], (Fig. 14.4). As a result, their F2 lambs exhibited elevated plasma glucose, insulin and cortisol at birth and also lacked the postnatal leptin peak exhibited by F2 lambs born to control fed F1 ewes indicating a probable multigenerational programming effect [55], (Fig. 14.2).

Chronic high-fat diets in a primate model resulted in increased serum levels of total triglycerides and glycerol but no change in leptin, insulin or free fatty acids in third-trimester fetuses of high-fat diet dams [37]. Thorn et al. [39] did not find any changes in fasting plasma glucose, glycerol,

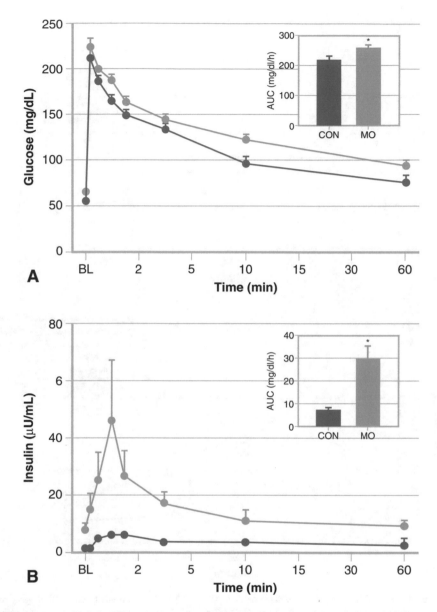

Fig. 14.3 Glucose (**a**) and insulin (**b**) concentrations prior to and after glucose bolus infusion (0.25 g/kg of 50% dextrose solution) during an intravenous glucose tolerance test on 75 days of gestation in F0 ewes fed 100% (control (CON), ○; $n = 6$) or 150% (obese group (MO), ●; $n = 6$) of NRC recommendations from 60 days before conception to day 75 of gestation. (**a**) Glucose concentrations; (**b**): insulin concentrations. Area under curve (AUC) is shown as insets. *Means ± SE differ ($P < 0.05$) (Adapted with permission from Ref. [40])

triglycerides and non-esterified fatty acid concentrations in juvenile offspring of HFD mothers despite of presence of insulin resistance and increased hepatic lipid accumulation in the offspring. In another study, elevated cortisol levels were reported in offspring of HFD mothers without any changes in circulating ACTH levels [48]. Dietary challenge in vervet monkeys (*Chlorocebus aethiops sabaeus*) using high fat diets, however, resulted in increased blood levels of glucose, fructosamine, insulin, triglycerides and cholesterol. Heritability's for these traits in subsequent generations were significant except for blood glucose elevation [59].

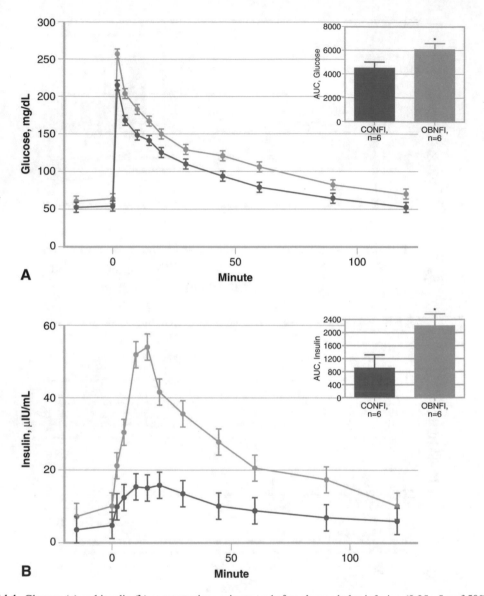

Fig. 14.4 Glucose (**a**) and insulin (**b**) concentrations prior to and after glucose bolus infusion (0.25 g/kg of 50% dextrose solution) during an intravenous glucose tolerance test at day 135 of gestation in female offspring born to obese (OBF1: ●) or control (CONF1: ○) dams, and fed at only 100% NRC recommendations throughout gestation. Area under the curve (AUC) is located in the top right corner of each panel. *Means ± SEM differ ($P < 0.05$) (Adapted with permission from Ref. [55])

Impact of Maternal Obesity on Tissue and Organ Structure and Function

The previous section has highlighted biochemical and hormonal phenotypes associated with maternal overnutrition/obesity in prenatal and postnatal offspring. Most of the changes were apparent during fetal development. Therefore, a crucial unanswered question remaining is whether these changes in the fetal stage will persist into postnatal life and further on into adulthood and consequently impact long-term disease risk.

The long-term consequences on the adult progeny due to consumption of a HFD diet by female rats include impaired glucose homeostasis, cardiovascular dysfunction, and alterations in hypothalamic energy circuitry and liver lipid metabolism. Bayol et al. [57] demonstrated that maternal cafeteria diet during gestation and lactation resulted in increased transcriptional activity in perirenal fat pads leading to greater adipose tissue mass in the female offspring than in males. Further, hepatic steatosis, hepatocyte ballooning and oxidative stress response was observed on offspring of rat dams on the cafeteria diet throughout pregnancy and maintained on the cafeteria diet after weaning. These changes were apparent in offspring of cafeteria diet fed mothers returned to a balanced chow diet after weaning indicating irreversibility of these pathologies once they occur [60]. Offspring of rats exposed to high fat feeding during gestation exhibit pancreatic β-cell hypertrophy early in life leading to an increase in glucose stimulated insulin secretion [51]. However, later in adult life these offspring exhibit declining functional β-cell mass and/or β-cell exhaustion leading to reduction in glucose stimulated insulin secretion. Gender-related cardiovascular dysfunction has also been reported on adult offspring of rats fed diets rich in lard during pregnancy despite being raised on normal chow after weaning, with an elevation of blood pressure (both systolic and diastolic blood pressures) being confined only to female offspring [42, 61]. These female specific effects could be due to glucocorticoid effects of the hypothalamic-pituitary-adrenal (HPA) axis. Indeed, permanent female specific offspring alteration in the HPA axis has been observed in pregnant rats exposed to glucocorticoid excess [61].

In our sheep model of maternal obesity we have also reported similar offspring effects to that observed in the rodent studies. Dysregulation in glucose/insulin dynamics during gestation is linked to pancreatic β-cell hyperplasia at mid-gestation and a decrease in β-cell number due to increased apoptosis in late-gestation (Fig. 14.5) and leading to insulin resistance later in life [40, 54]. In the liver, we have observed upregulation of genes associated with lipogenesis [62], as wells as increased expression of 11β-hydroxysteroid dehydrogenase type 1 (11ß-HSD1) and its cofactor hexose-6-phosphate dehydrogenase (H6PDH), these enzymes are responsible for tissue regulation of cortisol metabolism (Tuersunjiang et al., unpublished observations). Cardiovascular effects reported in our studies included left ventricular hypertrophy [46], fibrosis in myocardium of sheep [63, 64] and decreased insulin signaling pathways leading to insulin resistance and cardiac dysfunction [65]. Insulin signaling was also impaired in skeletal muscles of offspring of obese ewes leading to increased adiposity and fibrosis [63, 66]. Further, maternal obesity induced inflammation was also demonstrated in fetal skeletal muscles in late gestation [66]. During myopathy, inflammation is known to induce expression of cytokines which in turn induces connective tissue expansion necessary for muscle regeneration [63]. Because muscle regeneration involves processes similar to fetal muscle development, it is plausible to suggest that inflammation might alter the normal progression of regenerative events leading to adipogenesis and fibrogenesis in fetal muscle.

In primate studies, fetal offspring of HFD mothers have been shown to exhibit liver related pathologies including nonalcoholic fatty liver disease (NAFLD), hepatic inflammation, oxidative stress and/or damage, triglyceride accumulation and premature gluconeogenic gene expression [37]. Further, the increased risk for fetal NAFLD persisted in the postnatal period predisposing the adult offspring to similar effects even after switching the offspring to a healthy diet after weaning [39]. This fatty liver risk persisted despite the absence of maternal obesity or diabetes [37] or postnatal obesity, insulin resistance, or systemic or local adipose tissue inflammation [39]. Therefore, one can speculate that NAFLD phenotype is due to direct transfer of maternal lipids to the fetus and that this risk might not be reversed by postnatal diet. It is plausible to speculate that the potential adverse effects of excess lipids on the fetal liver during development relates to lack of white adipose tissue (WAT) during critical periods of exposure. Indeed, it is well accepted that WAT is critical for storage of excess lipids and that lack of WAT results in whole body insulin resistance and susceptibility to fatty liver. In most species, WAT develops relatively late in pregnancy [67], therefore, it is plausible that the adverse effects of excess lipids on fetal development may be due to lack of WAT at critical periods of exposure.

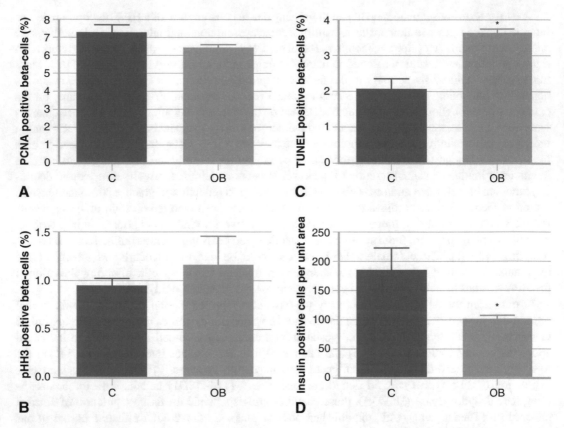

Fig. 14.5 Percentage of fetal pancreatic β-cells proliferating (*panels A* and *B*) and undergoing apoptosis (*panel C*), and insulin positive cells per unit area (mm²) (*panel D*), in fetal pancreatic islet tissue from Control (CON) and Obese (OB) ewes on day 135 of gestation. *Means ± SEM differ between treatment groups (*P* < 0.05) (Adapted with permission from Ref. [54])

Increased myocardial fibrosis was observed in fetal hearts of baboons fed a HFD diet during pregnancy [38]. The authors attributed this to upregulation of cardiac miRNAs involved in enhancing fibrosis and down regulation of miRNAs responsive for normal cardiac development. Proinflammatory conditions in the developing fetus of HFD mothers can have significant effects in brain development and function. For example, the hypothalamic melanocortin system in third trimester offspring was altered by chronic exposure to HFD in Japanese macaques [48]. The melanocortin system is pivotal to regulation of energy homeostasis; therefore, perturbations to this system during critical periods of development could predispose the offspring to hyperphagia and obesity [48].

Conclusion

To our knowledge, our studies in the sheep are the only studies in a precocial large animal species that have attempted to mimic human clinical findings demonstrating that both maternal obesity prior to conception, and excessive weight gain during pregnancy have the greatest impact on increasing childhood obesity and metabolic dysregulation in their offspring. Table 14.1 depicts the impacts on our model of diet-induced pre-pregnancy maternal obesity followed by excess maternal weight gain on altering metabolic, hormonal, and organ and tissue changes of fetal, neonatal, and adult offspring. We have reported that alterations in fetal metabolism, and organ and tissue development and function,

Table 14.1 Comparison of fetal, neonatal and adult offspring characteristics
of overfed-obese (MO) to ewes fed only to requirements

	MO offspring
Mid-gestation fetus	
Fetal weight	+
Crown rump length	+
Liver wt	+
Pancreatic â-cell numbers	+
Cardiac ventricular wt/fetal wt	+
Adiposity	+
Plasma glucose	+
Plasma insulin	+
Plasma cortisol	+
Plasma cholesterol	+
Plasma triglycerides	+
Late-gestation fetus	
Fetal wt	ND
Crown rump length	ND
Liver wt	ND
Pancreatic â-cell numbers	−
Cardiac ventricular wt./fetal wt	+
Adiposity	+
Plasma glucose	+
Plasma insulin	+
Plasma cortisol	+
Plasma cholesterol	+
Plasma triglycerides	+
Newborn lambs unsuckled	
Birth wt	ND
Crown rump length	ND
Plasma glucose	+
Plasma insulin	+
Plasma cortisol	+
Plasma leptin	−
Adult offspring	
Appetite	+
Plasma glucose to ad. lib. feeding	+
Plasma insulin to ad. lib. feeding	−
Plasma leptin	+
Wt. gain to ad. lib. feeding	+
Adiposity to ad. lib. feeding	+
Left ventricular wall thickness	+

From Refs. [40, 41, 45–47, 54, 55, 58, 62–66]
"+" indicates an increase ($P < 0.05$) and "−" indicates a decrease ($P < 0.05$) relative to controls, while *ND* indicates no difference

are associated with a proinflammatory milieu in the placenta creating an inflammatory environment for the fetus. This proinflammatory condition in the developing fetus leads to systemic effects on the brain, liver, heart, pancreas, adipose tissue, and skeletal muscles resulting in metabolic dysregulation in the postnatal offspring of overfed obese ewes. Outside of our studies, most chronic biomedical studies have been conducted in rodents, an altricial species quite different from the human.

There is a pressing need for additional data from models that extrapolate more directly to clinical human obesity. There are differences in many physiological systems between precocial (sheep, NHP, and humans) and altricial (rodents) species, especially in development, duration of gestation and offspring maturity at birth. For example, rats are polytocous and products of conception have a large biomass. A rat with 16 pups nurtures a biomass of nearly 100 g, equivalent to the weight adjusted nutritional challenge to a pregnant woman nurturing a 30 kg baby. These differences are important when it comes to translating metabolic and growth data obtained in rat pregnancy to precocial species including humans. The stage of organ development at birth is another important difference between sheep and NHP versus rodents used in programming studies – i.e., the developmental stage at which fetuses are exposed to air/nutrients, microbiome changes via the gut and other sources, and the stage of development at which placental support is removed. Each species has strengths, however, and addresses different developmental trajectories. Animals provide readily controllable experimental models, while even the best human case control studies can only provide evidence of associations. Specifically, animal studies (1) permit access to fresh fetal and maternal tissues, (2) allow better control of dependent variables, (3) provide clear answers more rapidly and (4) allow a greater burden of investigation on individual mothers and offspring than tolerated by humans.

References

1. Ng M, Fleming T, Robinson M, Thomson B, Graetz N, Margono C, et al. Global regional and national prevalence of overweight and obesity in children and adults during 1980–2013: a systematic analysis for the global burden of disease study 2014. Lancet. 2014;384:766–81.
2. Callaway LK, Prins JB, Chamng AM, McIntyre HD. The prevalence and impact of overweight and obesity in the Australian obstetric population. Med J Aust. 2006;184(2):56–9.
3. Visscher TLS, Seidell JC. The public health impact of obesity. Annu Rev Public Health. 2001;22:355–75.
4. Taylor VH, Forhan M, Vigod SN, McIntyre RS, Morrison KM. The impact of obesity on quality of life. Best Pract Res Clin Endocrinol Metab. 2013;27:139–46.
5. Boney CM, Verma A, Tucker R, Vohr BR. Metabolic syndrome in childhood: association with birth weight, maternal obesity, and gestational diabetes mellitus. Pediatrics. 2005;115:e290–6.
6. Catalano PM, Farrell K, Thomas A, Huston-Presley L, Mencin P, de Mouzon SH, et al. Perinatal risk factors for childhood obesity and metabolic dysregulation. Am J Clin Nutr. 2009;90:1303–13.
7. Catalano PM. Management of obesity in pregnancy. Obstet Gynecol. 2007;109:419–33.
8. Surkin PJ, Hsieh CC, Johansson AL, Diceman PW, Cnattingius S. Reasons for increasing trends in large for gestational age births. Obstet Gynecol. 2004;104:720–6.
9. Ananth CV, Wen SW. Trends in fetal growth among singleton gestation in the United States and Canada. Semin Perinatol. 2002;26(4):260–7.
10. Sewell MF, Huston-Presley L, Super DM, Catalano PM. Increased neonatal fat mass, is associated with maternal obesity. AJOG. 2006;195:1100–3.
11. Gottlieb AG, Galan HL. Shoulder dystocia: an update. Obstet Gynecol Clin N Am. 2007;34:501–31.
12. Catalano P, Presley L, Minium J, Hauguel-de MS. Fetuses of obese mothers develop insulin resistance in utero. Diabetes Care. 2009;32:1076–80.
13. Whitaker RC. Predicting preschooler obesity at birth: the role of maternal obesity in early pregnancy. Pediatrics. 2004;114:e29–36.
14. Mingrone G, Manco M, Mora ME, Guidone C, Laconelli A, Gniuli D, et al. Influence of maternal obesity on insulin sensitivity and secretion of the offspring. Diabetes Care. 2008;31:1872–6.
15. Gillman MW, Rifas-Shiman SL, Kleinman K, Oken E, Rich-Edwards JW, Taveras EM. Developmental origins of childhood overweight: potential public health impact. Obesity. 2008;16(7):1651–6.
16. Wen X, Triche EW, Hogan JW, Shenassa ED, Buka SL. Prenatal factors for childhood blood pressure mediated by intrauterine and/or childhood growth? Pediatrics. 2011;127:e713–21.
17. Mamun AA, O'Callaghan M, Callaway L, Williams G, Najman J, Lawler DA. Associations of gestational weight gain with offspring body mass index and blood pressure at 21 years of age: evidence from a birth cohort study. Circulation. 2009;119:1720–7.
18. Poston L, Bell R, Croker H, Flynn AC, Godfrey KM, Goff L, et al. Effect of behavioral intervention in obese pregnant women (the UPBEAT study): a multicenter, randomized controlled trial. Lancet Diabetes Endocrinol. 2015;3(10):767–77.

19. Hoet JJ, Hanson MA. Intrauterine nutrition: its importance during critical periods for cardiovascular and endocrine development. J Physiol. 1999;514:617–27.

20. Hoet JJ, Ozanne S, Reusens B. Influences of pre- and postnatal nutritional exposures on vascular/endocrine systems in animals. Environ Health Perspect. 2000;108(Suppl 3):563–8.

21. Nathanielsz PW. Life in the womb: the origin of health and disease. Ithaca: Promethean Press; 1999. p. 1–363.

22. Kitagawa T, Owada M, Urakami T, Yamauchi K. Increased incidence of non-insulin dependent diabetes mellitus among Japanese schoolchildren correlates with an increased intake of animal protein and fat. Clin Pediatr (Phila). 1998;37:111–5.

23. Skinner MK. What is an epigenetic transgenerational phenotype? F3 or F2. Reprod Toxicol. 2008;25(1):2–6.

24. Daxinger L, Whitelaw E. Understanding transgenerational epigenetic inheritance via the gametes in mammals. Nat Rev Genet. 2012;13(3):153–62.

25. Gluckman PD, Hanson MA, Cooper C, Thornburg KI. Effect of in utero and early-life conditions on adult health and disease. N Engl J Med. 2008;359(1):61–73.

26. Ferguson-Smith AC, Patti ME. You are what your dad ate. Cell Metab. 2010;13:115–7.

27. Verier-Mine O. Outcomes in women with a history of gestational diabetes. Screening and prevention of type 2 diabetes. Literature review. Diabetes Metab. 2010;6(Pt2):595–616.

28. Bilhartz TD, Bilhartz PA, Bilhartz TN, Bilhartz RD. Making use of a natural stress test: pregnancy and cardiovascular risk. J Womens Health (Larchmt). 2011;5:695–701.

29. Aerts L, Van Assche FA. Animal evidence for the transgenerational development of diabetes mellitus. Int J Biochem Cell Biol. 2006;38:894–903.

30. Gauguier D, Bihoreau MT, Ktorza A, Berthault MF, Picon L. Inheritance of diabetes mellitus as consequence of gestational hyperglycemia in rats. Diabetes. 1990;6:734–9.

31. Theys N, Bouckenooghe T, Ahn MT, Remacle C, Reusens B. Maternal low-protein diet alters pancreatic islet mitochondrial function in a sex-specific manner in the adult rat. Am J Physiol Regul Integr Comp Physiol. 2009;5:R1516–25.

32. Cummins JM. The role of maternal mitochondria during oogenesis, fertilization and embryogenesis. Reprod Biomed Online. 2002;2:176–82.

33. Polley DC, Spicer MT, Knight AP, Hartley BL. Intrafamilial correlates of overweight and obesity in African-American and native-American grandparents, parents, and children in rural Oklahoma. J Am Diet Assoc. 2005;105:262–5.

34. Davis MM, McGonagle K, Schoeni RF, Stafford F. Grandparental and parental obesity influences on childhood overweight: implications for primary care practice. J Am Board Fam Med. 2008;21:549–54.

35. Tamashiro KL, Terrillion CE, Hyun J, Koenig JI, Moran TH. Prenatal stress or high-fat diet increases susceptibility to diet-induced obesity in rat offspring. Diabetes. 2009;58(5):1116–25.

36. Lagisz M, Blair H, Kenyon P, Uller T, Raubenheimer D, Nakagawa S. Little appetite for obesity: meta-analysis of the effects of maternal obesogenic diets on offspring food intake and body mass in rodents. Int J Obes. 2015;39(12):1669–78. Review.

37. McCurdy CE, Bishop JM, Williams SM, Grayson BE, Smith MS, Friedman JE, et al. Maternal high-fat diet triggers lipotoxicity in the fetal livers of nonhuman primates. J Clin Invest. 2009;119(2):323–35.

38. Maloyan A, Muralimanoharan S, Huffman S, Cox LA, Nathanielsz PW, Myatt L, et al. Identification and comparative analyses of myocardial miRNAs involved in the fetal response to maternal obesity. Physiol Genomics. 2013;45(19):889–900.

39. Thorn SR, Baquero KC, Newsom SA, El Kasmi KC, Bergman BC, Shulman GI, et al. Early life exposure to maternal insulin resistance has persistent effects on hepatic NAFLD in juvenile nonhuman primates. Diabetes. 2014;63(8):2702–13.

40. Ford SP, Zhang L, Zhu M, Miller MM, Smith DT, Hess BW, et al. Maternal obesity accelerates fetal pancreatic β-cell but not α-cell development in sheep: prenatal consequences. Am J Physiol Regul Integr Comp Physiol. 2009;297(3):R835–43.

41. Long NM, George LA, Uthlaut AB, Smith DT, Nijland MJ, Nathanielsz PW, et al. Maternal obesity and increased nutrient intake before and during gestation in the ewe results in altered growth, adiposity, and glucose tolerance in adult offspring. J Anim Sci. 2010;88(11):3546–53.

42. Khan I, Dekou V, Hanson M, Poston L, Taylor P. Predictive adaptive responses to maternal high-fat diet prevent endothelial dysfunction but not hypertension in adult rat offspring. Circulation. 2004;110(9):1097–102.

43. Liang C, Oest ME, Prater MR. Intrauterine exposure to high saturated fat diet elevates risk of adult-onset chronic diseases in C57BL/6 mice. Birth Defects Res B Dev Reprod Toxicol. 2009;86(5):377–84.

44. Howie GJ, Sloboda DM, Kamal T, Vickers MH. Maternal nutritional history predicts obesity in adult offspring independent of postnatal diet. J Physiol. 2009;587(Pt 4):905–15.

45. Zhu MJ, Du M, Nathanielsz PW, Ford SP. Maternal obesity up-regulates inflammatory signaling pathways and enhances cytokine expression in the mid-gestation sheep placenta. Placenta. 2010;31(5):387–91.

46. Tuersunjiang N, Odhiambo JF, Long NM, Shasa DR, Nathanielsz PW, Ford SP. Diet reduction to requirements in obese/overfed ewes from early gestation prevents glucose/insulin dysregulation and returns fetal adiposity and organ development to control levels. Am J Physiol Endocrinol Metab. 2013;305(7):E868–78.

47. George LA, Uthlaut AB, Long NM, Zhang L, Ma Y, Smith DT, et al. Different levels of overnutrition and weight gain during pregnancy have differential effects on fetal growth and organ development. Reprod Biol Endocrinol. 2010;8:75.
48. Grayson BE, Levasseur PR, Williams SM, Smith MS, Marks DL, Grove KL. Changes in melanocortin expression and inflammatory pathways in fetal offspring of nonhuman primates fed a high-fat diet. Endocrinology. 2010;151(4):1622–32.
49. Rivera HM, Kievit P, Kirigiti MA, Bauman LA, Baquero K, Blundell P, et al. Maternal high-fat diet and obesity impact palatable food intake and dopamine signaling in nonhuman primate offspring. Obesity. 2015;23(11):2157–64.
50. Guo F, Jen KL. High-fat feeding during pregnancy and lactation affects offspring metabolism in rats. Physiol Behav. 1995;57(4):681–6.
51. Srinivasan M, Katewa SD, Palaniyappan A, Pandya JD, Patel MS. Maternal high-fat diet consumption results in fetal malprogramming predisposing to the onset of metabolic syndrome-like phenotype in adulthood. Am J Physiol Endocrinol Metab. 2006;291(4):E792–9.
52. Rajia S, Chen H, Morris MJ. Maternal overnutrition impacts offspring adiposity and brain appetite markers-modulation by postweaning diet. J Neuroendocrinol. 2010;22(8):905–14.
53. Chen H, Simar D, Lambert K, Mercier J, Morris MJ. Maternal and postnatal overnutrition differentially impact appetite regulators and fuel metabolism. Endocrinology. 2008;149(11):5348–56.
54. Zhang L, Long NM, Hein SM, Ma Y, Nathanielsz PW, Ford SP. Maternal obesity in ewes results in reduced fetal pancreatic β-cell numbers in late gestation and decreased circulating insulin concentration at term. Domest Anim Endocrinol. 2011;40(1):30–9.
55. Shasa DR, Odhiambo JF, Long NM, Tuersunjiang N, Nathanielsz PW, Ford SP. Multigenerational impact of maternal overnutrition/obesity in the sheep on the neonatal leptin surge in granddaughters. Int J Obes. 2015;39(4):695–701.
56. Fan L, Lindsley SR, Comstock SM, Takahashi DL, Evans AE, He G-W, et al. Maternal high-fat diet impacts endothelial function in nonhuman primate offspring. Int J Obes. 2005;37(2):254–62.
57. Bayol SA, Simbi BH, Bertrand JA, Stickland NC. Offspring from mothers fed a "junk food" diet in pregnancy and lactation exhibit exacerbated adiposity that is more pronounced in females. J Physiol. 2008;586(Pt 13):3219–30.
58. Long NM, Ford SP, Nathanielsz PW. Maternal obesity eliminates the neonatal lamb plasma leptin peak. J Physiol. 2011;589(Pt 6):1455–62.
59. Voruganti VS, Jorgensen MJ, Kaplan JR, Kavanagh K, Rudel LL, Temel R, et al. Significant genotype by diet (GxD) interaction effects on cardiometabolic responses to a pedigree-wide, dietary challenge in vervet monkeys (*Chlorocebus aethiops* sabaeus). Am J Primatol. 2013;75(5):491–9.
60. Bayol SA, Simbi BH, Fowkes RC, Stickland NC. A maternal "Junk Food" diet in pregnancy and lactation promotes nonalcoholic fatty liver disease in rat offspring. Endocrinology. 2010;151(4):1451–61.
61. Khan IY, Taylor PD, Dekou V, Seed PT, Lakasing L, Graham D, et al. Gender-linked hypertension in offspring of lard-fed pregnant rats. Hypertension. 2003;41(1):168–75.
62. Guida SM, Ghnenis AB, Odhiambo JF, Bell CJ, Nathanielsz PW, Ford SP. Maternal obesity (MO) increases acetyl-CoA carboxylase alpha (ACCα) mRNA and protein expression and alters ACACA gene methylation in day 135 sheep fetal liver. Society for Reproductive Investigation, 63rd Annual Meeting. 2016. Abstract.
63. Huang Y, Yan X, Zhao JX, Zhu MJ, McCormick RJ, Ford SP, et al. Maternal obesity induces fibrosis in fetal myocardium of sheep. Am J Physiol Endocrinol Metab. 2010;299(6):E968–75.
64. Ghnenis AB, Odhiambo JF, McCormick RJ, Ford SP. Maternal obesity (MO) during ovine pregnancy leads to increased collagen content and cross-linking in the myocardium of adult F1 but not F2 offspring. J Anim Sci. 2015;93:Suppl. s3/J. Dairy Sci. 2015;98:Suppl. 2. Abstract # 422.
65. Wang J, Ma H, Tong C, Zhang H, Lawlis GB, Li Y, et al. Overnutrition and maternal obesity in sheep pregnancy alter the JNK-IRS-1 signaling cascades and cardiac function in the fetal heart. FASEB J. 2010;24(6):2066–76.
66. Yan X, Zhu MJ, Xu W, Tong JF, Ford SP, Nathanielsz PW, et al. Up-regulation of toll-like receptor 4/nuclear factor-κB signaling is associated with enhanced Adipogenesis and insulin resistance in fetal skeletal muscle of obese sheep at late gestation. Endocrinology. 2010;151(1):380–7.
67. Symonds ME, Mostyn A, Pearce S, Budge H, Stephenson T. Endocrine and nutritional regulation of fetal adipose tissue development. J Endocrinol. 2003;179(3):293–9. Review.

Chapter 15
Ethnicity, Obesity, and Pregnancy Outcomes on Fetal Programming

Miranda Davies-Tuck, Mary-Ann Davey, Joel A. Fernandez, Maya Reddy, Marina G. Caulfield, and Euan Wallace

Key Points

- Cardiovascular disease, diabetes, asthma, cancer, allergies, and neurocognitive impairment occur at differing rates among people of different ethnicities.
- Pregnancy conditions such as gestational diabetes mellitus and hypertensive conditions and pregnancy outcomes such as preterm birth, low birth weight/small for gestational age, and cesarean birth occur at differing rates among people of different ethnicities.
- The associations between obesity, adverse pregnancy outcomes, and life course diseases may also be additive in some ethnicities.
- A combination of increasing obesity rates and migration may compound the risk of life course disease among people of different ethnicities via fetal programming effects.

Keywords Maternal ethnicity • Pregnancy complications • Pregnancy outcomes • Obesity • Fetal programing

Abbreviations

BMI   Body mass index
CVD   Cardiovascular disease

M. Davies-Tuck (✉)
The Ritchie Centre, Hudson Institute of Medical Research, 27-31 Wright Street, Clayton, VIC 3168, Australia
e-mail: miranda.davies@hudson.org.au

M.-A. Davey
Department of Obstetrics and Gynaecology, School of Clinical Sciences, Monash University, 246 Clayton Rd, Clayton, VIC 3168, Australia

J.A. Fernandez, BMedSc (Hons)
Department of Obstetrics and Gynaecology, Monash Medical Centre, Melbourne, VIC, Australia

M. Reddy
Monash Health, Monash Medical Centre, Clayton, Australia

M.G. Caulfield, MBBS (Hons), BMedSc (Hons) • E. Wallace
Department of Obstetrics and Gynecology, Monash University, Clayton, VIC, Australia

© Springer International Publishing AG 2017
R. Rajendram et al. (eds.), *Diet, Nutrition, and Fetal Programming*,
Nutrition and Health, DOI 10.1007/978-3-319-60289-9_15

DM   Diabetes mellitus
GDM   Gestational diabetes mellitus
HIC   High-income country
NICU   Neonatal intensive care unit
PE   Preeclampsia
UK   United Kingdom

Introduction

Cardiovascular disease, diabetes, and asthma all occur at differing prevalence among people of different ethnicities. Coronary artery disease is up to two times more common among South Asians compared to Europeans [1], and type 2 diabetes is almost four times more common [2]. Diabetes is also more common in Filipino, Hispanic, Chinese, Middle Eastern, north African, South and Central American, and people from the western Pacific region [2, 3]. "Black" individuals have a consistently higher prevalence of hypertension, diabetes [3], and stroke [4]. Interestingly, the etiology of stroke also differs according to ethnicity. Western populations are more likely to experience emboli originating from the heart or extracranial large arteries compared to Asian populations where small-vessel occlusion or intracranial atherosclerosis occurs more frequently [5]. Rates of asthma differ by ethnicity. Puerto Rican children have 2.4 and Black/African-American children 1.6-fold greater asthma prevalence than White children [6]. Aboriginal populations (Canadian Aboriginals, Native Americans, and New Zealand Maoris) are 40% more likely to report having asthma than non-Aboriginal populations [7]. While it is likely that some of the elevated risks relate to social disadvantage and poor lifestyle exposures, there is evidence to suggest that they are a consequence of the in utero environments in which the fetus develops.

Fetal Programming

Over 30 years ago, an epidemiologist, David Barker, first reported an association between early life nutrition, either in the womb or the perinatal period, and the risk of cardiovascular disease in later life [8]. Since that time a number of animal and epidemiological studies have demonstrated associations between early life exposures and rates of adult diseases. Termed the "Barker hypothesis" and now also referred to as "Developmental Origins of Health and Disease" [9], the premise is that exposures such as undernutrition, toxins, or stress during this window of fetal development or early perinatal period can alter genes leading to a greater predisposition to cardiovascular disease, diabetes, asthma, cancer, and neuropsychological conditions in later life [9]. The biological mechanism by which in utero exposures shape long-term childhood and adult health consequences is thought to be via epigenetic changes [10]. Epigenetics is the branch of genetics that deals with the suppression or expression of certain genes. It is a way of passing phenotypic information to the next generation without altering the DNA sequence itself [11, 12]. The environment that a fetus is exposed to can affect epigenetic processes to either increase or decrease the expression of different genes. It is thought that this confers an evolutionary advantage to a fetus by adapting the expression of the genome to a phenotype that is suited to the external environment [12]. On the flip side however, this may also predispose the fetus to certain noncommunicable diseases over their life course [13].

Maternal Ethnicity, Pregnancy Complications, and Fetal Programming

Gestational diabetes mellitus (GDM) and hypertensive conditions in pregnancy such as gestational hypertension and preeclampsia both affect the environment under which the fetus develops and have been shown to be associated with increased risks of disease for the offspring in later life. Interestingly both of these conditions also occur at elevated rates in women of certain ethnicities and may explain, via fetal programming effects, the differing prevalence and incidence of many life course diseases among people of different ethnicities.

Gestational Diabetes Mellitus

Gestational diabetes mellitus (GDM) occurs most frequently in South or Southeast Asian women and is also experienced in high rates in Hispanic, African-American, Native American, Pacific Islander, and Indigenous Australian women [14–18].

The impact of GDM has been widely studied. GDM is characterized by hyperglycemia, hyperinsulinemia, and hyperlipidemia [19, 20]. Alterations in the placental transport of nutrients as a result of GDM lead to the fetus experiencing an increased supply of glucose, amino acids, triglycerides, and cholesterol compared to when the mother does not have GDM [20]. It is well documented that offspring born in pregnancies complicated by GDM are at increased risk of type 2 diabetes, metabolic syndrome, and cardiovascular and renal disease [21, 22]. In a study of ~600 predominantly Caucasian women, those with GDM had offspring that experienced type 2 diabetes at almost eight times the rate of the background population [22]. The same offspring also experienced increased rates of obesity, metabolic syndrome, and reduced insulin sensitivity compared to the background population [21, 22]. Among American infants born to women with GDM, 15% of them had three or more components of the metabolic syndrome at age 11 compared to only 3% off offspring who were not exposed to GDM [23]. Chinese offspring born to women with GDM had significantly higher blood pressure and lower high-density lipoprotein cholesterol at 11 years of age. Highest umbilical cord insulin levels were also associated with abnormal glucose tolerance [24]. Studies in animals have shown that diabetes in pregnancy impairs nephrogenesis [25] and is associated with salt-sensitive hypertension and decreased renal function [26]. Whether the same impacts are true in humans is not yet known; however given the association between GDM and CVD in the offspring, it seems plausible. The immediate impacts of GDM on the infant have been found to vary by ethnicity. A retrospective study of women with GDM in Hawaii from 1995 to 2005 found that babies born to Native Hawaiian/Pacific Islander mothers and Filipino mothers had four and two times the prevalence of macrosomia, respectively, compared with neonates born to Japanese, Chinese, and Caucasian mothers. Differences in neonatal hypoglycemia and hyperbilirubinemia were also observed [27]. Similarly, in a study of ~20,000 Southeast Asian and ~33,000 White women with GDM, macrosomia was more likely in Cambodian and Laotian women compared to Japanese women, but overall Southeast Asian women had reduced odds of GDM [28]. Whether the long-term impacts of fetal programing also differ by ethnicity is not yet fully clear. A summary of these associations is presented in Fig. 15.1.

Hypertensive Conditions of Pregnancy

Hypertensive conditions in pregnancy, such as gestational hypertension and preeclampsia (PE) , occur more frequently in Black, Hispanic, Caucasian, Filipino women, sub-Saharan African, Latin America, and the Caribbean [29–31] and significantly less frequently in Chinese and Indian women [30]. The

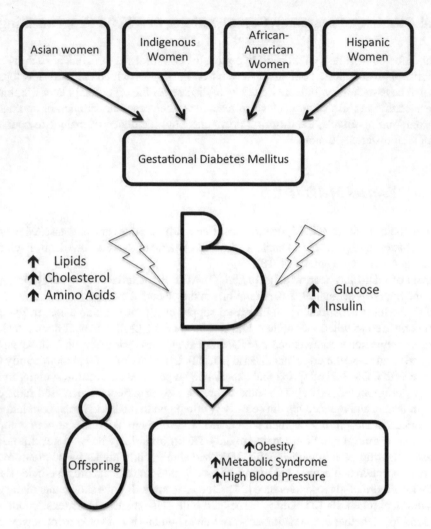

Fig. 15.1 Schematic diagram of associations between maternal ethnicity, gestational diabetes, and fetal programming effects generated from references in text

babies in these pregnancies are exposed to systemic inflammation [32] and elevated glucocorticosteroids [33]. They may also experience insufficient nutrition and hypoxia [34].

Infants from pregnancies affected by hypertensive disorders have been shown to be at increased risk of hypertension and other CVD in later life (reviewed in [35]), type 1 diabetes [36], and reduced cognitive abilities [37]. Adult children born to 2608 Australian women in the early 1980s who had a diastolic blood pressure over 90 mmHG on at least two occasions beyond 20 weeks' gestation associated with proteinuria and/or fluid retention had 3.46 mmHG greater systolic and 3.02 mmHg greater diastolic blood pressure 21 years later [38]. Offspring of women in Finland between 1934 and 1944 with gestational hypertension (*n* = 1592) or PE (*n* = 284) had 1.4 and 1.9 times the risk of stroke, respectively [39]. The association with type 1 diabetes is less consistent [40]; however, a case-control study of 602 children with type 1 diabetes and 1490 controls in Denmark did find that maternal PE was associated with type 1 diabetes in the offspring; however this association was only seen in boys [36].

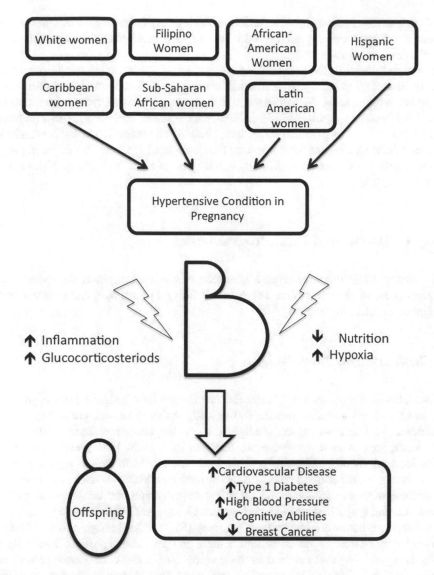

Fig. 15.2 Schematic diagram of associations between maternal ethnicity, hypertensive conditions in pregnancy, and fetal programming effects generated from references in text

As early as the 1960s, the association between hypertensive conditions and cognitive outcomes was documented [41]. In a sibling study, children from pregnancies affected by PE scored lower on verbal reasoning at 11 years of age compared to their unaffected sibling adjusting for birth rank [41]. More recently a systematic review of 19 studies concluded that maternal hypertensive disorders are associated with lower cognitive abilities in the offspring [37]. Babies born to mothers with hypertensive conditions are also more likely to be growth restricted and born preterm, both of which in themselves have fetal programming effects. There is evidence however to suggest that the associations between hypertension in pregnancy and life course disease are independent of fetal growth restriction and preterm birth [42].

Intriguingly, positive fetal programming effects have also been observed. A systematic review that assessed six studies published between 1980 and 2007 found that overall, there was a 52% decreased risk (95% CI 0.3–0.78) of breast cancer in female offspring born from pregnancies complicated by PE or eclampsia [43]. It has been suggested that this may relate to reduced estrogen concentrations which are observed in PE pregnancies [44].

Like gestational diabetes, the perinatal complications of hypertensive conditions of pregnancy also differ by maternal ethnicity. In the same study of ~20,000 Southeast Asian women, [28] Southeast Asian women with PE had increased odds for preterm delivery when compared with Japanese and White women with PE [28]. A New York study of birth certificate data from 1988 to 1994 showed that among hypertensive mothers, the risk of having a low birth weight baby was highest among White women and lowest among Black women [31]. Whether the fetal programming effects of hypertensive conditions also differ by ethnicity is not clear. A summary of these associations is presented in Fig. 15.2.

Pregnancy Outcomes and Fetal Programming

Women of different ethnicities experience higher rates of adverse pregnancy outcomes and interventions including preterm birth, low birth weight/small for gestational age, and cesarean birth, which have been linked to fetal programming.

Preterm Birth and Low Birth Weight

African, Asian, South American, and Middle Eastern women have a significantly higher rate of preterm birth compared to Caucasian women [30, 45–47]. Asian (Chinese, Vietnamese, Filipino, and Indian), African, Middle Eastern, and Indigenous (Native Hawaiian, Indigenous Mexican, and Indigenous Australian) women are also more likely to have a low birth weight baby [30, 48–50]. Many of the fetal programing effects of preterm birth and low birth weight appear to be the same, likely due to the two outcomes often coinciding. Low birth weight and preterm birth have been associated with adverse outcomes in adulthood including hypertension and cardiovascular disease [51], insulin resistance and type 2 diabetes [51, 52], reduced language development [53], asthma [54], and more recently reduced bone mass and knee arthroplasty [55]. The fetal programming effects attributed to preterm birth may be a consequence of both in utero and postnatal exposures. They may reflect the adverse pregnancy event(s) that resulted in the preterm birth such as infection, growth restriction, preeclampsia, smoking, chronic illness, or placental conditions. Alternatively they may be a consequence of the NICU stay, treatments, and feeding practices.

The first evidence of low birth weight having fetal programming effects was through studies on the Dutch famine. Smaller singleton babies, a consequence of nutritional deficits, had increased risks of obesity, cardiovascular disease, and mental health conditions [56–58]. Since then, many other studies have followed. Among babies born in the UK, the lower the birth weight of a baby, the greater its' odds were of developing diabetes mellitus or metabolic syndrome as an adult [59, 60]. A systematic review and meta-analysis of ten observational studies of 1342 preterm or LBW and 1738 full-term participants from eight countries found that those who were preterm or very low birth weight had a significantly higher systolic blood pressure at 18 years of age [61]. Among 52 adults aged 34–38 years, those who were born preterm were also less insulin sensitive than those born at term [52]. Consistent findings were observed in a case-control study of very preterm compared to healthy controls; those born very preterm had reduced insulin sensitivity at 23 years [62]. When considering this from ethnic-specific angle, Indian babies, when compared to Caucasian controls, are generally smaller in terms of size and weight but have a higher adipose percentage leading to the concept of the "thin-fat" baby [63, 64].

The consequence of this is a more adipose body composition which is thought to predispose these infants to development of diabetes (both type 2 and gestational diabetes) as well as other cardiovascular diseases in the future. Whether this is a product of transgenerational fetal programming effects is not known. It is well documented though that his body composition is considered the "thrifty phenotype" where reduced nutrition in utero impairs the development of the pancreas. The nutrient-poor intrauterine environment causes the fetus to reduce its production of insulin and increase its resistance to insulin to maximize circulating glucose. This is done with the expectation of living in an environment where food sources are scarce. Insulin is also a fetal growth factor which explains why these babies are smaller. After birth, living in an environment with ample provision of food, these susceptible babies go on to develop obesity and DM [59, 60, 64].

Beyond metabolic effects, asthma diagnosed in mid childhood that persists through adolescence was significantly more likely among teenagers who were of low birth weight compared to those who were of normal weight, more so if that child was male and White [54]. Findings from a meta-analysis of 17 studies including 874,710 children found that wheezing disorders were 46% more likely in preterm and almost three times more likely in very preterm children (<32 weeks' gestation) [65]. It has been proposed that underlying mechanism may be poor growth in utero leading to low birth weight also leads to impaired airway development or immunological mechanisms [66, 67]. Therapeutic interventions after birth, such as ventilation approaches, may also be involved [67]. The effects of preterm birth on asthma development may differ by ethnicity. A systematic review and meta-analysis reported a stronger association between preterm birth and asthma in studies done in non-European compared to European countries [68]. Bias may explain this finding; however low birth weight, preterm birth, and asthma are all more common in certain ethnic groups, warranting further investigation.

Low birth weight and preterm birth are also associated with musculoskeletal conditions in later life. Among almost 4000 participants in the Australian Diabetes, Obesity, and Lifestyle Study, those born preterm were 2.5 and those of low birth weight 2.0 times more likely to require a knee arthroscopy [55]. Unfortunately in this study, ethnicity was not reported. Preterm birth has been associated with acetabular dysplasia, which in turn increases the incidence of hip OA [69]. It has been suggested this may reflect a reprogramming of the insulin-like growth factor 1 (IGF-1) axis [70] which is involved in osteoblastic differentiation of mesenchymal stem cells and new bone formation [71]. Consistent with that, a case-control study of very preterm compared to healthy controls showed that those born very preterm had reduced peak bone mass at 23 years [62].

There is growing evidence to link preterm birth and low birth weight to neurodevelopmental outcomes. The association between preterm birth, particularly early preterm birth and neurocognitive effects, is well known. Among school-age children, cognitive delay is very prevalent (40%) in children born at less than 28 weeks [72] even when there is no severe disability [73]. This association is also true for less preterm infants. A systematic review of 14 studies of long-term cognitive and education outcomes among those who were late preterm births found that even at the late preterm period (34–36 weeks), they underperformed in all cognitive outcomes, and the effect persisted into adulthood [74]. Interestingly, there is some evidence to suggest that the association between prematurity and cognitive outcomes differs by ethnicity [75]. In a retrospective cohort study of 865 children born <28 weeks, there were no differences in cognitive domains assessed by the Bayley Scales of Infant Development among children of different ethnicities; however, both Blacks and Hispanic-Whites scored significantly lower than Whites in regard to the language domains with Hispanic-Whites scoring the lowest [75]. Further research is needed to confirm this and also to assess this and other domains of neurocognitive development among other ethnicities independent of important confounding factors. The association between being born small for gestational age and neurocognitive effects is less consistent. In a population-based study of 515 infants born before 32 weeks' gestation, being SGA was not significantly associated with cognitive ability at 5 years of age [76]. In contrast, a recent systematic review found that independent of prematurity, babies born small for gestational age were at higher risk of cognitive deficits, hyperactivity, or attention-deficit disorders at 5 years and 8 years of

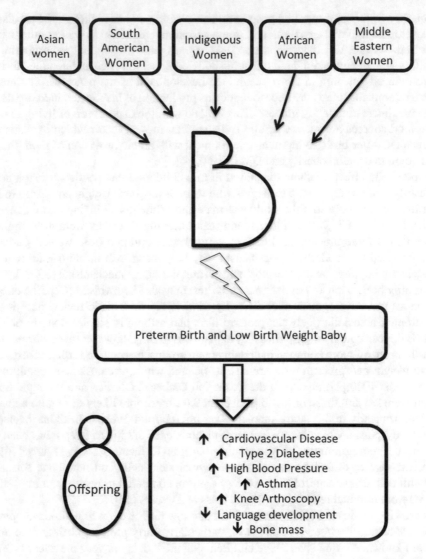

Fig. 15.3 Schematic diagram of associations between maternal ethnicity, preterm birth and low birth weight baby, and fetal programming effects generated from references in text

age [77]. To our knowledge there are no studies that have assessed the interaction between maternal ethnicity and being born small on neurocognitive outcomes in later life. However there is some evidence that childhood intelligence at age 14 differs by parental ethnicity [78], and small babies are more common in Asian, African, Middle Eastern, and Indigenous women [30, 48–50]. Exploring the potential interaction is therefore warranted. A summary of these associations is presented in Fig. 15.3.

Caesarean Birth

The rates of obstetric interventions experienced also differ by maternal ethnicity [79–82]. Black and Asian women in the USA experience higher rates of cesarean delivery [79, 80]. Indian, Bangladeshi, and Pakistani low-risk primiparous women had a twofold higher rate of emergency cesarean

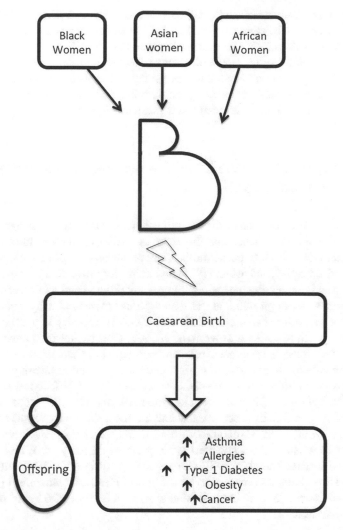

Fig. 15.4 Schematic diagram of associations between maternal ethnicity cesarean and fetal programming effects generated from references in text

section compared to their Caucasian counterparts in England [81]. Primiparous East African women also had higher rates of unplanned cesarean in an Australian population [83]. Indian women giving birth in New Zealand have been shown to have higher rates of emergency cesarean than others [82]. A number of epidemiological studies have found that where a baby is born by cesarean, it is at greater risk of developing asthma, allergies, type 1 diabetes, celiac disease, obesity, and cancer in later life. Among over 2000 8-year-old children, those born by cesarean were significantly more likely to report wheezing and asthma and be atopic compared to those born vaginally. The association between cesarean and atopy was also stronger in those children born in Cyprus with a family history [84]. A systematic review of 20 studies also identified an overall 20% increase in risk of type 1 diabetes following cesarean delivery; however no consideration for maternal ethnicity was made [85]. A case-control study of almost 2000 children found that those with celiac disease were 80% more likely to have been born by cesarean compared to those without celiac disease [86]. Caesarean birth was also associated with an increased likelihood of obesity by age 11; however babies born by cesarean were significantly smaller than those born vaginally so this may reflect the fetal programming effects of low birth weight rather than mode of birth [87]. In a Swedish case-control study, children who developed myeloid leukemia were 2.5 times more likely to have been born by cesarean [88]. Similarly in an American case-control study of testicular germ cell tumors, those with cancer were twice as likely to have been born by cesarean [89]. It has been suggested that the association with cesarean birth may reflect fetal programming events associated with the complication leading to the cesarean such as gestational diabetes, preeclampsia, and/or growth restriction or may be a consequence of altered gut microbiota and immune system function and/or perinatal stress [85]. A summary of these associations is presented in Fig. 15.4.

Maternal Obesity Influences the Ethnicity-Associated Pregnancy Conditions and Fetal Programming Effects

Maternal obesity has emerged as one of the key contributors to adverse pregnancy outcomes in high-income nations [90], with no evidence that this trend is likely to reverse in the near future. It is also well established that babies born to obese mothers are at elevated risk of developing type 2 diabetes [91], metabolic syndrome [92], and asthma [93] and having cognitive deficits, attention-deficit/hyperactivity disorders, and internalizing psychopathology in childhood and adolescence [94].

Emerging evidence has suggested that the associations between obesity and adverse pregnancy outcomes may also be additive in some ethnicities [95–98]. Obesity is a stronger risk factor for GDM in Asian compared to Caucasian women [96, 97]. Obesity has also been shown to be more strongly associated with PE development in Latina compared to Caucasian women [98]. The association between obesity, preterm birth, low birth weight baby, and cesarean also appears to differ by ethnicity. A cross-sectional study of ~24,000 women in the UK found that the association between obesity and cesarean birth was weaker in Black and Oriental women and protective in Asian women. The association between obesity and having a low birth weight baby was protective in White and Asian women, but associated with an increased risk in Black and Oriental women. Obesity was also most strongly associated with preterm delivery in White women and least strongly associated in Black women [97]. Consequently, differential BMI cutoffs for people of Asian background have been recommended by the World Health Organization [99]. Where a BMI of ≥ 30 kg/m^2 is considered "obese" in Caucasian women, a BMI of ≥ 26 kg/m^2 is considered obese in a woman of Asian descent.

Conclusion

Over the last 20 years, there have been big changes to the characteristics of women giving birth in high-income countries [4]. Two maternal characteristics for which there have been dramatic changes are maternal obesity and ethnicity. According to the 2011–2012 National Health and Nutrition Examination Survey, 32% of women of reproductive age are obese, and almost half of women entering pregnancy now have a body mass index (BMI) of 25 or more [90] in contrast to 24% in 1983 [100].Over the same period, increasing rates of migration have also meant that the number of women giving birth in HIC who themselves were born overseas is increasing. This is important because both ethnicity and obesity are associated with a range of health consequences, both in pregnancy and later life via fetal programming mechanisms, and likely act synergistically to increase the risk of disease over the life course.

References

1. Fernando E, et al. Cardiovascular disease in South Asian migrants. Can J Cardiol. 2015;31(9):1139–50.
2. Meeks KA, et al. Disparities in type 2 diabetes prevalence among ethnic minority groups resident in Europe: a systematic review and meta-analysis. Intern Emerg Med. 2016;11(3):327–40.
3. Gasevic D, Ross ES, Lear SA. Ethnic differences in cardiovascular disease risk factors: a systematic review of North American evidence. Can J Cardiol. 2015;31(9):1169–79.
4. Hicks LS, et al. Determinants of JNC VI guideline adherence, intensity of drug therapy, and blood pressure control by race and ethnicity. Hypertension. 2004;44(4):429–34.
5. Kim BJ, Kim JS. Ischemic stroke subtype classification: an Asian viewpoint. J Stroke. 2014;16:1.
6. Akinbami LJ. Status of childhood asthma in the United States 1980–2007. Pediatrics. 2009;123(Suppl 3):S131–45.
7. Ospina MB, et al. Prevalence of asthma and chronic obstructive pulmonary disease in aboriginal and non-aboriginal populations: a systematic review and meta-analysis of epidemiological studies. Can Respir J. 2012;19(6):355–60.
8. Barker DJ, Osmond C. Infant mortality, childhood nutrition, and ischaemic heart disease in England and Wales. Lancet. 2016;1(8489):1077–81.
9. Gillman MW. Developmental origins of health and disease. N Engl J Med. 2005;353(11):1984–50.
10. Burdge GC, et al. Epigenetic regulation of transcription: a mechanism for inducing variations in phenotype (fetal programming) by differences in nutrition during early life? Br J Nutr. 2007;97(6):1036–46.
11. Grandjean P, et al. Life-long implications of developmental exposure to environmental stressors: new perspectives. Endocrinology. 2015;156(10):3408–15.
12. Hanson M, et al. Developmental plasticity and developmental origins of non-communicable disease: theoretical considerations and epigenetic mechanisms. Prog Biophys Mol Biol. 2011;106(1):272–80.
13. Entringer S, Buss C, Wadhwa PD. Prenatal stress, telomere biology, and fetal programming of health and disease risk. Sci Signal. 2012;5(248):pt12.
14. Retnakaran R, et al. Ethnicity modifies the effect of obesity on insulin resistance in pregnancy: a comparison of Asian, South Asian, and Caucasian women. J Clin Endocrinol Metab. 2006;91(1):93–7.
15. Jenum AK, et al. Impact of ethnicity on gestational diabetes identified with the WHO and the modified International Association of Diabetes and Pregnancy Study Groups criteria: a population-based cohort study. Eur J Endocrinol Eur Fed Endocr Soc. 2012;166(2):317–24.
16. Dornhorst A, et al. High prevalence of gestational diabetes in women from ethnic minority groups. Diabet Med. 1992;9(9):820–5.
17. Schwartz N, Nachum Z, Green MS. The prevalence of gestational diabetes mellitus recurrence – effect of ethnicity and parity: a metaanalysis. Am J Obstet Gynecol. 2015;213(3):310–7.
18. Kjos SL, Buchanan TA. Gestational diabetes mellitus. N Engl J Med. 1999;341:1749–56.
19. American Diabetes Association. Classification and diagnosis of diabetes. Diabetes Care. 2015;38:S8–16.
20. Brett KE, et al. Maternal-fetal nutrient transport in pregnancy pathologies: the role of the placenta. Int J Mol Sci. 2014;15(9):16153–85.
21. Kelstrup L, et al. Insulin resistance and impaired pancreatic β-cell function in adult offspring of women with diabetes in pregnancy. J Clin Endocrinol Metab. 2013;98(9):3793–801.
22. Clausen TD, et al. High prevalence of type 2 diabetes and pre-diabetes in adult offspring of women with gestational diabetes mellitus or type 1 diabetes: the role of intrauterine hyperglycemia. Diabetes Care. 2008;31(2):340–6.
23. Boney CM, et al. Metabolic syndrome in childhood: association with birth weight, maternal obesity, and gestational diabetes. Pediatrics. 2005;115:290–6.
24. Tam WH, et al. Glucose intolerance and cardiometabolic risk in children exposed to maternal gestational diabetes mellitus in utero. Pediatrics. 2008;122(6):1229–34.
25. Amri K, et al. Adverse effects of hyperglycemia on kidney development in rats: in vivo and in vitro studies. Diabetes. 1999;48(11):2240–5.
26. Nehiri T, et al. Exposure to maternal diabetes induces salt-sensitive hypertension and impairs renal function in adult rat offspring. Diabetes. 2008;57(8):2167–75.
27. Silva JK, et al. Ethnic differences in perinatal outcome of gestational diabetes mellitus. Diabetes Care. 2006;29(9):2058–63.
28. Cripe SM, et al. Perinatal outcomes of Southeast Asians with pregnancies complicated by gestational diabetes mellitus or preeclampsia. J Immigr Minor Health. 2012;14(5):747–53.
29. Urquia ML, et al. Disparities in pre-eclampsia and eclampsia among immigrant women giving birth in six industrialised countries. BJOG. 2014;121(12):1492–500.
30. Dahlen HG, et al. Rates of obstetric intervention during birth and selected maternal and perinatal outcomes for low risk women born in Australia compared to those born overseas. BMC Pregnancy Childbirth. 2013;13:100.
31. Fang J, Madhavan S, Alderman MH. The influence of maternal hypertension on low birth weight: differences among ethnic populations. Ethn Dis. 1999;9(3):369–76.

32. Redman CW, Sargent IL. Immunology of pre-eclampsia. Am J Reprod Immunol. 2010;63:534–54.
33. Aufdenblatten M, et al. Prematurity is related to high placental cortisol in preeclampsia. Pediatr Res. 2009;65:198–202.
34. Newnham JP, et al. Nutrition and the early origins of adult disease. Asia Pac J Clin Nutr. 2002;11(Suppl 3):S537–42.
35. Davis EF, et al. Cardiovascular risk factors in children and young adults born to preeclamptic pregnancies: a systematic review. Pediatrics. 2012;129(6):e1552–61.
36. Svensson J, et al. Early childhood risk factors associated with type 1 diabetes – is gender important? Eur J Epidemiol. 2005;20(5):429–34.
37. Tuovinen S, et al. Maternal hypertensive pregnancy disorders and cognitive functioning of the offspring: a systematic review. J Am Soc Hypertens. 2014;8(11):832–47.
38. Mamun AA, et al. Does hypertensive disorder of pregnancy predict offspring blood pressure at 21 years? Evidence from a birth cohort study. J Hum Hypertens. 2012;26(5):288–94.
39. Kajantie E, et al. Pre-eclampsia is associated with increased risk of stroke in the adult offspring: the Helsinki birth cohort study. Stroke. 2009;40(4):1176–80.
40. Henry EB, Patterson CC, Cardwell CR. A meta-analysis of the association between pre-eclampsia and childhood-onset Type 1 diabetes mellitus. Diabet Med. 2011;28(8):900–5.
41. Barker DJ, Edwards JH. Obstetric complications and school performance. Br Med J. 1967;3:695–9.
42. Wu CS, et al. Health of children born to mothers who had preeclampsia: a population-based cohort study. Am J Obstet Gynecol. 2009;201(3):269.
43. Xue F, Michels KB. Intrauterine factors and risk of breast cancer: a systematic review and meta-analysis of current evidence. Lancet Oncol. 2007;8:1088–100.
44. Zeisler H, et al. Concentrations of estrogens in patients with preeclampsia. Wien Klin Wochenschr. 2002;114:446–58.
45. Park AL, Urquia ML, Ray JG. Risk of preterm birth according to maternal and paternal country of birth: a population-based study. J Obstet Gynaecol Can. 2015;37(12):1053–62.
46. Leon DA, Moser KA. Low birth weight persists in South Asian babies born in England and Wales regardless of maternal country of birth. Slow pace of acculturation, physiological constraint or both? Analysis of routine data. J Epidemiol Community Health. 2012;66(6):544–51.
47. Oftedal AM, et al. Socio-economic risk factors for preterm birth in Norway 1999–2009. Scand J Public Health. 2016;44:587–92. Epub ahead of print.
48. Servan-Mori E, et al. Timeliness, frequency and content of antenatal care: which is most important to reducing indigenous disparities in birth weight in Mexico? Health Policy Plan. 2016;3(4):444–53.
49. Chang AL, et al. Maternal risk factors and perinatal outcomes among pacific islander groups in Hawaii: a retrospective cohort study using statewide hospital data. BMC Pregnancy Childbirth. 2015;15:239.
50. Kildea S, et al. The maternal and neonatal outcomes for an urban indigenous population compared with their non-indigenous counterparts and a trend analysis over four triennia. BMC Pregnancy Childbirth. 2013;13:167.
51. Alexander BT, Dasinger JH, Intapad S. Fetal programming and cardiovascular pathology. Compr Physiol. 2015;5(2):997–1025.
52. Mathai S, et al. Insulin sensitivity and β-cell function in adults born preterm and their children. Diabetes. 2012;61(10):2479–83.
53. Zerbeto AB, Cortelo FM, Filho ÉB C. Association between gestational age and birth weight on the language development of Brazilian children: a systematic review. J Pediatr. 2015;91:4.
54. Johnson CC, et al. Birth weight and asthma incidence by asthma phenotype pattern in a racially diverse cohort followed through adolescence. J Asthma. 2015;52(10):1006–12.
55. Hussain SM, et al. Association of low birth weight and preterm birth with the incidence of knee and hip arthroplasty for osteoarthritis. Arthritis Care Res. 2015;67(4):502–8.
56. El Hajj N, et al. Epigenetics and life-long consequences of an adverse nutritional and diabetic intrauterine environment. Reproduction (Cambridge, England). 2014;148(6):R111–20.
57. Roseboom T, de Rooij S, Painter R. The Dutch famine and its long-term consequences for adult health. Early Hum Dev. 2006;82(8):485–91.
58. Yajnik CS. Transmission of obesity-adiposity and related disorders from the mother to the baby. Ann Nutr Metab. 2014;64(Suppl 1):8–17.
59. Hales CN, Barker DJ. Type 2 (non-insulin-dependent) diabetes mellitus: the thrifty phenotype hypothesis. Diabetologia. 1992;35(7):595–601.
60. Hales CN, Barker DJ. The thrifty phenotype hypothesis. Br Med Bull. 2001;60:5–20.
61. de Jong F, et al. Systematic review and meta-analysis of preterm birth and later systolic blood pressure. Hypertension. 2012;59(2):226–34.
62. Smith CM, et al. Very low birth weight survivors have reduced peak bone mass and reduced insulin sensitivity. Clin Endocrinol. 2011;75(4):443–9.
63. Yajnik CS, Deshmukh US. Maternal nutrition, intrauterine programming and consequential risks in the offspring. Rev Endocr Metab Disord. 2008;9(3):203–11.

64. Yajnik CS, et al. Neonatal anthropometry: the thin-fat Indian baby. The Pune Maternal Nutrition Study. Int J Obes Relat Metab Disord: J Int Assoc Stud Obes. 2003;27(2):173–80.

65. Been JV, et al. Preterm birth and childhood wheezing disorders: a systematic review and meta-analysis. PLoS Med. 2014;11:1.

66. Barker DJ, et al. Foetal and childhood growth and asthma in adult life. Acta Paediatr. 2013;102(7):732–8.

67. Duijts L, et al. Early origins of chronic obstructive lung diseases across the life course. Eur J Epidemiol. 2014;29(12):871–85.

68. Jaakkola JJ, et al. Preterm delivery and asthma: a systematic review and meta-analysis. Allergy Clin Immunol. 2006;118(4):823–30.

69. Simić S, et al. Does the gestation age of newborn babies influence the ultrasonic assessment of hip condition? Srp Arh Celok Lek. 2009;137(7):402–8.

70. Meas T. Fetal origins of insulin resistance and the metabolic syndrome: a key role for adipose tissue? Diabete Metab. 2010;36(1):11–20.

71. Xian L, et al. Matrix IGF-1 maintains bone mass by activation of mTOR in mesenchymal stem cells. Nat Med. 2012;18(7):1095–101.

72. Anderson P, Doyle LW. Neurobehavioral outcomes of school-age children born extremely low birth weight or very preterm in the 1990s. JAMA. 2003;289(24):3264–72.

73. Bhutta AT, et al. Cognitive and behavioral outcomes of school-aged children who were born preterm: a meta-analysis. JAMA. 2002;288(6):728–37.

74. Chan E, et al. Long-term cognitive and school outcomes of late-preterm and early-term births: a systematic review. Child Care Health Dev. 2016;42(3):297–312.

75. Duncan AF, et al. Effect of ethnicity and race on cognitive and language testing at age 18–22 months in extremely preterm infants. J Pediatr. 2012;160(6):966–71.

76. Bickle Graz M, Tolsa JF, Fischer Fumeaux CJ. Being small for gestational age: does it matter for the neurodevelopment of premature infants? A Cohort Study. PLoS One. 2015;10:5.

77. Gascoin G, Flamant C. Long-term outcome in context of intra uterine growth restriction and/or small for gestational age newborns. J Gynecol Obstet Biol Reprod (Paris). 2013;42(8):911–20.

78. Lawlor DA, et al. Early life predictors of childhood intelligence: findings from the Mater-University study of pregnancy and its outcomes. Paediatr Perinat Epidemiol. 2006;20(2):148–62.

79. Edmonds JK, et al. Racial and ethnic differences in primary, unscheduled cesarean deliveries among low-risk primiparous women at an academic medical center: a retrospective cohort study. BMC Pregnancy Childbirth. 2013;13:168.

80. Janevic T, et al. Disparities in cesarean delivery by ethnicity and nativity in New York City. Matern Child Health J. 2014;18(1):250–7.

81. Ibison JM. Ethnicity and mode of delivery in 'low-risk' first-time mothers, East London, 1988–1997. Eur J Obstet Gynecol Reprod Biol. 2005;118(2):199–205.

82. Anderson NH, et al. Ethnicity and risk of caesarean section in a term, nulliparous New Zealand obstetric cohort. Aust N Z J Obstet Gynaecol. 2013;53(3):258–64.

83. Belihu FB, Small R, Davey MA. Variations in first-time caesarean birth between Eastern African immigrants and Australian-born women in public care: a population-based investigation in Victoria. BMC Pregnancy Childbirth. 2016;16:86. doi:10.1186/s12884-016-0886-z.

84. Kolokotroni O, et al. Asthma and atopy in children born by caesarean section: effect modification by family history of allergies – a population based cross-sectional study. BMC Pediatr. 2012;12:179.

85. Cardwell CR, et al. Caesarean section is associated with an increased risk of childhood-onset type 1 diabetes mellitus: a meta-analysis of observational studies. Diabetologia. 2008;51(5):726–35.

86. Decker E, et al. Cesarean delivery is associated with celiac disease but not inflammatory bowel disease in children. Pediatrics. 2010;125(6):1433–40.

87. Blustein J, et al. Association of caesarean delivery with child adiposity from age 6 weeks to 15 years. Int J Obes. 2013;37(7):900–6.

88. Cnattingius S, et al. Prenatal and neonatal risk factors for childhood myeloid leukemia. Cancer Epidemiol Biomark Prev. 1995;4(5):441–5.

89. Cook MB, et al. Perinatal factors and the risk of testicular germ cell tumors. Int J Cancer. 2008;122(11):2600–6.

90. Marchi J, et al. Risks associated with obesity in pregnancy, for the mother and baby: a systematic review of reviews. Obes Rev. 2015;16:621–38.

91. Shaw J. Epidemiology of childhood type 2 diabetes and obesity. Pediatr Diabetes. 2007;8(Suppl 9):7–15.

92. Fall C. Evidence for the intra-uterine programming of adiposity in later life. Ann Hum Biol. 2011;38(4):410–28.

93. Rizzo GS, Sen S. Maternal obesity and immune dysregulation in mother and infant: a review of the evidence. Paediatr Respir Rev. 2015;16(4):251–7.

94. Van Lieshout RJ. Role of maternal adiposity prior to and during pregnancy in cognitive and psychiatric problems in offspring. Nutr Rev. 2013;71(Suppl 1):S95–101.
95. Penn N, et al. Ethnic variation in stillbirth risk and the role of maternal obesity: analysis of routine data from the London maternity unit. BMC Pregnancy Childbirth. 2014;14:404.
96. Makgoba M, Savvidou MD, Steer PJ. An analysis of the interrelationship between maternal age, body mass index and racial origin in the development of gestational diabetes mellitus. BJOG. 2011;119:276–82.
97. Oteng-Ntim E, et al. Impact of obesity on pregnancy outcome in different ethnic groups: calculating population attributable fractions. PLoS One. 2013;8:1.
98. Ramos GA, Caughey AB. The interrelationship between ethnicity and obesity on obstetric outcomes. Am J Obstet Gynecol. 2005;193(3, Supplement):1089–93.
99. Consultation, We. Appropriate body-mass index for Asian populations and its implications for policy and intervention strategies. Lancet. 2004;363:157–63.
100. Reinold C, Dalenius K, Brindley P, Smith B, Grummer-Strawn L. Pregnancy Nutrition Surveillance 2009 Report. Atlanta: U.S. Department of Health and Human Services, Centers for Disease Control and Prevention; 2011.

Chapter 16
Obesogenic Programming of Foetal Hepatic Metabolism by microRNAs

Laís Angélica de Paula Simino, Marcio Alberto Torsoni, and Adriana Souza Torsoni

Key Points

- Maternal obesity can promote deleterious effects on adult life of offspring due to metabolic programming;
- Consumption of a high-fat diet by obese dams have been associated with increased adiposity, fatty liver, insulin resistance, endoplasmic reticulum stress and decreased autophagy and cholinergic anti-inflammatory pathway in the liver of offspring.
- MicroRNAs expression could be responsible for permanent changes in the expression profile of genes related to hepatic lipid metabolism in offspring of obese mothers.
- The gestational period by itself, disregarding the lactation period, can promote important epigenetic alterations in offspring.
- miR-122 seems to be a central controller of hepatic lipid metabolism in both health and disease.

Keywords microRNAs • High-fat diet • Hepatic metabolism • Fatty liver • Offspring • Maternal programming • Pregnancy • Lactation • Epigenetic

Abbreviations

Acadvl	Acyl-CoA dehydrogenase, very long chain
Acc1	Acetyl-CoA carboxylase 1
Agpat1	Acylglycerol-3-phosphate O-acyltransferase 1
C/EBP-β	CCAAT/enhancer-binding protein-β
Cpt1-α	Carnitine palmitoyltransferase 1
DAG	Diacylglycerol
Dgat1	Diacylglycerol acyltransferase 1
Fas	Fatty acid synthase
G6pc	Glucose-6-phosphatase
GPAM	Glycerol-3-phosphate acyltransferase mitochondrial

L.A. de Paula Simino, MSc • M.A. Torsoni, PhD • A.S. Torsoni, PhD (✉)
Laboratory of Metabolic Disorders, School of Applied Sciences, University of Campinas, Limeira, SP, Brazil
e-mail: adriana.torsoni@fca.unicamp.br

© Springer International Publishing AG 2017
R. Rajendram et al. (eds.), *Diet, Nutrition, and Fetal Programming*,
Nutrition and Health, DOI 10.1007/978-3-319-60289-9_16

GPAT	Glycerol-3-phosphate acyltransferase
HCC	Hepatocellular carcinoma
HFD	High-fat diet
HIC2	Hypermethylated in cancer 2
IKK	IkB kinase
Lclat1	Lysocardiolipin acyltransferase 1
MAG	Monoacylglycerol
MAP K1	Mitogen-activated protein kinase 1
MECP2	Methyl-CpG binding protein 2
miR/miRNA	microRNA
Mogat2	Monoacylglycerol acyltransferase 2
mTOR	Mechanistic target of rapamycin
NAFLD	Non-alcoholic fatty liver disease
NASH	Non-alcoholic steatohepatitis
ncRNA	Non-coding RNA
NFkB	Nuclear factor kappa B
p-JNK	c-Jun N-terminal kinase phosphorylated
Ppar-α	Peroxisome proliferator-activated receptor- α
Ppar-γ	Peroxisome proliferator-activated receptor-γ
RISC	RNA-induced silencing complex
Scd1	Stearoyl-CoA desaturase 1
Srebp-1c	Sterol regulatory element-binding protein 1c
TAG	Triacylglycerol
TNFα	Tumor necrosis factor α
UTR	Untranslated region

Introduction

The prevalence of obesity worldwide has increased. Human and animal studies have shown that environment in early life can have deleterious effects on adult life. The increase in the prevalence of obesity in women of reproductive age [1, 2] and children is worrying because both can contribute to increasing the risk of later metabolic disease. This condition has increased the interest in the effects of maternal obesity on the risk of disease in offspring [3–5].

The effect of overnutrition during foetal development is critical in increasing the risk of adult-onset ill health outcome. Different types of stress during critical periods of early development permanently alter an organism's physiology and metabolism. This phenomenon is called "metabolic programming" and it originated from the foetal hypothesis proposed by Baker [6].

Maternal obesity and consumption of a high-fat diet have been associated with increased adiposity [5, 7–11], fatty liver [8, 12], insulin resistance [7], endoplasmic reticulum stress and autophagy disturbance [9, 10] and impairment of the cholinergic anti-inflammatory pathway [11] in post-weaning and adult life of offspring (Fig. 16.1).

Maternal obesity and dietary fat consumption during pregnancy/lactation also alter the blood level of hormones (leptin and insulin), nutrients (fatty acids and glucose) and inflammatory cytokines [7, 8, 10, 11, 13] in both dams and offspring. This new biochemical condition can affect the environment of the developing offspring, imposing molecular and physiological adaptations.

Epigenetic modifications that regulate gene machinery transcriptionally (through histone and DNA modification) and post-transcriptionally (through non-coding RNA expression) could be responsible for permanent changes in the expression profile of genes related to metabolism and energy homeostasis in offspring of obese mothers.

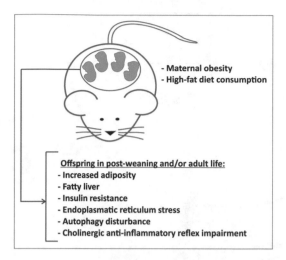

Fig. 16.1 Effect of maternal high-fat diet consumption and obesity on post-weaning and/or adult offspring. Maternal obesity induced by the consumption of a high-fat diet prior to conception and during gestation and lactation leads off-spring to fatty liver development, insulin resistance, endoplasmic reticulum stress, autophagy disturbances and cholinergic anti-inflammatory reflex impairment in post-weaning and/or adult life

According to the ENCODE project,[1] only 1–2% of the genome encodes for proteins, suggesting that a large proportion of the transcripts in the cell represents non-coding RNA (also called ncRNA) that seems to modulate gene expression [14]. ncRNAs are grouped into two classes: long ncRNAs (>200 nucleotides) and small or short ncRNAs (<200 nucleotides). Short ncRNAs include microR-NAs (miRNAs), small interfering RNAs and piwi-interacting RNAs.

Functionally, long ncRNAs can modulate gene transcription through recruitment of histone modifying complexes to the DNA whereas short ncRNAs induce mRNA degradation and/or translational repression [11]. Among ncRNAs, emphasis has been attributed to miRNAs in the regulation of gene expression.

A summary of the biogenesis of microRNAs is presented in Fig. 16.2.

The present chapter aims to point out the main and recent findings on the role of microRNAs in modulating the hepatic metabolism in the offspring of obese mothers or mothers consuming a high-fat diet during important periods of development, such as pregnancy and lactation.

Hepatic microRNAs in Foetal Programming Induced by Dietary Fat and/or Obesity

The liver is a multifunctional organ that regulates many vital physiological processes. These include processing nutrients after intestinal absorption, synthesis and excretion of metabolites, detoxification of xenobiotics, modulation of lipid and glucose metabolism and energy homeostasis [15].

Disruption of hepatic lipid metabolism is often associated with metabolic disturbances. In human and animal models, obesity is closely related to inflammation and insulin resistance and this condition leads to ectopic lipid storage in metabolically active tissues, such as the liver. Excessive lipid storage within hepatocytes characterizes non-alcoholic fatty-liver disease (NAFLD) [16]. Fatty liver is caused by an imbalance in lipid metabolism pathways involved in triacylglycerol (TAG) synthesis, export, delivery and oxidation [17] (Fig. 16.3).

---

[1] The ENCODE project started in September 2003 and was completed in 2012. It brought together an international group of scientists with the goal of identifying all functional elements in the human genome sequence.

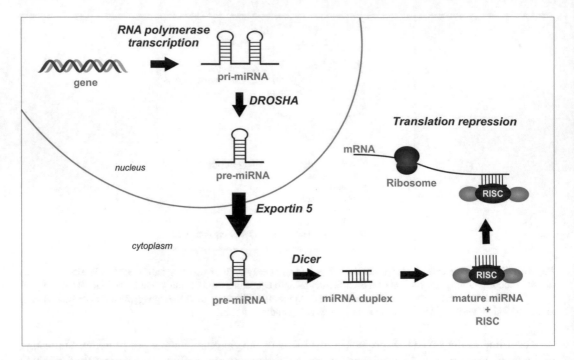

Fig. 16.2 microRNA biogenesis. miRNA biogenesis starts in the nucleus, where the gene is transcribed by RNA polymerase II in a primary hairpin structure (pri-miRNA), which is cleaved by the DROSHA enzyme yielding precursors (pre-miRNA) of ~70 nucleotides. Pre-miRNA hairpins are exported to cytoplasm by EXPORTIN 5 and, thereafter, are cleaved by the DICER enzyme, producing the miRNA duplex. One of the strands is usually cleaved and the other, the functional strand of miRNA, is incorporated into the RISC. The complex RISC-miRNA interacts with its target by cleaving and degrading the mRNA or by inhibiting protein synthesis. *miRNA* microRNA, *RISC* RNA-induced silencing complex

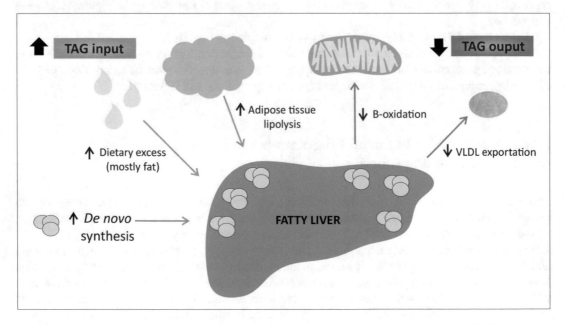

Fig. 16.3 Mechanisms for fat accumulation in the liver. Fatty liver can be caused by increased TAG input through increased de novo synthesis, dietary excess and adipose tissue lipolysis as well as by a decrease in TAG output, through impairment of mitochondrial β-oxidation and VLDL exportation of liver triglycerides. Ordinarily, fatty liver is caused by a combination of more than one of these factors. *TAG* triacylglycerol

Under normal conditions, hepatic fat represents about 5% of total liver weight. Obesity and consumption of a high-fat or high-calorie diet favour ectopic hepatic fat accumulation, through the supply of free fatty acids to the liver and stimulation of synthesis and storage of TAG [18]. It is known that NAFLD can progress to non-alcoholic steatohepatitis (NASH), fibrosis and hepatocellular carcinoma (HCC). However, the mechanism involved in its progression and individual characteristics that protect from the evolution of the disease, even under consumption of a high-fat diet, are still not fully understood. It has been proposed that more than a single hepatic insult is necessary to promote the progression of NAFLD. The hypothesis to explain this phenomenon was postulated as the "two-hits hypothesis" or "multiple-hits hypothesis" [19–21].

In this context, exposure to deleterious conditions *in uterus* has been considered a determining factor in predisposing offspring to the development of liver diseases in later life [18, 19], and could represent the "first hit" (Fig. 16.4). An elegant study conducted in 2009 by McCurdy and colleagues with non-human primates showed that foetuses of dams fed an HFD developed NAFLD characteristics in the gestational third trimester. The authors observed lipid accumulation, oxidative stress and inflammation markers in the foetuses' liver [12].

In another study, Glavas et al. (2010) used a mice model of early overnutrition by reducing litter size during lactation to induce the "first hit" in offspring, since lactation also represents an important period of tissue immaturity and plasticity.

Interestingly the authors observed that when offspring were maintained on a chow diet after weaning but submitted to HFD in adult life (which could be interpreted as a "second hit"), mice exhibited extensive and severe fat accumulation, compared to the respective control, suggesting permanent molecular alterations [22].

Some important questions emerge regarding metabolic imprinting. How do gestation and lactation contribute to the outcome observed? What might be the molecular trigger that connects maternal overnutrition to metabolic disturbances in offspring?

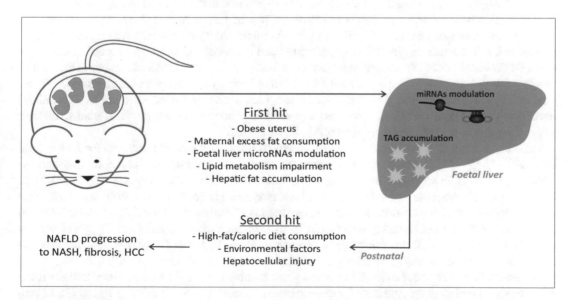

Fig. 16.4 microRNAs influences in "two-hits hypothesis" in the development of liver diseases. It is hypothesized that, for NAFLD to progress to other liver diseases such as NASH, more than one hepatic insult is necessary. The "first hit" can be induced by the intra-uterine environment, where maternal obesity and excess fat consumption could programme foetal liver to display alterations in important microRNA expression, leading to impairments in lipid metabolism and ectopic fat accumulation. Afterwards, in post-natal life, a "second hit", such as consumption of a high-fat diet, environmental factors or hepatocellular injuries, could trigger inflammation and the progression of NAFLD to NASH and HCC. *miRNA* microRNA, *TAG* triacylglycerol, *NAFLD* non-alcoholic fatty liver disease, *NASH* non-alcoholic steatohepatitis, *HCC* hepatocellular carcinoma

Authors have hypothesized that maternal consumption of HFD increases the transfer of lipids to foetuses through the placenta. Subcutaneous adipose tissue at early gestational stages is not available to store nutrient excess and, consequently, other organs, such as the liver, are required for depositing fat [18, 23]. Furthermore, maternal obesity during pregnancy increases placental inflammation and leads to altered genes in both placental [24] and foetal liver [25, 26]. However, although the contribution of maternal HFD consumption to impaired liver metabolism is a well-described phenomenon, the underlying mechanisms are still unclear.

A substantial number of studies in the literature have highlighted epigenetic changes as determinants of differential expression of genes in health and disease conditions [27–31].

Among the epigenetic changes, miRNA expression seems to be a promising approach to explain the effects of metabolic programming in the development of hepatic disorders in adult offspring. However, few studies have been conducted on the role of miRNAs in liver diseases.

Zhang and co-workers conducted the first study showing miRNA modulation in the liver of offspring of obese dams, in 2009. In this study the authors used an HFD to induce obesity in female mice prior to conception and during gestation and lactation. After weaning, offspring were fed a chow diet until adulthood when microarray analysis was performed. They identified several miRNAs (about 5.7% from a total of 579 evaluated) differentially expressed in offspring of obese dams compared to lean dams (Table 16.1). In total, ten miRNAs were increased 1.5–2.0-fold whereas 23 miRNAs were reduced 1.5–4.9-fold, some of them participating in the modulation of key hepatic genes involved in fat metabolism, such as miR-122, miR-709 and let-7c [32].

Since offspring from both HFD- and chow-fed dams were weaned onto the same chow diet and maintained on a chow diet until adulthood, changes in the expression of key metabolic genes and miRNAs in adult offspring were likely to occur prior to weaning, resulting from changes in the maternal diet.

Zhang and co-authors from Byrne's Lab used two different algorithms (TargetScan and miRanda) for in silico analysis. According to the authors, several important genes involved in epigenetics were predicted targets for those miRNAs showing altered expression in the HFD offspring. They found that methyl-CpG binding domain protein 6 and methyl-CpG binding protein 2 (MECP2) are targets for miR-709, an abundantly expressed miRNA in the liver detected by microarray. Among the predicted targets of let-7c are proteins including hypermethylated in cancer 2 (HIC2), chromodomain helicase 4 and DOT1-like histone H3 methyltransferase (Fig. 16.5). Moreover, the authors observed that reduction in miR-122 expression in the maternal HFD adult offspring was consistent with increased expression of Pparα (peroxisome proliferator-activated receptor-α) and Cpt1-α (carnitine palmitoyl transferase 1α). Pparα and Cpt1-α are two key molecules regulating hepatic fatty acid oxidation, suggesting that they could be targeted by miR-122 (Fig. 16.5).

miR-122 is a highly conserved liver-specific microRNA and its expression accounts for 70% of total liver miRNAs [33–35]. Recent studies have shown that miR-122 expression is essential for liver homeostasis once it plays an important anti-inflammatory role and acts as a tumour suppressor [35, 36]. Mice lacking miR-122 present altered expression of several enzymes related to lipid metabolism and this leads to the development of hepatosteatosis, hepatitis and hepatocellular carcinoma (HCC) [33]. Moreover, in silico analysis reveals that some key enzymes in TAG synthesis, such as Agpat1 (1-acylglycerol-3-phosphate O-acyltransferase), Dgat1 (diacylglycerol acyltransferase 1), Lclat1 (lysocardiolipin acyltransferase 1) and Mogat2 (monoacylglycerol acyltransferase 2), are predicted targets of miR-122.

However, literature about miR-122 contains some contradictory information, since initially miR-122 was appointed as an upregulator of lipogenic gene expression, activating Srebp-1c and Dgat2 and, subsequently, Fas and Acc1. Experiments using antisense for miR-122 showed that its inhibition downregulated the enzymes diacylglycerol acyltransferase-2 (Dgat2), fatty acid synthase (Fas) and acyl-CoA carboxylase 1 (Acc1), which regulate fatty acid and triglyceride biosynthesis [37, 38].

In the following year of Byrne's Lab publication, Iliopoulos and colleagues [39], using adenovirus dominant negative to cJun in mice, verified increased plasma cholesterol and triglyceride levels in those animals. These findings prompted them to investigate its effects on the regulation of genes implicated in hepatic fatty acid and triglyceride metabolism and the potential involvement of miRNAs [39].

Table 16.1 miRNAs differentially expressed in liver of maternal HFD-fed offspring vs control, represented by fold change

miR	Fold change (HFD vs Control Offspring)	
miR-503*	1,5	↑
miR-379	1,51	
miR-770-3p	1,56	
miR-369-3p	1,58	
miR-197	1,6	
miR-21*	1,6	
miR-328	1,62	
miR-471	1,62	
miR-207	1,78	
miR-667	2,04	
miR-410	1.51	↓
miR-804	1.51	
miR-323-5p	1.51	
let-7c	1.52	
miR-302a*	1.54	
miR-711	1.61	
miR-26a	1.61	
miR-122	1.68	
miR-216b	1.71	
miR-294*	1.71	
miR-185	1.76	
miR-192	1.79	
miR-29a	1.84	
miR-194	1.85	
miR-145	1.89	
miR-126-3p	2.09	
miR-762	2.32	
miR-16	2.55	
miR-1224	2.85	
miR-22	2.94	
miR-30c-2*	3.28	
miR-494	3.61	
miR-483	4.93	

The authors found that among 365 miRNAs evaluated by microarray, miR-370 was significantly increased. This miRNA targets the 3' untranslated region (UTR) of Cpt1-α, downregulating the expression of this important enzyme to fatty acid β oxidation. Iliopoulos and co-workers also suggested that miR-370 could promote lipogenesis indirectly through upregulation of miR-122, indicating that extracellular stimuli that trigger upregulation of miR-370 and indirectly miR-122 may have a causative role in the accumulation of hepatic triglycerides by promoting lipogenesis and inhibiting β oxidation.

In 2014, Benatti and colleagues published a study focused on the two microRNAs predicted to control liver lipid metabolism, miR-122 and miR-370, which had been described by Zhang et al. [32] and Iliopoulos et al. [39]. Using the same experimental model developed by Zhang in 2009, the authors conducted evaluations in offspring of obese dams 10 days after weaning and exclusively consuming a chow diet [8]. At day 28, offspring from obese dams presented higher body weight, white adipose mass and food intake than mice from control dams. In addition, they showed an altered serum lipid profile, i.e. higher cholesterol, free fatty acids and triacylglycerol content than the control group.

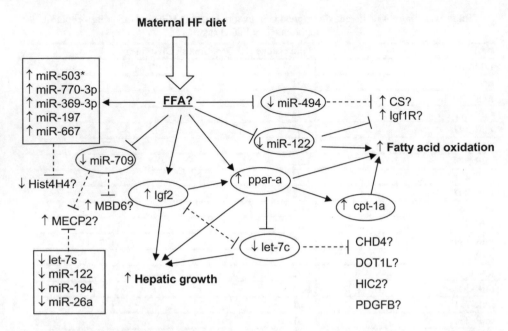

Fig. 16.5 Maternal high fat diet during gestation and lactation alters hepatic expression of key genes and miRNAs in the offspring. A maternal HF diet during gestation and lactation increased hepatic Igf2 expression in the offspring, which may be required for the up-regulation of ppar-α/cpt-1a by HF diet. Increased ppar-α suppresses expression of let-7c, facilitates hepatic growth. Igf2 could down regulate let-7c through increased expression of ppar-α. Increased expression of ppar-α and reduced expression of miR-122 may increase hepatic fatty acid oxidation in the offspring. Igf1 receptor (Igf1R) and citrate synthase (CS) are predicted targets shared by both miR-122 and miR-494. Similar to miR-122, maternal HF offspring have reduced miR-494 levels, which favour increased Igf1R and CS activities. Several key proteins involved in epigenetics are predicted targets for miRNAs, in particular, methyl-CpG binding protein 2 are predicted targets for 5 miRNAs (miR-709, let-7s, miR-122, miR-194 and miR-26a) showing reduced levels in maternal HF fed offspring. Histone 4 H4 are predicted targets for 5 miRNAs (miR-503*, miR-770-3p, miR-369-3p, miR-197 and miR-667) showing increased levels in maternal HF fed offspring. Arrows suggest stimulatory and blocked arrows inhibitory effects. Solid lines represent established relationships whereas broken lines represent relationships not yet confirmed experimentally. *FFA* free fatty acids, *CS* citrate synthase, *ppar-a* peroxisome proliferator activated receptor-alpha, *cpt* carnitine pamitoyltransferase, *MBD* methyl-CpG binding domain protein, *MECP2* methyl-CpG-binding protein 2, *CHD4* chromodomain helicase DNA binding protein 4, *DOT1L* DOT1-like, histone H3 methyltransferase, *HIC2* hypermethylated in cancer 2, *Hist4H4* histone 4 H4) (Figure was reproduced and legend was modified from Zhang et al. [32])

Interestingly, in addition to elevated content of inflammation-related proteins, such as p-IKK, p-JNK and NFκB, offspring from obese dams presented higher lipid vacuole accumulation accompanied by increased Agpat1 and Scd1 (stearoyl-CoA desaturase 1) and a decrease in Cpt1a and Acadvl (acyl-CoA dehydrogenase, very long chain) expression in liver. Agpat is a key enzyme in TAG synthesis, responsible for converting lysophosphatidate into phosphatidate, a substrate for diacylglycerol and TAG biosynthesis [40]. Furthermore, Agpat expression is usually altered in lipid-associated diseases in the liver, such as non-alcoholic fatty-liver disease (NAFLD) (Fig. 16.6). Scd1, in turn, is a desaturase responsible for monounsaturated fatty acids which serve as substrate for new TAG molecules [41]. The increased expression of these enzymes in the liver of recently weaned offspring from obese dams was consistent with their elevated hepatic TAG content. Interestingly, miR-122 seems to be related to this phenomenon, since its expression was concomitantly downregulated – the same behaviour observed by Zhang and colleagues.

Moreover, the authors demonstrated an increased expression of miR-370 in this model that may also play a role in the ectopic fat accumulation in the liver. This miRNA is known to control the expression of miR-122 and, in addition, it directly targets Cpt1-α. Long-chain fatty acids constitute

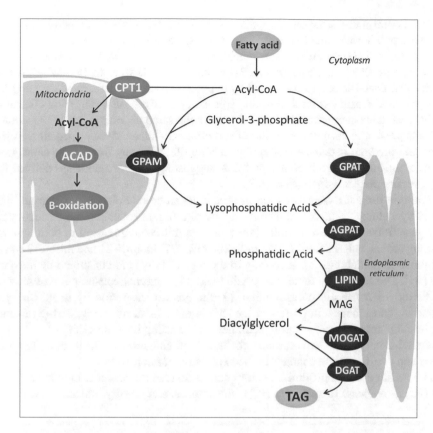

Fig. 16.6 Fatty acid metabolism: triacylglycerol synthesis and β-oxidation. Triacylglycerol synthesis starts with the releasing of Acyl-CoA from free fatty acids, which, with glycerol-3-phosphate, is converted to lysophosphatidic acid by GPAT (at the endoplasmatic reticulum) or GPAM (mitochondrial form of GPAT). Next, at the endoplasmatic reticulum, AGPAT, LIPIN and DGAT act to form TAG molecules. Monoacylglycerol molecules in cytoplasm can also form TAG by MOGAT conversion of MAG and diacylglycerol (DAG) into TAG. Otherwise, Acyl-CoA present in cytoplasm can be driven to mitochondria by CPT1 and start β-oxidation, where the first step is mediated by ACAD. *CPT1* carnitine palmitoyl transferase 1, *ACAD* Acyl-CoA dehydrogenase, *GPAM* glycerol-3-phosphate acyltransferase mitochondrial, *GPAT* glycerol-3-phosphate acyltransferase, *AGPAT* acylglycerol-3-phosphate O-acyltransferase 1, *MOGAT* monoacylglycerol acyltransferase, *DGAT* diacylglycerol acyltransferase, *MAG* monoacylglycerol, *DAG* diacylglycerol, *TAG* triacylglycerol

the majority of the fatty acids available to cells but they are not able to cross the mitochondrial membrane. Cpt1-α is the enzyme responsible for the translocation of these fatty acids into the mitochondria, providing substrate for β-oxidation. In addition, Acadvl, the enzyme that catalyses the first step of β-oxidation (Fig. 16.6), is also downregulated in offspring from obese dams. Thus changes in the oxidative pathway are associated with the differential expression of miR-370 and miR-122 that could be responsible for liver injury triggered by hepatic lipid accumulation in the offspring of obese dams.

Recently, another study showed that consumption of a high-calorie, fat-rich diet during gestation and lactation leads to modulation in several miRNAs in the liver of offspring. Among them, miR-615, miR-124 and miR-101b were downregulated and miR-143 was upregulated. Bioinformatic analysis showed that miR-101b targets genes of inflammatory pathways and miR-143 targets genes involved in adipogenesis. As a consequence, an increase in both the mRNA and protein content of TNFα and MAPK1 can be seen, as well as higher body weight and impaired glucose homeostasis at weaning age [42].

Thus, it is possible to conclude that maternal consumption of an HFD during critical periods of development, such as gestation and lactation, leads to modulation in key miRNAs, which, in turn, alters the hepatic lipid metabolism in young offspring. Furthermore, adult offspring from obese dams, even

208 L.A. de Paula Simino et al.

when fed just a control diet after weaning, display the same phenotype as recently weaned offspring: reduced sensitivity to insulin, and increased body weight, white adipose mass, expression of inflammation-related proteins, TAG content and lipid vacuoles, compared to offspring from lean dams.

Recently, Simino et al. observed that miR-122 and miR-370 were modulated earlier at birth in offspring from HFD-fed dams, accompanied by hyperinsulinaemia, decreased Cpt1a and Acadvl and increased Agpat and Gpam expression in the liver and, moreover, offspring from control dams fostered to HFD-fed dams in the lactation period present the same phenotype [43]. These findings suggest that lipids present in both maternal blood and milk can independently programme offspring for impairments in lipid homeostasis. Additionally, in adult life, offspring from obese dams present modulation of liver miR-122 and miR-370 expression, suggesting that the alterations derived from metabolic programming are permanent (Fig. 16.7).

The hypothesis that miRNA expression in offspring can be modulated by maternal lipids is also strengthened by a study that shows that consumption of different sources of fatty acids by mothers in the first 12 gestational days differentially influences the miRNA expression in both mother and offspring. Among others, miR-215, miR-10b, miR-26, miR-377-3p, miR-21 and miR-192 were differentially modulated in adult offspring according to the type of fatty acid consumed by the dam in early pregnancy [44]. The results reinforce three main ideas: (1) maternal consumption of fatty acids is an important factor for metabolic programming, (2) the gestational period by itself, disregarding the lactation period, can promote important epigenetic alterations in offspring, and (3) metabolic programming by fatty acids is a permanent phenomenon, persisting into adult life.

An excess of dietary lipids and chronic subclinical inflammation seems to be a common point of most studies and could mediate changes in the expression of microRNAs.

Some authors have shown pro-inflammatory components in the placenta in humans [24], rats [45] and sheep [46] in response to maternal HFD consumption and obesity. Indeed it seems that uterine

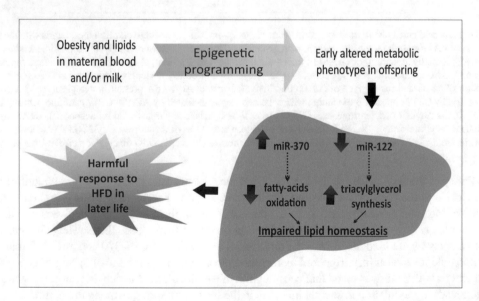

Fig. 16.7 Impaired lipid homeostasis by microRNA modulation in foetal metabolic programming. Maternal obesity and consumption of a high-fat diet programme foetal metabolism through epigenetic mechanisms and lead offspring to an altered phenotype and modulation of key liver microRNA expression. Hepatic miR-370 is upregulated while miR-122 is downregulated, inducing a decrease in fatty acid oxidation and increase in triacylglycerol synthesis, respectively. These alterations impair lipid metabolism and, as a consequence, offspring present a harmful response when exposed to a high-fat diet in later life. *HFD* high-fat diet

changes and embryonic inflammation precede placentation. Blastocyst gene expression at day 4.5 post-coitum was clearly influenced by maternal obesity in rats. In the same study, increased inflammation in the uterus, ectopic lipid accumulation and altered expression of lipid metabolic genes were also observed [47].

These effects can be related to the increase in placental transport of amino acids, glucose and fatty acids [48] observed in pregnancy associated with HFD consumption.

Although controversial, the increase of circulating lipids seems to be a mediator of foetal programming [49–51].

Nevertheless, fatty acids are not the only nutrient that can lead to foetal programming by hepatic miRNA modulation in offspring. Studies have shown that a maternal low-protein diet induces epigenetic changes through differential miRNA expression. In 2012, Jia and colleagues demonstrated that maternal malnutrition through consumption of a low-protein diet during pregnancy impairs epigenetic mechanisms, including hepatic miRNA expression, in a gender-dependent manner in newborn piglets, leading to altered G6PC (glucose-6-phosphatase) gene expression [52]. A maternal low-protein diet also increases miR-130b and miR-374b in recently weaned piglets, modulating the hepatic expression of PPAR-γ (peroxisome proliferator-activated receptor-γ) and C/EBP-β (CCAAT/enhancer-binding protein β), respectively and, thus, regulating lipid metabolism and adipogenesis [53]. Additionally, protein restriction during pregnancy also induces miRNA modulation (miR-199a-3p and miR-342) in β cells in newborn mice, downregulating mTOR (mechanistic target of rapamycin) expression in this cells and modulating insulin secretion and global glucose homeostasis [54].

In addition to the effects of the maternal diet in the expression of miRNAs in offspring, the paternal diet may also affect miRNA expression. Recently, a study published by French researchers supported the evidence of paternal heredity of diet-induced obesity and metabolic disorders [55]. The authors showed that microinjection of total RNA (including several microRNAs) from testis or sperm transcriptome of male mice fed a Western-like diet into naive one-cell embryos leads to the establishment of a Western-like diet-induced metabolic phenotype in the resulting progenies, represented by glucose intolerance and insulin resistance. On the other hand, RNAs prepared from healthy controls did not promote the same effect. Importantly, injection of miR-19b induced metabolic alterations that were similar to the obese phenotype and were inherited by the offspring after crosses with healthy partners [55].

Interestingly, recent evidence from a swine model of maternal obesity suggests that increased risk of liver disease can be programmed transgenerationally, since early post-natal increases in adiposity and markers of paediatric liver disease are found in male piglets of obese grandmothers [56].

Although all the above-mentioned studies were conducted in non-human models, probably due to experimental difficulties and ethical issues surrounding research in humans, particularly in foetuses and newborns, there is a lot of evidence to suggest that the studies of foetal metabolic programming involving miRNA expression are promising and the differential expression of these molecules is already being correlated with gestational obesity and used to predict gestational diabetes in plasma from pregnant women [57, 58].

Conclusion

In summary, nutritional and weight gain monitoring during pregnancy is an important prophylactic action aimed at preventing metabolic disorders in later life in offspring. Importantly, the research of dietary interventions or supplementation for preventing placental inflammation in obese mothers and metabolic complications among offspring is also very exciting.

References

1. Guelinckx I, Devlieger R, Beckers K, Vansant G. Maternal obesity: pregnancy complications, gestational weight gain and nutrition. Obes Rev. 2008;9(2):140–50.
2. Hamad R, Cohen AK, Rehkopf DH. Changing national guidelines is not enough: the impact of 1990 IOM recommendations on gestational weight gain among US women. Int J Obes. 2016;40:1529–34.
3. Drake AJ, Reynolds RM. Impact of maternal obesity on offspring obesity and cardiometabolic disease risk. Reproduction. 2010;140(3):387–98.
4. Dyer JS, Rosenfeld CR. Metabolic imprinting by prenatal, perinatal, and postnatal overnutrition: a review. Semin Reprod Med. 2011;29(3):266–76.
5. Penfold NC, Ozanne SE. Developmental programming by maternal obesity in 2015: outcomes, mechanisms, and potential interventions. Horm Behav. 2015;76:143–52.
6. Barker D. Infant mortality, childhood nutrition, and ischaemic heart disease in England and Wales. Lancet. 1986;327(8489):1077–81.
7. Ashino NG, Saito KN, Souza FD, et al. Maternal high-fat feeding through pregnancy and lactation predisposes mouse offspring to molecular insulin resistance and fatty liver. J Nutr Biochem. 2012;23(4):341–8.
8. Benatti RO, Melo AM, Borges FO, et al. Maternal high-fat diet consumption modulates hepatic lipid metabolism and microRNA-122 (miR-122) and microRNA-370 (miR-370) expression in offspring. Br J Nutr. 2014;111(12):2112–22.
9. Melo AM, Benatti RO, Ignacio-Souza LM, et al. Hypothalamic endoplasmic reticulum stress and insulin resistance in offspring of mice dams fed high-fat diet during pregnancy and lactation. Metabolism. 2014;63(5):682–92.
10. Reginato A, de Fante T, Portovedo M, et al. Autophagy proteins are modulated in the liver and hypothalamus of the offspring of mice with diet-induced obesity. J Nutr Biochem. 2016;34:30–41.
11. Payolla TB, Lemes SF, de Fante T, et al. High-fat diet during pregnancy and lactation impairs the cholinergic anti-inflammatory pathway in the liver and white adipose tissue of mouse offspring. Mol Cell Endocrinol. 2016;422:192–202.
12. McCurdy CE, Bishop JM, Williams SM, et al. Maternal high-fat diet triggers lipotoxicity in the fetal livers of nonhuman primates. J Clin Invest. 2009;119(2):323–35.
13. Kępczyńska MA, Wargent ET, Cawthorne MA, Arch JRS, O'Dowd JF, Stocker CJ. Circulating levels of the cytokines IL10, IFNγ and resistin in an obese mouse model of developmental programming. J Dev Orig Health Dis. 2013;4(6):491–8.
14. Djebali S, Davis CA, Merkel A, et al. Landscape of transcription in human cells. Nature. 2012;489(7414):101–8.
15. Rui L. Energy metabolism in the liver. Compr Physiol. 2014;4(1):177–97.
16. Samuel VT, Liu Z-X, Qu X, et al. Mechanism of hepatic insulin resistance in non-alcoholic fatty liver disease. J Biol Chem. 2004;279(31):32345–53.
17. Yamaguchi K, Yang L, McCall S, et al. Inhibiting triglyceride synthesis improves hepatic steatosis but exacerbates liver damage and fibrosis in obese mice with nonalcoholic steatohepatitis. Hepatology. 2007;45(6):1366–74.
18. Brumbaugh DE, Friedman JE. Developmental origins of nonalcoholic fatty liver disease. Pediatr Res. 2014;75(1–2):140–7.
19. Stewart MS, Heerwagen MJ, Friedman JE. Developmental programming of pediatric non-alcoholic fatty liver disease: redefining the "first-hit.". Clin Obstet Gynecol. 2013;56(3):577–90.
20. Day CP, James OF. Steatohepatitis: a tale of two "hits"? Gastroenterology. 1998;114(4):842–5.
21. Tilg H, Moschen AR. Evolution of inflammation in nonalcoholic fatty liver disease: the multiple parallel hits hypothesis. Hepatology. 2010;52(5):1836–46.
22. Glavas MM, Kirigiti MA, Xiao XQ, et al. Early overnutrition results in early-onset arcuate leptin resistance and increased sensitivity to high-fat diet. Endocrinology. 2010;151(4):1598–610.
23. Bernstein IM, Goran MI, Amini SB, Catalano PM. Differential growth of fetal tissues during the second half of pregnancy. Am J Obstet Gynecol. 1997;176(1 Pt 1):28–32.
24. Challier JC, Basu S, Bintein T, et al. Obesity in pregnancy stimulates macrophage accumulation and inflammation in the placenta. Placenta. 2008;29(3):274–81.
25. Frias AE, Morgan TK, Evans AE, et al. Maternal high-fat diet disturbs uteroplacental hemodynamics and increases the frequency of stillbirth in a nonhuman primate model of excess nutrition. Endocrinology. 2011;152(6):2456–64.
26. Panchenko PE, Voisin S, Jouin M, et al. Expression of epigenetic machinery genes is sensitive to maternal obesity and weight loss in relation to fetal growth in mice. Clin Epigenetics. 2016;8(1):22.
27. Ceccarelli S, Panera N, Gnani D, Nobili V. Dual role of microRNAs in NAFLD. Int J Mol Sci. 2013;14(4):8437–55.
28. Moore GE, Oakey R. The role of imprinted genes in humans. Genome Biol. 2011;12(3):106.
29. Pogribny IP, Starlard-Davenport A, Tryndyak VP, et al. Difference in expression of hepatic microRNAs miR-29c, miR-34a, miR-155, and miR-200b is associated with strain-specific susceptibility to dietary nonalcoholic steatohepatitis in mice. Lab Invest. 2010;90(10):1437–46.

30. Xie H, Lim B, Lodish HF. MicroRNAs induced during adipogenesis that accelerate fat cell development are down-regulated in obesity. Diabetes. 2009;58(5):1050–7.
31. Desai M, Jellyman JK, Han G, Beall M, Lane RH, Ross MG. Rat maternal obesity and high-fat diet program offspring metabolic syndrome. Am J Obstet Gynecol. 2014;211(3):237.e1–237.e13.
32. Zhang J, Zhang F, Didelot X, et al. Maternal high fat diet during pregnancy and lactation alters hepatic expression of insulin like growth factor-2 and key microRNAs in the adult offspring. BMC Genomics. 2009;10:478.
33. Hsu SH, Wang B, Kota J, et al. Essential metabolic, anti-inflammatory, and anti-tumorigenic functions of miR-122 in liver. J Clin Invest. 2012;122(8):2871–83.
34. Miyaaki H, Ichikawa T, Kamo Y, et al. Significance of serum and hepatic microRNA-122 levels in patients with non-alcoholic fatty liver disease. Liver Int. 2014;34(7):e302–7.
35. Nakao K, Miyaaki H, Ichikawa T. Antitumor function of microRNA-122 against hepatocellular carcinoma. J Gastroenterol. 2014;49(4):589–93.
36. Tsai W-C, Hsu S-D, Hsu C-S, et al. MicroRNA-122 plays a critical role in liver homeostasis and hepatocarcinogenesis. J Clin Invest. 2012;122(8):2884–97.
37. Esau C, Davis S, Murray SF, et al. miR-122 regulation of lipid metabolism revealed by in vivo antisense targeting. Cell Metab. 2006;3(2):87–98.
38. Cheung O, Sanyal AJ. Role of microRNAs in non-alcoholic steatohepatitis. Curr Pharm Des. 2010;16:1952–7.
39. Iliopoulos D, Drosatos K, Hiyama Y, Goldberg IJ, Zannis VI. MicroRNA-370 controls the expression of MicroRNA-122 and Cpt1 and affects lipid metabolism. J Lipid Res. 2010;51(6):1513–23.
40. Takeuchi K, Reue K. Biochemistry, physiology, and genetics of GPAT, AGPAT, and lipin enzymes in triglyceride synthesis. Am J Physiol Endocrinol Metab. 2009;296(6):E1195–209.
41. Cohen P, Miyazaki M, Socci ND, et al. Role for stearoyl-CoA desaturase-1 in leptin-mediated weight loss. Science. 2002;297(5579):240–3.
42. Zheng J, Zhang Q, Mul JD, et al. Maternal high-calorie diet is associated with altered hepatic microRNA expression and impaired metabolic health in offspring at weaning age. Endocrine. 2016;54(1):70–80.
43. de Paula Simini LA, de Fante T, Figueiredo Fontana M, Oliveira Borges F, Torsoni MA, Milanski M, Velooso LA, Souza TA. Lipid overload during gestation and lactation can independently alter lipid homeostasis in offspring and promote metabolic impairment after new challenge to high-fat diet. Nutr Metab. 2017;20(14):16.
44. Casas-Agustench P, Fernandes FS, Tavares Do Carmo MG, Visioli F, Herrera E, Dávalos A. Consumption of distinct dietary lipids during early pregnancy differentially modulates the expression of microRNAs in mothers and offspring. PLoS One. 2015;10(2):1–17.
45. Shankar K, Zhong Y, Kang P, et al. Maternal obesity promotes a proinflammatory signature in rat uterus and blastocyst. Endocrinology. 2011;152(11):4158–70.
46. Zhu MJ, Ma Y, Long NM, Du M, Ford SP. Maternal obesity markedly increases placental fatty acid transporter expression and fetal blood triglycerides at midgestation in the ewe. Am J Phys Regul Integr Comp Phys. 2010;299(5):R1224–31.
47. Shankar K, Kang P, Harrell A, et al. Maternal overweight programs insulin and adiponectin signaling in the offspring. Endocrinology. 2010;151(6):2577–89.
48. Sferruzzi-Perri AN, Camm EJ. The programming power of the placenta. Front Physiol. 2016;14(7):33.
49. Krasnow SM, Nguyen MLT, Marks DL. Increased maternal fat consumption during pregnancy alters body composition in neonatal mice. Am J Physiol Endocrinol Metab. 2011;301(6):E1243–53.
50. Strakovsky RS, Zhang X, Zhou D, Pan Y-X. Gestational high fat diet programs hepatic phosphoenolpyruvate carboxykinase gene expression and histone modification in neonatal offspring rats. J Physiol. 2011;589(Pt 11):2707–17.
51. Masuyama H, Hiramatsu Y. Effects of a high-fat diet exposure in utero on the metabolic syndrome-like phenomenon in mouse offspring through epigenetic changes in adipocytokine gene expression. Endocrinology. 2012;153(6):2823–30.
52. Jia Y, Cong R, Li R, et al. Maternal low-protein diet induces gender-dependent changes in epigenetic regulation of the glucose-6-phosphatase gene in newborn piglet liver. J Nutr. 2012;142(9):1659–65.
53. Pan S, Zheng Y, Zhao R, Yang X. MicroRNA-130b and microRNA-374b mediate the effect of maternal dietary protein on offspring lipid metabolism in Meishan pigs. Br J Nutr. 2013;109(10):1731–8.
54. Alejandro EU, Gregg B, Wallen T, et al. Maternal diet-induced microRNAs and mTOR underlie β cell dysfunction in offspring. J Clin Invest. 2014;124(10):4395–410.
55. Grandjean V, Fourré S, De Abreu DAF, Derieppe M-A, Remy J-J, Rassoulzadegan M. RNA-mediated paternal heredity of diet-induced obesity and metabolic disorders. Sci Rep. 2015;14(5):18193.
56. Gonzalez-Bulnes A, Astiz S, Ovilo C, et al. Early-postnatal changes in adiposity and lipids profile by transgenerational developmental programming in swine with obesity/leptin resistance. J Endocrinol. 2014;223(1):M17–29.
57. Carreras-Badosa G, Bonmatí A, Ortega F-J, et al. Altered circulating miRNA expression profile in Pregestational and gestational obesity. J Clin Endocrinol Metab. 2015;100(11):E1446–56.
58. Zhu Y, Tian F, Li H, Zhou Y, Lu J, Ge Q. Profiling maternal plasma microRNA expression in early pregnancy to predict gestational diabetes mellitus. Int J Gynaecol Obstet. 2015;130(1):49–53.

Chapter 17
Impacts of Maternal High-Fat Diet on Stress-Related Behaviour and the Endocrine Response to Stress in Offspring

Sameera Abuaish and Patrick O. McGowan

Key Points

- Maternal obesity is induced by diets high in fat; however variations of the diet warrant caution when comparing results from different studies.
- Timing of the HFD exposure has differential effects on offspring weight, physiology and behaviour.
- Some studies have reported that HFD alters the maternal HPA axis, maternal behaviour and milk production.
- Developmental exposure to HFD programmes offspring HPA axis physiology by altering basal and stress-induced levels of corticosterone.
- Offspring of HFD litters exhibit increased anxiety-like behaviour.
- Epigenetic modifications in offspring exposed to maternal HFD may contribute to phenotype.

Keywords Maternal obesity • High-fat diet • Gestation • Lactation • Developmental programming • Hypothalamic-pituitary-adrenal axis • Corticosterone • Anxiety • Stress • Epigenetics • DNA methylation

Abbreviations

11β-HSD	11beta-hydroxysteroid dehydrogenase
α-MSH	α-Melanocyte-stimulating hormone
ACTH	Adrenocorticotropic hormone
ADHD	Attention deficit hyperactivity disorder
BDNF	Brain-derived neurotrophic factor

S. Abuaish, MSc • P.O. McGowan, PhD (✉)
Department of Biological Sciences and Center for Environmental Epigenetics and Development, University of Toronto Scarborough, Toronto, ON, Canada

Department of Cell and Systems Biology, University of Toronto, Toronto, ON, Canada
e-mail: patrick.mcgowan@utoronto.ca

© Springer International Publishing AG 2017
R. Rajendram et al. (eds.), *Diet, Nutrition, and Fetal Programming*,
Nutrition and Health, DOI 10.1007/978-3-319-60289-9_17

Cort	Corticosterone
CRH	Corticotropin-releasing hormone
DNMT1	DNA methyltransferase
DOHaD	Developmental Origins of Health and Disease
E	Embryonic day
GADD45b	Growth arrest and DNA damage-inducible beta
GR	Glucocorticoid receptor
HFD	High-fat diet
HPA	Hypothalamic-pituitary-adrenal
MR	Mineralocorticoid receptor
NFκB	Nuclear factor κB
PFC	Prefrontal cortex
PND	Postnatal day
POMC	Proopiomelanocortin
PVN	Paraventicular nucleus

Introduction

Obesity is recognized as a major threat to public health and a risk factor for many chronic diseases. The prevalence of obesity has risen dramatically worldwide in the last 30 years, including in women of reproductive age [1, 2]. A number of studies in humans have indicated that maternal obesity is a major factor in predisposing the offspring to develop metabolic disorders [3]. There is also evidence linking maternal obesity to the development of a number of neuropsychological disorders in the offspring including anxiety and depression, schizophrenia, ADHD and cognitive impairments [4]. It is important to acknowledge that psychosocial stress is a risk factor for obesity and, as such, may influence physiological systems and behaviours related to poor metabolic outcomes. For example, chronic stress due to job demand and low socioeconomic position is associated with obesity [5]. It has been proposed that the influence of stress on the regulation of food intake could be explained in part by effects on shared neurocircuitry and by shared effects on the hypothalamic-pituitary-adrenal (HPA) axis, mediating the endocrine response to stress (Fig. 17.1) [6, 7]. For example, in rodent models, obesity and chronic stress are associated with a hyperactivated HPA axis and elevated glucocorticoid levels [8, 9]. Prenatal and early postnatal psychological or nutritional environments can cause persistent alterations in the HPA axis, leading to the development of stress-related cognitive, emotional and social adaptations in human and animal models [10–16]. Adaptations to early life events through stable alterations in phenotype are typically referred to as "early life programming" [17]. Several studies have reported that epigenetic modifications, which regulate gene expression, could help to explain these long-lasting changes [18–20]. In this review, we will focus our discussion on rodent models of the effects of maternal overnutrition in the form of high-fat diet (HFD) on offspring mental health, more specifically HPA axis-mediated behaviours.

Rodent Models of Maternal HFD

A number of rodent models have been used to study the Developmental Origins of Health and Disease (DOHaD), including the impact of the early life nutritional environment on behaviour, physiology and gene regulatory mechanisms. Generally, increasing the fat content of a diet to over 30% has been

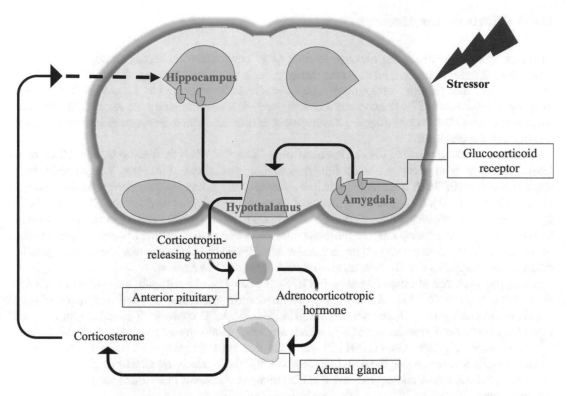

Fig. 17.1 The hypothalamic-pituitary-adrenal axis. The hypothalamic-pituitary-adrenal (HPA) axis orchestrates a hormonal cascade to regulate the endocrine stress response and maintain homeostatic equilibrium. Upon exposure to a stressor, the paraventricular nucleus (PVN) of the hypothalamus receives coordinated neuronal inputs from different stress monitoring brain regions, leading to the release of corticotropin-releasing hormone (CRH) that reaches the anterior pituitary gland and induces the release of adrenocorticotropic hormone (ACTH). Through systemic circulation, ACTH reaches the adrenal cortex, stimulating the release of the downstream effecter of the HPA axis, corticosterone. Corticosterone has a wide range of effects on the body in response to stress and leads to feedback through its interaction with corticosteroid receptors, including the glucocorticoid receptor (GR) (Modified from Robert Sanders. *New neurons help us remember fear.* Adapted from http://news.berkeley.edu/2011/06/14/new-neurons-help-to-remember-fear/)

demonstrated to induce obesity in rodents, which is also associated with a dysfunctional HPA axis and related behavioural dysfunction [21–23]. However, several variations of the diet exist under the broad umbrella of HFD, which likely contribute to the variability in results found in the field of HFD-induced obesity. For example, commercially available diets offer a number of purified HFDs with a range of between 20% and 60% fat content. In addition, there is a substantial variation in the type of fatty acid in the diet, ranging from primarily animal sources (i.e. lard, beef tallow, fish oil) to plant sources (i.e. corn, soybean, olive) [23–25]. For example, a recent report [26] has shown that saturated and monounsaturated fat have different effects on mesolimbic function in rats. Another paradigm that has been used to induce obesity in rodents is "cafeteria diet" or "junk food diet", where a combination of highly palatable human food (i.e. potato chips, cookies, chocolate, cheese, etc.) is given to the animal with ad libitum access to the regular chow diet. This type of diet has received some criticism due to the difficulty of accurately measuring nutrient intake and the variation in caloric content and type [25]. While acknowledging the different types of HFD regimen used to study diet-induced obesity in the literature and their possible contribution to variation in the results across studies, here we will explore the effects of maternal consumption of HFD on the development of HPA axis and emotionality in the offspring. However, we will begin by discussing the effects of the HFD on the mothers, who are the first level of interface between the offspring and their environment.

HFD Effects on the Mothers

In many species, offspring are exposed to their early environment primarily through the mother. Therefore, in order to understand how early environments affect the offspring, the effects of environmental factors that influence offspring development should be examined in the mother. There are a number of paradigms of HFD exposure that have been developed to study the effect of the time of exposure of this diet during offspring development and to distinguish between effects of maternal obesity and the diet itself.

One way in which maternal obesity has been modelled in rodents is by feeding females HFD for at least 4 weeks prior to gestation and continued throughout gestation and lactation. The pregestational exposure to the HFD leads to an increase in body weight of the females and an increase in their caloric intake [13, 14, 27–31]. Also, there is evidence of an increase in glucose levels in the blood and development of insulin resistance [28]. In our laboratory, we have shown [21] that adult females exposed to HFD for 8 weeks develop anxiety-like behaviour and a decrease in glucocorticoid receptors in the brain, while others have shown [32] an increase in basal levels of Cort in plasma. These findings indicate that these animals already have an altered HPA axis prior to gestation.

Once pregnant and still maintained on the HFD, the dams continue to gain more weight and consume more calories [13, 33]. In addition, obese dams show a decrease in basal locomotor activity which could contribute to their body weight gain [29, 34]. HFD consumption leads to an elevated basal Cort levels during gestation [29, 35], which was accompanied by a decrease in placental 11beta-hydroxysteroid dehydrogenase (11β-HSD) type 2, an enzyme that rapidly metabolizes maternal Cort to deactivate it before entering the foetal circulation [29]. These effects are similar to effects of prenatal stress [36], which could suggest that HFD is acting as a stressor during this sensitive period of development.

Obese dams have been reported in some studies [15, 30, 33, 37] to lose weight during lactation – a finding that is not fully understood. However, one study [15] suggested an increased investment in energy in milk production in these dams compared to control dams could explain the higher weight loss. Indeed, in studies of milk composition [38–40], it was found that maternal milk is higher in energy provided by higher fat and protein content in obese dams compared to those on a control diet. One study reported [41] that HFD dams are more active during the dark phase of the circadian cycle during lactation. Thus, the increase in locomotor activity during the dark phase might account, in part, for the weight loss observed in obese dams. Further, dams during late gestation and lactation become hyperphagic and accumulate visceral fat in order to meet the demands of lactation, and this is regulated in part by an increase in prolactin, a key hormone for milk production, during this period [42]. A recent study [37] indicated that obese HFD mice are unresponsive to prolactin signalling in both mammary glands and the hypothalamus during lactation and that this unresponsiveness is mediated by the high levels of leptin in obese animals, a common feature seen in obese dams [27, 37]. Interestingly, one study [20] reported that HFD dams' weight loss during lactation was correlated with demethylation of the proopiomelanocortin (POMC) gene in the arcuate nucleus where it functions to inhibit food intake. In addition, the weight loss was also correlated with the increased expression of the growth arrest and DNA damage-inducible beta (GADD45b) gene, which has been associated with the active demethylation of DNA [20].

A few studies that use mice to study maternal HFD have reported increased pup cannibalism, reduced lactation and reduced maternal retrieval behaviour, all of which contribute to a lower survival rate of litters. These effects may also be explained in part by the insensitivity to prolactin, which plays a role in maternal behaviour and pup retrieval [29, 37, 43, 44]. HFD mouse dams also show lower c-fos expression in the olfactory bulb during gestation, which could explain the increased cannibalism and reduced retrieval of their pups, since olfaction plays an important role in identifying the pup and initiating maternal behaviour [29, 45]. On the other hand, at least two studies in rats [40, 41] have reported increased maternal behaviour in HFD dams, seen by an increase in arched back nursing and a decrease in time away from the pups. HFD rat dams have shown delayed lactation during a weigh-suckle-weigh test, where the pups were separated from their dams for 4 h and weighed then returned to their mothers for 30 min and weighed again to measure milk yield. The HFD dams had lower milk yield compared to controls on postnatal day (PND) 1; however by PND 2, the milk yield was comparable to between HFD and control dams [46]. This was accompanied by an increase in inflammatory cytokine production in mammary glands. An earlier study [27] showed that HFD dams have higher pro-inflammatory cytokine in their plasma during lactation, indicating a systemic inflammation. Inflammation is highly influenced by altered HPA axis as we will discuss below. Alterations in the HPA axis in lactating HFD dams have recently been reported, where the dams showed a low basal Cort level, an increase in their reactivity to adrenocorticotropin-releasing hormone (ACTH) injection and increased anxiety-like behaviour compared to control dams [47]. This was associated with an alteration adrenal lipid supply and steroidogenesis. As evident by the results discussed above, HFD and maternal obesity alter several aspects of maternal physiology and behaviour, which in turn appear to contribute to the programming of offspring phenotype.

Maternal Obesity Effects on Offspring HPA Axis and Stress-Related Behaviours

Work in our laboratory and others [13, 27, 35, 48, 49] has demonstrated that maternal obesity leads to an increase in anxiety-like behaviour in adult offspring in novelty-induced approach/avoidance tasks. We found [13] that the increase in anxiety-like behaviour was accompanied by an increase in GR gene expression in the amygdala, a brain region where GR activation potentiates the HPA response to stress [50]. In tandem, we found that adult female offspring exhibited a more reactive HPA axis, as they released higher levels of Cort in response to restraint stress. A recent study [51] measuring HPA axis reactivity to a repeated restraint stress reported a higher Cort response in HFD adult offspring of HFD dams and showed an impaired habituation of the HPA response to repeated restraint after four restraint trials compared to the controls. The same study also measured depressive-like behaviour in the adult offspring after 14 days of chronic unpredictable mild stress, where the animals were randomly exposed to nine different mild stressors, and found an increase in anhedonia and learned helplessness in offspring, which was also present prior to the chronic unpredictable mild stress in young adult HFD offspring. Corticotropin-releasing hormone (CRH), a key activator of the HPA axis, was highly expressed in the paraventicular nucleus (PVN) of the hypothalamus of adult offspring exposed to HFD during development [52].

Perinatal HFD effects may lead to a differential anxiety-like behaviour profiles between adolescents and adults, where a decrease in anxiety-like behaviour and an accompanying increase in GR levels in the hippocampus were observed in adolescent offspring [14]. The hippocampus is a primary region through which GR inhibits HPA axis activity, which could explain the decrease in anxiety-like behaviour in adolescent animals [14]. The decrease in anxiety-like behaviour in adolescents has been reported previously in several studies investigating other forms of early life stress and could potentially be an indication of an increased impulsivity in these animals [14]. Risk-taking behaviour is considered one of the hallmarks of adolescent behaviour, and it has been suggested that early life environment could augment the display of this behaviour [14, 53]. A recent study [54] showed that adult offspring of obese dams had an increased impulsivity when tested on a five-choice serial reaction time test.

An examination of Cort levels in offspring of obese dams at different ages revealed low basal Cort level at birth compared to control animals that later changed to higher basal Cort levels at 3 weeks of age and in adulthood in HFD offspring compared to control offspring. However, these animals also had higher weights in adulthood compared to controls, a finding that is not always observed [13, 55, 56] and could potentially explain the high basal Cort levels. In contrast, we have previously found evidence of [13] low basal Cort levels in the HFD offspring and an increase in mineralocorticoid receptor (MR) in the amygdala. At basal levels, MR binds Cort with high affinity, which might explain the decreased basal Cort levels seen in the HFD offspring [50]. Anxious behaviour was also seen in HFD juvenile female offspring of non-human primates [11].

Cort and GR expression are believed to modulate inflammatory responses in the body and the brain, which are upregulated as mentioned above in response to developmental HFD exposure [13, 27, 31, 57]. Consequently, some work has revealed [13, 27, 31, 49] an increase in inflammation in the brains of HFD offspring, revealed by an activation in microglia and increased pro-inflammatory cytokines. In addition, increased inflammation in the limbic regions of the brain has been linked to anxiety and depression [58]. Increased oxidative damage has been observed in HFD offspring [31, 59]. Nuclear factor κB (NFκB), a pro-inflammatory transcription factor, which was upregulated in the amygdala of HFD offspring, is known to induce oxidative stress in neurons [13, 60].

Oxidative stress has also been reported in a number of anxiety disorders in humans [60]. An oxidative stress-mediated reduction in brain-derived neurotrophic factor (BDNF) in the hippocampus of HFD offspring has been reported, which was associated with decreased neurogenesis and impaired arborization of hippocampal neurons [59]. Hippocampal plasticity that is governed by BDNF levels is highly sensitive to the HPA axis and is altered in anxiety disorders and depression [61, 62].

Overall, this evidence suggests that developmental exposure to maternal obesity has an impact on the HPA axis of the offspring, reflected at least in part in an alteration in their behaviour, HPA axis physiology and stress-related gene expression, though additional mechanisms are also involved. Procedural variations in the timing of HFD exposure during development can lead to differential effects on the offspring HPA axis and behaviour, as we will discuss below.

Timing of HFD Exposure During Development and Its Effects on the Offspring

Other dietary paradigms have been developed to try to understand the effects of maternal HFD consumption in the presence or absence of maternal obesity at different developmental stages, during gestation and/or lactation (Fig. 17.2). For instance, in one study [63], the authors investigated whether obesity prior to conception and not during gestation and lactation could programme the offspring brain. Using embryo transfer from obese or lean donor mice into obese or lean pseudopregnant dams, pregestational obesity alone was found to alter gene expression of the μ-opioid receptor, which plays a role in reward signalling in the nucleus accumbens. However, obesity during gestation and lactation had a more pronounced impact on increasing gene expression in other brain regions in the same study. Others also showed [15] that pregestational obesity alone could impact behaviour in the offspring seen by reduced activity in the elevated plus maze and open field tests.

Two procedures that have been used to examine the effect of gestational and/or lactational HFD effects on offspring are diet intervention during gestation or lactation and cross-fostering. In the diet intervention procedure, the dams are switched from HFD in gestation to control diet in lactation or from control diet in gestation to HFD in lactation. In the cross-fostering procedure, offspring from HFD dams are cross-fostered to control diet dams and vice versa. While these study designs have been used in a number of studies investigating metabolic programming in the offspring (see [3] for review), there are limited studies looking at the effect of these manipulations on behavioural outcomes in offspring. One study [56] investigating the effects of maternal HFD on offspring HPA axis has shown that gestational HFD was shown to cause an elevation of basal Cort levels in the offspring that was not rescued by control diet during lactation. Another study [49] found that gestational HFD leads to increased anxiety-like behaviour in female offspring that was not observed in offspring exposed to the HFD during lactation alone. In addition, while increased microglial activation and pro-inflammatory cytokine levels were observed in female offspring of dam exposed to gestational HFD, offspring switched onto control diet during the dams' lactational period did not show this inflammatory response

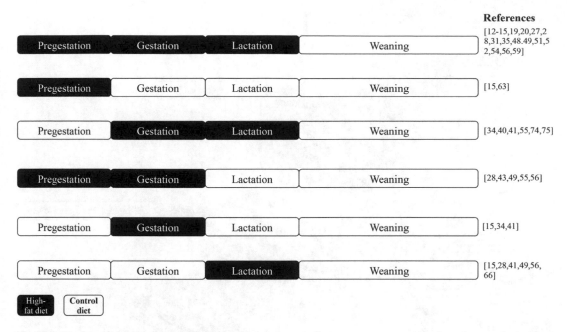

Fig. 17.2 Timing of high-fat diet exposure. Timeline of common dietary exposure protocols throughout early development along with selected references

[49]. Further, there is evidence suggesting that adult male offspring exposed to maternal HFD during the dams' lactational period alone exhibit reduced anxiety-like behaviour [15]. Another report [64] found reduced anxiety-like behaviour in adult male offspring when exposed to HFD during the dams' gestational period alone. However, at 12 months of age, offspring had an increase in anxiety-like behaviour due to the gestational HFD exposure [64]. Lactational exposure to HFD alone leads to a blunted HPA axis response to stress in neonates from HFD litters, which was suggested to be mediated via the high levels of leptin in the offspring, as earlier reports indicated that leptin inhibits the ACTH response to stress in neonatal rats [65]. However, in adolescence, the offspring had a heightened HPA axis response to stress compared to control rats, and their leptin levels were normalized at that age [66]. Leptin, in addition to its role in food intake and energy homeostasis, plays a role in regulating the HPA axis, where it downregulates CRH mRNA levels in the PNV and increases GR levels in the hippocampus and hypothalamus [7, 65, 66]. At the same time, at high levels, Cort is believed to stimulate the secretion of leptin, indicating a reciprocal relationship between the two hormones [67]. It is clear that HFD has differential effects depending on the developmental timing of exposure. More research is necessary to disentangle the mechanisms by which these effects occur, especially given the complex relationship between the HPA axis and hormones that regulate diet and energy homeostasis. In the next section, we discuss evidence suggesting that the long-term effects of maternal HFD on offspring behavioural phenotype may, at least in part, involve epigenetic modifications.

Epigenetic Mechanisms of Maternal Programming in Offspring

Epigenetic modifications cause an alteration in the expression patterns of genes without changing the underlying sequences [68]. These epigenetic regulations include DNA modifications, histone modifications and non-coding RNA (Fig. 17.3) [68]. DNA methylation has been extensively studied and has been considered a relatively stable epigenetic modification. Recent research has indicated that, in certain conditions, this mark may remain dynamic throughout the lifespan [68]. DNA methylation of

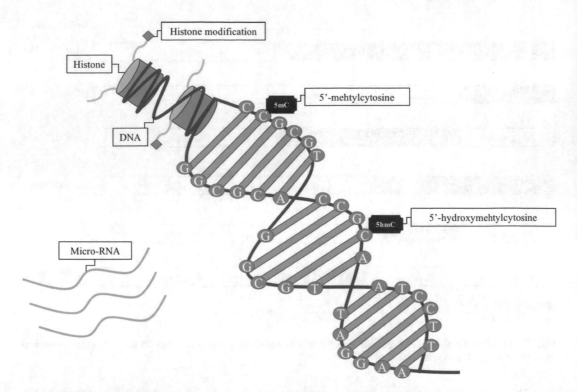

Fig. 17.3 Epigenetic regulation of transcription. There are a number of epigenetic mechanisms the cell uses to regulate gene expression. These include the modification of histone tails, DNA methylation modifications at the 5' end of cytosines in cytosine- and guanine-rich regions and the expression of non-coding RNAs

cytosine and guanine (CpG)-rich sites at gene promoters, where a methyl group is added to the 5' cytosines, leads, in many cases, to repression of gene expression [69]. Recently, 5-hydroxymethylcytosine (5-hmC), thought to be an intermediary DNA modification between fully methylated and unmethylated DNA, may contribute to the dynamic nature of DNA modifications [68]. As discussed above, the HPA axis appears to be highly impacted by and act as a sensor of early life environment that later shapes the organism's response to stress and consequently modulating its mental health [17]. Methylation of GR in the brain's limbic regions has been shown to be involved in HPA axis programming seen in many models of early life stress [68].

There is evidence that the maternal diet is associated with alterations in the epigenome of the offspring and offspring phenotype. For instance, supplementing obese agouti dams, an animal model of obesity, with methyl donors in their diet led to the methylation and silencing of the agouti gene in offspring, sparing them the obese phenotype [70]. Maternal HFD has also been reported to impact the offspring epigenome. Adult offspring of HFD dams exhibited global DNA hypomethylation in the hypothalamus and the prefrontal cortex (PFC) compared to control offspring, which was reversed when dams were supplemented with methyl donors in their diets [71, 72]. This was associated with an overexpression in the DNA methyltransferase DNMT1 in the PFC, which was positively correlated with impulsive behaviour in adult offspring [54]. Increased methylation was observed in the POMC gene promoter, a precursor to ACTH, and α-melanocyte-stimulating hormone (α-MSH), an anorexigenic neuropeptide, in the arcuate nucleus of the hypothalamus of HFD offspring [20]. This reduction could indirectly affect the HPA axis. For example, POMC is also a precursor to β-endorphin which has an inhibitory effect on CRH release [73]. Global hypomethylation was observed in HFD female placentas, associated with a downregulation of DNMT3l, a de novo DNA methyltransferase [74, 75]. This exciting field is still in its infancy, and future work will help elucidate the epigenetic alterations associated with maternal HFD in brain regions and genes regulating HPA axis function.

Consideration of Relevance of Rodent Models as Translational Models: Strengths and Limitations

Animal models have been successful in recapitulating some aspects of maternal obesity effects in human offspring, such as the alteration in metabolic outcomes [3]. More work is needed to characterize the emotional and behavioural phenotypes in both human and animal models; however, important parallels have emerged between the human and animal literature. Maternal obesity in humans is associated with emotional dysregulation, as children from obese mothers were reported to have increased fear and sadness [4]. In animals, as discussed above, offspring from HFD dams exhibit increased anxiety and depression-like behaviours in a number of studies [13, 48, 52]. However, a few considerations need to be taken into account when comparing studies of animal models of maternal HFD consumption. First, the timing of exposure varies across studies. For example, many of the studies start HFD feeding in the dam prior to gestation. However, the duration of the pregestational exposure varies among studies, ranging from HFD exposure from weaning age to mating to a few weeks prior to mating. This difference in the duration of maternal exposure might yield different outcomes. For instance, starting the HFD regimen from the weaning period in the prospective dams was reported to result in higher body weights in the offspring that were maintained until adulthood along with elevated Cort levels [56], a result not found by a number of studies using more restricted maternal exposures to HFD [13, 19, 55]. Second, as discussed earlier, lactational compared to gestational exposure to HFD is associated with differential behavioural outcomes. Maternal metabolic hormones such as insulin and leptin, which depend on the duration of HFD feeding in the dams, are either unreported or variable across studies. Insulin and leptin act as growth factors in the brain and could influence the development and maturation of neurocircuitry in the brain of the offspring, which in turn could influence the behaviour and physiology of the offspring [3, 28]. In order to better characterize the phenotype of the offspring, we suggest measuring and reporting maternal leptin and insulin levels as a way to validate the HFD exposure protocol used in the study and to help compare the results across models of maternal HFD. Consequently, this will help improve our understanding of how these maternal hormones could play a role in mediating the effects of the HFD on the offspring.

It is essential to acknowledge the difference in brain development when translating rodent finding to humans. For example, the prenatal period is a time of heightened neurogenesis, while important milestones in neurocircuit development and changes in connectivity occur during the early postnatal period of development in rodents and during the third trimester in humans [3, 28]. Thus, the early postnatal period in rodents diverges from conditions during human development, where these milestones occur in utero.

The timing of the developmental expression of GR in the brain between the rodent and humans is also different. In the foetal rat brain, GR is first detected at embryonic day (E) 13 at low levels that increase rapidly after birth [17]; however, GR expression in humans is detected in the hippocampus between 23 and 34 weeks of gestation, and its level stays stable in the early postpartum period [17]. It is important to be cognizant of limitations in directly translating the results from rodent studies to humans, despite the obvious advantages of rodent studies vis-à-vis a causal and mechanistic understanding of dietary effects.

Conclusions

There is evidence that maternal nutritional status is an important contributor to programming the offspring HPA axis and behavioural outcomes. Here, we have reviewed behavioural and physiological outcomes of HFD feeding in both mothers and their offspring (Fig. 17.4). A number of reports suggest that mothers consuming a HFD display altered HPA axis physiology and maternal behaviour. We and

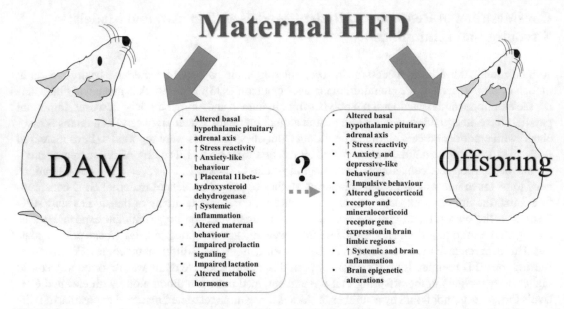

Fig. 17.4 Summary of reported effects of maternal high-fat diet. High-fat diet consumption in the dams causes a number of effects in the dams and the offspring. The altered behaviour and physiology in the dams may directly or indirectly influence behavioural and physiological outcomes in the offspring

others have found that offspring develop abnormal emotionality along with alterations in stress reactivity and gene expression of stress-related genes. It is possible that epigenetic modifications may underlie some of these effects. The limitations of animal models of maternal HFD effects include differences in the diets and timing of exposure that have distinct consequences for the phenotype, and important differences exist between humans and rodent models of maternal HFD. Future research in this area may benefit from the use of endocrine measures including circulating levels of leptin and insulin to validate the consequences of maternal HFD exposures on dams when examining their offspring.

References

1. Ng M, Fleming T, Robinson M, et al. Global, regional, and national prevalence of overweight and obesity in children and adults during 1980–2013: a systematic analysis for the Global Burden of Disease Study 2013. Lancet. 2014;384(9945):766–81. doi:10.1016/S0140-6736(14)60460-8.
2. Fisher SC, Kim SY, Sharma AJ, Rochat R, Morrow B. Is obesity still increasing among pregnant women? Prepregnancy obesity trends in 20 states, 2003–2009. Prev Med (Baltim). 2013;56(6):372–8. doi:10.1016/j.ypmed.2013.02.015.
3. Dearden L, Ozanne SE. Early life origins of metabolic disease: developmental programming of hypothalamic pathways controlling energy homeostasis. Front Neuroendocrinol. 2015;39:3–16. doi:10.1016/j.yfrne.2015.08.001.
4. Rivera HM, Christiansen KJ, Sullivan EL. The role of maternal obesity in the risk of neuropsychiatric disorders. Front Neurosci. 2015;9:1–16. doi:10.3389/fnins.2015.00194.
5. Rosmond R, Björntorp P. Psychosocial and socio-economic factors in women and their relationship to obesity and regional body fat distribution. Int J Obes Relat Metab Disord. 1999;23:138–45.
6. Warne JP. Shaping the stress response: interplay of palatable food choices, glucocorticoids, insulin and abdominal obesity. Mol Cell Endocrinol. 2009;300(1–2):137–46. doi:10.1016/j.mce.2008.09.036.
7. Spencer SJ. Perinatal programming of neuroendocrine mechanisms connecting feeding behavior and stress. Front Neurosci. 2013;7(June):109. doi:10.3389/fnins.2013.00109.
8. Rosmond R, Chagnon YC, Holm G, et al. A glucocorticoid receptor gene marker is associated with abdominal obesity, leptin, and dysregulation of the hypothalamic-pituitary-adrenal axis. Obes Res. 2000;8(3):211–8. doi:10.1038/oby.2000.24.

9. Dallman MF, Akana SF, Strack AM, et al. Chronic stress-induced effects of corticosterone on brain: direct and indirect. Ann N Y Acad Sci. 2004;1018:141–50. doi:10.1196/annals.1296.017.

10. Richardson HN, Zorrilla EP, Mandyam CD, Rivier CL. Exposure to repetitive versus varied stress during prenatal development generates two distinct anxiogenic and neuroendocrine profiles in adulthood. Endocrinology. 2006;147(5):2506–17. doi:10.1210/en.2005-1054.

11. Sullivan EL, Grayson B, Takahashi D, et al. Chronic consumption of a high-fat diet during pregnancy causes perturbations in the serotonergic system and increased anxiety-like behavior in nonhuman primate offspring. J Neurosci. 2010;30(10):3826–30. doi:10.1523/JNEUROSCI.5560-09.2010.

12. Raygada M, Cho E, Hilakivi-Clarke L. High maternal intake of polyunsaturated fatty acids during pregnancy in mice alters offsprings' aggressive behavior, immobility in the swim test, locomotor activity and brain protein kinase C activity. J Nutr. 1998;128(12):2505–11.

13. Sasaki A, de Vega WC, St-Cyr S, Pan P, McGowan PO. Perinatal high fat diet alters glucocorticoid signaling and anxiety behavior in adulthood. Neuroscience. 2013;240:1–12. Available at: http://www.ncbi.nlm.nih.gov/pubmed/23454542.

14. Sasaki A, de Vega W, Sivanathan S, St-Cyr S, McGowan PO. Maternal high-fat diet alters anxiety behavior and glucocorticoid signaling in adolescent offspring. Neuroscience. 2014;272:92–101. doi:10.1016/j.neuroscience.2014.04.012.

15. Wright T, Langley-Evans SC, Voigt J-P. The impact of maternal cafeteria diet on anxiety-related behaviour and exploration in the offspring. Physiol Behav. 2011;103(2):164–72. doi:10.1016/j.physbeh.2011.01.008.

16. Painter RC, Roseboom TJ, Bleker OP. Prenatal exposure to the Dutch famine and disease in later life: an overview. Reprod Toxicol. 2005;20(3):345–52. doi:10.1016/j.reprotox.2005.04.005.

17. Xiong F, Zhang L. Role of the hypothalamic-pituitary-adrenal axis in developmental programming of health and disease. Front Neuroendocrinol. 2013;34(1):27–46. doi:10.1016/j.yfrne.2012.11.002.

18. McGowan PO, Sasaki A, D'Alessio AC, et al. Epigenetic regulation of the glucocorticoid receptor in human brain associates with childhood abuse. Nat Neurosci. 2009;12(3):342–8. doi:nn.2270 [pii]\r10.1038/nn.2270.

19. Vucetic Z, Carlin JL, Totoki K, Reyes TM. Epigenetic dysregulation of the dopamine system in diet-induced obesity. J Neurochem. 2012;120(6):891–8. doi:10.1111/j.1471-4159.2012.07649.x.

20. Marco A, Kisliouk T, Tabachnik T, Meiri N, Weller A. Overweight and CpG methylation of the Pomc promoter in offspring of high-fat-diet-fed dams are not "reprogrammed" by regular chow diet in rats. FASEB J. 2014;28(9):4148–57. doi:10.1096/fj.14-255620.

21. Sivanathan S, Thavartnam K, Arif S, Elegino T, McGowan PO. Chronic high fat feeding increases anxiety-like behaviour and reduces transcript abundance of glucocorticoid signalling genes in the hippocampus of female rats. Behav Brain Res. 2015;286:265–70. doi:10.1016/j.bbr.2015.02.036.

22. Sharma S, Fulton S. Diet-induced obesity promotes depressive-like behaviour that is associated with neural adaptations in brain reward circuitry. Int J Obes. 2013;37(3):382–9. doi:10.1038/ijo.2012.48.

23. Hariri N, Thibault L. High-fat diet-induced obesity in animal models. Nutr Res Rev. 2010;23(2):270–99. doi:10.1017/S0954422410000168.

24. Lai M, Chandrasekera PC, Barnard ND. You are what you eat, or are you? The challenges of translating high-fat-fed rodents to human obesity and diabetes. Nutr Diabetes. 2014;4(9):e135. doi:10.1038/nutd.2014.30.

25. Buettner R, Schölmerich J, Bollheimer LC. High-fat diets: modeling the metabolic disorders of human obesity in rodents. Obesity (Silver Spring). 2007;15(4):798–808. doi:10.1038/oby.2007.608.

26. Hryhorczuk C, Florea M, Rodaros D, et al. Dampened mesolimbic dopamine function and signaling by saturated but not monounsaturated dietary lipids. Neuropsychopharmacology. 2015;41(July):1–11. doi:10.1038/npp.2015.207.

27. Bilbo SD, Tsang V. Enduring consequences of maternal obesity for brain inflammation and behavior of offspring. FASEB J. 2010;24(6):2104–15. doi:10.1096/fj.09-144014.

28. Vogt MC, Paeger L, Hess S, et al. Neonatal insulin action impairs hypothalamic neurocircuit formation in response to maternal high-fat feeding. Cell. 2014;156(3):495–509. doi: 10.1016/j.cell.2014.01.008.

29. Bellisario V, Panetta P, Balsevich G, et al. Maternal high-fat diet acts as a stressor increasing maternal glucocorticoids' signaling to the fetus and disrupting maternal behavior and brain activation in C57BL/6J mice. Psychoneuroendocrinology. 2015;60:138–50. doi:10.1016/j.psyneuen.2015.06.012.

30. Rolls BJ, Rowe EA. Pregnancy and lactation in the obese rat: effects on maternal and pup weights. Physiol Behav. 1982;28(3):393–400. doi:10.1016/0031-9384(82)90130-5.

31. White CL, Pistell PJ, Purpera MN, et al. Effects of high fat diet on Morris maze performance, oxidative stress, and inflammation in rats: contributions of maternal diet. Neurobiol Dis. 2009;35(1):3–13. doi:10.1016/j.nbd.2009.04.002.

32. Ressler IB, Grayson BE, Ulrich-Lai YM, Seeley RJ. Diet-induced obesity exacerbates metabolic and behavioral effects of polycystic ovary syndrome in a rodent model. Am J Physiol Endocrinol Metab. 2015;308(12):E1076–84. doi:10.1152/ajpendo.00182.2014.

33. Rolls BJ, van Duijvenvoorde PM, Rowe EA. Effects of diet and obesity on body weight regulation during pregnancy and lactation in the rat. Physiol Behav. 1984;32(2):161–8. Available at: http://www.ncbi.nlm.nih.gov/pubmed/6718543.

34. Bayol SA, Farrington SJ, Stickland NC. A maternal "junk food" diet in pregnancy and lactation promotes an exac-
    erbated taste for "junk food" and a greater propensity for obesity in rat offspring. Br J Nutr. 2007;98(4):843–51.
    doi:10.1017/S0007114507812037.
35. Rodriguez JS, Rodríguez-González GL, Reyes-Castro LA, et al. Maternal obesity in the rat programs male off-
    spring exploratory, learning and motivation behavior: prevention by dietary intervention pre-gestation or in gesta-
    tion. Int J Dev Neurosci. 2012;30(2):75–81. doi:10.1016/j.ijdevneu.2011.12.012.
36. Jensen Peña C, Monk C, Champagne FA. Epigenetic effects of prenatal stress on 11β-hydroxysteroid dehydroge-
    nase-2 in the placenta and fetal brain. PLoS One. 2012;7(6):e39791. doi:10.1371/journal.pone.0039791.
37. Buonfiglio DC, Ramos-Lobo AM, Freitas VM, et al. Obesity impairs lactation performance in mice by inducing
    prolactin resistance. Sci Report. 2016;6:22421. doi:10.1038/srep22421.
38. Rolls BA, Gurr MI, van Duijvenvoorde PM, Rolls BJ, Rowe EA. Lactation in lean and obese rats: effect of cafeteria
    feeding and of dietary obesity on milk composition. Physiol Behav. 1986;38(2):185–90. Available at: http://www.
    ncbi.nlm.nih.gov/pubmed/3797485.
39. Sun B, Purcell RH, Terrillion CE, Yan J, Moran TH, Tamashiro KLK. Maternal high-fat diet during gestation or
    suckling differentially affects offspring leptin sensitivity and obesity. Diabetes. 2012;61(11):2833–41. doi:10.2337/
    db11-0957.
40. Purcell RH, Sun B, Pass LL, Power ML, Moran TH, Tamashiro KLK. Maternal stress and high-fat diet effect on
    maternal behavior, milk composition, and pup ingestive behavior. Physiol Behav. 2011;104(3):474–9. doi:10.1016/j.
    physbeh.2011.05.012.
41. Bertino M. Effect of high fat, protein supplemented diets on maternal behavior in rats. Physiol Behav.
    1982;29(6):999–1005. Available at: http://ovidsp.ovid.com/ovidweb.cgi?T=JS&PAGE=reference&D=med2&NE
    WS=N&AN=7163403.
42. Woodside B. Prolactin and the hyperphagia of lactation. Physiol Behav. 2007;91(4):375–82. doi:10.1016/j.
    physbeh.2007.04.015.
43. Bellisario V, Berry A, Capoccia S, et al. Gender-dependent resiliency to stressful and metabolic challenges following
    prenatal exposure to high-fat diet in the p66(Shc−/−) mouse. Front Behav Neurosci. 2014;8:285. doi:10.3389/
    fnbeh.2014.00285.
44. Terkel J, Bridges RS, Sawyer CH. Effects of transecting lateral neural connections of the medial preoptic area on
    maternal behavior in the rat: nest building, pup retrieval and prolactin secretion. Brain Res. 1979;169(2):369–80.
    doi:10.1016/0006-8993(79)91037-0.
45. Fleming AS, Rosenblatt JS. Olfactory regulation of maternal behavior in rats. I. Effects of olfactory bulb removal
    in experienced and inexperienced lactating and cycling females. J Comp Physiol Psychol. 1974;86(2):221–32.
    doi:10.1037/h0035937.
46. Hernandez LL, Grayson BE, Yadav E, Seeley RJ, Horseman ND. High fat diet alters lactation outcomes: pos-
    sible involvement of inflammatory and serotonergic pathways. PLoS One. 2012;7(3):3–10. doi:10.1371/journal.
    pone.0032598.
47. Perani CV, Neumann ID, Reber SO, Slattery DA. High-fat diet prevents adaptive peripartum-associated adrenal
    gland plasticity and anxiolysis. Sci Report. 2015;5:14821. doi:10.1038/srep14821.
48. Peleg-Raibstein D, Luca E, Wolfrum C. Maternal high-fat diet in mice programs emotional behavior in adulthood.
    Behav Brain Res. 2012;233(2):398–404. doi:10.1016/j.bbr.2012.05.027.
49. Kang SS, Kurti A, Fair DA, Fryer JD. Dietary intervention rescues maternal obesity induced behavior deficits and
    neuroinflammation in offspring. J Neuroinflammation. 2014;11(1):156. doi:10.1186/s12974-014-0156-9.
50. Joels M, Karst H, DeRijk R, de Kloet ER. The coming out of the brain mineralocorticoid receptor. Trends Neurosci.
    2008;31(1):1–7. doi:10.1016/j.tins.2007.10.005.
51. Lin C, Shao B, Huang H, Zhou Y, Lin Y. Maternal high fat diet programs stress-induced behavioral disorder in adult
    offspring. Physiol Behav. 2015;152:119–27. doi:10.1016/j.physbeh.2015.09.023.
52. Chen H, Simar D, Morris MJ. Hypothalamic neuroendocrine circuitry is programmed by maternal obesity: interac-
    tion with postnatal nutritional environment. PLoS One. 2009;4(7):e6259. doi:10.1371/journal.pone.0006259.
53. Jacobson-Pick S, Richter-Levin G. Differential impact of juvenile stress and corticosterone in juvenility and in
    adulthood, in male and female rats. Behav Brain Res. 2010;214(2):268–76. doi:10.1016/j.bbr.2010.05.036.
54. Grissom NM, Herdt CT, Desilets J, Lidsky-Everson J, Reyes TM. Dissociable deficits of executive func-
    tion caused by gestational adversity are linked to specific transcriptional changes in the prefrontal cortex.
    Neuropsychopharmacology. 2015;40:1353–1363. doi: 10.1038/npp.2014.313.
55. Tamashiro K, Terrillion C, Hyun J. Prenatal stress or high-fat diet increases susceptibility to diet-induced obesity in
    rat offspring. Diabetes. 2009;58(5):1116–25. doi:10.2337/db08-1129.
56. Desai M, Jellyman JK, Han G, Beall M, Lane RH, Ross MG. Rat maternal obesity and high-fat diet program off-
    spring metabolic syndrome. Am J Obstet Gynecol. 2014;211(3):237.e1–237.e13. doi:10.1016/j.ajog.2014.03.025.
57. Sorrells SF, Munhoz CD, Manley NC, Yen S, Sapolsky RM. Glucocorticoids increase excitotoxic injury and inflam-
    mation in the hippocampus of adult male rats. Neuroendocrinology. 2014;100:129–40. doi:10.1159/000367849.

58. Maes M, Verkerk R, Bonaccorso S, Ombelet W, Bosmans E, Scharpé S. Depressive and anxiety symptoms in the early puerperium are related to increased degradation of tryptophan into kynurenine, a phenomenon which is related to immune activation. Life Sci. 2002;71(16):1837–48. doi:10.1016/S0024-3205(02)01853-2.
59. Tozuka Y, Kumon M, Wada E, Onodera M, Mochizuki H, Wada K. Maternal obesity impairs hippocampal BDNF production and spatial learning performance in young mouse offspring. Neurochem Int. 2010;57(3):235–47. doi:10.1016/j.neuint.2010.05.015.
60. Hovatta I, Juhila J, Donner J. Oxidative stress in anxiety and comorbid disorders. Neurosci Res. 2010;68(4):261–75. doi:10.1016/j.neures.2010.08.007.
61. Lupien SJ, Mcewen BS, Gunnar MR, Heim C. Effects of stress throughout the lifespan on the brain, behaviour and cognition. Nat Rev Neurosci. 2009;10:434. doi:10.1038/nrn2639.
62. Roth TL, Zoladz PR, Sweatt JD, Diamond DM. Epigenetic modification of hippocampal Bdnf DNA in adult rats in an animal model of post-traumatic stress disorder. J Psychiatr Res. 2011;45(7):919–26. doi:10.1016/j.jpsychires.2011.01.013.
63. Grissom NM, Lyde R, Christ L, et al. Obesity at conception programs the opioid system in the offspring brain. Neuropsychopharmacology. 2014;39(4):801–10. doi:10.1038/npp.2013.193.
64. Balsevich G, Baumann V, Uribe A, Chen A, Schmidt MV. Prenatal exposure to maternal obesity alters anxiety and stress-coping behaviors in aged mice. Neuroendocrinology. 2015; doi:10.1159/000439087.
65. Oates M, Woodside B, Walker CD. Chronic leptin administration in developing rats reduces stress responsiveness partly through changes in maternal behavior. Horm Behav. 2000;37(4):366–76. doi:10.1006/hbeh.2000.1578.
66. Trottier G, Koski KG, Brun T, Toufexis DJ, Richard D, Walker CD. Increased fat intake during lactation modifies hypothalamic-pituitary-adrenal responsiveness in developing rat pups: a possible role for leptin. Endocrinology. 1998;139(9):3704–11. doi:10.1210/endo.139.9.6208.
67. Slieker LJ, Sloop KW, Surface PL, et al. Regulation of expression of ob mRNA and protein by glucocorticoids and cAMP. J Biol Chem. 1996;271(10):5301–4. doi:10.1074/jbc.271.10.5301.
68. McGowan PO, Roth TL. Epigenetic pathways through which experiences become linked with biology. Dev Psychopathol. 2015;27:637–48. doi:10.1017/s0954579415000206.
69. Bird A. DNA methylation patterns and epigenetic memory DNA methylation patterns and epigenetic memory. Genes Dev. 2002;16:6–21. doi:10.1101/gad.947102.
70. Waterland RA, Travisano M, Tahiliani KG, Rached MT, Mirza S. Methyl donor supplementation prevents transgenerational amplification of obesity. Int J Obes. 2008;32(9):1373–9. doi:10.1038/ijo.2008.100.
71. Vucetic Z, Kimmel J, Totoki K, Hollenbeck E, Reyes TM. Maternal high-fat diet alters methylation and gene expression of dopamine and opioid-related genes. Endocrinology. 2010;151(10):4756–64. doi:10.1210/en.2010-0505.
72. Carlin JL, George R, Reyes TM. Methyl donor supplementation blocks the adverse effects of maternal high fat diet on offspring physiology. PLoS One. 2013;8(5):e63549. doi:10.1371/journal.pone.0063549.
73. Weinstock M. Does prenatal stress impair coping and regulation of hypothalamic–pituitary-adrenal axis? Neurosci Biobehav Rev. 1997;21(1):1–10.
74. Gabory A, Ferry L, Fajardy I, et al. Maternal diets trigger sex-specific divergent trajectories of gene expression and epigenetic systems in mouse placenta. PLoS One. 2012;7(11):e47986. doi:10.1371/journal.pone.0047986.
75. Gallou-Kabani C, Gabory A, Tost J, et al. Sex- and diet-specific changes of imprinted gene expression and DNA methylation in mouse placenta under a high-fat diet. PLoS One. 2010;5(12):e14398. doi:10.1371/journal.pone.0014398.

Chapter 18
Maternal Junk Food Diets: The Effects on Offspring Fat Mass and Food Preferences

Beverly S. Muhlhausler, Jessica R. Gugusheff, and Simon C. Langley-Evans

Key Points

- Excess maternal junk food intake during pregnancy and/or lactation is associated with an increased fat mass and increased preference for high-fat/high-sugar foods in the offspring.
- These effects are present from the time of weaning and persist through the life course.
- Excess maternal junk food intake results in altered development of a large number of physiological systems in the offspring, including key systems regulating fat deposition, food intake!! and food preferences.
- Altered development of the fat cells and central reward pathways in the offspring are thought to underlie the increased fat mass and increased preference for fat and sugar in these offspring.
- The impact of maternal junk food diets on the offspring is often different between males and females, and it is therefore important to consider the sex of the offspring in these studies.

Keywords Reward • Opioid • Dopamine • Obesity • High-fat diet

Abbreviations

C	Control
CAF	Cafeteria diet-fed
DAT	Dopamine active transporter
GABA	Gamma amino butyric acid
IGF-1	Insulin-like growth factor
NAc	Nucleus accumbens
PPARγ	Peroxisome proliferator receptor gamma
VTA	Ventral tegmental area

B.S. Muhlhausler, PhD (✉) • J.R. Gugusheff, PhD
FOODplus Research Centre, School of Agriculture Food and Wine, The University of Adelaide, Urrbrae, SA, Australia
e-mail: beverly.muhlhausler@adelaide.edu.au

S.C. Langley-Evans, PhD
School of Biosciences, University of Nottingham, Loughborough, UK

© Springer International Publishing AG 2017
R. Rajendram et al. (eds.), *Diet, Nutrition, and Fetal Programming*,
Nutrition and Health, DOI 10.1007/978-3-319-60289-9_18

Introduction

The increased availability and consumption of high-fat, high-sugar, highly palatable 'junk foods' in conjunction with decreased levels of physical activity over the past three to four decades has been cited as a major contributor to the current worldwide epidemic of obesity, poor cardiometabolic health and cancer [1–3]. It is also clear, however, that an individual's susceptibility to developing obesity and its associated comorbidities is critically dependent on environmental exposures they experience before birth and/or in early postnatal life [4]. Exposure to an excessive nutrient supply, as a consequence of maternal obesity, maternal diabetes!! and/or maternal overnutrition, is particularly detrimental for the future metabolic health of the offspring [5]. This has created an intergenerational cycle in which women who enter pregnancy overweight or obese give birth to infants who are typically, though not always, heavier at birth and go on to be at increased risk of obesity and cardiometabolic disease as children, adolescents!! and adults (Fig. 18.1). More recent research has attempted to define the biological mechanisms through which exposure to an increased nutrient supply in general, and exposure to excess maternal junk food intake in particular, acts to predispose the offspring to later obesity. These studies have demonstrated that perinatal junk food exposure has negative effects on the development of almost all organs and physiological systems investigated to date, including those regulating insulin signalling in skeletal muscle, hepatic lipid metabolism!! and pancreatic insulin secretion [6–9].

Two of the major targets of metabolic programming by perinatal junk food exposure are the developing fat cell, or adipocyte, and the central neural networks regulating appetite and the response to reward. A number of studies have demonstrated that maternal overnutrition is associated with a precocial activation of lipogenic pathways in foetal and neonatal fat depots, which leads to early accumulation of excess fat tissue and persistently increases the capacity of the fat depots for fat storage [6]. Perinatal exposure to nutritional excess, in particular high levels of fat and/or sugar, also leads to permanent alteration in the structure and function of the appetite and reward pathways in the brain, resulting in increased appetite drive and a shift in food preferences towards highly palatable (high-fat, high-sugar) foods in the offspring through the life course [7, 10].

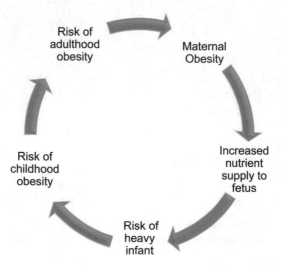

Fig. 18.1 Schematic representation of the intergenerational cycle of obesity. Maternal overnutrition during pregnancy can predispose the offspring towards increased fat consumption and diet-induced obesity (Adapted from McMillen et al. [59])

This chapter will summarise the evidence from both human and animal studies which has supported the critical role of maternal overnutrition, in particular excess intake of junk foods, in the programming of fat mass and food preferences in the offspring. It will describe our current understanding of the underlying mechanisms, highlight the sex-specific nature of the effects and identify the key knowledge gaps which remain to be addressed.

Definition of the 'Junk Food' Diet

While junk food is a term in mainstream use, and there is a general concept of what foods it refers to, it is important to define its meaning in the context of this chapter. In the context of developmental programming by excess maternal junk food intake, the junk food label is applied to any food which is high in fat, sugar and/or salt, energy dense, nutrient poor as well as highly palatable [11]. In some healthcare and public health settings, these foods will be referred to as non-core foods. Junk food is clearly a broad label; however, the key feature is the lack of nutrient density in relation to energy content. In animal models, junk food diets are often referred to as cafeteria diets. These diets typically include a range of human junk foods (examples of the cafeteria diet composition are included in Table 18.1) and have been used extensively in rodents to model the effects of overconsumption of junk food in humans. Cafeteria diet protocols were initially developed by Rothwell and Stock [12] to induce obesity in rodents and explore their impact on thermogenesis.

Cafeteria diets are designed to replicate some aspects of poor quality western style diets, but are generally somewhat more extreme (i.e., with a higher caloric density and poorer nutritional quality) than the typical western diets consumed by humans. It is therefore important to note that the phenotypes produced by feeding animals such diets are more pronounced, and manifest more quickly, than the response to the consumption of typical western style diets. Nevertheless, the use of junk food or cafeteria diets in animal research has been shown to produce a phenotype more comparable to the features of diet-induced obesity in humans, than experimental rodent diets which are based on standard rodent feeds with the addition of extra fat or sugar [13, 14]. Studies which utilise junk food/cafeteria diets also take advantage of the ability of highly palatable foods to act as natural rewards, by activating central reward processing pathways. The main disadvantage of the junk food protocol is that food and nutrient intake is not consistent between animals, or sometimes between experiments. However, models based on junk food feeding have been reported as being superior to other approaches to inducing obesity in rodents [15]. While experimental high-fat and high-sugar diets have the advantage of a defined and consistent nutritional composition, they do not replicate the increased palatability created by combining fat and sugar as well as including a variety of different foods and can induce profiles of fatty acid intake that are of little relevance to human diets and which may have extreme metabolic and physiological consequences [15].

Table 18.1 Examples of the composition of 'junk food' diets used in studies which have investigated the effect of maternal 'junk food' diets on the programming of food preferences and diet-induced obesity in the offspring

Study	Diet composition
Bayol et al. (2007)	Biscuits, flapjacks, cheese, crisps, doughnuts, muffins, chocolate, marshmallows
Wright et al. (2011)	Biscuits, potato chips, fruit and nut chocolate, Mars bars, cheddar cheese, golden syrup cake, pork pie, cocktail sausages, liver and bacon pate, strawberry jam and peanuts
Ong et al. (2011)	Peanut butter, hazelnut spread, chocolate biscuits, cheese and bacon balls, Fruit Loops, lard and chow mix

Maternal Junk Food Consumption and Offspring Outcomes

Pregnancy and Neonatal Outcomes

Most of the studies to date which have investigated the impact of maternal junk food diets have randomly assigned dams to consume either a nutritionally balanced, standard rodent feed or a cafeteria diet (as defined above) prior to or from mating until the end of lactation. In most studies, the cafeteria diet has been provided to dams for at least 2 weeks prior to mating and then continued through pregnancy and lactation. While longer periods of maternal junk food consumption prior to mating can be associated with greater differences in maternal body weight/fat mass between dietary groups at the time of mating, and during pregnancy and lactation, prolonged periods of junk food feeding and/or excess weight gain can reduce fertility, leading to difficulties in achieving and maintaining pregnancy. This is consistent with what is observed clinically, where maternal obesity is associated with an increase in the risk of pregnancy complications, including stillbirth [16]. Studies in which pre-feeding of cafeteria diet lasts for 8 weeks prior to mating have found that fertility is impaired, although neonatal survival is not consistently impacted upon [17–19].

The effect of maternal junk food diets on birth weight of the offspring differs between studies; with some studies reporting reductions in birth weight of the offspring [20–22], while other studies have reported either increases [23] or no differences [10] in the birth weight of offspring of junk food dams compared to controls. It has been suggested that these different outcomes could be related to differences in the composition of the cafeteria diets used in these studies, particularly the protein content, as studies in which protein intakes in the cafeteria group are reduced typically report reductions in birth weight of the offspring. Differences in the content of key micronutrients between diets may also play an important role in driving these differential effects.

Offspring Growth and Fat Mass

There are also differences between studies in the effects of maternal cafeteria diets on body weight of the offspring after birth. Some studies have reported an increase in bodyweight from birth and continuing throughout the life course [24], while others have reported either no difference or reduced body weights at weaning in the offspring of junk food-fed dams [17, 25, 26]. The reduction in body weight at weaning in offspring exposed to a junk food diet is perhaps counterintuitive, given that the increased amount of energy being consumed by junk food dams in most of these studies. However, the deficits in pup growth may be related to reductions in the quality or quantity of the dam's milk, since maternal junk food consumption and obesity have been associated with impaired milk production/lactation performance in both humans and animals [27–29] or impacts of the cafeteria diet on maternal care [30].

Despite differences between studies in the observed effects on offspring body weight, however, all studies have consistently demonstrated that offspring of junk food-fed dams have a significantly higher percentage body fat at weaning compared to offspring of control dams [10, 31]. Thus, irrespective of effects on body weight, perinatal junk food exposure is associated with increased fat deposition in early life. In addition, studies in which the offspring have been provided with access to a cafeteria or high-fat/high-sugar diet after weaning have demonstrated that offspring of junk food dams have an increased susceptibility to diet-induced obesity and that this persists throughout the life course.

Offspring Food Preferences

Over the past few years, a series of studies have demonstrated that maternal junk food consumption is associated with altered food preferences in the offspring, in particular an increased preference for fat and sugar. In these studies, food preferences are typically assessed by providing the offspring with free access to both a cafeteria diet and control diet (standard rodent feed) and monitoring their food choices over a period of time. These studies have demonstrated that both male and female offspring of junk food dams consume a greater amount of junk food compared to their control counterparts, and this effect is observed from the time the animals are weaned until at least 3 months of age in these studies [10].

It has also been established that the increased preference for junk food persists even when offspring are provided with a nutritionally balanced diet after weaning, in an attempt to 'wash out' the effects of the earlier junk food exposure. In one study, offspring of dams fed a junk food diet during pregnancy and lactation were provided with a nutritionally balanced standard rodent feed from weaning until 6 weeks of age, after which their access to the cafeteria diet was reinstated and food preferences in all offspring monitored over the subsequent 14 days. It was demonstrated that both male and female offspring of junk food dams consumed significantly more of the cafeteria diet, both in relation to the total amount and as a proportion of their total energy intake, and more dietary fat compared to controls [32]. They also gained more weight and had a higher fat mass than control offspring, indicating a higher propensity to diet-induced obesity [32]. Similar results have been obtained in other rodent studies in which offspring of junk food-fed dams are weaned onto a standard feed, yet still exhibit an increased preference for fat/sucrose when tested as adults [33, 34]. A study in which cafeteria feeding was focused upon lactation found that adult female offspring exhibited an aberrant behavioural satiety sequence [19].

The Relative Role of Junk Food Exposure During the Foetal and Suckling Periods

There has been a growing interest in determining whether exposure to a junk food diet during different periods of development, i.e. before birth vs the suckling period, has differential effects on food preferences and fat deposition in the offspring. The relative impact of maternal junk food consumption in these periods has been evaluated in a number of studies in which offspring born to junk food-fed dams are cross-fostered onto dams provided a control diet, or vice versa, within 24 h of birth. This approach allows analysis of the effects of junk food diet exposure in each period without any lingering effects associated with switching the dam's diet.

A cross-fostering study conducted by the authors of this chapter provided clear evidence of the importance of the suckling period in the programming of both fat mass and food preferences. In this study, offspring fat mass at the end of the suckling period was approximately twofold higher in pups who were cross-fostered to a cafeteria diet-fed dam compared to those cross-fostered onto a control dam, independent of whether they were born to a control or cafeteria diet-fed dam (Fig. 18.2, Vithayathil et al. unpublished). Exposure to the junk food diet during the suckling period also has consequences for fat deposition and food preferences in the adult offspring. Male pups cross-fostered onto a junk food dam exhibited an increased preference for dietary fat, and female pups exhibited a higher fat mass when all pups had free access to both standard rat feed and cafeteria diet from 2 to 4 months of age [35]. Similarly, Chang and colleagues reported that offspring of an obesity-resistant breed of rats who were cross-fostered onto an obesity-prone breed exhibited a significantly higher energy intake when given free access to a high-energy diet between 8 and 12 weeks of age compared to those cross-fostered to another obesity-resistant dam [22].

While cross-fostering studies make it possible to clearly separate prenatal and postnatal environmental exposures, a limitation of the approach is that the cross-fostering itself may impact on metabolic outcomes in the offspring. There have been some reports that placing pups with a foster mother

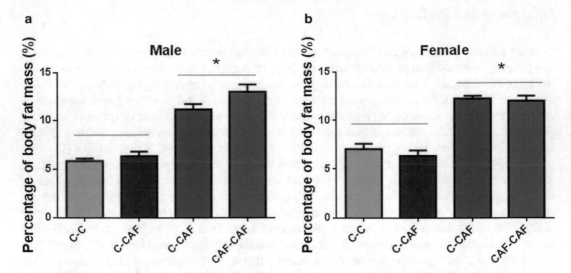

Fig. 18.2 Fat mass at weaning of offspring suckled by control and cafeteria diet-fed dams. Body fat mass (expressed as a percentage of total body weight) at weaning (3 weeks of age) of male (**a**) and female (**b**) offspring born to and suckled by control dams (*C-C, yellow* bars), born to cafeteria diet-fed dams and suckled by control dams (*CAF-C, blue* bars), born to control dams and suckled by cafeteria diet-fed dams (*C-CAF, green* bars) and born to and suckled by cafeteria diet-fed dams (*CAF-CAF, purple* bars). Values are expressed as mean ± SEM. ***denotes significance at $P < 0.001$

at birth, even if she is consuming the same diet, alters the subsequent growth, metabolic profile and behaviour of the offspring, potentially due to subtle effects on maternal/pup interaction [36]. However, the importance of the suckling period for the programming of increased fat mass and altered food preferences in rodent models has also been shown in studies in which pups remained with their natural mother. In one such study, the offspring of dams fed a junk food diet both before birth and during the suckling period had an increased food intake and higher body mass index after weaning than offspring of mothers who were fed a junk food diet during pregnancy, but were switched to a control diet after delivery [25]. Similarly, a separate study reported that rat pups whose mothers were fed a junk food diet only after giving birth exhibited more robust feeding behaviour in adulthood, compared to pups in the same experiment whose dams had continued on the control diet after delivery [37].

As with many areas of science, however, not all studies are consistent. A study by Chang and colleagues, for example, reported that offspring who had been exposed to a high-fat diet in utero exhibited an increased body weight, increased body fat mass and increased fat preference, independent of whether they were suckled by a dam consuming a control or high-fat diet [38]. These authors therefore concluded that exposure to a high-fat diet before birth was both necessary and sufficient for the programming of adverse metabolic outcomes in the offspring. Thus, further work is required in order to fully disentangle the relative impact of exposure to a junk food diet during the prenatal and sucking periods.

Maternal Junk Food and Offspring Outcomes: The Underlying Mechanisms

Fat Deposition

There is clear evidence from studies in both humans and animal models that nutritional perturbations, including exposure to a maternal junk food diet, before birth and in the early postnatal period have significant long-term impacts for adipose tissue function and, consequently, adipose tissue

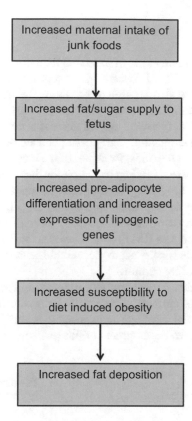

Fig. 18.3 Schematic representation of the potential mechanism through which maternal junk food diet consumption programmes obesity. Maternal junk food consumption leads to an oversupply of fat and sugar to the foetus. This leads to an increase adipocyte pre-differentiation and overexpression of lipogenic genes, predisposing the offspring towards diet-induced obesity in adulthood

mass [39, 40] (Fig. 18.3). The transcription factor peroxisome proliferator-activated receptor gamma (PPARγ) and insulin-like growth factor 1 (IGF-1), both of which are involved in promoting adipocyte differentiation, are two key targets identified to date [6, 41, 42]. Increased mRNA expression of PPARγ in the major foetal/neonatal fat depot has been reported both in pups of rat dams fed a junk food diet during pregnancy and lactation [41] and in foetuses of well-fed ewes (fed at ~55% above their maintenance energy requirements) in late gestation [42]. In addition to adipocyte differentiation, PPARγ is a major regulator of the uptake and storage of lipids in mature adipocytes. Indeed, the increase in PPARγ mRNA expression in response to maternal overnutrition in foetal sheep was also associated with an upregulation of key lipogenic genes, including lipoprotein lipase, in the same fat depots [42].

A rodent study of maternal cafeteria feeding demonstrated that mRNA expression of IGF-1 in the perinatal adipose depots was also increased in female offspring of junk food-fed dams, in conjunction with an increased mass of this fat depot [39]. Overall, the available evidence suggests that the programming of obesity by maternal nutritional excess (in particular junk food diets) is the result of altered expression of key regulatory factors within the adipose tissue, which persist after birth and which drive an increase in both the number of adipocytes that initially form, and also the capacity of these individual adipocytes for storing lipid. As discussed above, rats following a cafeteria diet often select a diet that is low in protein, but more energy dense. There is an extensive literature on the effects of protein restriction in pregnancy upon offspring development, and these studies include evidence of programming of the expression of genes which regulate lipid oxidation and lipogenesis [43].

Food Preferences

The drive to consume junk foods or any kind of palatable food has a biological basis that goes beyond the requirement to satisfy hunger. This is because junk foods, in addition to activating the appetite regulating regions of the brain, are also capable of activating the neural circuits that regulate reward processes in a similar way as alcohol and drugs of abuse [44–46]. Two of the most important brain areas involved in regulating reward response are the nucleus accumbens (NAc) in the forebrain and the ventral tegmental area (VTA) in the midbrain. These brain areas, together with key neurotransmitters including dopamine and opioid peptides, form part of the mesolimbic reward pathway. Activation of this pathway results in the release of endogenous opioids that bind to opioid receptors in the VTA [47, 48] and ultimately decreases GABAergic inhibition of dopamine synthesis. These dopaminergic neurons project to the NAc where the dopamine is released [49] (Fig. 18.4). Termination of dopamine signalling occurs through active reuptake of dopamine through high affinity membrane carriers, known as dopamine active transporters (DAT) [50]. These increases in extracellular dopamine in the NAc are thought to be responsible for the acute pleasurable sensation associated with the consumption of junk food and other rewarding stimuli.

Given the role of the mesolimbic reward pathway in regulating junk food intake, this pathway has been the primary subject of studies aiming to identify the neural mechanisms behind the programming of the preference for palatable food in offspring exposed to a junk food diet in the perinatal period, and there is clear evidence of altered development of this pathway in offspring born to and/or suckled

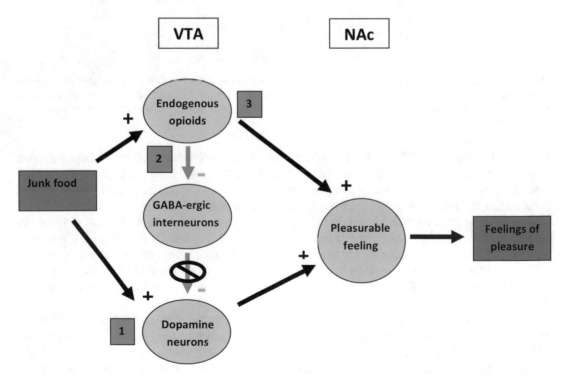

Fig. 18.4 Simplified version of the activation of the mesolimbic reward system. (*1*) A rewarding stimulus such as drugs and palatable foods can stimulate the dopamine neurons at the VTA, resulting in the release of dopamine at the NAc. (*2*) The rewarding stimulus can activate the release of endogenous opioids at the VTA, which inhibits GABA-ergic inter-neurons. GABA normally inhibits dopamine release. Therefore, this inhibition of GABA release disinhibits dopamine neurons resulting in increased dopamine release at the NAc. (*3*) Opioids can also bind to their receptors located at the NAc. The activation of efferent target neurons at the NAc through (*1*), (*2*) and (*3*) creates a pleasurable feeling associated with the rewarding stimuli. *Black* and *grey arrows* indicate neuronal activation and inhibition, respectively. Neurons are represented in *circles* (This figure has been previously published in Ong et al. [60])

by dams consuming a junk food diet. Maternal junk food consumption during pregnancy and lactation has been reported to result in increased expression of the mu-opioid receptor and decreases the expression of the dopamine active transporter (DAT), at 6 weeks of age [10]. Interestingly, when the offspring's access to the junk food diet was maintained beyond 6 weeks of age, these changes appeared to reverse, such that expression of the mu-opioid receptor was decreased and DAT expression was increased compared to controls by 3 months of age [30]. Feeding dams a cafeteria diet only during lactation has also been associated with perturbed hypothalamic dopamine metabolism [51]. These observations imply that the effects of maternal junk food diet consumption on the reward pathway of the offspring may not be set at birth, but that reward pathway development is also susceptible to nutritional/environmental influences in early postnatal life, and this is an important area for future research.

Sex Differences in the Response to a Maternal Junk Food Diet

Despite evidence from adult rodents showing that the response to fat consumption is different between males and females, there are few studies that have considered sex differences in the impact of a maternal junk food diet on offspring outcomes (Table 18.2). Historically, males have been studied in preference to females in order to avoid the potential complications introduced by the hormonal fluctuations as part of the estrous cycle in females [52]. However, it is now clear that male and female offspring often respond very differently to early life nutritional insults and therefore inappropriately to assume that findings obtained in males can be extrapolated to females. Indeed, studies which have compared the effects of maternal junk food exposure on male and female offspring provide clear evidence of significant differences in the response to maternal junk food intake in male and female offspring. By way of example, two studies examining the effects of maternal 'cafeteria diets' and 'lard-based' diet respectively on offspring fat mass both reported that the increase in fat mass was more pronounced in female offspring than in males [39, 53] and the effect of cafeteria diet during lactation upon satiety was specific to females [51].

It is also important to note that, even when the phenotype is similar between males and females, the underlying mechanisms may be very different. In one study, for example, it was demonstrated that female but not male offspring of junk food-fed dams up-regulating the expression of dopamine receptor 1 and 2 and DAT in response to a junk food challenge in adolescence, even though both sexes exhibited the same significant increase in junk food intake [22]. These results suggest that future studies investigating the effects of maternal diet on the food preferences need to consider each sex separately.

Clinical Studies

Although the vast majority of studies looking the programming of obesity and food preference have been performed in animal models, a number of clinical studies have also demonstrated a clear association between maternal obesity and obesity in the infant/child. A retrospective cohort study involving

Table 18.2 A summary of sex-specific changes in fat deposition and food preference in offspring exposed to a maternal junk food diet identified in response to a maternal junk food diet

	Male	Female	Study
4 weeks	Increased subcutaneous fat mass	Increased preference for dietary fat	Gugusheff et al. (2013)
10 weeks*	No difference in adipocyte size	Increase in adipocyte size	Bayol et al. (2008)
6 months*	No difference in body fat mass	Higher total body fat mass	Ong and Muhlhausler (2014)

*10-week-old offspring weaned onto chow
*6-month offspring weaned onto chow, but challenged for 3 weeks with a junk food diet from 12 to 15 weeks of age

8400 participants conducted by Whitaker and colleagues, for example, showed that the children of obese mothers were twice as likely to be obese by age two, than those born to mothers in a healthy weight range [54]. Similarly, a longitudinal cohort study suggested that the children of obese mothers who also had gestational diabetes had a 3.6 times greater risk of being obese at age 11 if they were born large for gestational age [55]. Importantly, a study conducted on a northern Finland birth cohort, in which data from the mother during pregnancy as well as measurements from the child at birth and at 1, 14 and 31 years of age were collected, identified maternal obesity both during adolescence and immediately prior to pregnancy as significant predictors of obesity in her adult children [56].

Clinical studies which evaluate the effect of maternal diet during pregnancy and breastfeeding on later food preferences in the child are complicated by difficulty of obtaining reliable food intake data and the confounding effects of shared food environments/parental influences over child feeding behaviour. Nevertheless, a study in 5717 mother-child pairs and 3009 father-child pairs from the Avon Longitudinal Study of Parents and Children (ALSPAC) demonstrated a strong correlation between maternal fat intake during pregnancy and the child's preference for fat at 10 years of age [57]. Importantly, the child's food preferences were not related to paternal diet at any time, or to maternal fat intake after pregnancy. In support of this, a smaller study involving 428 children from the United Kingdom showed that the children of obese parents have a higher preference for junk food and lower preference for vegetables than those born to lean parents [58]. Despite the paucity of studies conducted to date, the available data is consistent with the results from animal models, reinforcing the importance of maternal diet for the child's later food preferences.

Conclusions

The vast impact of rising obesity rates on the health of the general population is undisputed, and it is becoming increasingly evident that maternal diet and weight status during pregnancy and while breast-feeding play an important role in facilitating what has become an intergenerational cycle of obesity. Evidence from animal and clinical studies has shown that both maternal junk food diet consumption and maternal obesity during pregnancy and lactation can programme increased fat deposition, a greater preference for dietary fat as well as glucose intolerance and increased appetite in juvenile and adult offspring. Exploration into the biological mechanisms behind these effects has also begun, with a focus on adipocyte function/molecular biology and the mesolimbic reward pathway. Sex differences in the response to maternal junk food diet exposure have been identified. Continued investigations into the critical windows for the programming of food preferences and obesity, as well as the improved understanding of the mechanisms driving this programming, will ultimately enable the design of targeted interventions to prevent the spread of poor metabolic health from mother to child.

References

1. Haslam DW, James WPT. Obesity. Lancet. 2005;366:1197–209.
2. Rosenheck R. Fast food consumption and increased caloric intake: a systematic review of a trajectory towards weight gain and obesity risk. Obes Rev. 2008;9:535–47.
3. Hu F. Sedentary lifestyle and risk of obesity and type 2 diabetes. Lipids. 2003;38:103–8.
4. Langley-Evans SC. Nutrition in early life and the programming of adult disease: a review. J Hum Nutr Diet. 2015;28(Suppl 1):1–14.
5. Rkhzay-Jaf J, O'Dowd JF, Stocker CJ. Maternal obesity and the fetal origins of the metabolic Syndrome. Curr Cardiovasc Risk Rep. 2012;6:487–95.
6. Muhlhausler B, Smith SR. Early-life origins of metabolic dysfunction: role of the adipocyte. Trends Endocrinol Metab. 2009;20:51–7.

7. Muhlhausler BS, Adam CL, McMillen IC. Maternal nutrition and the programming of obesity: the brain. Organogenesis. 2008;4:144–52.

8. Poston L. Intergenerational transmission of insulin resistance and type 2 diabetes. Prog Biophys Mol Biol. 2011;106:315–22.

9. Muhlhausler BS, Ong ZY. The fetal origins of obesity: early origins of altered food intake. Endocr Metab Immune Disord Drug Targets. 2011;11:189–97.

10. Ong ZY, Muhlhausler BS. Maternal "junk-food" feeding of rat dams alters food choices and development of the mesolimbic reward pathway in the offspring. FASEB J. 2011;25:2167–79.

11. Anderson JW, Patterson K. Snack foods: comparing nutrition values of excellent choices and "junk foods". J Am Coll Nutr. 2005;24:155–6.

12. Rothwell NJ, Stock MJ, Warwick BP. The effect of high fat and high carbohydrate cafeteria diets on diet-induced thermogenesis in the rat. Int J Obes. 1983;7:263–70.

13. Johnson PM, Kenny PJ. Dopamine D2 receptors in addiction-like reward dysfunction and compulsive eating in obese rats. Nat Neurosci. 2010;13:635–41.

14. Martire SI, Holmes N, Westbrook RF, Morris MJ. Altered feeding patterns in rats exposed to a palatable cafeteria diet: increased snacking and its implications for development of obesity. PLoS One. 2013;8:e60407.

15. Sampey BP, Vanhoose AM, Winfield HM, Freemerman AJ, Muehlbauer MJ, Fueger PT, Newgard CB, Makowski L. Cafeteria diet is a robust model of human metabolic syndrome with liver and adipose inflammation: comparison to high-fat diet. Obesity. 2011;19:1109–17.

16. Aviram A, Hod M, Yogev Y. Maternal obesity: implications for pregnancy outcome and long-term risks-a link to maternal nutrition. Int J Gynaecol Obstet. 2011;115(Suppl 1):S6–10.

17. Akyol A, Langley-Evans SC, McMullen S. Obesity induced by cafeteria feeding and pregnancy outcome in the rat. Br J Nutr. 2009;102:1601–10.

18. Akyol A, McMullen S, Langley-Evans SC. Glucose intolerance associated with early-life exposure to maternal cafeteria feeding is dependent upon post-weaning diet. Br J Nutr. 2012;107:964–78.

19. Wright T, Langley-Evans SC, Voigt JP. The impact of maternal cafeteria diet on anxiety-related behaviour and exploration in the offspring. Physiol Behav. 2011;103:164–72.

20. Nivoit P, Morens C, Van Assche F, Jansen E, Poston L, Remacle C, Reusens B. Established diet-induced obesity in female rats leads to offspring hyperphagia, adiposity and insulin resistance. Diabetologia. 2009;52:1133–42.

21. Gugusheff JR, Ong ZY, Muhlhausler BS. A maternal "junk-food" diet reduces sensitivity to the opioid antagonist naloxone in offspring postweaning. FASEB J. 2013;27:1275–84.

22. Ong ZY, Muhlhausler BS. Consuming a low-fat diet from weaning to adulthood reverses the programming of food preferences in male, but not female, offspring of 'junk food'-fed rat dams. Acta Physiol. 2013;210:127–41.

23. Akyol A, McMullen S, Langley-Evans SC. Glucose intolerance associated with early-life exposure to maternal cafeteria feeding is dependent upon post-weaning diet. Br J Nutr. 2012;107: 964–78.

24. Kirk SL, Samuelsson A-M, Argenton M, Dhonye H, Kalamatianos T, Poston L, Taylor PD, Coen CW. Maternal obesity induced by diet in rats permanently influences central processes regulating food intake in offspring. PLoS One. 2009;4:e5870.

25. Bayol SA, Farrington SJ, Stickland NC. A maternal "junk food" diet in pregnancy and lactation promotes an exacerbated taste for "junk food" and a greater propensity for obesity in rat offspring. Br J Nutr. 2007;98:843–51.

26. Férézou-Viala J, Roy AF, Sérougne C, Gripois D, Parquet M, Bailleux V, Gertler A, Delplanque B, Djiane J, Riottot M. Long-term consequences of maternal high-fat feeding on hypothalamic leptin sensitivity and diet-induced obesity in the offspring. Am J Phys Regul Integr Comp Phys. 2007;293:R1056.

27. Donath S, Amir L. Does maternal obesity adversely affect breastfeeding initiation and duration? J Paediatr Child Health. 2000;36:482–6.

28. Hilson JA, Rasmussen KM, Kjolhede CL. High prepregnant body mass index is associated with poor lactation outcomes among white, rural women independent of psychosocial and demographic correlates. J Hum Lact. 2004;20:18–29.

29. Agius L, Rolls B, Rowe E, Williamson D. Impaired lipogenesis in mammary glands of lactating rats fed on a cafeteria diet. Reversal of inhibition of glucose metabolism in vitro by insulin. Biochem J. 1980;186:1005.

30. Connor KL, Vickers MH, Beltrand J, Meaney MJ, Sloboda DM. Nature, nurture or nutrition? Impact of maternal nutrition on maternal care, offspring development and reproductive function. J Physiol. 2012;590:2167–80.

31. Sun B, Purcell RH, Terrillion CE, Yan J, Moran TH, Tamashiro KLK. Maternal high-fat diet during gestation or suckling differentially affects offspring leptin sensitivity and obesity. Diabetes. 2012;61:2833.

32. Bayol SA, Farrington SJ, Stickland NC. A maternal 'junk food' diet in pregnancy and lactation promotes an exacerbated taste for 'junk food' and a greater propensity for obesity in rat offspring. Br J Nutr. 2007;98:843–51.

33. Teegarden SL, Scotta AN, Bale TL. Early life exposure to a high fat diet promotes long-term changes in dietary preferences and central reward signaling. Neuroscience. 2009;162:924–32.

34. Vucetic Z, Kimmel J, Totoki K, Hollenbeck E, Reyes TM. Maternal high-fat diet alters methylation and gene expression of dopamine and opioid-related genes. Endocrinology. 2010;151:4756–64.

35. Gugusheff JR, Vithayathil M, Ong ZY, Muhlhausler BS. The effects of prenatal exposure to a 'junk food' diet on offspring food preferences and fat deposition can be mitigated by improved nutrition during lactation. J Dev Orig Health Dis. 2013.;FirstView:1–10.;4:348–57.

36. Matthews PA, Samuelsson AM, Seed P, Pombo J, Oben JA, Poston L, Taylor PD. Fostering in mice induces cardiovascular and metabolic dysfunction in adulthood. J Physiol. 2011;589:3969–81.

37. Wright TM, Fone KCF, Langley-Evans SC, Voigt J-PW. Exposure to maternal consumption of cafeteria diet during the lactation period programmes feeding behaviour in the rat. Int J Dev Neurosci. 2011;29:785–93.

38. Chang G-Q, Gaysinskaya V, Karatayev O, Leibowitz SF. Maternal high-fat diet and fetal programming: increased proliferation of hypothalamic peptide-producing neurons that increase risk for overeating and obesity. J Neurosci. 2008;28:12107–19.

39. Bayol S, Simbi B, Bertrand J, Stickland N. Offspring from mothers fed a 'junk food'diet in pregnancy and lactation exhibit exacerbated adiposity that is more pronounced in females. J Physiol. 2008;586:3219–30.

40. Martin R, Hausman G, Hausman D: Regulation of adipose cell development in utero. R Soc Med. 1998;219:200–10.

41. Bayol SA, Simbi BH, Bertrand JA, Stickland NC. Offspring from mothers fed a 'junk food' diet in pregnancy and lactation exhibit exacerbated adiposity that is more pronounced in females. J Physiol. 2008;586:3219–30.

42. Muhlhausler BS, Duffield JA, McMillen IC. Increased maternal nutrition stimulates peroxisome proliferator activated receptor-{gamma} (PPAR{gamma}), adiponectin and leptin mRNA expression in adipose tissue before birth. Endocrinology. 2007;148:878–85.

43. Erhuma A, Salter AM, Sculley DV, Langley-Evans SC, Bennett AJ. Prenatal exposure to a low-protein diet programs disordered regulation of lipid metabolism in the aging rat. Am J Physiol Endocrinol Metab. 2007;292:E1702–14.

44. Nestler EJ. Is there a common molecular pathway for addiction? Nat Neurosci. 2005;8:1445–9.

45. Berridge KC. Food reward: brain substrates of wanting and liking. Neurosci Biobehav Rev. 1996;20:1–25.

46. Davis C, Patte K, Levitan R, Reid C, Tweed S, Curtis C. From motivation to behaviour: a model of reward sensitivity, overeating, and food preferences in the risk profile for obesity. Appetite. 2007;48:12–9.

47. Bodnar RJ, Glass MJ, Ragnauth A, Cooper ML. General, [mu] and [kappa] opioid antagonists in the nucleus accumbens alter food intake under deprivation, glucoprivic and palatable conditions. Brain Res. 1995;700:205–12.

48. Bakshi VP, Kelley AE. Feeding induced by opioid stimulation of the ventral striatum: role of opiate receptor subtypes. J Pharmacol Exp Ther. 1993;265:1253–60.

49. Bergevin A, Girardot D, Bourque M-J, Trudeau L-E. Presynaptic [mu]-opioid receptors regulate a late step of the secretory process in rat ventral tegmental area GABAergic neurons. Neuropharmacology. 2002;42:1065–78.

50. Gainetdinov RR, Jones SR, Fumagalli F, Wightman RM, Caron MG. Re-evaluation of the role of the dopamine transporter in dopamine system homeostasis. Brain Res Rev. 1998;26:148–53.

51. Wright TM, Fone KC, Langley-Evans SC, Voigt JP. Exposure to maternal consumption of cafeteria diet during the lactation period programmes feeding behaviour in the rat. Int J Dev Neurosci. 2011;29:785–93.

52. Asarian L, Geary N. Modulation of appetite by gonadal steroid hormones. Philos Trans Royal Soc B: Biol Sci. 2006;361:1251–63.

53. Khan IY, Taylor PD, Dekou V, Seed PT, Lakasing L, Graham D, Dominiczak AF, Hanson MA, Poston L. Gender-linked hypertension in offspring of lard-fed pregnant rats. Hypertension. 2003;41:168–75.

54. Whitaker RC. Predicting preschooler obesity at birth: the role of maternal obesity in early pregnancy. Pediatrics. 2004;114:e29–36.

55. Boney CM, Verma A, Tucker R, Vohr BR. Metabolic syndrome in childhood: association with birth weight, maternal obesity, and gestational diabetes mellitus. Pediatrics. 2005;115:e290–6.

56. Laitinen J, Power C, Järvelin M-R. Family social class, maternal body mass index, childhood body mass index, and age at menarche as predictors of adult obesity. Am J Clin Nutr. 2001;74:287–94.

57. Brion M-JA, Ness AR, Rogers I, Emmett P, Cribb V, Davey Smith G, Lawlor DA. Maternal macronutrient and energy intakes in pregnancy and offspring intake at 10 y: exploring parental comparisons and prenatal effects. Am J Clin Nutr. 2010;91:748–56.

58. Wardle J, Guthrie C, Sanderson S, Birch L, Plomin R. Food and activity preferences in children of lean and obese parents. Int J Obes. 2001;25:971–7.

59. McMillen IC, Rattanatray L, Duffield JA, Morrison JL, MacLaughlin SM, Gentili S, Muhlhausler BS. The early origins of later obesity: pathways and mechanisms. In: Kolatzko B, Decsi T, Molnar D, DeLaHunty A, editors. Early nutrition programming and health outcomes in later life: obesity and beyond, Advances in Experimental Medicine and Biology. Springer, Dordrecht vol. 646; 2009, p. 71–81.

60. Ong ZY, Gugusheff JR, Muhlhausler BS. Perinatal overnutrition and the programming of food preferences: pathways and mechanisms. J Dev Orig Health Dis. 2012;3:299–308.

Part IV
Specific Dietary Components

Chapter 19
Maternal Fish Intake During Pregnancy and Effects on the Offspring

Leda Chatzi and Nikos Stratakis

Key Points

- Fish is the primary dietary source of n-3 long-chain polyunsaturated fatty acids and a rich source of other beneficial nutrients such as selenium, iodine, and vitamin D.
- Fish is also a common route of exposure to environmental contaminants such as methylmercury, polychlorinated biphenyls, and dioxins.
- In utero exposure to nutrients and toxicants found in the same fish might act on the exact same end points at an opposite direction.
- The overall effect of fish consumption during pregnancy on child health outcomes, incorporating the risks as well as the benefits, remains uncertain.
- To usefully inform policy, it is essential that future studies of maternal fish consumption assess and carefully account for fetal exposure to contaminants.

Keywords Fish • Pregnancy • N-3 fatty acids • Methylmercury • Pollutants • Birth weight • Childhood obesity • Asthma • Allergy • Neurodevelopment

Abbreviations

BMI	Body mass index
DHA	Docosahexaenoic acid
EPA	Eicosapentaenoic acid
LCPUFAs	Long-chain polyunsaturated fatty acids

L. Chatzi, MD, PhD (✉)
Keck School of Medicine, Division of Environmental Health, University of Southern California, 2001 North Soto St. 230-07, Los Angeles, California 90032, USA

Department of Social Medicine, Faculty of Medicine, University of Crete, Heraklion, Crete, Greece

Department of Genetics & Cell Biology Faculty of Health, Medicine and Life Sciences Maastricht University, The Netherlands
e-mail: chatzi@usc.edu

N. Stratakis, MSc
NUTRIM School of Nutrition and Translational Research in Metabolism, Faculty of Health, Medicine and Life Sciences, Maastricht University Medical Centre, Maastricht, The Netherlands

© Springer International Publishing AG 2017
R. Rajendram et al. (eds.), *Diet, Nutrition, and Fetal Programming*,
Nutrition and Health, DOI 10.1007/978-3-319-60289-9_19

MeHg	Methylmercury
PCBs	Polychlorinated biphenyls
SGA	Small for gestational age

Introduction

Intrauterine life is a critical period of developmental plasticity. A nutritional stress or stimulus encountered during this period could elicit permanent alterations in body physiology and metabolism that have important long-term consequences for later health and disease susceptibility [1]. In this context, fish constitutes a complex exposure. It is a rich source of protein, selenium, iodine, and vitamin D and the primary dietary source of the n-3 long-chain polyunsaturated fatty acids (LCPUFAs), including eicosapentaenoic acid (EPA) and docosahexaenoic acid (DHA), which are considered beneficial for growth and development [2]. In contrast, fish is also a well-known route of exposure to pollutants such as methylmercury (MeHg), polychlorinated biphenyls (PCBs), and dioxins, which may adversely affect child development [3].

Hence, the effect of fish intake by pregnant women remains an important issue, especially in populations that consume fish frequently. In June 2014, the US Food and Drug Administration (FDA) and Environmental Protection Agency updated their advice on fish consumption for women of childbearing age, encouraging women who are pregnant, breastfeeding, or likely to become pregnant to consume more fish, but no more than three servings per week to limit fetal exposure to MeHg [4]. The European Food Safety Authority (EFSA) has also reported recently that the benefits from fish consumption of up to three to four servings per week during pregnancy could outweigh the risks associated with MeHg exposure [5]. Fish advisories have focused so far on potential neurocognitive harms from MeHg exposure but have not considered other childhood outcomes including growth and asthma occurrence. Furthermore, pregnant women are faced with conflicting messages about the health effects of fish consumption, which result in confusion concerning the place of fish in a healthy prenatal diet.

We aimed in this chapter to examine the association of fish intake during pregnancy with offspring health outcomes, including fetal growth and preterm birth, childhood obesity, neurodevelopment, and allergic diseases.

Fish, Fetal Growth, and Preterm Birth

The failure of the fetus to reach its full growth potential is an important predictor of short- and long-term health. Growth-restricted fetuses are at increased risk of infant mortality and morbidity [6] and have a higher risk of developing chronic diseases in adulthood, such type 2 diabetes and coronary heart disease [7, 8]. Anthropometric measurements at birth (i.e., birth weight, birth length, and head circumference) and the index small for gestational age (SGA; defined as a neonate whose birth size is below the tenth percentile for a given reference growth chart for sex and gestational age) are widely used to assess fetal growth. Preterm birth, defined as a gestational age of less than 37 completed weeks, is an established risk factor for later morbidity and mortality [9].

Early observations showing that gestation length and birth weight are increased among populations with a high habitual fish intake [10] generated a lot of interest in the scientific literature regarding the association of fish intake during pregnancy with fetal growth. It has been hypothesized that the n-3 LCUFAs found in fish can prolong gestation by decreasing the production of eicosanoids that play a role in the initiation of delivery and increasing the production for prostacyclins (PGI_2 and PGI_3) that exert myometrial relaxant properties [11]. n-3 LCPUFAs can also increase fetal growth rate by raising the prostacyclin-to-thromboxane ratio and reducing blood viscosity, thereby enhancing placental blood flow [12]. However, reports from human trials have not shown a clear and consistent benefit of fish oil supplementation in birth weight and duration of gestation [13, 14].

To date, several observational cohort studies have been conducted to assess the association of pre-natal fish intake with measures of fetal growth and have produced puzzling results (Table 19.1). In the British Avon Longitudinal Study of Parents and Children (ALSPAC) of 11,585 mother and child pairs, women consuming rarely fish in late pregnancy had an increased risk of intrauterine growth retarda-tion (defined as birth weight adjusted for sex and gestational age below the tenth percentile) compared with those with a mean consumption of four portions per week [15]. Similarly, the Danish Aarhus Birth Cohort involving 8729 mother-child pairs showed that low consumption of fish in early preg-nancy was a strong risk factor for low birth weight and preterm delivery, with the strongest associa-tions being observed at a daily intake of less than 15 g of fish [16]. In seemingly contrast to these results, Oken et al. [17], using data from 2109 mother-child pairs of the US Project Viva birth cohort, reported an inverse association of first-trimester seafood consumption with birth weight and fetal growth, while no effect was found on the length of gestation or risk of preterm birth.

In the Danish National Birth Cohort (DNBC) including 44,824 mother-child pairs, Halldorsson et al. [18] examined the separate effects of the types of fish consumed in midpregnancy and showed that fatty fish intake more than four times per month was associated with a higher risk of giving birth to children who were SGA, while no association was found for lean fish. By way of contrast, Brantsæter et al. [19], in the Norwegian Mother and Child Cohort Study (MoBa) including 62,099 mother-child pairs, showed that increasing midpregnancy seafood consumption was associated with increased birth weight and head circumference. This positive association was mainly driven by con-sumption of lean fish, while fatty fish was not associated with any birth size measures [19]. Ramon et al. [20] used data from a Spanish cohort of 554 mother-child pairs to assess associations of the type of fish consumed, cord blood mercury levels, and birth outcomes. As anticipated, higher fish con-sumption in pregnancy was associated with higher cord blood mercury levels. The authors showed that after adjusting for prenatal exposure to mercury, weekly consumption of more than two portions of lean fish and canned tuna consumption was associated with a lower risk of being born SGA, while large oily fish consumption was associated with a higher risk [20]. The differential influence by dif-ferent types of seafood on fetal growth might be indirect evidence of harmful contaminants found in fish [21]. MeHg can inhibit the antioxidant systems and stimulate the production of free radicals, which in turn can adversely affect fetal growth [20]. Many studies, but not all, have reported associa-tions of higher prenatal concentrations of mercury with reduced birth weight and an increased risk of SGA (reviewed in [22]). Additionally, persistent organic pollutants commonly found in fish, such as PCBs, can exert endocrine-disrupting properties and affect fetal growth through effects on sex steroid and thyroid hormone function [23]. In the DNBC, intake of fatty fish was associated with levels of PCBs in maternal plasma, and exposure to these pollutants was found to be inversely associated with low birth weight [24]. Several other studies [23, 25], but not all [26, 27], have also reported an associa-tion between exposure to persistent organic pollutants and low birth weight.

Because the balance between the potential beneficial effect of n-3 LCPUFAs and deleterious effect of contaminants in fish intake is determined by the relative exposure, results may differ across popula-tions consuming different types of seafood.

Direct comparison between individual studies is also complicated by small sample sizes, exposure misclassification, exposure profile heterogeneity, or differences in adjustment for confounding variables.

In an effort to assess the strength and consistency of the association of fish intake during pregnancy with fetal growth, a Europe-wide study harmonized and pooled individual data from 151,880 mother-child pairs participating in 19 birth cohort studies [28]. The study showed that, compared to fish consumption of less than one time per week, moderate intake of more than one time per week was

Table 19.1 Summary of prospective studies on fish intake during pregnancy in association with fetal growth and preterm birth

Authors, year	Country; number of participants	Maternal exposure during pregnancy	Outcomes	Results
Brantsæter et al. (2012) [19]	Norway; *n* = 62,099	Total fish, fatty fish, lean fish, and shellfish intake. Intakes of total fish and different fish types were treated as continuous variables (in g/day). Total fish intake was also divided as 0–5, >5–20, >20–40, >40–60, and >60 g/day	Birth weight, length, and head circumference	Total fish intake was positively associated with birth weight (P trend = <0.001) and head circumference (P trend = <0.001). Lean fish was positively associated with all birth size measures; shellfish was positively associated with birth weight, while fatty fish was not associated with any birth size measures
Halldorsson et al. (2007) [18]	Denmark; *n* = 44,824	Total fish, fatty fish, and lean fish intake in midpregnancy. Total fish intake was divided as 0–5, >5–20, >20–40, >40–60, and >60 g/day and lean and fatty fish intake as 0, 1, 2–3, and ≥4 meals/month	Birth weight, birth length, head circumference, gestational age, and SGA (defined as infants whose z scores, standardized for gestational age and gender, for birth weight, birth length, and head circumference were below the tenth percentile of growth reference curves)	Fish consumption >60 g/day, as compared with women who consumed 0–5 g/day, was associated with an increased risk of giving birth to SGA newborns for birth weight (OR 1.24, 95% CI 1.03–1.49), for head circumference (OR 1.21, 95% CI 1.01–1.43), and for birth length (OR 1.20, 95% CI 1.00–1.45). The inverse association for total fish consumption could be explained by consumption of fatty fish, while no association was found for lean fish
Leventakou et al. (2014) [28]	Multicenter; *n* = 151,880	Total fish, fatty fish, lean fish, and shellfish consumption. Intakes of total fish and different fish types were treated as continuous variables (in times/week). Total fish intake was also divided as ≤1, >1–<3, and ≥3 times/week	Birth weight, birth length, head circumference, gestational age, and SGA for weight, length, or head circumference (defined as a neonate being below the tenth percentile of the cohort-specific growth curve stratified by gestational length and sex)	Consumption of fish >1 time/week during pregnancy was associated with lower risk of preterm birth, as compared with intake ≤1 time/week; the RR of fish intake >1–<3 times/week was 0.87 (95% CI 0.82–0.92), and for intake ≥3 times/week, the adjusted RR was 0.89 (95% CI 0.84–0.96). Higher fish intake was also associated with a higher birth weight by 8.9 g (95% CI 3.3–14.6) for >1–<3 times/week and 15.2 g (95% CI 8.9–21.5 g) for ≥3 times/week. Increased fatty fish intake was associated with higher birth weight, while lean and shellfish were not associated with any outcome

Oken et al. (2004) [17]	US; n = 2109	Total fish intake in first and second trimester. One group of women with less than one serving of seafood/month, while the remaining participants were divided into tertiles of monthly fish consumption	Birth weight, birth-weight-for-gestational-age z value (fetal growth), length of gestation, and SGA (defined as birth weight below the tenth percentile of a standard US reference group for sex and gestational age)	There was an inverse association of first-trimester fish intake with birth weight (P trend = 0.05) and fetal growth (P trend = 0.02). No associations were found for fish consumption in the second trimester of pregnancy
Olsen and Secher (2002) [16]	Denmark; n = 8729	Total fish consumption in early pregnancy; four categories with mean daily intakes of 0, 3.1, 12.4, and 44.3 g, respectively	Preterm delivery, low birth weight, and IUGR (defined as below the tenth centile and birth weight expected from gestational age from the infant's birth weight, gestational age, and sex, on the basis of a Danish standard)	The OR for preterm delivery was 3.6 (95% CI 1.2–11.2) in the zero consumption group compared with the highest consumption group. Estimates for low birth weight were similar to those for preterm delivery. No association was found with IUGR
Ramon et al. (2009) [20]	Spain; n = 554	Canned tuna, lean fish, and oily fish intake during the second and part of the third trimester, up to 28–32 weeks; four categories: <1 portion/month, 1–3 portions/month, 1 portion/week, and ≥2 portions/week	Birth weight, birth length, and SGA (defined as birth weight and length below the tenth percentile according to Spanish population reference growth charts for sex and gestational age)	After adjustment for prenatal mercury exposure, consumption of ≥2 portions of canned tuna per week was associated with higher birth weight (P for trend = 0.03) and a lower risk of being born SGA for weight (P for trend = 0.01). Compared with consumption of <1 portion/month, consumption of ≥2 portions of oily fish per week was associated with a higher risk of SGA for weight (OR 4.6, 95% CI 1.4–15.4) and consumption of lean fish with a lower risk of SGA for length (OR 0.1, 95% CI 0.0–0.6)
Rogers et al. (2004) [15]	England; n = 11,585	Total fish consumption in late pregnancy; four categories with mean weekly intakes of 0, 0.74, 2.29, and 4.44 portions, respectively	Low birth weight, preterm delivery, and IUGR (defined as a birth weight for gestational age and sex below the tenth centile of the cohort-specific reference curve)	The frequency of IUGR decreased with increasing fish intake—the OR (95% CI) of IUGR in those eating no fish was 1.37 (1.02–1.84) compared with those in the highest fish intake group

Abbreviations: CI confidence interval, *IUGR* intrauterine growth retardation, *OR* odds ratio, *RR* relative risk, and *SGA* small for gestational age

associated with a lower risk of preterm birth and a small but significant increase in birth weight (Fig. 19.1). The most pronounced effect on birth weight was observed for fatty fish types, while no association was observed with lean fish or shellfish intake. Notably, the protective effect of fish intake on preterm birth was shown only in the categorical analysis and not in the continuous analysis, suggesting that for very high amounts of fish intake, the protective effect is attenuated (U-shaped association) [28].

Further analyses using biomarker information on both the amounts of fatty acids and environmental chemicals contained within fish will be helpful for refining estimates of the influence of prenatal fish intake on fetal growth.

Fish and Childhood Obesity

Childhood overweight and obesity is considered a major public health issue [29]. Evidence suggests that a high body mass index (BMI), used as a surrogate measure of excess adiposity, in childhood tends to track into adulthood [30]. It has been argued that efforts to prevent obesity should begin early in life and even before birth [31].

Intrauterine life is a critical period, during which the proliferation of mesenchymal precursor cells and their differentiation into adipocytes are highly sensitive to alterations of the nutritional environment [32]. Evidence from in vitro and animal studies suggests that early exposure to n-3 LCPUFAs has the potential to reduce adipose tissue deposition by inhibiting adipocyte formation [33].

Few human trials have been conducted to date to assess the effect of fish oil supplementation in early life on body composition later in life and have shown limited support for a benefit [34]. Likewise, birth cohort studies on early n-3 LCPUFA exposure and later adiposity have produced discrepant results [35, 36]. Table 19.2 provides an overview of prospective studies assessing fish intake during pregnancy and child somatic growth. In the Project Viva cohort, Donahue et al. [35] demonstrated that higher midpregnancy fish intake was associated with lower odds of obesity at age 3. In contrast, the Dutch Prevention and Incidence of Asthma and Mite Allergy (PIAMA) birth cohort study failed to find an effect of maternal fish consumption on child BMI values from birth up to 14 years of age [37]. Reasons for the divergent results may be small sample sizes, exposure heterogeneity, or differences in adjustment.

Recently, we harmonized and pooled individual data of repeated follow-ups until the age of 6 years from 26,184 pregnant women and their children participating in 15 European and US cohort studies to assess the strength and consistency of the associations of fish intake during pregnancy with BMI growth trajectories and the risk of childhood overweight and obesity [38]. We found that children of mothers consuming fish more than three times a week during pregnancy exhibited consistently higher BMI values from infancy up to age 6 than did those of mothers with an intake of less than one time a week (Fig. 19.2) . High fish intake during pregnancy was also associated with an increased risk of rapid infant growth from birth to 2 years and increased risk of offspring overweight or obesity at 4 years and 6 years of age. Results indicated a non-detrimental effect of fish consumption of more than one time but less than three times per week on childhood somatic growth [38].

Contamination by environmental pollutants in fish could provide an explanation for the association between high fish intake in pregnancy and increased childhood adiposity. Mixtures of organochlorine pesticides, PCBs, and dioxins found in fish have been shown to increase fat storage in cultured adipocytes, as well as weight gain in animals [39]. It has been proposed that these toxicants may perturb signaling of several nuclear receptors and, through altered gene expression, influence adipocyte differentiation and fat metabolism [40]. Many cohort studies [41], but not all [42], have shown that exposure to these pollutants during the intrauterine period is associated with an increased risk of childhood overweight or obesity.

| Cohort | ≤1 times/week | Fish intake during pregnancy | | ≥3 times/week | |
| | N | 1<times/week<3 | | | |
		β (95% CI)	N	β (95% CI)	N
ABCD, NL	4309	2.14 (-18.60, 22.87)	2783	-13.40 (-49.62, 22.83)	627
DNBC, DK	13232	12.82 (-3.75, 21.89)	27642	20.85 (10.86, 30.84)	17047
EDEN, FR	684	-2.38 (-41.81, 37.05)	783	-13.77 (-65.83, 38.29)	298
GASPII, IT	58	-30.62 (-140.34, 79.10)	317	19.89 (-98.62, 138.40)	161
HUMIS, NO	382	55.45 (-0.30, 111.19)	923	44.03 (-30.18, 118.24)	250
INMA, ES	127	16.30 (-59.00, 91.61)	392	-2.89 (-70.90, 65.12)	1776
KOALA, NL	1420	-2.62 (-34.42, 29.17)	1151	-14.79 (-86.27, 56.68)	136
Lifeways, IR	505	51.37 (-47.39, 150.13)	96	1.62 (-120.74, 123.98)	61
LucKi, NL	336	5.65 (-75.82, 87.13)	169	56.51 (-89.56, 202.57)	38
MoBa, NO	13935	7.94 (-0.89, 16.76)	24709	14.74 (5.53, 23.95)	20282
NINFEA, IT	894	-11.02 (-45.36, 23.32)	1093	-15.88 (-72.62, 40.85)	226
REPRO_PL, PL	342	18.65 (-46.40, 83.70)	289	41.79 (-24.50, 108.08)	271
SWS, UK	870	6.08 (-30.32, 42.49)	1017	-3.77 (-43.63, 36.09)	709
All subjects	37094	**Overall estimate** 8.93 (3.31, 14.56) p-heter = 0.835 $I^2 = 0.0\%$	61364	**Overall estimate** 15.2 (8.86, 21.54) p-heter = 0.672 $I^2 = 0.0\%$	41882

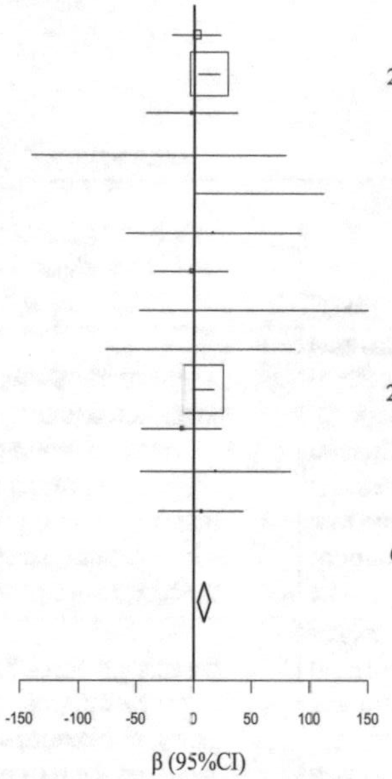

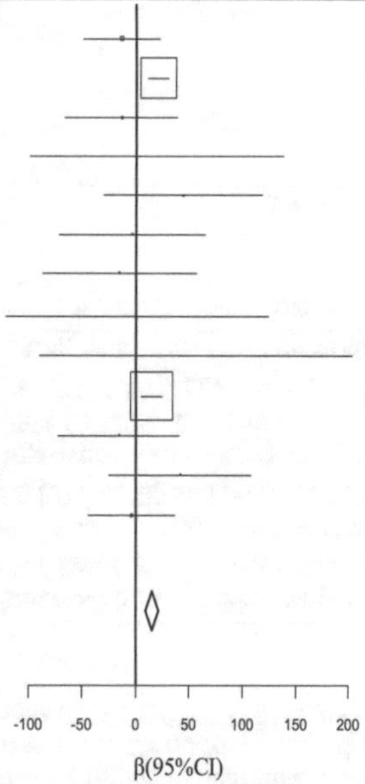

Fig. 19.1 Fish intake during pregnancy and birth weight: a meta-analysis of 19 European birth cohort studies. β coefficients (95% CIs) by cohort were obtained by using linear regression models adjusted for maternal age, prepregnancy BMI, maternal height, education level, smoking during pregnancy, parity, infant sex, gestational age, and gestational age squared. Reference category was ≤1 time/week. Overall estimates were obtained by using a random- or fixed-effects meta-analysis. p-heter values were estimated by using Cochran's Q test. *ABCD* Amsterdam Born Children and their Development study, *DK* Denmark, *DNBC* Danish National Birth Cohort, *EDEN* study on the pre- and early postnatal determinants of child health and development, *ES* Spain, *FR* France, *GASPII* Genetic and Environment: Prospective Study on Infancy in Italy, *HUMIS* Norwegian Human Milk Study, *INMA* Infancia y Medio Ambiente—Environment and Childhood Project, *IR* Ireland, *IT* Italy, *KOALA* Kind, Ouders en gezondheid: Aandacht voor Leefstijl en Aanleg Birth Cohort Study, *Lifeways* Lifeways Cross-Generation Cohort Study, *LucKi* Luchtwegklachten bij Kinderen Cohort Study, *MoBa* Norwegian Mother and Child Cohort Study, *NINFEA* Nascita e INFanzia: gli Effetti dell'Ambiente, *NL* Netherlands, *NO* Norway, *p-heter* P-heterogeneity, *PL* Poland, *REPRO-PL* Polish Mother and Child Cohort Study, *SWS* Southampton Women's Survey, *UK* United Kingdom (Reproduced with permission from Leventakou et al. [28], American Society for Nutrition)

Table 19.2 Summary of prospective studies on fish intake during pregnancy in association with child growth and adiposity

Authors, year	Country; number of participants	Maternal exposure during pregnancy	Outcomes	Results
Donahue et al. (2011) [35]	US; $n = 1120$	Total fish intake in mid- and late pregnancy. Fish intake expressed as continuous in servings/week and in two categories: ≤ 2 and >2 servings/week	BMI z score and obesity (defined as BMI $\geq$95th percentile of a standard US reference group for age and sex) at age 3	Higher midpregnancy fish intake was associated with lower risk for obesity; the OR per serving/week was 0.77 (95% CI 0.62–0.95)
Stratakis et al. (2016) [38]	Multicenter; $n = 26,184$	Total fish, fatty fish, lean fish, and shellfish consumption. Intakes of total fish and different fish types were treated as continuous variables (in times/week). Total fish intake was also divided as ≤ 1, >1–≤ 3, and >3 times/week	Rapid infant growth (defined as a z score change in weight >0.67) and BMI z scores and overweight/obesity (defined as BMI $\geq$85th percentile of WHO reference curves for age and sex) up to age 6	Fish intake >3 times/week, compared with an intake $\leq$1 time/week, was associated with increased risk of rapid infant growth (OR 1.22, 95% CI 1.05–1.42) and increased risk of offspring overweight/obesity at 4 years (OR, 1.14, 95% CI 0.99–1.32) and 6 years (OR 1.22, 95% CI 1.01–1.47). The effect of high fish intake during pregnancy was more pronounced in girls
van den Berg et al. (2015) [37]	Netherlands; $n = 3684$	Total fish intake in late pregnancy; three categories: never, 1–3 times/month, and >1 time/week	BMI z scores up to age 14	No overall association was found

Abbreviations: BMI body mass index, *CI* confidence interval, and *OR* odds ratio

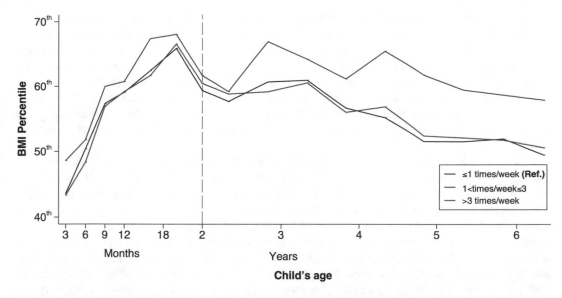

Fig. 19.2 Body mass index (BMI) percentile trajectories from 3 months to 6 years according to different levels of fish intake in pregnancy: a pooled analysis of 15 European and US birth cohort studies. BMI percentile values indicate the place of children in the corresponding growth chart of the WHO reference population and were derived by using mixed-effects linear regression models fitted with fish intake, an interaction term for fish intake and child age, maternal age, maternal education, prepregnancy BMI, smoking during pregnancy, and birth weight as fixed-effects parameters; random cohort and child intercepts; and a random slope for child age (Reproduced with permission from Stratakis et al. [38])

Notably, none of the studies of maternal fish intake controlled for, or took into account, related exposure to persistent organic pollutants. Hence, the hypothesis that contaminants contained with fish may play a role in the influence of prenatal fish intake on later somatic growth remains speculative. Further studies that use direct measurements of fat mass and incorporate biomarker information on both the amounts of fatty acids and environmental chemicals potentially contained within fish will contribute to a clearer picture of the influence of fish intake during pregnancy on child growth.

Fish and Neurodevelopment in Childhood

The effect of prenatal nutrition on later brain and cognitive development is receiving increasing attention. Most of the scientific literature regarding fish consumption during pregnancy and later neurodevelopment has placed emphasis on the opposing neurodevelopmental effects of n-3 LCPUFAs and MeHg contained within fish.

n-3 LCPUFAs, especially DHA, are important components of neural membranes and have several influences on brain development [43]. They seem to affect membrane fluidity and speed of signal transmission, gene expression, and neurogenesis [44]. Accumulation of DHA in the human brain starts in utero, with marked deposition occurring in the later part of gestation when the brain undergoes a period of rapid growth [45]. Hence, it has been hypothesized that increasing n-3 LCPUFA intake during pregnancy can benefit neurodevelopment of the offspring. Systematic reviews of randomized controlled trials have concluded that the evidence does not support or refute the hypothesis that n-3 LCPUFA supplementation in pregnancy improves child cognitive or visual development (reviewed in [46, 47]).

Animal studies have shown that ingested MeHg can cross the placenta and blood-brain barrier [48] and exert neurotoxic effects by promoting the production of free radicals and inhibiting antioxidant mechanisms through binding to thiol-containing molecules [49]. Reports from prospective studies of prenatal mercury exposure and neurodevelopment in infants are mixed, whereas, for older children, there has been a more consistent association with adverse neurodevelopmental outcomes (reviewed in [22]).

In terms of fish consumption, a dilemma arises of whether the potential beneficial effects of n-3 LCPUFAs on child neurocognitive development can counteract or outweigh the neurotoxic effects of MeHg. Several observational cohort studies have attempted to understand this benefit-risk trade-off (Table 19.3).

Few studies have assessed the association of prenatal fish intake with cognitive development in infancy, and they all showed positive results. In the DNBC, Oken et al. [50] showed that higher fish consumption in midpregnancy was associated with increased scores of motor, social, and cognitive developmental milestones at 6 and 18 months of age. Similarly, the Project Viva cohort study found that greater fish consumption during the second trimester of pregnancy was associated with higher infant scores on the visual recognition memory test (an assessment of visual memory that is correlated with later IQ) at 6 months of age [51]. Additional adjustment for mercury levels strengthened the beneficial association of fish consumption with infant cognition [51]. In the ALSPAC cohort, Daniels et al. [52] showed that fish consumption of more than one serving per week in pregnancy had modest but significant improvements in developmental scores of the offspring for language and communication skills at 15 and 18 months of age. This association remained but was not strengthened when additional adjustment was made for cord blood mercury levels [52].

Several studies have evaluated the effect of fish intake during pregnancy on various measures of cognitive performance in later childhood. Oken et al. [53], in a follow-up of the Project Viva cohort at 3 years, showed that second-trimester fish intake of more than twice a week was associated with higher scores on tests of language and visual motor skills, with further adjustment for maternal erythrocyte mercury levels strengthening the estimates of the benefits. Similarly, four other studies reported an association of higher maternal fish intake with higher neurodevelopmental scores [54–56] and a lower risk for attention-deficit/hyperactivity disorder-related behaviors in childhood [57]. In three studies, moderate levels of fish intake during pregnancy were associated with improved child neurocognitive function, while a dilution of this benefit was observed at the highest intake levels [58–60].

To date, several observational cohort studies suggest that fish consumption during pregnancy can confer a neurodevelopmental benefit in the offspring. In some studies, there was a light attenuation of this benefit at the highest levels of fish consumption, which may be indicative of a counterbalancing association due to the potential harm of related contaminants. Findings from studies using biomarker information also indicate that women should avoid fish most highly contaminated with MeHg to gain the greatest possible benefit.

Fish and Allergic Diseases in Childhood

Black and Sharpe hypothesized that the observed increase in the prevalence of allergic disease in Western countries over the last decades has been preceded and then paralleled with a shift in the consumption of fatty acids toward a lower intake of n-3 LCPUFAs and fish and an increased intake of vegetable oils containing n-6 fatty acids [61]. In support of this hypothesis, animal and in vitro studies have shown that n-3 LCPUFAs can exert anti-inflammatory properties and modulate immune responses [62]. Intrauterine life is a critical period for the development of the immune system; hence, the role of prenatal n-3 LCPUFA and fish intakes in the etiology of allergic diseases has gained considerable interest [62]. Many intervention studies, but not all, suggest a beneficial effect of fish oil supplementation during pregnancy on the incidence of allergic disease symptoms in childhood

Table 19.3 Summary of prospective studies on fish intake during pregnancy in association with child neurodevelopment

Authors, year	Country; number of participants	Maternal exposure during pregnancy	Outcomes	Results
Budtz-Jorgensen et al. (2007) [54]	Faroe Islands; n = 917	Total fish intake; expressed as number of dinners per week	NES2 finger tapping and hand-eye coordination tests and Boston Naming Test at age 7 and NES2-CPT (average reaction time, number of false positives and false negatives), the CATSYS system, NES2 finger tapping test, block design and digit span from the WISC-R and WAIS-R, spatial pan from the WMS-III, Stanford-Binet Copying Test, Boston Naming Test, and California Verbal Learning Test at age 14	Higher fish intake was associated with improved motor function at 7 and 14 years and improved spatial function at 14 years
Daniels et al. (2004) [52]	UK; n = 7421	Total fish intake; four categories: rarely or never, once per 2 weeks, 1–3 times/week, and ≥4 times/week	MCDI at 15 months and ALSPAC-adapted DDST at 18 months	Higher fish intake was associated with higher mean developmental scores. The adjusted mean MCDI comprehension scores for children whose mothers consumed fish ≥4 times/week was 72 (95% CI 71–74), compared with 68 (95% CI 66–71) among those whose mothers did not consume fish
Gale et al. (2008) [58]	UK; n = 217	Total fish and oily fish intake in early and late pregnancy. Intake of total fish was divided as 0, <1, 1–2, and ≥3 times/week and oily fish as 0, <1, and ≥1 time/week	SDQ and WASI at age 9	Consumption of fish (whether oily or non-oily) in late pregnancy up to 2 times/week, but not greater, was associated with a higher full scale IQ. Consumption of oily fish <1 time/week (whether in early or late pregnancy) was associated with reduced risk of child hyperactivity
Hibbeln et al. (2007) [55]	UK; n = 8801	Total fish intake in late pregnancy; three categories: none, 1–340, and >340 g/week	ALSPAC-adapted DDST at 6, 18, 30, and 42 months of age, SDQ at 81 months, IQ scores from the WISC-III at 8 years	For each outcome, the lower the intake of fish, the higher the risk of suboptimum development

(continued)

Table 19.3 (continued)

Authors, year	Country; number of participants	Maternal exposure during pregnancy	Outcomes	Results
Julvez et al. (2016) [59]	Spain; n = 1892	Total fish, fatty fish, lean fish, and shellfish intake in first trimester. Median intakes in specific quantiles, in g/week: total seafood, Q1, 195; Q2, 338; Q3, 461; Q4, 600; and Q5, 854; large fatty fish, Q1, none; Q2, 48; Q3, 92; and Q4, 238; small fatty fish, Q1, none; Q2, 37; Q3, 69; and Q4, 147; lean fish, Q1, 90; Q2, 192; Q3, 286; Q4, 382; and Q5, 557; and shellfish, Q1, none; Q2, 27; Q3, 49; Q4, 76; and Q5, 139	BSID at 14 months and MCSA and the Childhood Asperger Syndrome Test at 5 years	There were positive associations between fish consumption during pregnancy and child neuropsychological scores, particularly at 5 years. Intake of small fatty fish explained part of the positive associations at 14 months of age, and lean and large fatty fish were the main predictors of child neuropsychological function at age 5. A dilution of the associations was observed at the highest fish intake levels
Lederman et al. (2008) [56]	US; n = 329	Total fish intake; two categories: non-fish and fish eaters	MDI and PDI scores from the BSID-II at 1, 2, and 3 years and performance, verbal, and full IQ scores from the WPPSI-R at 4 years	Fish consumption was associated with increases in 3-year PDI, and 4-year verbal and full IQ scores, after controlling for cord blood mercury
Mendez et al. (2009) [60]	Spain; n = 392	Total fish intake; four categories: ≤1, >1–2, >2–3, and >3 times/week	MCSA at 4 years	Among children breastfed for <6 months, maternal fish intake of >2–3 times/week, but not greater, was associated with significantly higher scores on several MCSA subscales compared with intakes ≤1 time/week. There was no association among children breastfed for longer periods
Oken et al. (2005) [51]	US; n = 135	Total fish intake in second trimester; expressed in number of weekly servings (range, 0–5.5 servings/week)	Visual recognition memory at 6 months	Higher fish intake was associated with higher infant cognition. This association strengthened after adjustment for maternal hair mercury level; each additional weekly fish serving increased visual recognition memory score by 4.0 points (95% CI 1.3–6.7)

Oken et al. (2008) [50]	Denmark; n = 25,446	Total fish intake in midpregnancy. Median intakes in specific quantiles, in g/day: Q1, 5.9; Q2, 14.5; Q3, 22.2; Q4, 32.2; and Q5, 50.8	Milestones of motor, social, or cognitive and total development at 6 and 18 months	Higher maternal fish was associated with higher developmental score at 18 months; for the highest (50.8 g/day) versus the lowest (5.9 g/day) quintile of intake, the OR for total development was 1.29 (95% CI 1.20–1.38). Associations were similar for development at 6 months
Oken et al. (2008) [53]	US; n = 341	Total fish intake in second trimester; three categories: never, ≤2, and >2 servings/week	PPVT and WRAVMA at 3 years	Higher fish intake was associated with better cognitive performance. After adjustment for maternal erythrocyte mercury levels, the effect estimates for fish intake of >2 servings/week versus never were 2.2 (95% CI 2.6–7.0) for the PPVT and 6.4 (95% CI 2.0–10.8) for the WRAVMA
Sagiv et al. (2012) [57]	US; n = 515	Total fish intake; two categories: ≤2 and >2 servings/week	DSM-IV inattentive, hyperactive-impulsive, and total subscales from the CRS-T, processing speed and freedom from distractibility from the WISC-III, and mean reaction time, reaction time variability, errors of omission, and errors of commission from the NES2-CPT at 8 years	Fish intake >2 serving per week was associated with improved CRS-T outcomes, particularly for DSM-IV impulsivity/hyperactivity (RR for a score greater than the 86th percentile 0.4, 95% CI, 0.2–0.6). After adjusting for maternal hair mercury level, fish consumption was also associated with higher scores for the WISC-III outcomes

Abbreviations: AvLSPAC the Avon Longitudinal Study of Parents and Children, *BSID* Bayley Scales of Infant Development, *CRS-T* Conners Rating Scale—Teachers, *DDST* the Denver Developmental Screening Test, *DSM-IV* Diagnostic and Statistical Manual of Mental Disorders (Fourth Edition), *IQ* intelligence quotient, *MDI* Mental Development Index, *MCDI* the MacArthur Communicative Development Inventory, *MCSA* the McCarthy Scales of Children's Abilities test, *NES2-CPT* the Neurobehavioral Evaluation System 2 Continuous Performance Test, *PDI* Psychomotor Development Index, *PPVT* the Peabody Picture Vocabulary Test, *SDQ* the Strengths and Difficulties Questionnaire, *WAIS-R* the Wechsler Adult Intelligence Scale-Revised, *WASI* the Wechsler Abbreviated Scale of Intelligence, *WISC-R* the Wechsler Intelligence Scale for Children-Revised, *WISC-III* the Wechsler Intelligence Scale for Children III, *WMS-III* the Wechsler Memory Scale III, *WPPSI-R* the Wechsler Preschool and Primary Scale of Intelligence-Revised, and *WRAVMA* the Wide Range Assessment of Visual Motor Abilities (reviewed in [63]). Similarly, findings from birth cohort studies assessing n-3 LCPUFA intake or biomarker levels in pregnancy and childhood allergic disease are discrepant, with reports of either beneficial (i.e., lower incidence) [64, 65] or null [66, 67] associations.

Finding from prospective studies on the association of fish intake during pregnancy and the occurrence of eczema have been discrepant (Table 19.4). A Spanish study showed that increasing fish intake from once per week to 2.5 times per week in pregnancy was associated with a reduced risk of eczema among 12-month-year-old infants [68]. Fish intake of more than one to two times per week in late pregnancy was inversely associated with parent-reported, doctor-diagnosed eczema at 2 years in a German study [69], and fish intake of once or more a week was associated with a decreased risk of doctor-confirmed eczema and currently treated eczema at 5 years in a UK study [70]. In contrast to these results, studies conducted in Norway [71], France [72], and Spain and Greece [73] found no association of maternal fish intake with eczema occurrence. The Generation R study showed a harmful effect of first-trimester fatty fish and shellfish consumption (but not total or lean fish consumption) on eczema occurrence in the first 4 years of life [74]. The authors speculated that potential toxicant contamination in these fish species could provide an explanation for their findings [74].

Three studies have assessed symptoms of childhood allergic rhinitis in association with fish intake in pregnancy (Table 19.4). One UK study found that higher maternal intake of oily fish intake was protective against hay fever at 5 years [70], while two studies conducted in Denmark [75] and Finland [76] found no association. Likewise, results from prospective studies assessing sensitization to inhalant and food allergens have been conflicting (Table 19.4). One Spanish study showed that an increase in maternal fish intake from once per week to 2.5 times per week during pregnancy was protective against sensitization to house dust mite at age 6, while a study in Germany [69] failed to find any effect. A French study showed that pre-parturition shellfish intake, but not total fish intake, at least once a month compared with a lower intake was associated with a higher risk of food allergy before age 2 [72].

Several prospective studies have examined the association of fish intake during pregnancy with the occurrence of wheezing or asthma in childhood and have produced mixed results (Table 19.4). Fish intake of 2.5 times per week or more during pregnancy was associated with a reduced risk of wheezing in school-aged children in two separate Spanish studies [68, 77]. Similarly, the DNBC study showed that children whose mothers never consumed fish in pregnancy were more likely to have a parent report of physician diagnosis of asthma at 18 months and clinically established asthma by the age of 7 years, as compared with those whose mothers consumed fish more than two to three times per week [75]. In contrast, the Generation R study reported an association of first-trimester shellfish consumption, but not total, lean or fatty fish consumption, during pregnancy with wheezing occurrence by the age of 4 years [74]. Other prospective studies conducted in the Netherlands [78], Finland [64, 76], Norway [71], and France [72] failed to find an association of prenatal fish consumption with the occurrence of wheeze or asthma in childhood.

Inconsistencies in the results may be due to inadequate sample sizes, heterogeneity in exposure (e.g., population level of fish consumption), exposure misclassification, or differences in adjustment for confounding variables. Most notably, none of the studies examining the impact of prenatal fish intake on allergic symptoms controlled for prenatal exposure to environmental pollutants. Emerging evidence suggests that persistent organic pollutants potentially contained within fish can exert adverse immunomodulatory effects and increase the risk of developing allergic disease symptoms [79, 80].

Currently, there is conflicting evidence on the association between maternal fish intake during pregnancy and childhood allergic diseases, with reports of beneficial, null, or even harmful effects. Further large-scale epidemiological studies incorporating information on fish-related toxicant exposures are warranted before any conclusions can be drawn regarding the effects of prenatal fish intake on the developing respiratory and immune systems in children.

Table 19.4 Summary of prospective studies on fish intake during pregnancy in association with child asthma and allergic diseases

Authors, year	Country; number of participants	Maternal exposure during pregnancy	Outcomes	Results
Chatzi et al. (2008) [77]	Spain; n = 468	Total fish intake; two categories: ≤2.5 and >2.5 times/week	Parent-reported persistent wheeze at 6.5 years (>1 episode at this age and in preceding years), atopy (based on skin prick test response), and atopic wheeze (defined as current wheeze and atopy) at 6.5 years	Maternal fish intake of >2.5 times/week was inversely associated with persistent wheeze (OR 0.34, 95% CI 0.13–0.84)
Chatzi et al. (2013) [73]	Multicenter; n = 2516	Total fish intake; consumption was divided in tertiles of daily intake	Parent-reported wheeze and doctor-diagnosed eczema up to 1 year	No associations were found
Erkolla et al. (2012) [76]	Finland; n = 2441	Total fish intake; three categories according to quartiles of intake (second and third quartiles were combined): <10.9, 10.9–33.27, and 33.28–254.8 g/day	Parent-reported wheeze, allergic rhinitis, and doctor diagnosis of asthma at 5 years	No associations were found
Leermakers et al. (2013) [74]	Netherlands; n = 2976	Total fish, fatty fish, lean fish, and shellfish intake in first trimester. Total fish consumption was divided as 0, 1–69, 70–139, 140–209, and >210 gr/week; fatty and lean fish consumption as 0, 1–34, 35–69, and >70 gr/week; and shellfish consumption as 0, 1–13, and >14 g/week	Parent-reported wheeze and doctor-diagnosed eczema up to 4 years	Maternal shellfish consumption of 1–13 g/week compared with no intake was associated with overall increased risks of childhood wheezing and eczema (OR 1.20, 95% CI 1.04–1.40, and 1.18, 95% CI 1.01–1.37, respectively). Maternal fatty fish consumption of 35–69 g/week, compared with no intake, was associated with increased overall risks of childhood eczema (OR 1.17, 95% CI 1.00–1.38)
Maslova et al. (2013) [75]	Denmark; n = 28,936	Total fish intake in midpregnancy; five categories: zero intake, monthly or less, more than monthly, weekly at low frequency (<1–2 times), and weekly at high frequency (>2–3 times)	Ever wheeze, recurrent wheeze (>3 episodes), ever asthma and allergic rhinitis, and current asthma, assessed at 18 months and 7 years using parent-reported data of doctor diagnosis and registry data	No fish intake, compared with high frequency of intake, was associated with higher risk of child asthma diagnosis at 18 months (OR 1.30, 95% CI 1.05–1.63), ever admitted asthma (OR 1.46, 95% CI 0.99–2.13), and ever prescribed asthma (OR 1.37, 95% CI 1.10–1.71)
Oien et al. (2010) [71]	Norway; n = 3086	Total fish consumption; two categories: never or <1 and ≥1 time/week	Parent-reported or medical diagnosis of asthma and eczema at 2 years	No associations were found with any outcome

(continued)

Table 19.4 (continued)

Authors, year	Country; number of participants	Maternal exposure during pregnancy	Outcomes	Results
Pele et al. (2013) [72]	France; $n = 1500$	Fish and shellfish intake before pregnancy. Three categories for fish: <1, 1–4, and >4 times/month. Two categories for shellfish: <1 and ≥1 time/month	Parent-reported or medical diagnosis of wheeze, eczema, and food allergy up to 2 years	No associations were found for fish intake. Shellfish intake ≥1 time/month, compared to <1, was associated with a higher risk of food allergy (OR 1.62, 95% CI 1.11–2.37)
Romieu et al. (2007) [68]	Spain; $n = 468$	Total fish consumption; expressed as times/week	Diagnosis of eczema at 1 year, atopy at 4 and 6 years, skin test positivity to HDM, persistent wheeze (wheeze at 6 years and in any preceding years), and atopic wheeze (defined as atopy and wheeze) at 6 years	Fish intake 2.5 times/week, compared to once, was protective against risk of eczema at age 1 (OR 0.73, 95% CI 0.55–0.98). No significant association was found between fish intake and atopy at 4 years. Fish intake 2.5 times/week, compared to once, was protective against skin test positivity to HDM and atopic wheeze (OR 0.68, 95% CI 0.46–1.01, and 0.55, 95% CI 0.31–0.96, respectively) at age 6
Sausenthaler et al. (2007) [69]	Germany; $n = 2641$	Total fish consumption in late pregnancy; two categories: <1 and 1–2 times/week	Doctor-diagnosed eczema and total and specific atopic sensitization at 2 years	High compared with low maternal fish intake was associated with reduced risk of eczema (OR 0.75, 95% CI 0.57–0.98)
Willers et al. (2007) [70]	UK; $n = 1212$	Total and oily fish consumption in late pregnancy; three categories: never, <1, and ≥1 time/week	Parent-reported or medical diagnosis of wheeze, asthma, eczema and hay fever at 5 years, and spirometry, atopic sensitization, bronchodilator response, and exhaled nitric oxide at 5 years	Higher maternal fish was associated with decreased risk of doctor-confirmed eczema (P trend = 0.008) and currently treated eczema (P trend = 0.028). Consumption of oily fish >1 time/week, compared with never, was associated with reduced risk of ever having hay fever (OR 0.37, 95% CI 0.14–0.98)
Willers et al. (2008) [78]	Netherlands; $n = 2832$	Total fish intake; three categories: never to 1–3 times/month and >1 time/week	Parent-reported wheeze, dyspnea, steroid use and asthma symptoms, and doctor-diagnosed asthma up to 8 years	No associations were found

Abbreviations: CI confidence interval, *HDM* house dust mite, and *OR* odds ratio

Conclusion

Fish provides n-3 LCPUFAs and other nutrients but is also a common route of exposure to methylmercury and other pollutants. As a consequence, fish advisories generally suggest pregnant women to limit consumption up to three to four servings per week. Both nutrients and toxicants found in the same fish might act on the exact same end points at an opposite direction; it is therefore reasonable to presume that depending on the content of nutrients and pollutants, the health effect of a given fish type will vary. To date, several prospective studies have been conducted to assess the health effects of prenatal fish intake. Overall, the evidence on the association of maternal fish consumption during pregnancy with child health outcomes such as fetal growth, child neurodevelopment, and the occurrence of allergic diseases has been largely inconsistent.

There is a need for well-designed intervention studies targeting maternal fish intake rather than supplement use, which may exert different mechanistic effects. To usefully inform policy, it is essential that future studies of maternal fish consumption assess and carefully account for fetal exposure to contaminants.

References

1. Gluckman PD, Hanson MA, Cooper C, Thornburg KL. Effect of in utero and early-life conditions on adult health and disease. N Engl J Med. 2008;359:61–73.
2. Gil A, Gil F. Fish, a Mediterranean source of n-3 PUFA: benefits do not justify limiting consumption. Br J Nutr. 2015;113(Suppl 2):S58–67.
3. Food and Agriculture Organization of the United Nations (FAO) and World Health Organization (WHO). Joint FAO/WHO expert consultation on the risks and benefits of fish consumption FAO fisheries and aquaculture report no. 978. Roma: FAO/WHO; 2010.
4. Fish: What Pregnant Women and Parents Should Know. Draft updated advice by FDA and EPA. 2014. http://www.fda.gov/Food/FoodborneIllnessContaminants/Metals/ucm393070.htm. Accessed 26 Feb 2016.
5. EFSA Scientific Committee. Statement on the benefits of fish/seafood consumption compared to the risks of methylmercury in fish/seafood. EFSA J. 2015;13:3982.
6. McIntire DD, Bloom SL, Casey BM, Leveno KJ. Birth weight in relation to morbidity and mortality among newborn infants. N Engl J Med. 1999;340:1234–8.
7. Barker DJP. Fetal origins of coronary heart-disease. Br Med J. 1995;311:171–4.
8. Barker DJ, Hales CN, Fall CH, Osmond C, Phipps K, Clark PM. Type 2 (non-insulin-dependent) diabetes mellitus, hypertension and hyperlipidaemia (syndrome X): relation to reduced fetal growth. Diabetologia. 1993;36:62–7.
9. Beck S, Wojdyla D, Say L, Betran AP, Merialdi M, Requejo JH, et al. The worldwide incidence of preterm birth: a systematic review of maternal mortality and morbidity. Bull World Health Organ. 2010;88:31–8.
10. Olsen SF, Hansen HS, Sorensen TI, Jensen B, Secher NJ, Sommer S, et al. Intake of marine fat, rich in (n-3)-polyunsaturated fatty acids, may increase birthweight by prolonging gestation. Lancet. 1986;2:367–9.
11. Hansen HS, Olsen SF. Dietary (n-3)-fatty acids, prostaglandins, and prolonged gestation in humans. Prog Clin Biol Res. 1988;282:305–17.
12. Sorensen JD, Olsen SF, Pedersen AK, Boris J, Secher NJ, FitzGerald GA. Effects of fish oil supplementation in the third trimester of pregnancy on prostacyclin and thromboxane production. Am J Obstet Gynecol. 1993;168:915–22.
13. Makrides M, Duley L, Olsen SF. Marine oil, and other prostaglandin precursor, supplementation for pregnancy uncomplicated by pre-eclampsia or intrauterine growth restriction. Cochrane Database Syst Rev. 2006;3:CD003402.
14. Saccone G, Berghella V. Omega-3 long chain polyunsaturated fatty acids to prevent preterm birth: a systematic review and meta-analysis. Obstet Gynecol. 2015;125:663–72.
15. Rogers I, Emmett P, Ness A, Golding J. Maternal fish intake in late pregnancy and the frequency of low birth weight and intrauterine growth retardation in a cohort of British infants. J Epidemiol Community Health. 2004;58:486–92.
16. Olsen SF, Secher NJ. Low consumption of seafood in early pregnancy as a risk factor for preterm delivery: prospective cohort study. BMJ. 2002;324:447.
17. Oken E, Kleinman KP, Olsen SF, Rich-Edwards JW, Gillman MW. Associations of seafood and elongated n-3 fatty acid intake with fetal growth and length of gestation: results from a US pregnancy cohort. Am J Epidemiol. 2004;160:774–83.

18. Halldorsson TI, Meltzer HM, Thorsdottir I, Knudsen V, Olsen SF. Is high consumption of fatty fish during pregnancy a risk factor for fetal growth retardation? A study of 44,824 Danish pregnant women. Am J Epidemiol. 2007;166:687–96.
19. Brantsaeter AL, Birgisdottir BE, Meltzer HM, Kvalem HE, Alexander J, Magnus P, et al. Maternal seafood consumption and infant birth weight, length and head circumference in the Norwegian Mother and Child Cohort Study. Br J Nutr. 2012;107:436–44.
20. Ramon R, Ballester F, Aguinagalde X, Amurrio A, Vioque J, Lacasana M, et al. Fish consumption during pregnancy, prenatal mercury exposure, and anthropometric measures at birth in a prospective mother-infant cohort study in Spain. Am J Clin Nutr. 2009;90:1047–55.
21. Lee DH, Jacobs DR. Inconsistent epidemiological findings on fish consumption may be indirect evidence of harmful contaminants in fish. J Epidemiol Community Health. 2010;64:190–2.
22. Karagas MR, Choi AL, Oken E, Horvat M, Schoeny R, Kamai E, et al. Evidence on the human health effects of low-level methylmercury exposure. Environ Health Perspect. 2012;120:799–806.
23. Vafeiadi M, Vrijheid M, Fthenou E, Chalkiadaki G, Rantakokko P, Kiviranta H, et al. Persistent organic pollutants exposure during pregnancy, maternal gestational weight gain, and birth outcomes in the mother-child cohort in Crete, Greece (RHEA study). Environ Int. 2014;64:116–23.
24. Halldorsson TI, Thorsdottir I, Meltzer HM, Nielsen F, Olsen SF. Linking exposure to polychlorinated biphenyls with fatty fish consumption and reduced fetal growth among Danish pregnant women: a cause for concern? Am J Epidemiol. 2008;168:958–65.
25. Govarts E, Nieuwenhuijsen M, Schoeters G, Ballester F, Bloemen K, de Boer M, et al. Birth weight and prenatal exposure to polychlorinated biphenyls (PCBs) and dichlorodiphenyldichloroethylene (DDE): a meta-analysis within 12 European birth cohorts. Environ Health Perspect. 2012;120:162–70.
26. Farhang L, Weintraub JM, Petreas M, Eskenazi B, Bhatia R. Association of DDT and DDE with birth weight and length of gestation in the Child Health and Development Studies, 1959-1967. Am J Epidemiol. 2005;162:717–25.
27. Khanjani N, Sim MR. Maternal contamination with dichlorodiphenyltrichloroethane and reproductive outcomes in an Australian population. Environ Res. 2006;101:373–9.
28. Leventakou V, Roumeliotaki T, Martinez D, Barros H, Brantsaeter AL, Casas M, et al. Fish intake during pregnancy, fetal growth, and gestational length in 19 European birth cohort studies. Am J Clin Nutr. 2014;99:506–16.
29. Gluckman P, Nishtar S, Armstrong T. Ending childhood obesity: a multidimensional challenge. Lancet. 2015;385:1048–50.
30. Singh AS, Mulder C, Twisk JW, van Mechelen W, Chinapaw MJ. Tracking of childhood overweight into adulthood: a systematic review of the literature. Obes Rev. 2008;9:474–88.
31. Gillman MW, Ludwig DS. How early should obesity prevention start? N Engl J Med. 2013;369:2173–5.
32. Symonds ME, Mostyn A, Pearce S, Budge H, Stephenson T. Endocrine and nutritional regulation of fetal adipose tissue development. J Endocrinol. 2003;179:293–9.
33. Ailhaud G, Massiera F, Weill P, Legrand P, Alessandri JM, Guesnet P. Temporal changes in dietary fats: role of n-6 polyunsaturated fatty acids in excessive adipose tissue development and relationship to obesity. Prog Lipid Res. 2006;45:203–36.
34. Stratakis N, Gielen M, Chatzi L, Zeegers MP. Effect of maternal n-3 long-chain polyunsaturated fatty acid supplementation during pregnancy and/or lactation on adiposity in childhood: a systematic review and meta-analysis of randomized controlled trials. Eur J Clin Nutr. 2014;68:1277–87.
35. Donahue SMA, Rifas-Shiman SL, Gold DR, Jouni ZE, Gillman MW, Oken E. Prenatal fatty acid status and child adiposity at age 3 y: results from a US pregnancy cohort. Am J Clin Nutr. 2011;93:780–8.
36. Moon RJ, Harvey NC, Robinson SM, Ntani G, Davies JH, Inskip HM, et al. Maternal plasma polyunsaturated fatty acid status in late pregnancy is associated with offspring body composition in childhood. J Clin Endocrinol Metab. 2013;98:299–307.
37. van den Berg SW, Wijga AH, van Rossem L, Gehring U, Koppelman GH, Smit HA, et al. Maternal fish consumption during pregnancy and BMI in children from birth up to age 14 years: the PIAMA cohort study. Eur J Nutr. 2016;55(2):799–808.
38. Stratakis N, Roumeliotaki T, Oken E, Barros H, Basterrechea M, Charles MA, et al. Fish intake in pregnancy and child growth: a pooled analysis of 15 European and US birth cohorts. JAMA Pediatr. 2016;170(4):381–90.
39. Ibrahim MM, Fjaere E, Lock EJ, Naville D, Amlund H, Meugnier E, et al. Chronic consumption of farmed salmon containing persistent organic pollutants causes insulin resistance and obesity in mice. PLoS One. 2011;6(9):e25170.
40. Grun F, Blumberg B. Endocrine disrupters as obesogens. Mol Cell Endocrinol. 2009;304:19–29.
41. Vafeiadi M, Georgiou V, Chalkiadaki G, Rantakokko P, Kiviranta H, Karachaliou M, et al. Association of prenatal exposure to persistent organic pollutants with obesity and cardiometabolic traits in early childhood: the Rhea mother-child cohort (Crete, Greece). Environ Health Perspect. 2015;123:1015–21.
42. Cupul-Uicab LA, Klebanoff MA, Brock JW, Longnecker MP. Prenatal exposure to persistent organochlorines and childhood obesity in the US collaborative perinatal project. Environ Health Perspect. 2013;121:1103–9.

43. Hadders-Algra M. Prenatal and early postnatal supplementation with long-chain polyunsaturated fatty acids: neurodevelopmental considerations. Am J Clin Nutr. 2011;94:1874S–9S.

44. Uauy R, Mena P, Rojas C. Essential fatty acids in early life: structural and functional role. Proc Nutr Soc. 2000;59:3–15.

45. Martinez M. Tissue levels of polyunsaturated fatty acids during early human development. J Pediatr. 1992;120: S129–38.

46. Gould JF, Smithers LG, Makrides M. The effect of maternal omega-3 (n-3) LCPUFA supplementation during pregnancy on early childhood cognitive and visual development: a systematic review and meta-analysis of randomized controlled trials. Am J Clin Nutr. 2013;97:531–44.

47. Campoy C, Escolano-Margarit MV, Anjos T, Szajewska H, Uauy R. Omega 3 fatty acids on child growth, visual acuity and neurodevelopment. Br J Nutr. 2012;107(Suppl 2):S85–106.

48. Bridges CC, Zalups RK. Transport of inorganic mercury and methylmercury in target tissues and organs. J Toxicol Environ Health B Crit Rev. 2010;13:385–410.

49. Fretham SJB, Caito S, Martinez-Finley EJ, Aschner M. Mechanisms and modifiers of methylmercury-induced neurotoxicity. Toxicology Research. 2012;1:32–8.

50. Oken E, Osterdal ML, Gillman MW, Knudsen VK, Halldorsson TI, Strom M, et al. Associations of maternal fish intake during pregnancy and breastfeeding duration with attainment of developmental milestones in early childhood: a study from the Danish National Birth Cohort. Am J Clin Nutr. 2008;88:789–96.

51. Oken E, Wright RO, Kleinman KP, Bellinger D, Amarasiriwardena CJ, Hu H, et al. Maternal fish consumption, hair mercury, and infant cognition in a US cohort. Environ Health Perspect. 2005;113:1376–80.

52. Daniels JL, Longnecker MP, Rowland AS, Golding J, Health ASTUoBIoC. Fish intake during pregnancy and early cognitive development of offspring. Epidemiology. 2004;15:394–402.

53. Oken E, Radesky JS, Wright RO, Bellinger DC, Amarasiriwardena CJ, Kleinman KP, et al. Maternal fish intake during pregnancy, blood mercury levels, and child cognition at age 3 years in a US cohort. Am J Epidemiol. 2008; 167:1171–81.

54. Budtz-Jorgensen E, Grandjean P, Weihe P. Separation of risks and benefits of seafood intake. Environ Health Perspect. 2007;115:323–7.

55. Hibbeln JR, Davis JM, Steer C, Emmett P, Rogers I, Williams C, et al. Maternal seafood consumption in pregnancy and neurodevelopmental outcomes in childhood (ALSPAC study): an observational cohort study. Lancet. 2007;369:578–85.

56. Lederman SA, Jones RL, Caldwell KL, Rauh V, Sheets SE, Tang D, et al. Relation between cord blood mercury levels and early child development in a World Trade Center cohort. Environ Health Perspect. 2008;116:1085–91.

57. Sagiv SK, Thurston SW, Bellinger DC, Amarasiriwardena C, Korrick SA. Prenatal exposure to mercury and fish consumption during pregnancy and attention-deficit/hyperactivity disorder-related behavior in children. Arch Pediatr Adolesc Med. 2012;166:1123–31.

58. Gale CR, Robinson SM, Godfrey KM, Law CM, Schlotz W, O'Callaghan FJ. Oily fish intake during pregnancy – association with lower hyperactivity but not with higher full-scale IQ in offspring. J Child Psychol Psychiatry. 2008;49:1061–8.

59. Julvez J, Mendez M, Fernandez-Barres S, Romaguera D, Vioque J, Llop S, et al. Maternal consumption of seafood in pregnancy and child neuropsychological development: a longitudinal study based on a population with high consumption levels. Am J Epidemiol. 2016;183:169–82.

60. Mendez MA, Torrent M, Julvez J, Ribas-Fito N, Kogevinas M, Sunyer J. Maternal fish and other seafood intakes during pregnancy and child neurodevelopment at age 4 years. Public Health Nutr. 2009;12:1702–10.

61. Black PN, Sharpe S. Dietary fat and asthma: is there a connection? Eur Respir J. 1997;10:6–12.

62. Calder PC, Kremmyda LS, Vlachava M, Noakes PS, Miles EA. Is there a role for fatty acids in early life programming of the immune system? Proc Nutr Soc. 2010;69:373–80.

63. Best KP, Gold M, Kennedy D, Martin J, Makrides M. Omega-3 long-chain PUFA intake during pregnancy and allergic disease outcomes in the offspring: a systematic review and meta-analysis of observational studies and randomized controlled trials. Am J Clin Nutr. 2016;103:128–43.

64. Lumia M, Luukkainen P, Tapanainen H, Kaila M, Erkkola M, Uusitalo L, et al. Dietary fatty acid composition during pregnancy and the risk of asthma in the offspring. Pediatr Allergy Immunol. 2011;22:827–35.

65. Pike KC, Calder PC, Inskip HM, Robinson SM, Roberts GC, Cooper C, et al. Maternal plasma phosphatidylcholine fatty acids and atopy and wheeze in the offspring at age of 6 years. Clin Dev Immunol. 2012;2012:474613.

66. Newson RB, Shaheen SO, Henderson AJ, Emmett PM, Sherriff A, Calder PC. Umbilical cord and maternal blood red cell fatty acids and early childhood wheezing and eczema. J Allergy Clin Immunol. 2004;114:531–7.

67. Standl M, Demmelmair H, Koletzko B, Heinrich J. Cord blood LC-PUFA composition and allergic diseases during the first 10 yr. results from the LISAplus study. Pediatr Allergy Immunol. 2014;25:344–50.

68. Romieu I, Torrent M, Garcia-Esteban R, Ferrer C, Ribas-Fito N, Anto JM, et al. Maternal fish intake during pregnancy and atopy and asthma in infancy. Clin Exp Allergy. 2007;37:518–25.

69. Sausenthaler S, Koletzko S, Schaaf B, Lehmann I, Borte M, Herbarth O, et al. Maternal diet during pregnancy in relation to eczema and allergic sensitization in the offspring at 2 y of age. Am J Clin Nutr. 2007;85:530–7.

70. Willers SM, Devereux G, Craig LC, McNeill G, Wijga AH, Abou El-Magd W, et al. Maternal food consumption during pregnancy and asthma, respiratory and atopic symptoms in 5-year-old children. Thorax. 2007;62:773–9.

71. Oien T, Storro O, Johnsen R. Do early intake of fish and fish oil protect against eczema and doctor-diagnosed asthma at 2 years of age? A cohort study. J Epidemiol Community Health. 2010;64:124–9.

72. Pele F, Bajeux E, Gendron H, Monfort C, Rouget F, Multigner L, et al. Maternal fish and shellfish consumption and wheeze, eczema and food allergy at age two: a prospective cohort study in Brittany. France Environ Health. 2013;12:102.

73. Chatzi L, Garcia R, Roumeliotaki T, Basterrechea M, Begiristain H, Iniguez C, et al. Mediterranean diet adherence during pregnancy and risk of wheeze and eczema in the first year of life: INMA (Spain) and RHEA (Greece) mother-child cohort studies. Br J Nutr. 2013;110:2058–68.

74. Leermakers ET, Sonnenschein-van der Voort AM, Heppe DH, de Jongste JC, Moll HA, Franco OH, et al. Maternal fish consumption during pregnancy and risks of wheezing and eczema in childhood: the Generation R Study. Eur J Clin Nutr. 2013;67:353–9.

75. Maslova E, Strom M, Oken E, Campos H, Lange C, Gold D, et al. Fish intake during pregnancy and the risk of child asthma and allergic rhinitis – longitudinal evidence from the Danish National Birth Cohort. Br J Nutr. 2013;110:1313–25.

76. Erkkola M, Nwaru BI, Kaila M, Kronberg-Kippila C, Ilonen J, Simell O, et al. Risk of asthma and allergic outcomes in the offspring in relation to maternal food consumption during pregnancy: a Finnish birth cohort study. Pediatr Allergy Immunol. 2012;23:186–94.

77. Chatzi L, Torrent M, Romieu I, Garcia-Esteban R, Ferrer C, Vioque J, et al. Mediterranean diet in pregnancy is protective for wheeze and atopy in childhood. Thorax. 2008;63:507–13.

78. Willers SM, Wijga AH, Brunekreef B, Kerkhof M, Gerritsen J, Hoekstra MO, et al. Maternal food consumption during pregnancy and the longitudinal development of childhood asthma. Am J Respir Crit Care Med. 2008;178:124–31.

79. Gascon M, Sunyer J, Casas M, Martinez D, Ballester F, Basterrechea M, et al. Prenatal exposure to DDE and PCB 153 and respiratory health in early childhood: a meta-analysis. Epidemiology. 2014;25:544–53.

80. Hansen S, Strom M, Olsen SF, Maslova E, Rantakokko P, Kiviranta H, et al. Maternal concentrations of persistent organochlorine pollutants and the risk of asthma in offspring: results from a prospective cohort with 20 years of follow-up. Environ Health Perspect. 2014;122:93–9.

Chapter 20
Maternal Fish Oil Intake and Insulin Resistance in the Offspring

Emilio Herrera, Patricia Casas-Agustench, and Alberto Dávalos

Key Points

- Fish oil is the most common dietary supplement in many countries, and this chapter focuses on its effects during pregnancy and its long-term consequences for insulin sensitivity in offspring.
- Although the intake of fish oil during pregnancy has benefits for the neonates, some harmful effects have also been reported.
- The intake of fish oil has been associated with reduced insulin resistance in metabolic syndrome, but contradictory results have been described.
- The long-term effects of fish oil during the perinatal stages are variable in both humans and experimental animals, depending on the dose and time-window used.
- The intake of moderate doses of fish oil during the first half of pregnancy in rats increases insulin sensitivity in 1-year-old male pups, and, among the epigenetic mechanisms involved, the effect has been related to the modulation of microRNA expression.

Keywords Long-chain polyunsaturated fatty acids • Insulin sensitivity • Programmed effects • Fish oil supplements • Pregnancy • Epigenome • Noncoding RNA • miRNA

Abbreviations

AA	Arachidonic acid
ALA	α-Linolenic acid
AUC	Area under the curve
DHA	Docosahexaenoic acid
EFA	Essential fatty acids
EPA	Eicosapentaenoic acid
FO	Fish oil

E. Herrera, PhD (✉)
Department of Biochemistry and Chemistry, University CEU San Pablo, Madrid, Spain
e-mail: eherrera@ceu.es

P. Casas-Agustench, PhD • A. Dávalos, PhD
Laboratory of Disorders of Lipid Metabolism and Molecular Nutrition, IMDEA Food Institute, Madrid, Spain

© Springer International Publishing AG 2017
R. Rajendram et al. (eds.), *Diet, Nutrition, and Fetal Programming*,
Nutrition and Health, DOI 10.1007/978-3-319-60289-9_20

HOMA	Homeostasis model assessment of insulin resistance
LA	Linoleic acid
LCPUFA	Long-chain polyunsaturated fatty acids
LO	Linseed oil
miRNA	microRNA
miRNAome	Whole-genome microRNA
ncRNA	Noncoding RNA
NF-Y	Nuclear factor Y
OO	Olive oil
PA	Palm oil
PPAR-α and PPAR-γ	Peroxisome proliferator-activated receptor α and γ
SO	Soy oil
Sp1	Specificity protein 1
siRNA	Small interfering RNA
snoRNA	Small nucleolar RNA
SREBP-1	Sterol regulatory element binding protein-1
stRNA	Sperm transfer RNA
tiRNA	Transcription initiation RNA

Introduction

Fatty acids are used as structural tissue components, precursors of eicosanoids (e.g., prostacyclins, prostaglandins, thromboxanes, and leukotrienes), a source of energy, and regulators of transcription factors. Of these, structural and metabolic regulatory functions mainly require polyunsaturated fatty acids (PUFA), which are essential for intrauterine and postnatal development; during the perinatal stage, their supply depends upon the mother. During gestation, a reduced maternal intake of the essential fatty acids (EFA), linoleic acid (LA, 18:2 ω-6), and α-linolenic acid (ALA, 18:3 ω-3) has been correlated with reduced neonatal growth. Maternal plasma concentrations of long-chain PUFA (LCPUFA) during pregnancy correlate with those in the fetus and newborn. Furthermore, there is a lot of evidence to suggest that ω-3 LCPUFA have a positive impact on health in humans and in animal models, including the improvement of insulin sensitivity and the reduction in risk factors for several diseases; however, the response is quite variable, probably depending on the time and dose window used. These considerations have been used to justify the advice that maternal diets should be supplemented with oils rich in ω-3 LCPUFA like the fish oil, which is rich in eicosapentaenoic acid (EPA, 20:5 ω-3) and docosahexaenoic acid (DHA, 22:6 ω-3), during pregnancy or lactation. There is now evidence that fatty acids may alter the epigenome, although studies in healthy humans and experiments in animals have shown variable long-term metabolic and gene function responses to fish oil supplementation during pregnancy.

The purpose of this chapter is to review the long-term implications of consuming fish oil supplements during pregnancy or lactation on insulin sensitivity in the offspring, analyzing also the potential epigenetic modifications that could be involved, especially those corresponding to the expression of microRNAs (miRNAs).

Fish Oil Intake During Pregnancy

Dietary Fatty Acids During Pregnancy and Lactation

During pregnancy, fetal development needs the availability of both EFA and their LCPUFA derivatives, like DHA and arachidonic acid (AA, 20:4 ω-6) which are essential to support the synthesis of structural lipids and for intrauterine and postnatal development. Both term and preterm infants have been shown to synthesize AA and DHA from their respective EFA precursors, but the actual endogenous synthesis is low and appears to contribute very little to their plasma levels [1]. Therefore during intrauterine life, EFA and LCPUFA must be obtained from maternal circulation by passage across the placenta. This process is carried out with high efficiency and as shown in Fig. 20.1, whereas the proportion of both DHA and AA in maternal circulation declines in the third trimester of pregnancy compared to values in the first trimester, the percentage values of these two fatty acids in the neonate at birth are higher than in the mother indicating that their placental transfer is even more efficient than that of other fatty acids. In healthy women maternal plasma concentrations of LCPUFA have been shown to correlate with those in the fetus and newborn in both humans [2] and rats [3]; after the supplementation of maternal diet with fish oil (rich in DHA) during late pregnancy, there are increases in the concentrations of DHA in the plasma of both mothers and newborns [4]. These findings form the basis of advice that maternal diets should be supplemented with fish oil during the third trimester of pregnancy. Increased ω-3 LCPUFA intake during pregnancy has been shown to increase the duration of pregnancy, to reduce the incidence of premature delivery and intrauterine growth retardation, and to increase neonatal birth weight [5]. However, some harmful effects of high maternal doses of fish oil or DHA supplements have also been reported in both women [6] and rats [7]. Certain specific fatty acids inhibit the Δ^6- and Δ^5-desaturases that catalyze key reactions in the synthesis of LCPUFA from EFA; thus, an excess of one fatty acid may inhibit the synthesis of another that could be essential

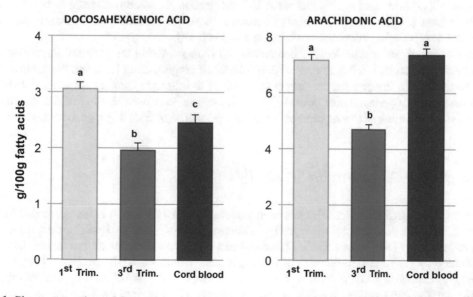

Fig. 20.1 Plasma proportions of docosahexaenoic acid (22:6 ω-3) and arachidonic acid (20:4 ω-6) in pregnant women at first and third trimester of pregnancy and in umbilical cord blood. Different lowercase letters over the bars mean statistically significant differences ($P < 0.05$) (Data (mean ± SE) are from Ref. [57])

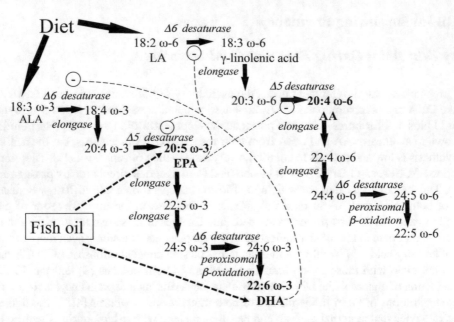

Fig. 20.2 Schematic view of major pathways of the biosynthesis of ω-6 and ω-3 long-chain polyunsaturated fatty acids from their respective dietary-derived essential fatty acid precursor, linoleic acid (*LA*), and α-linolenic acid (*ALA*) through desaturation and elongation. The role of the intake of fish oil, rich in eicosapentanoic acid (EPA) and docosahexaenoic acid (*DHA*), in the inhibition of delta-6 and delta-5 desaturases, and the synthesis of arachidonic acid (*AA*) is also shown

for the fetus. In fact, DHA inhibits Δ^6-desaturase, which is the rate-limiting enzyme for LCPUFA biosynthesis from EFA, and EPA inhibits Δ^5-desaturase, which also contributes to the biosynthesis of LCPUFA (Fig. 20.2). Thus, when a fish oil supplement is consumed during pregnancy and lactation, low levels of AA are found in both the plasma and breast milk of the mother, fetus, or newborns, both in humans [8, 9] and rats [7, 10]. Plasma AA concentration has been correlated to body weight in preterm infants [11], and adverse effects of marine oil supplementation on growth, related to low plasma AA levels during infancy, have been reported [11, 12].

The concept of "critical periods," when nutritional changes during the perinatal stage have effects on the health of adults, is a key feature of developmental programming [13], and the same argument could be applied to the quantitative aspect (or size) of the change. Thus, as for other nutrients, the long-term effects of perinatal nutritional LCPUFA imbalance have been shown to differ depending on the dose and the timing of the supplementation during specific periods of pregnancy and lactation.

Effects of Fish Oil on Insulin Sensitivity

The intake of ω-3 LCPUFA from fish has been associated with a reduction in the major risk factors of the metabolic syndrome, including adiposity, inflammation, dyslipidemia, hypertension, insulin resistance, and diabetes [14]. In rats, fish oil has also been shown to prevent insulin resistance induced by high-fat feeding [15] and to improve systemic and muscle insulin sensitivity in obesity [16]. However, prospective studies in humans have shown mixed findings in the association of fish oil intake and reductions in the incidence of type 2 diabetes, and a systematic search of multiple literature databases does not support benefits of fish/seafood or EPA + DHA on the development of diabetes mellitus [17]. In a prospective study based on middle-aged and older men, serum ω-3 LCPUFA concentration was associated with a lower incidence of type 2 diabetes [18]. Since there were significant differences in the results based on the region of the study population, the possibility that differences in genetic background, gene-diet interactions, geographic (other environmental) effects, or the type of fish consumed could be responsible for the heterogenic response.

The molecular mechanisms, through which ω-3 LCPUFA could increase insulin sensitivity, seem to be very diverse. These fatty acids could suppress lipid synthesis in the liver and upregulate fatty acid oxidation in the liver and skeletal muscle and thereby decrease circulating and tissue lipids, which could improve insulin sensitivity. Some of the beneficial effects of LCPUFA are also due to changes in membrane phospholipid composition and consequent changes in hormonal signaling [19]. Additionally, LCPUFA can exert their beneficial effects directly by upregulating the expression of genes encoding proteins that control fatty acid oxidation. This is achieved by activating the transcription factor peroxisome proliferator-activated receptor α (PPAR-α) and consequently remodeling lipid metabolism to increase fat catabolism. They also suppress the genes involved in lipid synthesis, in particular the expression and abundance of sterol regulatory element binding protein-1 (SREBP-1), and simultaneously reduce the DNA-binding activities of transcription factors like nuclear factor Y (NF-Y) and specificity protein 1 (Sp1) [20]. These complex mechanisms of inhibiting transcription factors seem to contribute to the ω-3 LCPUFA-mediated increase in insulin sensitivity.

Intake of Fish Oil During Pregnancy: Consequences for the Mother and Fetus

With the exception of vitamins and minerals, fish oils constitute the most common dietary supplements in many countries. The evidence supporting claimed maternal and offspring benefits is however poor. The evidence of the benefits of ω-3 fatty acid supplementation during pregnancy on maternal and offspring outcomes originated from observational studies, but randomized controlled trials have produced contradictory results, as recently reviewed [21]. Despite numerous clinical investigations designed to determine the benefits of fish oil supplementation during pregnancy on neurodevelopment, the evidence is still in its infancy and warrants further research. In animal studies, however, it has been shown that excessive consumption of fish oil during pregnancy and lactation can cause adverse effects on offspring body and neurological development [7]. Some studies evaluated the effects of ω-3 fatty acid supplementation on the incidence of preterm birth, but found no significant reduction in the number of preterm births and no significantly improved neonatal outcome [22]. Other studies have evaluated the efficacy of fish oil supplementation during pregnancy in the prevention of pre-eclampsia and intrauterine growth restriction or small-for-gestational-age births. An increase in the length of gestation and a consequent increase in birth weight were consistently found, but there was little evidence to support an improvement in pre-eclampsia associated with ω-3 supplementation [21].

With reference to the potential effects of fish oil reducing the risk of gestational diabetes, there is evidence in animal studies that such supplementation decreases the high rate of macrosomia induced by diabetic pregnancy [23]. However, from randomized controlled human trials, it can be concluded that supplementation with fish oil during the second or third trimester of pregnancy is not associated with reduced risk of gestational diabetes mellitus and related pathologies like hypertension and pre-eclampsia [24].

On the basis of these and other experiments, and given that fetal development is highly vulnerable to external factors, there is not enough evidence to support the routine use of ω-3 fatty acid supplementation during pregnancy. One factor that could be responsible for the variable response to fish oil supplements during pregnancy could be the degree of oxidation. The chain of ω-3 PUFA contains a large number of double bonds, which are highly prone to oxidation producing a variety of lipid peroxides and secondary oxidation products like aldehydes and ketones. Intake of oxidized fish oil could increase lipid peroxidation and reduce antioxidant capacity. Analysis of commercial fish oil preparations has shown that most of them do not meet content of ω-3 LCPUFA claimed on the label and exceed the recommended levels of oxidation markers [25]. This is probably the reason why plasma levels of vitamin E, the main lipophilic antioxidant vitamin, is decreased in both maternal plasma and fetal plasma and fetal tissues in rats given fish oil diet; it contributes to their delayed postnatal development compared to controls given an olive oil diet [7], the monounsaturated fatty acids of which are much more resistant to lipid peroxidation and don't cause such reductions in vitamin E. Oxidative stress during pregnancy in humans has also been shown to be associated with adverse effects both in the mother and in the offspring [26].

Programmed Effects of Maternal Fish Oil Intake on Metabolic Function in Offspring

Clinical studies in humans indicate that adverse prenatal and early postnatal nutritional status may contribute to the programming of (sometimes distant) future events like the susceptibility to impaired glucose tolerance, obesity, and cardiovascular disease [27]. In experimental animals, it has also been shown that perinatal nutritional disturbances may program the fetus for susceptibility to the later development of several chronic diseases including altered functioning of the adult insulin axis, the response being specific to the time-window of exposure in a sex-dependent manner [28]. As recently reviewed [29], currently there is experimental support for the suggestion that dietary fatty acids, particularly PUFA during pregnancy and lactation, affect the development of the fetus and newborn and alter the risk of developing diseases such as obesity, diabetes, cancer, and cardiovascular or liver disorders in adults, probably as result of modifying the epigenome.

The evidence for programming from fish oil intake during the perinatal stage in human trials on later changes in body composition or on the glucose-insulin axis is limited. In a longitudinal pre-birth cohort study, it was found that increased maternal-fetal ω-3 PUFA status was associated with lower adiposity in 3-year-old children [30], and, in a population-based case control study, it was found that the use of cod liver oil during pregnancy was associated with reduced risk of type I diabetes in the children before they reach 15 years of age [31]. However, in a randomized controlled trial of daily supplementation with fish oil capsules versus those containing olive oil during the third trimester of pregnancy, no association with differences in adiposity, plasma insulin, and glucose or "homeostasis model assessment of insulin resistance" (HOMA) values in 19-year-old offspring [32] was found.

The data on long-term effects of fish oil intake during fetal or early life on the glucose-insulin axis from animal studies are too scarce and have been shown to be variable in rodents, results showing that the dose and time-window of supplementation are of importance. Mice given a fish-based diet during pregnancy and lactation showed reduced body fat mass of male offspring at 9 or 21 weeks of age, and those mice given fish after weaning had increased insulin sensitivity at 15 weeks of age [33]. There were no differences in rats of either sex at 6 or 11 months of age, in terms of plasma glucose, insulin, and body weight, whether they were born of dams that were given a 7% fish oil supplement or control diets throughout pregnancy [34]. In 105-day-old male offspring of maternal rats that were given a diet supplemented with 10% fish oil starting 90 days preconception and throughout gestation and lactation, insulin sensitivity (as measured by plasma insulin and area under the curve (AUC) of glucose and insulin after an oral glucose load) did not differ from other groups being given isocaloric diets supplemented with other oils (e.g., safflower seed, palm, or groundnut) [35a]. In offspring of rats given a diet during gestation containing 10% fish oil compared to those containing the same dose of olive oil, we found that at 2 months of age, the AUC of glucose after an oral glucose load did not differ between the two groups, whereas the AUC of plasma insulin was lower in the fish oil group, indicating an increased insulin sensitivity. At 4 months there were no differences in these variables, and at 18 months there was a higher AUC for glucose without change in insulin, indicating a decreased insulin sensitivity in the fish oil group [35b].

By feeding pregnant sows with a diet containing 10% of extra energy derived from either fish oil or olive oil during just the first half of gestation, we found that dietary fatty acid composition influenced the fatty acid composition in the milk of lactating sows and in the plasma of newborn piglets [36]. This finding indicates the important role of maternal adipose tissue store of dietary-derived LCPUFA during the anabolic stage of gestation; these are mobilized around parturition becoming available for milk synthesis and suckling the newborn. A similar protocol of dietary oil supplement was applied during just the first 12 days of pregnancy in the rat showing that dietary fatty acids during early pregnancy influence fatty acid content in maternal fat stores, which are released into the blood during late pregnancy and are available for milk production and to the newborn offspring [37, 38]. Thus it was proposed that maternal fat depots laid down during early pregnancy may function as a mediator in the transfer of dietary LCPUFA to the milk and tissues of pups and have major repercussions on their development.

Based on the foregoing evidence, we chose to study whether changes in maternal dietary status during just the first 12 days (roughly first half) of pregnancy in rats had long-term consequences in adiposity and insulin sensitivity in male and female offspring [39]. During those days of early pregnancy, rats were given isocaloric diets containing 9% of fat based on soybean, olive, fish, linseed, or palm oil; then all groups were changed onto a standard laboratory diet from day 13 onward. Figure 20.3a shows that for female offspring, at 12 months of age, body weight and lumbar adipose tissue weights did not differ between the groups. However, Fig. 20.3b shows a different story for male offspring (also at 12-month-old) of the same dams; the corresponding values were lower in those from the fish oil group compared to the other groups. As shown in Fig. 20.4 in these same pups, at 8 months of age, the insulin sensitivity index assessed after oral glucose load was higher only in males of dams given the fish oil supplement during the only first 12 days of pregnancy; once again no differences between the groups were found in female offspring.

These findings contrast with the lack of effect on insulin sensitivity in offspring at 12 weeks of age of dams given a diet containing 18% fish oil during the 2 weeks prior to mating and continued through pregnancy and lactation that have been reported; nevertheless, an increased number of pancreatic islets was also reported in the experimental group [40]. This study also reported an increase in resorptions, lower body weight in male offspring, and a higher incidence of dead pups in the first 3 weeks of life in the group receiving the fish oil diet compared to controls, indicating a perinatal offspring selection that could have influenced the results. Thus although these findings indicate that nutritional intake of fish oil during pregnancy and lactation may program pancreatic responsiveness in the offspring, the results were disrupted by the negative effects on development probably as a consequence of the high dose applied and possibly also the prolonged treatment.

Therefore it seems that, in rats, exposure to a moderate amount of fish oil intake during early pregnancy, rather than high doses, is needed to reduce both insulin resistance and adipose tissue mass in the adult male, but not female, offspring. The fact that the potential mark in the embryo caused by the increased fish oil intake during early pregnancy occurred before the sexual differentiation of the gonads suggests that the differential hormonal environment in adult males versus females may be responsible for the differential gender response of adult insulin sensitivity to the diet.

The mechanism of the effects of fish oil intake during early pregnancy on adult insulin sensitivity is epigenetic and, as we discuss below, could be explained by their influence on miRNA expression as we recently reported [41].

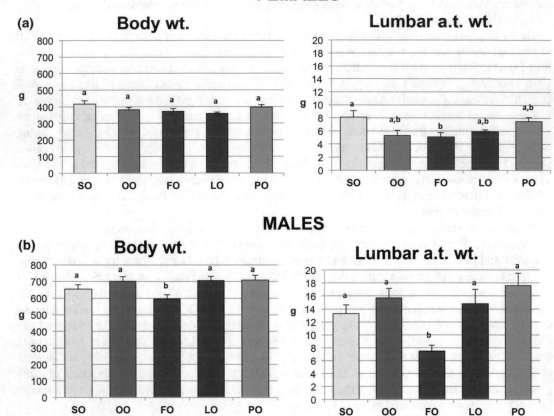

Fig. 20.3 Body and lumbar adipose tissue weights at the age of 12 months in female (**a**) and male (**b**) offspring of rat dams that were given diets containing 9% as non-vitamin fat based on soybean (*SO*), olive (*OO*), fish (*FO*), linseed (*LO*), or palm (*PO*) oil during the first 12 days of pregnancy. Different lowercase letters over the bars mean statistically significant differences ($P < 0.05$) (Results (mean ± SE) correspond to a previously published study [39])

Fetal Metabolic Programming and Epigenetic Modifications: Role of Noncoding RNAs

Understanding Epigenetics and Noncoding Sequences

Epigenetics is popular in part because it contradicts some aspects of the central dogma of molecular biology, which holds that DNA maintains the information to encode all of our proteins and that three different types of RNA rather passively convert this code into polypeptides. Specifically, messenger RNA (mRNA) carries the protein blueprint from a cell's DNA to its ribosomes, which will drive protein synthesis. Transfer RNA (tRNA) then carries the appropriate amino acids into the ribosomes for inclusion in the new protein. Meanwhile, the ribosomes themselves consist largely of ribosomal RNA (rRNA) molecules. This notion is essentially true in prokaryotes, whose genomes are almost entirely composed of closely packed protein-coding sequences that are flanked by 5′ and 3′ cis-regulatory elements that contribute – either at the transcriptional or translational level – to control its expression. Exceptions to this rule are genes that encode structural RNAs that are required for protein synthesis (i.e., rRNAs or tRNAs) and certain genes (less than 1% of the genome sequence) that express noncoding RNAs (ncRNAs) with regulatory functions. Therefore, in prokaryotes at least, proteins comprise

Insulin sensitivity idex at 8 months of age

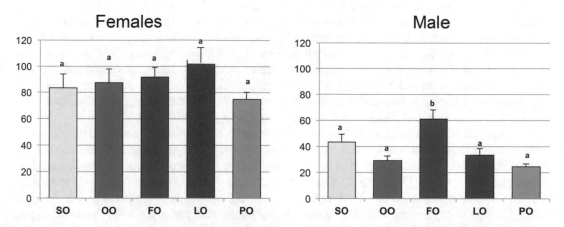

Fig. 20.4 Insulin sensitivity index (*ISI*) at the age of 8 months in female and male offspring of rat dams that were given diets containing 9% non-vitamin fat based on soybean (*SO*), olive (*OO*), fish (*FO*), linseed (*LO*), or palm (*PO*) oil during the first 12 days of pregnancy. ISI values were calculated from the plasma glucose and insulin values after an oral glucose tolerance test as previously described [39]. Values are expressed as mean ± SE. Different lowercase letters mean statistically significant differences ($P < 0.05$) between the groups of either female or male offspring

the primary functional and structural components of cells as well as the main agents by which cellular dynamics are controlled, in conjunction with cis-regulatory elements and environmental signals. This has long been assumed to be true in multicellular organisms.

Prior to the completion of the Human Genome Project, it was suggested that the number of protein-coding genes that an organism may use was a valid measure of its complexity. However, evidence from the post-genomic era, showing that the ratio of noncoding to protein-coding DNA rises as a function of the development of complex life, suggests that ncRNAs may be intimately involved in the evolution and maintenance of developmentally sophisticated multicellular complexity [42]. In fact, 98% of the human genome consists of non-protein-coding DNA, most of which was originally thought to be "junk DNA." Recent data from the "Encyclopedia of DNA Elements" (ENCODE) Consortium found that 80% of our human genome contain elements linked to biochemical functions, while about 75% of our full genome is transcribed at some point in certain cells [43]. The vast majority of the mammalian genome is differentially transcribed in precise cell-specific patterns [44] to produce a large suit of intergenic, interlacing, antisense, or intronic non-protein-coding RNAs transcripts, which show dynamic regulation during development, tissue differentiation, and disease [45]. Even regions previously described as "gene deserts" express specific transcripts in a tissue-controlled manner [46]. Moreover, there is increasing evidence of their functional relevance, including through epigenetic mechanisms, like guiding chromatin-modifying complexes to their sites of action [47]. This appears to comprise a far greater fraction of human genetic programming than expected in order to specify the architecture of the organism at a level of detail well beyond mere cell-type specification.

Noncoding RNAs

Different types of non-protein-coding RNAs have been described, and according to their size, they can be classified as short, including microRNAs (miRNAs), small interfering RNAs (siRNA), PIWI-interacting RNAs (piRNAs), transcription initiation RNAs (tiRNAs), or the newly described sperm transfer RNA-derived small RNAs (stRNAs); mid-size (small nucleolar RNAs (snoRNAs), PASRs, TSSa-RNAs, or PROMPTs); or long non-protein-coding RNAs (large intergenic non-coding RNAs (lincRNAs), T-UCRs, and other lncRNAs). Among the short RNAs, miRNAs are the most widely studied class of non-protein-coding RNAs and consist of approximately 22 nucleotides that mediate posttranscriptional gene silencing by controlling the translation of mRNA into proteins. MiRNAs are estimated to regulate the translation of more than 60% of protein-coding genes. They are involved in the regulation of different processes, including proliferation, differentiation, apoptosis, and development. In addition, some miRNAs regulate specific individual targets, others can function as master regulators of a process, so key miRNAs regulate the expression of hundreds of genes simultaneously, and many types of miRNAs regulate their targets cooperatively [48].

It is through different epigenetic "marks" – DNA methylation, histone modification, chromatin folding, and miRNA alterations – that our cells can respond quickly to environmental changes. In general terms, the addition of a methyl group (methylation) to a cytosine residue (converting it to 5-methylcytosine) on the DNA usually occurs at CpG sites, where cytosine (C) lies next to guanine (G). The state of methylation at CpG sites that are near the promoters of a gene is critical for gene activity and gene expression. Although there are exceptions, it is generally recognized that hypermethylation at CpG sites is associated with gene repression and vice versa.

The different epigenetic mechanisms may explain in part not only the effects of dietary factors at early critical developmental stages on the susceptibility to metabolic diseases in adulthood but also the means by which exposure to an altered intrauterine milieu or metabolic perturbation may influence gene expression and modulate the phenotype of the organism much later in life [49–51]. Nevertheless, whether the reported differences in miRNA expression levels are related to future disease susceptibility is still speculative. By targeting complex biological pathways, miRNAs contribute to diverse physiological and pathological processes including cardio-metabolic diseases and insulin sensitivity [52] (Fig. 20.5). However, the role of miRNAs in fetal programming remains largely understudied. Understanding the contribution of nutritionally modulated miRNAs during critical stages of development may open up new avenues for the pharmacological or dietary manipulation of miRNA action in offspring.

Small Noncoding RNAs and Epigenetic Consequences of Maternal Fish Oil Intake

Several studies conducted in animals have evaluated the effect of maternal diet on the modulation of the expression of miRNAs in the offspring that may lead to the development of metabolic and cardiovascular disease risk factors – such as obesity, inflammation, insulin resistance, hypertension, cardiac development, and artery remodeling – in young offspring or in later life [53]. Most of the studies evaluated the effect of either a high fat (HF), a low protein (LP), or an obesogenic diet compared to a standard diet on the expression of miRNAs. They use different species, diets, tissues, age of offspring, and metabolic consequences, all of which impairs our ability to make meaningful comparisons between studies. However, increasing evidence indicates that prenatal and postnatal nutritional status may influence adult susceptibility to the development of cardio-metabolic risk factors, in part through miRNA action; miRNAs may "fine-tune" cellular and biological processes by regulating the expression of genes related to cardio-metabolic risk factors, thereby modulating the phenotype of the organism much later in life. Therefore, dietary modulation of miRNA expression might theoretically be a viable option to accompany current pharmacological therapy targeting miRNAs, but further research is required to understand how the diet, and especially maternal fish oil intake, can epigenetically influence the development of insulin resistance and cardiovascular risk factors.

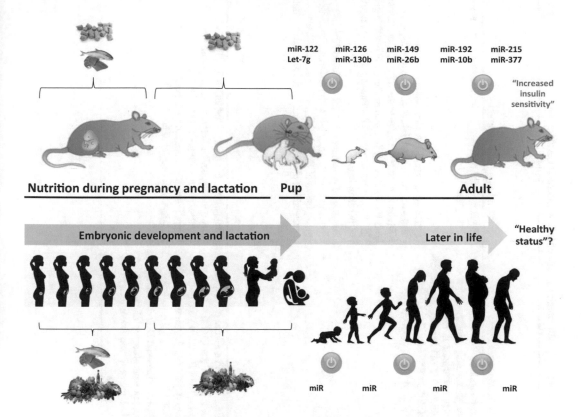

Fig. 20.5 Mother's fish oil intake and its miRNA legacy. Nutrition during pregnancy and its possible implications for the development of cardio-metabolic disease and insulin sensitivity in later life. Dietary supplementation with fish oil during the first half of pregnancy has been shown to increase insulin sensitivity in adult male offspring rats through noncoding mechanisms [39, 41]. The miRNAs ("miR-"; or "let-", which is also a class of miRNA) shown were reported to be either dysregulated in diabetes or target genes involved in glucose or insulin metabolism [41, 53]. These miRNAs were found to be modulated by fish supplementation in pregnant rats and their adult offspring [41]. Whether these molecular mechanisms also occur in humans remains unexplored

As summarized in Table 20.1, to our knowledge only two studies conducted in humans and two in rats have assessed the maternally induced epigenetic modifications of the offspring when there was significant fish oil intake during pregnancy. Of these, only our own studies in rats have related the intake of fish oil, specifically during early pregnancy only, with the modulation of miRNA and its relationship with insulin signaling in the offspring [41]. Following the protocol described above (paragraph 5 in the section "Programmed effects of maternal fish oil intake on metabolic function in offspring" and Figs. 20.3 and 20.4), we studied the effects of the consumption of different type of FAs – soy oil (SO), olive oil (OO), fish oil (FO), linseed oil (LO), and palm oil (PO) – in an isoenergetic diet during just the first 12 days of pregnancy on the expression of whole-genome miRNAs (miRNome) in adult offspring [41]. As shown in Fig. 20.6, the consumption of different fatty acids during early pregnancy induced changes in miRNA expression (only two miRNAs are shown) in the livers of adult offspring. One-year-old male offspring of rats that had received the FO diet during early pregnancy showed lower liver expression of miR-192 compared to SO, OO, LO, and PO diets; lower expressions of miR-10b-5p and miR-377-3p compared to SO, OO, and PO diets; reduced expression of miR-215 compared to OO and PO diets; and lower expression of miR-26b-5p compared to PO diet [41]. The reduced expression of liver miR-192, miR-215, and miR-10b resulted in a de-repression of their predicted targets, plasminogen activator inhibitor type 1 (serpine1), and Igf2. Other genes including PPAR- γ, Pck2, Pdpk1, and Dok1, which are genes corresponding to proteins involved in the

Table 20.1 Summary of literature showing maternal-induced ncRNAs or epigenetic modifications of fish oil intake in the offspring

Author, year	Sample	Experimental model	Offspring tissue and age (for epigenetic analysis)	Metabolic consequences	Gene and epigenetic expression
Hoile et al. (2013) [54]	Animal, Wistar rats	Given the following diets from 14 days before conception and throughout pregnancy and lactation: (a) 3.5% low fat (LF) diet with butter (predominately saturated and monounsaturated fatty acids) (b) 3.5% LF diet with fish oil (FO) (c) 7% adequate fat (AF) diet with butter (d) 7% AF diet with FO (e) 21% high fat (HF) with butter (f) 21% HF with FO	Male and female liver samples from offspring sacrificed at 77 days of age ($n = 6$, each group)	$20{:}4$ $\omega{-}6$ and $22{:}6$ $\omega{-}3$ levels were lower in liver phosphatidylcholine (PC) and phosphatidylethanolamine and plasma PC (all $P < 0.0001$) in offspring of dams fed 21% than 3.5% or 7% fat diets regardless of type	Hepatic *Fads2* expression related inversely to maternal dietary fat Fads2 messenger RNA expression correlated negatively with methylation of CpGs at -623, -394, -84, and -76 bases relative to the transcription start site (all $P < 0.005$). Methylation of these CpGs was higher in offspring of dam fed 21% than 3.5% or 7% fat; FO higher than butter Feeding adult female rats 7% fat reduced $20{:}4$ $\omega{-}6$ status in liver PC and *Fads2* expression and increased methylation of CpGs -623, -394, -84, and -76 that reversed in animals switched from 7% to 4% fat diets
Amarasekera et al. (2014) [55]	Human	Diet supplemented from 20 weeks of gestation until delivery with: (a) 3.7 g of fish oil (with 56.0% as DHA and 27.7% as EPA) (b) Placebo capsules	Cord blood mononuclear cells from neonatal blood samples ($n = 36$ and $n = 34$ from fish oil and control, respectively)	$\omega{-}3$ fatty acids in cord red blood cells increased significantly (FO = 17.8 and control = 13.6, $P < 0.001$) and $\omega{-}6$ decreased (FO = 25.2 and control = 29.6; $P < 0.001$) $\omega{-}3$ PUFAs (EPA and DHA) were higher in the treatment group, while $\omega{-}6$ PUFA (arachidonic acid) was lower than in the control group	Comparison of purified total CD4+ T cells DNA methylation profiles between the supplemented and control groups did not reveal any statistically significant differences in CpG methylation, at the single-CpG or regional level

Study	Model	Diet	Sample	Findings	Findings
Casas-Agustench et al. (2015) [41]	Animal, Sprague, Dawley rats	Isoenergetic diets with different non-vitamin lipid components during the first 12 days of pregnancy: (a) The soybean oil (SO) diet contained 9% soybean oil (b) The olive oil (OO) diet contained 9% olive oil (c) The fish oil (FO) diet contained 8% fish oil plus 1% sunflower oil (d) The linseed oil (LO) diet contained 8% linseed oil plus 1% sunflower oil (e) The palm oil (PO) diet contained 8% palm oil plus 1% soybean oil	Male liver sample of offspring sacrificed at 1 day of age and male adults at 12 months (n = 10–12, each group)	Body weight of offspring at birth was not different between dietary groups The fatty acid composition of liver tissues of rats fed the experimental diets during the first 12 days of pregnancy closely reflected the fatty acid composition of the diets eaten by each group. At day 1 after birth, the fatty acid composition of the liver of pups marginally reflected those of the respective experimental diets, given to their mothers during the first 12 days of pregnancy. However, the hepatic fatty acid profile of adults were the same FO group adults (12 months old) had lower concentrations of insulin at this age compared to other diet groups	Adult offspring of rats that were fed the FO diet during the first 12 days of pregnancy showed: (a) Lower liver expression of miR-192 (targeting Serpine1 and Igf2: insulin signaling) compared with SO, OO, LO, and PO diets (b) Lower liver expressions of miR-10b-5p (targeting Serpine1 and Igf2: insulin signaling) and miR-377-3p compared with SO, OO, and PO diets (c) Lower liver expression of miR-215 (targeting Serpine1 and Igf2: insulin signaling) compared with OO and PO diets (d) Lower liver expression of miR-26b-5p compared with PO diet
Lee et al. (2014) [56]	Human	Diets supplemented from 18 to 22 weeks of gestation until delivery with: (a) 400 mg of algal DHA (b) Mixture of corn and soy oil	Cord blood mononuclear cells from (n = ≈130, each group)	Quantitative profiling of DNA methylation states at IGF2 promoter 3 (P3), IGF2 differentially methylated region (DMR) and lncRNA H19 DMR	Compared to control group, DHA supplementation showed: (a) Higher DNA methylation level in IGF2 P3 (b) Higher IFG2 DMR methylation (c) Lower lncRNA H19 DMR methylation (d) Positive association between DNA methylation and maternal body mass index (BMI) (e) Methylation levels at IGF2/H19 imprinted regions were associated with maternal BMI

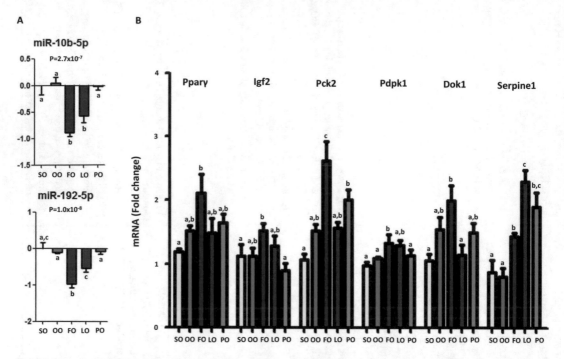

Fig. 20.6 Expression levels of small coding RNAs (miRNAs) (**a**) and of selected genes related to insulin signaling (**b**) in the liver of a 1-year-old male offspring according to their mother's dietary treatment during the first 12 days of pregnancy: diets contained 9% soybean (*SO*), olive (*OO*), fish (*FO*), linseed (*LO*), or palm oil (*PO*). Data is expressed as fold change (mean ± SD) relative to the SO diet group. SO diet, 1; OO diet, 2; FO diet, 3; LO diet, 4; PO diet, 5. Different letters in the same graph indicate statistical difference (*P* < 0.05) between dietary groups (Adapted from Ref. [41])

insulin signaling pathway, were also found to be modulated by FO. Whether these genes are regulated by other miRNAs not evaluated in this study remains unexplored. As previously described [39] and summarized in Fig. 20.4, the FO group of male adults had an increased insulin sensitivity index compared to the other dietary groups. Therefore, our findings of miRNA expression and of their target genes related to insulin sensitivity may explain epigenetically the long-term phenotypic changes of increasing insulin sensitivity observed in the male offspring of rats consuming a moderate amount of fish oil during early pregnancy.

These findings give an epigenetic explanation for the long-term increases in insulin sensitivity of male offspring of rat mothers given fish oil during early pregnancy through noncoding small RNAs (miRNAs). Understanding how the maternal nutritional status during pregnancy influences, through miRNAs or other epigenetic mechanisms, the susceptibility to disease in later life suggests new avenues for the prevention or treatment of the rampant epidemic of cardio-metabolic disease and warrants further research.

Conclusions

There is paucity of robust data from human studies showing that gestational supplementation with fish oil during the second and third trimester of pregnancy is associated with a reduction in the risks for metabolic syndrome or with increased insulin sensitivity in the adult offspring. Whether early supplementation of fish oil may affect insulin sensitivity in adults needs to be determined in the future. The existence of "critical periods" of pregnancy, when changes in dietary composition lead to effects that persist into adulthood, has been proposed. The potential for developmental programming affecting insulin sensitivity in adults as a result of modified maternal dietary fatty acid composition – such as the supplement with fish oil – is likely to be greatest when applied at key stages of cell growth and differentiation, as is the case during embryonic development. In rats the intake of fish oil supplement during early pregnancy reduced fat accretion and age-related decline in insulin sensitivity in male offspring. Although it is not known yet how dietary fatty acids modify the epigenome, several mechanisms – including noncoding RNAs – seem to be involved. Noncoding RNAs have been shown to modify DNA methylation and to change chromatin structure. Thus the finding that a high dietary supplement of fish oil during a specific developmental stage in rats decreased the expression of miR-NAs, and was accompanied by increased insulin sensitivity in the resulting adults, indicates a putative mechanism by which intake of ω-3 LCPUFA may alter specific epigenetic regulatory processes. Due to the great complexity of the human genome and epigenome, it is expected that many more molecular mechanisms will be discovered to explain these epigenetic processes; additional studies using different doses of fish oil or natural sources of ω-3 LCPUFA at specific periods of perinatal stage are warranted.

Acknowledgments   The authors thank pp.-science-editing.com for editing and linguistic revision of the manuscript. Preparation of this chapter was carried out in part with grants from the Universidad San Pablo–CEU and the Fundación Ramón Areces (CIVP16A1835) of Spain to EH.

References

1. Szitanyi P, Koletzko B, Mydlilova A, Demmelmair H. Metabolism of 13C-labeled linoleic acid in newborn infants during the first week of life. Pediatr Res. 1999;45(5 Pt 1):669–73.
2. Matorras R, Perteagudo L, Sanjurjo P, Ruiz JI. Intake of long chain w3 polyunsaturated fatty acids during pregnancy and the influence of levels in the mother on newborn levels. Eur J Obstet Gynecol Reprod Biol. 1999;83(2):179–84.
3. Herrera E, Amusquivar E. Lipid metabolism in the fetus and the newborn. Diabetes Metab Res Rev. 2000;16(3):202–10.
4. van Houwelingen AC, Sorensen JD, Hornstra G, et al. Essential fatty acid status in neonates after fish-oil supplementation during late pregnancy. Br J Nutr. 1995;74(5):723–31.
5. Olsen SF, Secher NJ. Low consumption of seafood in early pregnancy as a risk factor for preterm delivery: prospective cohort study. BMJ. 2002;324(7335):447.
6. Thorsdottir I, Birgisdottir BE, Halldorsdottir S, Geirsson RT. Association of fish and fish liver oil intake in pregnancy with infant size at birth among women of normal weight before pregnancy in a fishing community. Am J Epidemiol. 2004;160(5):460–5.
7. Amusquivar E, Ruperez FJ, Barbas C, Herrera E. Low arachidonic acid rather than alpha-tocopherol is responsible for the delayed postnatal development in offspring of rats fed fish oil instead of olive oil during pregnancy and lactation. J Nutr. 2000;130(11):2855–65.
8. van Goor SA, Dijck-Brouwer DA, Erwich JJ, Schaafsma A, Hadders-Algra M. The influence of supplemental docosahexaenoic and arachidonic acids during pregnancy and lactation on neurodevelopment at eighteen months. Prostaglandins Leukot Essent Fat Acids. 2011;84(5–6):139–46.
9. Helland IB, Smith L, Saarem K, Saugstad OD, Drevon CA. Maternal supplementation with very-long-chain n-3 fatty acids during pregnancy and lactation augments children's IQ at 4 years of age. Pediatrics. 2003;111(1):e39–44.
10. Jimenez MJ, Bocos C, Panadero M, Herrera E. Fish oil diet in pregnancy and lactation reduces pup weight and modifies newborn hepatic metabolic adaptations in rats. Eur J Nutr. 2015;56:409.
11. Carlson SE, Werkman SH, Peeples JM, Cooke RJ, Tolley EA. Arachidonic acid status correlates with first year growth in preterm infants. Proc Natl Acad Sci U S A. 1993;90(3):1073–7.
12. Koletzko B, Braun M. Arachidonic acid and early human growth: is there a relation? Ann Nutr Metab. 1991;35(3):128–31.
13. Innis SM. Metabolic programming of long-term outcomes due to fatty acid nutrition in early life. Matern Child Nutr. 2011;7(Suppl 2):112–23.
14. Poudyal H, Panchal SK, Diwan V, Brown L. Omega-3 fatty acids and metabolic syndrome: effects and emerging mechanisms of action. Prog Lipid Res. 2011;50(4):372–87.

15. Storlien LH, Kraegen EW, Chisholm DJ, Ford GL, Bruce DG, Pascoe WS. Fish oil prevents insulin resistance induced by high-fat feeding in rats. Science. 1987;237(4817):885–8.

16. Yamazaki RK, Brito GA, Coelho I, et al. Low fish oil intake improves insulin sensitivity, lipid profile and muscle metabolism on insulin resistant MSG-obese rats. Lipids Health Dis. 2011;10:66.

17. Wu JH, Micha R, Imamura F, et al. Omega-3 fatty acids and incident type 2 diabetes: a systematic review and meta-analysis. Br J Nutr. 2012;107(Suppl 2):S214–27.

18. Virtanen JK, Mursu J, Voutilainen S, Uusitupa M, Tuomainen TP. Serum omega-3 polyunsaturated fatty acids and risk of incident type 2 diabetes in men: the Kuopio Ischemic Heart Disease Risk Factor study. Diabetes Care. 2014;37(1):189–96.

19. Herrera E, Amusquivar E, Cacho J. Changes in dietary fatty acids modify the decreased lipolytic beta3-adrenergic response to hyperinsulinemia in adipocytes from pregnant and nonpregnant rats. Metabolism. 2000;49(9):1180–7.

20. Clarke SD. Polyunsaturated fatty acid regulation of gene transcription: a molecular mechanism to improve the metabolic syndrome. J Nutr. 2001;131(4):1129–32.

21. Saccone G, Saccone I, Berghella V. Omega-3 long-chain polyunsaturated fatty acids and fish oil supplementation during pregnancy: which evidence? J Matern Fetal Neonatal Med. 2016;29(15): 2389–97.

22. Saccone G, Berghella V. Omega-3 long chain polyunsaturated fatty acids to prevent preterm birth: a systematic review and meta-analysis. Obstet Gynecol. 2015;125(3):663–72.

23. Yessoufou A, Nekoua MP, Gbankoto A, Mashalla Y, Moutairou K. Beneficial effects of omega-3 polyunsaturated fatty acids in gestational diabetes: consequences in macrosomia and adulthood obesity. J Diabetes Res. 2015;2015:731434.

24. Chen B, Ji X, Zhang L, Hou Z, Li C, Tong Y. Fish oil supplementation does not reduce risks of gestational diabetes mellitus, pregnancy-induced hypertension, or pre-eclampsia: a meta-analysis of randomized controlled trials. Med Sci Monit. 2015;21:2322–30.

25. Albert BB, Derraik JG, Cameron-Smith D, et al. Fish oil supplements in New Zealand are highly oxidised and do not meet label content of n-3 PUFA. Sci Rep. 2015;5:7928.

26. Gitto E, Reiter RJ, Karbownik M, et al. Causes of oxidative stress in the pre- and perinatal period. Biol Neonate. 2002;81(3):146–57.

27. Lucas A. Programming by early nutrition in man. CIBA Found Symp. 1991;156:38–50. discussion 50-35.

28. Zambrano E, Bautista CJ, Deas M, et al. A low maternal protein diet during pregnancy and lactation has sex- and window of exposure-specific effects on offspring growth and food intake, glucose metabolism and serum leptin in the rat. J Physiol. 2006;571(Pt 1):221–30.

29. Mennitti LV, Oliveira JL, Morais CA, et al. Type of fatty acids in maternal diets during pregnancy and/or lactation and metabolic consequences of the offspring. J Nutr Biochem. 2015;26(2):99–111.

30. Donahue SM, Rifas-Shiman SL, Gold DR, Jouni ZE, Gillman MW, Oken E. Prenatal fatty acid status and child adiposity at age 3 y: results from a US pregnancy cohort. Am J Clin Nutr. 2011;93(4):780–8.

31. Stene LC, Ulriksen J, Magnus P, Joner G. Use of cod liver oil during pregnancy associated with lower risk of type I diabetes in the offspring. Diabetologia. 2000;43(9):1093–8.

32. Rytter D, Bech BH, Christensen JH, Schmidt EB, Henriksen TB, Olsen SF. Intake of fish oil during pregnancy and adiposity in 19-y-old offspring: follow-up on a randomized controlled trial. Am J Clin Nutr. 2011;94(3):701–8.

33. Hussain A, Nookaew I, Khoomrung S, et al. A maternal diet of fatty fish reduces body fat of offspring compared with a maternal diet of beef and a post-weaning diet of fish improves insulin sensitivity and lipid profile in adult C57BL/6 male mice. Acta Physiol. 2013;209(3):220–34.

34. Joshi S, Rao S, Golwilkar A, Patwardhan M, Bhonde R. Fish oil supplementation of rats during pregnancy reduces adult disease risks in their offspring. J Nutr. 2003;133(10):3170–4.

35a.Ibrahim A, Ghafoorunissa, Basak S, Ehtesham NZ. Impact of maternal dietary fatty acid composition on glucose and lipid metabolism in male rat offspring aged 105 d. Br J Nutr. 2009;102(2):233–41.

35b.López-Soldado I, Ortega-Senovilla H, Herrera E. Fish oil intake during pregnancy and lactation in rats has different long-term effects on glucose-insulin relationships in male pups depending on their age. Scientific Pages Diabetol 2016;1(1):1–5.

36. Amusquivar E, Laws J, Clarke L, Herrera E. Fatty acid composition of the maternal diet during the first or the second half of gestation influences the fatty acid composition of sows' milk and plasma, and plasma of their piglets. Lipids. 2010;45(5):409–18.

37. Fernandes FS, Tavares do Carmo M, Herrera E. Influence of maternal diet during early pregnancy on the fatty acid profile in the fetus at late pregnancy in rats. Lipids. 2012;47(5):505–17.

38. Fernandes FS, Sardinha FL, Badia-Villanueva M, Carulla P, Herrera E, Tavares do Carmo MG. Dietary lipids during early pregnancy differently influence adipose tissue metabolism and fatty acid composition in pregnant rats with repercussions on pup's development. Prostaglandins Leukot Essent Fat Acids. 2012;86(4–5):167–74.

39. Sardinha FL, Fernandes FS, Tavares do Carmo MG, Herrera E. Sex-dependent nutritional programming: fish oil intake during early pregnancy in rats reduces age-dependent insulin resistance in male, but not female, offspring. Am J Physiol Regul Integr CompPhysiol. 2013;304(4):R313–20.
40. Siemelink M, Verhoef A, Dormans JA, Span PN, Piersma AH. Dietary fatty acid composition during pregnancy and lactation in the rat programs growth and glucose metabolism in the offspring. Diabetologia. 2002;45(10):1397–403.
41. Casas-Agustench P, Fernandes FS, Tavares do Carmo MG, Visioli F, Herrera E, Davalos A. Consumption of distinct dietary lipids during early pregnancy differentially modulates the expression of microRNAs in mothers and offspring. PLoS One. 2015;10(2):e0117858.
42. Levine M, Tjian R. Transcription regulation and animal diversity. Nature. 2003;424(6945):147–51.
43. Djebali S, Davis CA, Merkel A, et al. Landscape of transcription in human cells. Nature. 2012;489(7414):101–8.
44. Mercer TR, Dinger ME, Sunkin SM, Mehler MF, Mattick JS. Specific expression of long noncoding RNAs in the mouse brain. Proc Natl Acad Sci U S A. 2008;105(2):716–21.
45. Ng SY, Johnson R, Stanton LW. Human long non-coding RNAs promote pluripotency and neuronal differentiation by association with chromatin modifiers and transcription factors. EMBO J. 2012;31(3):522–33.
46. Mercer SE, Cheng CH, Atkinson DL, et al. Multi-tissue microarray analysis identifies a molecular signature of regeneration. PLoS One. 2012;7(12):e52375.
47. Dinger ME, Amaral PP, Mercer TR, et al. Long noncoding RNAs in mouse embryonic stem cell pluripotency and differentiation. Genome Res. 2008;18(9):1433–45.
48. Mendell JT. MicroRNAs: critical regulators of development, cellular physiology and malignancy. Cell Cycle. 2005;4(9):1179–84.
49. Canani RB, Costanzo MD, Leone L, et al. Epigenetic mechanisms elicited by nutrition in early life. Nutr Res Rev. 2011;24(2):198–205.
50. Langley-Evans SC. Nutritional programming of disease: unravelling the mechanism. J Anat. 2009;215(1):36–51.
51. Simmons R. Epigenetics and maternal nutrition: nature v. nurture. Proc Nutr Soc. 2011;70(1):73–81.
52. Mendell JT, Olson EN. MicroRNAs in stress signaling and human disease. Cell. 2012;148(6):1172–87.
53. Casas-Agustench P, Iglesias-Gutierrez E, Davalos A. Mother's nutritional miRNA legacy: nutrition during pregnancy and its possible implications to develop cardiometabolic disease in later life. Pharmacol Res. 2015;100:322–34.
54. Hoile SP, Irvine NA, Kelsall CJ, et al. Maternal fat intake in rats alters 20:4n-6 and 22:6n-3 status and the epigenetic regulation of Fads2 in offspring liver. J Nutr Biochem. 2013;24(7):1213–20.
55. Amarasekera M, Noakes P, Strickland D, Saffery R, Martino DJ, Prescott SL. Epigenome-wide analysis of neonatal CD4(+) T-cell DNA methylation sites potentially affected by maternal fish oil supplementation. Epigenetics: official journal of the DNA Methylation Society. 2014;9(12):1570–6.
56. Lee IIS, Barraza-Villarreal A, Biessy C, et al. Dietary supplementation with polyunsaturated fatty acid during pregnancy modulates DNA methylation at IGF2/H19 imprinted genes and growth of infants. Physiol Genomics. 2014;46(23):851–7.
57. Herrera E, Ortega H, Alvino G, Giovannini N, Amusquivar E, Cetin I. Relationship between plasma fatty acid profile and antioxidant vitamins during normal pregnancy. Eur J Clin Nutr. 2004;58(9):1231–8.

Chapter 21
Maternal n-3 Fatty Acids and Blood Pressure in Children

Hasthi U.W. Dissanayake, Melinda Phang, and Michael R. Skilton

Key Points

- The potential for 'deprogramming' of hypertension and the underlying mechanisms are poorly understood.
- Animal studies indicate that long-chain omega-3 polyunsaturated fatty acid insufficiency in the perinatal period is associated with raised blood pressure in later life.
- Overall evidence for maternal omega-3 polyunsaturated fatty acid intake influencing offspring blood pressure in humans is inconclusive.
- Some cohort studies suggest an association between higher maternal omega-3 polyunsaturated fatty acid intake in late pregnancy with lower offspring blood pressure in childhood.
- Post hoc analyses of dietary interventions increasing maternal omega-3 polyunsaturated fatty acid intake during gestation or lactation have shown no effect on offspring blood pressure.
- There is a lack of evidence from prospective randomised trials of maternal omega-3 polyunsaturated fatty acid with offspring blood pressure as a prespecified outcome.
- There is a lack of evidence for associations of maternal omega-3 polyunsaturated fatty acid intake with offspring blood pressure in high-risk populations.

Keywords Omega-3 polyunsaturated fatty acids • Blood pressure • Developmental origins • Pregnancy • Lactation • Fetal programming • Life course

Abbreviations

ALA   Alpha-linolenic acid
BP   Blood pressure
DBP   Diastolic blood pressure
DHA   Docosahexaenoic acid
EPA   Eicosapentaenoic acid

H.U.W. Dissanayake, BSc, MPhil • M. Phang, BSc, PhD • M.R. Skilton, BSc, PhD (✉)
Boden Institute of Obesity, Nutrition, Exercise and Eating Disorders, Charles Perkins Centre,
Sydney Medical School, University of Sydney, NSW, Australia
e-mail: Michael.skilton@sydney.edu.au

© Springer International Publishing AG 2017
R. Rajendram et al. (eds.), *Diet, Nutrition, and Fetal Programming*,
Nutrition and Health, DOI 10.1007/978-3-319-60289-9_21

GA	Gestational age
LCPUFA	Long chain polyunsaturated fatty acids
MAP	Mean arterial pressure
n-3 PUFA	Omega-3 polyunsaturated fatty acids
n-6	Omega-6 polyunsaturated fatty acids
SBP	Systolic blood pressure

Introduction

High blood pressure (BP) is a major risk factor for cardiovascular and cerebrovascular diseases, which in turn are the leading cause of morbidity and mortality worldwide [1]. For each 20 mmHg increase in systolic BP (SBP) or 10 mmHg increase in diastolic BP (DBP) the risk of cardiovascular disease increases by twofold [2].

Physiological control of BP involves the complex, yet precise, interaction between different organs and the continuous actions of the cardiovascular, renal, neural and endocrine systems. Under normal function, BP is tightly regulated, maintaining sufficient pressure to ensure constant perfusion of end organs and tissues, without causing pressure related structural damage [3]. This tight regulation of BP is achieved through combination of local and systemic mechanisms, whereby local mechanisms acutely regulate blood flow via vasoconstriction and dilatation, and global mechanisms act via the autonomic nervous system. The sympathetic branch of the autonomic nervous system affects BP control via direct adjustments to cardiac output and total peripheral resistance, and indirect adjustments to blood volume via changes in renal function. In contrast, the renal endocrine system is a powerful long-term regulator of BP, principally achieved via water and salt excretion related changes in blood volume.

Pathophysiology of Programmed Hypertension

There is now an extensive body of experimental and clinical work demonstrating that the intrauterine environment is a predictor of BP, and describing the underlying mechanisms. Mechanisms implicated include the kidney – with evidence for critical periods of exposure [4]; the vasculature – with extensive evidence that various forms of maternal malnutrition can affect nitric oxide dependent vasodilatation and microvascular density [5], key local mechanisms influencing total peripheral resistance and thus BP; and the autonomic nervous system. A number of studies show increased sympathetic activity [6], decreased parasympathetic activity [7], and changes to autonomic function [8] in children born small for gestation age, a group with at risk of elevated BP from childhood through adulthood [9]. This is supported by experimental models showing autonomic and baroreflex dysfunction induced by a number of maternal nutritional manipulations [10]. Nonetheless, the fine details of these mechanisms driving programmed hypertension remain elusive, although may provide an indication of potential targets for interventions.

Programmed Hypertension: Potential for Prevention or Early Treatment

High BP is one of the most modifiable risk factors and strong evidence supports that it can be affected by pharmacological agents and lifestyle interventions, including dietary strategies [11]. Effective strategies to counter programmed hypertension remain poorly described. Due to potential risks to the developing fetus and infant, safety is a key consideration for interventions during this period. Accordingly, maternal nutritional interventions are likely a practicable means by which to prevent programmed hypertension, with omega-3 polyunsaturated fatty acids (n-3 PUFA) being one such nutritional hemodynamic agent.

n-3 PUFA, Metabolism and Physiology

Embedded in the phospholipids of cellular membranes, fatty acids play vital biochemical and physiological roles serving as lipid platforms to drive mechanistic and signalling pathways. In particular, the essential PUFAs, namely n-3 α-linolenic acid (ALA; C18:3n-3) and n-6 linoleic acid (C18:2n-6), which cannot be synthesised by mammalian cells and are essential for normal physiological function. ALA is on average the most readily consumed n-3 PUFA, obtained predominantly from plant sources, and can be endogenously converted into longer chain n-3 PUFAs, including eicosapentaenoic acid (EPA; C20:5n-3) and docosahexaenoic acid (DHA; C22:6n-3) via desaturase-mediated desaturation and elongation. Linoleic acid and ALA compete for the same enzyme systems for biosynthesis to long-chain PUFA (LCPUFA) and, importantly, for incorporation into membranes. Nonetheless, the conversation of ALA to EPA & DHA is relatively inefficient in humans, partly due to competition with n-6 linoleic acid for the rate-limiting enzyme for conversion into arachidonic acid [12]. Alternatively, EPA and DHA can be obtained directly from the diet by consuming oily fish such as salmon, tuna and mackerel.

LCPUFAs are precursors for eicosanoids which act as local and systemic mediators for coagulation, immune, allergic and inflammatory responses as well as having effects on BP and vascular reactivity. EPA is metabolized by the cyclooxygenase pathway into 3-series eicosanoids (prostaglandins, thromboxanes) and by 5-lipoxygenase into 5-series leukotrienes which have antagonistic physiological effects to the 2-series eicosanoids derived from arachidonic acid. DHA also gives rise to anti-inflammatory lipid mediators [13]. Leukotrienes and lipoxins derived from EPA and arachidonic acid are additional lipid mediators that modulate inflammation and serve as endogenous regulators of vascular tone and BP. Importantly, those derived from arachidonic acid are pro-inflammatory and pro-aggregatory agonists while those derived from EPA have opposing effects including anti-arrhythmic, hypolipidemic and hypotensive effects [14].

The beneficial effects of n-3 PUFAs have been explained by some authors in terms of a balance between total n-6 and n-3 FAs, rather than the absolute amount of each [15]. A high n-6/n-3 ratio has been hypothesized as being detrimental for human health, while conversely a ratio of ~1, estimated to be that consumed by our paleolithic forebears, is considered cardioprotective. During the last 150 years, a dramatic increase in the Western diet towards consumption of n-6 PUFAs paralleled with a decrease of n-3 PUFAs intake has resulted in a drastic shift resulting in average n-6/n-3 ratio between 15:1 and 20:1 [15].

Thus the dietary imbalance of LCPUFAs in favour of n-6 FAs can drive vascular and inflammatory responses, with consequent elevations of BP and other chronic diseases. Other vascular actions of n-3 PUFA are relatively poorly understood, but include changes in membrane structures, gene expression, and direct interactions with ion channels.

Anti-hypertensive Actions of n-3 PUFA

Studies have shown a number of antihypertensive effects of n-3 PUFA (Fig. 21.1). Consumption of n-3 PUFA reduces systolic and diastolic BP as well as resting heart rate in adults [16]. The reduced heart rate is thought to be due to direct effects on cardiac electrophysiology as well as indirect

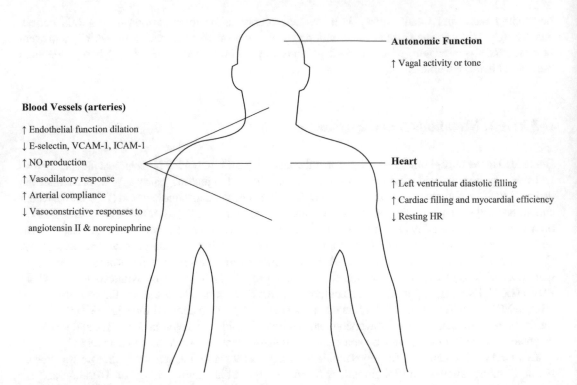

Fig. 21.1 Antihypertensive effects of omega-3 fatty acids: mechanistic evidence. n-3 polyunsaturated fatty acids have a number of antihypertensive effects, including improved arterial health, increased vagal activity and improved cardiac health. *ICAM-1* intercellular adhesion molecule-1, *NO* nitric oxide, *HR* heart rate, *VCAM-1* vascular cellular adhesion molecule-1

pathways [16], which include augmenting vagal tone and improving left ventricular diastolic filing [17]. Short-term trials indicate a number of vascular mechanisms of n-3 PUFAs including increased nitric oxide production, enhanced vasodilatory responses, attenuation of vasoconstrictive responses to angiotensin II and norepinephrine, improved arterial compliance and flow-mediated dilatation, a non-invasive marker of endothelial function [16]. N-3 LCPUFAs have beneficial effects on other aspects of endothelial health, including evidence that DHA decreases the expression of adhesion molecules on endothelial cells and monocytes, including E-selectin, intercellular cell-adhesion molecule-1 and vascular cell adhesion molecule-1. The magnitude of this effect is directly associated with the degree of incorporation of DHA into cellular phospholipids [18]. In human umbilical vein endothelial cells exposed to oxidized-LDL, EPA improves the balance between nitric oxide and reactive oxygen species [19]. Incubation with EPA also attenuates saturated fatty acid-induced generation of reactive oxygen species, expression of adhesion molecules and cytokines, activation of apoptosis-related proteins, and apoptosis in endothelial cells [20].

More recently, the cytochrome P450 enzymes have been proposed as targets of n-3 PUFAs to modulate vascular tone. It has become evident from several in vitro studies that n-3 PUFAs may exert potent vasodilatory effects as fatty epoxides metabolized by cytochrome P450 epoxygenase in the endothelium [21]. In isolated coronary arterial cells, DHA-derived epoxides were shown to activate calcium-activated potassium currents producing vasodilatation. Furthermore, the DHA-mediated dilatory effects were dose-dependent, increasing calcium-activated potassium currents by 5%, 170%, and 220% at 0.1, 0.3, and 1.0 mM DHA, respectively [22]. In recent experiments, n-3 PUFA-derived mono-epoxides was also reported to possess nearly 1000-fold greater potency than their precursors EPA or DHA in reducing effects of calcium overload in neonatal rat cardiomyocytes [23].

Observational studies and small trials suggest n-3 PUFA may improve autonomic function via augmentation of vagal activity or tone, although further studies are required to determine the appropriate dose required as either supplementation or as a component of dietary intake [16].

Taken together, these vascular and central mechanisms likely underpin the blood pressure lowering actions of n-3 PUFA.

Maternal n-3 PUFA and Offspring BP

The "fetal origins" hypothesis proposes that alterations in fetal nutrition result in developmental adaptations that permanently change structure, physiology, and metabolism, most likely influencing susceptibility to develop metabolic disorders, such as type 2 diabetes, cardiovascular disease, obesity and hypertension in later life [24]. It has been postulated that a deficiency in n-3 PUFAs in the perinatal period may be one such early life "insult" with hypertensive consequences.

Indeed, maternal DHA is readily transferred via the placenta, is an important component of breast milk, and is rapidly accumulated in the synapses during fetal development and early postnatal life. DHA comprise 30% of the phospholipid fatty acids within the cortex and 15% within the hypothalamus, a key brain centre that controls BP.

Maternal n-3 PUFA and Offspring BP: Experimental Animal Studies

To date, there is limited evidence from animal studies regarding the relationship between maternal n-3 PUFA and offspring BP. Armitage and colleagues [25] investigated the effects of maternal n-3 PUFA deficiency, in addition to the effects of post-weaning repletion of n-3 PUFA in the offspring, with subsequent offspring BP. Pregnant dams were given a diet either deficient in n-3 PUFA or supplemented with n-3 PUFA, throughout pregnancy and until weaning. At 9 weeks of age, half the supplemented offspring were crossed to the deficient diet and half the deficient offspring were subsequently supplemented, while the remainder continued to consume the diet to which their mother was originally allocated. In the adult offspring, mean arterial pressure (MAP) was highest in those fed the n-3 PUFA deficient diet throughout development and during post-weaning life (Fig. 21.2). Interestingly, the two groups with the lowest BP were those who were supplemented with n-3 PUFA throughout and those who were supplemented during pregnancy, but not post-weaning. This suggests that prenatal and early infancy is a critical period during which n-3 PUFA may modify adult BP in the rat, putatively via accumulation of n-3 PUFA in the developing nervous system.

A similar study investigating n-3 and n-6 PUFA, and their ratios, found that BP was elevated in the offspring of those dams fed either a diet enriched in n-3 or n-6 PUFA prenatally [26]. Only male offspring from dams given the diet containing both n-6 and n-3 PUFA had elevated blood pressure, suggesting that prenatal fatty acid balance may be important in influencing BP in a gender-specific manner.

Observations from Armitage and colleagues offer some clues as to mechanisms by which PUFA and its composition affect early development and BP control. Rats exposed to n-3 PUFA deficiency while in utero and during infancy were found to over ingest sodium and consequently consume lower amounts of water, as part of a sodium and water deprivation challenge [27]. Such behaviour is consistent with abnormalities in sodium and osmoreceptors as well as the renin angiotensin mechanism, both of which influence BP and hydromineral balance. N-3 PUFA deficiency is also found to affect phototransduction in the retina, which share similar receptor morphology as the angiotensin II receptor [25]. These changes may have emerged due to developmental changes in the membrane bound receptors.

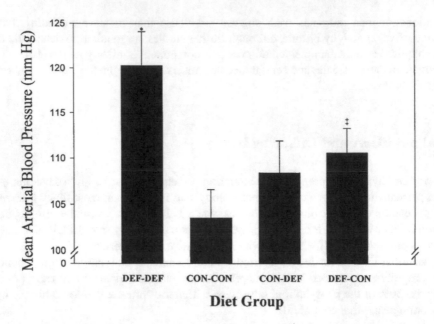

Fig. 21.2 Effect of dietary fatty acid supply on mean arterial blood pressure (MAP). Cross over diet was implemented at 9 weeks of age, where half the supplemented (CON) offspring were crossed to the deficient diet (CON-DEF) and half the DEF offspring were crossed to the control diet (DEF-CON). The remaining rats continued on their initial diets (CON-CON and DEF-DEF). This study demonstrated that (1) the highest MAP occurred in animals raised and maintained on a diet deficient in n-3 PUFA (DEF-DEF); and that (2) early n-3 PUFA deficiency with subsequent n-3 PUFA supplementation at 9 weeks of age (DEF-CON) still resulted in raised blood pressure when compared to those who received PUFA supplementation throughout (CON-CON). This is consistent with a deficiency in n-3 PUFA during the prenatal and perinatal period affecting adult hemodynamics. *Significantly higher than all other groups ($P < 0.05$); ‡ significantly higher than CON-CON ($P < 0.05$). n-3 PUFA, omega-3 polyunsaturated fatty acids (Reprinted from Armitage et al. [25] Copyright © 2003 by AOCS Press, with permission of Springer)

Maternal n-3 PUFA During Pregnancy and Offspring BP: Human Studies

All of the n-3 and n-6 PUFAs accumulated by the fetus must ultimately be derived from the mother by placental transfer and studies have demonstrated the preferential selectivity in the placental membrane binding sites for LCPUFAs, in particular DHA [28].

Despite the functions of n-3 PUFAs in fetal and newborn neurodevelopment and inflammation, there is only a relatively small body of evidence describing the associations of maternal n-3 PUFA intake with BP or measures of cardiovascular health in the offspring (Table 21.1).

In the Generation R Study, an observational cohort of 4455 mothers and children [29], higher maternal n-3 PUFA and lower n-6 PUFA concentration in the second trimester of pregnancy was associated with lower SBP but not with DBP in the offspring during childhood. In models adjusted for gestational age at sampling, pregnancy and childhood factors, and sex and age of the child, both higher total maternal n-3 PUFA concentration and DHA concentration were found to be associated with lower SBP in the children at 6 years of age (differences: −0.28 [95% CI −0.54, −0.03] and −0.29 mmHg [95% CI −0.54, −0.03] per SD increase of n-3 PUFAs [one SD is 1.5 wt%] and DHA [one SD is 1.1 wt%] respectively) [29]. Conversely, a higher maternal n-6 PUFA was associated with a higher childhood SBP (difference: 0.36 mmHg [95% CI 0.09, 0.62] per SD increase of total n-6 PUFA [2.5 wt%]). Furthermore, a higher n-6/n-3 ratio was associated with an increased childhood SBP, but not with DBP. In separate analyses of the Generation R cohort, a higher maternal n-6/n-3 PUFA ratio was associated with a higher childhood total body fat mass percentage, android:gynoid fat

Table 21.1 Outcomes of relevant studies examining the association between maternal n-3 PUFA intake and offspring BP

Ref no.	Study design	Subject details	Diet/intervention	Key outcomes
[33]	Randomised controlled trial	$n = 46$ pregnant women	Maternal DHA supplementation (600 mg/day; $n = 22$) or placebo ($n = 24$) from 14 weeks GA until birth	Weak evidence for lower fetal heart rate at 24, 32, and 36 weeks GA in mother supplemented with DHA compared to placebo ($P = 0.095$)
[34]	Randomised controlled trial	$n = 180$ mother-child pairs	Maternal supplementation with fish oil containing 2.7 g/day fish oil ($n = 108$) or olive oil ($n = 72$) or no supplementation ($n = 214$) from 30 weeks GA until birth	Maternal supplementation with fish oil during the last trimester of pregnancy was not associated with differences in BP, heart rate or heart rate variability in the offspring at 19 years of age, when compared to those assigned to olive oil [differences: 2 mmHg (95% CI: −1, 4) for SBP and 1 beat per minute (95% CI: −2, 4) for HR]
[29]	Cohort study (Generation R population-cohort study)	$n = 4455$ mother-child pairs	Maternal second trimester plasma concentrations of n-3 and n-6 PUFA (wt% total fatty acids)	Higher plasma concentrations of maternal n-3 PUFA and DHA was associated with lower SBP in the offspring at 6 years of age [differences: −0.28 mmHg (95% CI: −0.54, −0.03) and −0.29 mmHg (95% CI: −0.54, −0.03) per SD higher n-3 PUFAs and DHA respectively]
				Higher maternal n-6 PUFA was associated a higher childhood SBP [difference: 0.36 mmHg (95% CI: 0.09, 0.62) per SD higher n-6 PUFA] at 6 years of age
[31]	Cohort study (Avon Longitudinal Study of Parents and Children; ALSPAC)	$n = 6944$ mother-child pairs	Data from maternal Food Frequency Questionnaires based on the diet in pregnancy	In minimally adjusted models, maternal n-3PUFA intake based on the current diet in the last trimester of pregnancy was inversely associated with SBP in the children at 7.5 years of age ($P = 0.04$), effects were lost after adjusting for current anthropometry, maternal and social factors, birth weight and gestation ($P = 0.7$)
[32]	Cohort study (Southampton Women's Survey)	$n = 234$ mother-child pairs	Data from maternal Food Frequency Questionnaires based on diet in pregnancy	Higher oily fish consumption in late pregnancy was associated with reduced aortic pulse wave velocity in the offspring at 9 years of age (−0.084 m/s per portion per week; 95% CI, −0.137, −0.031)

(continued)

Table 21.1 (continued)

Ref no.	Study design	Subject details	Diet/intervention	Key outcomes
[35]	Cohort study	n = 443 mother-child pairs	Data from maternal Food Frequency Questionnaires based on diet in pregnancy	Maternal n-3 PUFA intakes expressed as quintiles in the second trimester of pregnancy was not associated with BP, heart rate, or heart rate variability in the offspring at 20 years of age
[45]	Randomised controlled trial	n = 98 mother-child pairs	Lactating mothers randomised to 4.5 g/day fish oil (n = 39) or olive oil (n = 30), or a non-randomized group consuming a high fish diet (n = 29) during the first 4 months after delivery	Blood pressure, pulse wave velocity, or heart rate variability did not differ between infants of mothers supplemented with fish oil or olive oil at 2.5 years of age
[46]	Randomised controlled trial	n = 147 newborn infants	Newborn infants randomised to a formula containing LCPUFA supplementation (n = 71) or nutritionally similar formula without LCPUFA (n = 76) for 4 months and followed up at 6 years	Mean BP was − 3.0 mmHg lower ([95%CI −5.4, −0.5]; P = 0.02) and DBP was −3.6 mmHg lower [95%CI −6.5, −0.6]; P = 0.02) than the non-supplemented group at 6 years of age
[47]	Randomised controlled trial	n = 83 term 9 month old infants	Infants randomised to 5 mL fish oil (n = 39) or no fish oil (n = 44) daily for 3 months	SBP was lower in the fish oil supplemented group at 12 months compared to those infants in the control group [mean difference−6.3 mmHg (95% CI, −0.9, 11.7 mmHg)]
[44]	Self-selected intervention study	n = 102 mother-child pairs	Breast milk (n = 31) vs. milk-based formula (n = 39) vs. soy-based formula without DHA (n = 12) vs. soy-based formula + DHA (n = 30) from birth to 6 months	Increased heart rate and decreased heart rate variability measures were observed in infants fed the DHA-deficient diet compared to the other diets

BP blood pressure, *DHA* docosahexaenoic acid, *GA* gestational age, *LCPUFA* long chain polyunsaturated fatty acids, *n-3 PUFA* omega-3 polyunsaturated fatty acids, *n-6 PUFA* omega-6 polyunsaturated fatty acids, *SBP* systolic blood pressure

mass ratio, and abdominal preperitoneal fat mass area adiposity at 3, 4 and 6 years of age [30], potentially driving the observed association with BP.

The Avon Longitudinal Study of Parents and Children reported an inverse association between maternal n-3 PUFA intake assessed during the third trimester of pregnancy with offspring SBP at 7.5 years of age in 6944 mother-child pairs ($P = 0.04$), although this effect was lost after adjusting for current anthropometry, maternal and social factors, birth weight and gestation ($P = 0.7$) [31]. There were no significant associations between maternal dietary n-3 PUFA intake and offspring DBP.

More recently, the Southampton Women's Survey reported that higher oily fish consumption in late pregnancy was associated with reduced aortic stiffness, assessed by pulse wave velocity, in the child at 9 years of age (-0.084 m/s per portion of oily fish consumed per week; 95% CI -0.137, -0.031) independent of the child's current oily fish consumption [32]; however there was no association with offspring BP or heart rate.

Promising findings on DHA supplementation and fetal heart rate have been reported. A randomised controlled trial involving maternal supplementation of 600 mg/day of DHA commenced at 14 weeks gestation was found to lower heart rate at 24, 32 and 36 weeks gestational age compared to placebo ($P = 0.095$) [33]. Furthermore, there was evidence that DHA intake during the last two trimesters of pregnancy results in more responsive autonomic function in the offspring.

Follow-up studies examining effects in adolescence have also yielded discrepant findings. A randomised controlled trial in which 180 pregnant women were supplemented with marine n-3 LCPUFAs in the last trimester of pregnancy showed no association with BP, heart rate or heart rate variability, a marker of autonomic function, in the offspring at 19 years or age [34]. Similarly, marine-derived dietary n-3 LCPUFA expressed as quintiles of energy-adjusted intake during the second trimester of pregnancy showed no association with SBP, DBP, heart rate or heart rate variability in 443 offspring at 20 years of age in a Danish cohort [35].

Maternal n-3 PUFA During Lactation and Offspring BP: Human Studies

For the infant, PUFAs are essential during the perinatal period where there is rapid growth and development of new tissues and organ systems, and is primarily sourced from breast milk in nursing infants. The lactating mammary tissue synthesises FAs intracellularly from a supply of substrates extracted from the maternal plasma. The lipid drops formed in the mammary epithelial cells are secreted into the milk by exocytosis or association with the plasma membrane bilayer [36]. While the level of n-6 arachidonic acid is relatively constant in human milk, the EPA and DHA levels are variable and dependent on the maternal nutritional habits [37], with maternal intake of fish oil, DHA, or DHA-enriched foods effectively increasing both maternal and neonatal n-3 PUFA status [38].

Studies linking breast milk intake in infancy to lower BP during childhood have been reported. Breastfeeding has also been associated with consistent reduction in obesity risk later in childhood [39], with likely benefits for BP, although the n-3 PUFA content of breast milk is likely not a major factor contributing to this lower risk of offspring adiposity. LCPUFAs are present in breast milk but were not routinely available in infant formula until the early 2000s. As infants have limited ability to synthesise DHA, infants fed unsupplemented formula may experience a relative deficiency of LCPUFAs compared to breast-fed infants [40].

Longitudinal observational studies in term infants have demonstrated that children who were breast-fed for at least 3 months have lower SBP and DBP during later childhood and adolescence compared to children who were formula fed [41, 42]. Fifteen year old children born preterm and randomised during infancy to being fed banked breast milk, had lower SBP and DBP compared to those who were randomised to infant formula [43].

Timing of n-3 PUFA intake   **Hemodynamic effects on offspring**

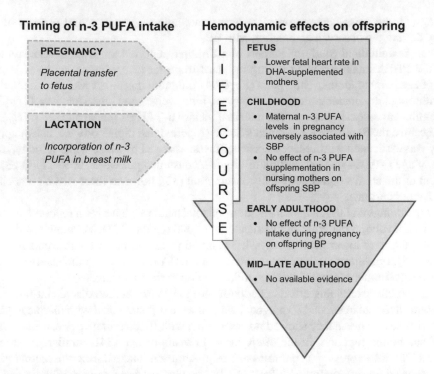

Fig. 21.3 Summary of evidence of maternal n-3 PUFA intake and offspring BP across the life course. Current evidence linking maternal intake of n-3 PUFA and lower offspring blood pressure is inconclusive. While some observational studies have shown inverse associations, others have not, and intervention studies have reported no effect. There is a lack of evidence from prospective randomised trials of maternal n-3 PUFA with offspring blood pressure as a prespecified outcome. *BP* blood pressure, *DHA* docosahexaenoic acid, *n-3 PUFA* omega-3 polyunsaturated fatty acids, *SBP* systolic blood pressure

Increased heart rate and decreased heart rate variability were found in infants fed a DHA-deficient milk formula compared to those fed DHA-supplemented formula or breast-fed infants [44]. In contrast, maternal supplementation with marine n-3 PUFAs during the first 4 months of lactation had no effect on BP, arterial stiffness or heart rate variability of the offspring at 2.5 years of age [45].

Postpartum intervention in infancy has proven effective in some randomised trials. A study of 71 newborn infants who were randomised to a formula with LCPUFAs reported a significantly lower DBP at 6 years of age compared to those children who were fed a nutritionally similar formula in infancy but devoid of LCPUFAs (mean difference −3.0 mmHg [95% CI −5.4, −0.5 mmHg]) [46]. The association was weaker for SBP (mean difference −2.3 mmHg [95% CI −5.3, 0.7 mmHg]). In late infancy supplementation with marine n-3 LCPUFA (924 mg/day) in 9 month old infants for 3 months resulted in a lower SBP compared to those infants that did not receive n-3 PUFA (mean difference −6.3 mmHg [95% CI −11.7, −0.9,mmHg]). No effects were observed for DBP or MAP [47]. Although these do not directly study the effect of maternal n-3 PUFA intake, these trials of formula supplemented with n-3 PUFA compared with deficient formula, can be used as proof-of-concept of the potential haemodynamic effects of n-3 PUFA intake during infancy per se. It is not unreasonable to posit that similar findings could result in breast-fed infants of mothers consuming an appropriate amount of n-3 PUFA. Importantly, these infants would also obtain the other well-described health benefits of being breast-fed, including reduced risk of later obesity (Fig. 21.3).

While there are currently no widely recognised guidelines for intake of n-3 PUFA during pregnancy and lactation, there are well established recommendations for the general population of two servings of oily fish per week providing an average of ~100 to 250 mg per day n-3 PUFAs of which

50–100 mg is from DHA [48]. It is likely that there are increased n-3 PUFA requirements during pregnancy, however most pregnant women likely do not meet the increased demand in part due to competing recommendations to limit oily fish consumption to a maximum of two servings per week due to concerns of their mercury content. For women consuming a solely or predominantly plant-based diet, there are other concerns in meeting these requirements. While plant-based foods can be rich in ALA, only a small amount of these short-chain n-3 PUFA appear to be endogenously converted to LCPUFA, and these dietary patterns provide only small amounts of EPA and DHA [48]. Accordingly, the use of supplements may be warranted in some women during pregnancy and lactation, who are otherwise unable to obtain sufficient n-3 LCPUFA from dietary sources.

The ability of n-3 PUFA in the fetus or during early infancy to reduce later BP may also depend on the background risk of the individual, particularly relating to the presence of other early life risk factors for hypertension. A recent randomized trial of fish oil supplementation over the first 5 years of life in children who were not considered to be at risk of cardiovascular disease, found evidence of interaction by birth weight, such that those with the lowest birth weight had less severe subclinical atherosclerosis if they had been allocated to receive the fish oil supplement [49]. Similar findings have since been demonstrated for BP, with intake of both plant and marine-derived n-3 PUFA being associated with lower BP [50]. It is plausible that those born with impaired fetal growth in particular, are a group in which sustained n-3 PUFA intake postnatally may be beneficial, given that birth weight is inversely associated with later BP, that on average children born with impaired fetal growth are more likely to have been exposed to lower n-3 PUFA in utero, and that impaired fetal growth is associated with lower serum DHA and EPA levels later in life [50] (Fig. 21.4). Indeed, the above studies reporting

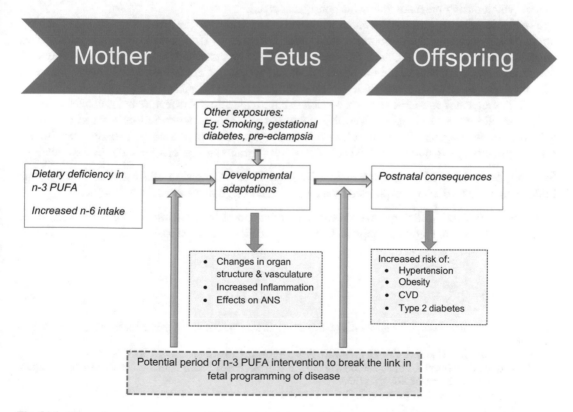

Fig. 21.4 Schematic proposed pathways linking n-3 deficiency with hypertensive disorders: potential timing for n-3 PUFA interventions. Theoretical time points, including while in utero and postnatal, during which n-3 PUFA interventions could be applied to reduce or prevent the chronic disease outcomes of fetal programming. *ANS* autonomic nervous system, *CVD* cardiovascular disease, *n-3 PUFA* omega-3 polyunsaturated fatty acids, *n-6* omega-6 polyunsaturated fatty acids

the association of n-3 PUFA intake and BP lowering properties in those born with impaired fetal growth, found that similar associations were either not present or markedly weaker in those born with healthy birth weight [50].

Conclusions

Accordingly, while a link between maternal intake of n-3 PUFAs and lower offspring BP is mechanistically plausible, the evidence thus far is mixed and inconclusive, and limited principally by the lack of prospective randomised trials with BP as a pre-specified outcome.

There are a number of issues that will need to be duly considered in the design of such trials, and any recommendations that flow therefrom. What is the best vehicle for n-3 PUFA interventions in pregnant women? Consuming oily fish is generally recommended outside of pregnancy, for cardiovascular disease prevention, predominantly due to the inherent substitution of such a meal for a likely less healthsome meal. However, mercury levels in consumed fish are an important consideration, particularly during pregnancy, and as such consumption of species including swordfish and shark should be limited.

Fish oil supplements may be more amenable to some women, due to food preferences and tolerances, and most of the widely available supplements are low-mercury or mercury-free. Algae-derived DHA preparations overcome these concerns, and are also a suitable source of n-3 LCPUFA for women adhering to a plant-based diet. People adhering to such diets have higher ALA intake on average, the role of which during pregnancy remains poorly described.

Finally, identifying groups of women whose offspring will have the greatest likelihood of achieving clinically meaningful reductions in BP resulting from n-3 PUFA intake during pregnancy is an on-going challenge. As noted, such offspring are likely to be those at the highest risk of elevated BP due to an adverse maternal-fetal environment, including but not limited to those born premature or with fetal growth restriction, although clinical identification of women at risk of these outcomes early enough in pregnancy to enable the intervention to have a meaningful effect, remains challenging.

Yet despite these challenges, given the global burden of hypertensive-disorders and the strong evidence for developmental origins of hypertension, maternal n-3 intake is a potentially powerful and meaningful strategy to normalize offspring BP which warrants further careful and robust evaluation.

Funding Sources MRS is supported by a National Heart Foundation of Australia Future Leader Fellowship (100419). HD is supported by an Australian Postgraduate Award (SC0042).

Conflicts of Interest MRS and MP receive research support from Swisse Wellness Pty Ltd. in the form of investigational product supplies. HD has no conflict of interest to declare.

References

1. World Health Organization. A global brief on hypertension: silent killer, global public health crisis: World Health Day 2013.
2. Franco V, Oparil S, Carretero OA. Hypertensive therapy: part II. Circulation. 2004;109(25):3081–8.
3. Dampney RA, Horiuchi J. Functional organisation of central cardiovascular pathways: studies using c-fos gene expression. Prog Neurobiol. 2003;71(5):359–84.
4. Vehaskari VM, Aviles DH, Manning J. Prenatal programming of adult hypertension in the rat. Kidney Int. 2001; 59(1):238–45.
5. Nuyt AM. Mechanisms underlying developmental programming of elevated blood pressure and vascular dysfunction: evidence from human studies and experimental animal models. Clin Sci. 2008;114(1):1–17.

6. IJzerman RG, Stehouwer CD, de Geus EJ, et al. Low birth weight is associated with increased sympathetic activity: dependence on genetic factors. Circulation. 2003;108(5):566–71.
7. Mathewson KJ, Van Lieshout RJ, Saigal S, Boyle MH, Schmidt LA. Reduced respiratory sinus arrhythmia in adults born at extremely low birth weight: evidence of premature parasympathetic decline? Int J Psychophysiol. 2014;93(2):198–203.
8. Rakow A, Katz-Salamon M, Ericson M, Edner A, Vanpee M. Decreased heart rate variability in children born with low birth weight. Pediatr Res. 2013;74(3):339–43.
9. Skilton MR, Pahkala K, Viikari JS, et al. The association of dietary alpha-linolenic acid with blood pressure and subclinical atherosclerosis in people born small for gestational age: the Special Turku Coronary Risk Factor Intervention Project study. J Pediatr. 2015;166(5):1252–7. e1252.
10. Rudyk O, Makra P, Jansen E, et al. Increased cardiovascular reactivity to acute stress and salt-loading in adult male offspring of fat fed non-obese rats. PLoS One. 2011;6(10):e25250.
11. Appel LJ, Brands MW, Daniels SR, et al. Dietary approaches to prevent and treat hypertension: a scientific statement from the American Heart Association. Hypertension. 2006;47(2):296–308.
12. Arterburn LM, Hall EB, Oken H. Distribution, interconversion, and dose response of n-3 fatty acids in humans. Am J Clin Nutr. 2006;83(6 Suppl):1467S–76S.
13. Bazan NG. Omega-3 fatty acids, pro-inflammatory signaling and neuroprotection. Curr Opin Clin Nutr Metab Care. 2007;10(2):136–41.
14. Grundt H, Nilsen DW. n-3 fatty acids and cardiovascular disease. Haematologica. 2008;93(6):807–12.
15. Simopoulos AP. Evolutionary aspects of diet, the omega-6/omega-3 ratio and genetic variation: nutritional implications for chronic diseases. Biomed Pharmacother. 2006;60(9):502–7.
16. Mozaffarian D, Wu JH. Omega-3 fatty acids and cardiovascular disease: effects on risk factors, molecular pathways, and clinical events. J Am Coll Cardiol. 2011;58(20):2047–67.
17. O'Keefe JH, Abuissa H, Sastre A, Steinhaus DM, Harris WS. Effects of omega-3 fatty acids on resting heart rate, heart rate recovery after exercise, and heart rate variability in men with healed myocardial infarctions and depressed ejection fractions. Am J Cardiol. 2006;97(8):1127–30.
18. De Caterina R, Liao JK, Libby P. Fatty acid modulation of endothelial activation. Am J C Nutr. Jan 2000;71(1 Suppl):213S–23S.
19. Mason PR, Jacob RF, Corbalan JJ, Malinski T. Combination eicosapentaenoic acid and statin treatment reversed endothelial dysfunction in HUVECs exposed to oxidized LDL. J Clin Lipidol. 2014;8(3):342–3.
20. Ishida T, Naoe S, Nakakuki M, Kawano H, Imada K. Eicosapentaenoic acid prevents saturated fatty acid-induced vascular endothelial dysfunction: involvement of long-chain acyl-CoA synthetase. J Atheroscler Thromb. 2015; 22(11):1172–85.
21. Fer M, Dreano Y, Lucas D, et al. Metabolism of eicosapentaenoic and docosahexaenoic acids by recombinant human cytochromes P450. Arch Biochem Biophys. 2008;471(2):116–25.
22. Wang RX, Chai Q, Lu T, Lee HC. Activation of vascular BK channels by docosahexaenoic acid is dependent on cytochrome P450 epoxygenase activity. Cardiovasc Res. 2011;90(2):344–52.
23. Arnold C, Markovic M, Blossey K, et al. Arachidonic acid-metabolizing cytochrome P450 enzymes are targets of {omega}-3 fatty acids. J Biol Chem. 2010;285(43):32720–33.
24. Barker DJ. Fetal origins of coronary heart disease. BMJ. 1995;311(6998):171–4.
25. Armitage JA, Pearce AD, Sinclair AJ, et al. Increased blood pressure later in life may be associated with perinatal n-3 fatty acid deficiency. Lipids. 2003;38(4):459–64.
26. Korotkova M, Gabrielsson BG, Holmäng A, et al. Gender-related long-term effects in adult rats by perinatal dietary ratio of n-6/n-3 fatty acids. Am J Phys Regul Integr Comp Phys. 2005;288(3):R575–9.
27. Weisinger HS, Armitage JA, Sinclair AJ, et al. Perinatal omega-3 fatty acid deficiency affects blood pressure later in life. Nat Med. 2001;7(3):258–9.
28. Hanebutt FL, Demmelmair H, Schiessl B, Larque E, Koletzko B. Long-chain polyunsaturated fatty acid (LC-PUFA) transfer across the placenta. Clin Nutr. 2008;27(5):685–93.
29. Vidakovic AJ, Gishti O, Steenweg-de Graaff J, et al. Higher maternal plasma n-3 PUFA and lower n-6 PUFA concentrations in pregnancy are associated with lower childhood systolic blood pressure. J Nutr. 2015;145(10):2362–8.
30. Vidakovic AJ, Gishti O, Voortman T, et al. Maternal plasma PUFA concentrations during pregnancy and childhood adiposity: the Generation R Study [published online ahead of print February 24, 2016]. Am J Clin Nutr. 2016;103 (4):1017–25
31. Leary SD, Ness AR, Emmett PM, et al. Maternal diet in pregnancy and offspring blood pressure. Arch Dis Child. 2005;90(5):492–3.
32. Bryant J, Hanson M, Peebles C, et al. Higher oily fish consumption in late pregnancy is associated with reduced aortic stiffness in the child at age 9 years. Circ Res. 2015;116(7):1202–5.
33. Gustafson KM, Carlson SE, Colombo J, et al. Effects of docosahexaenoic acid supplementation during pregnancy on fetal heart rate and variability: a randomized clinical trial. Prostaglandins Leukot Essent Fat Acids. 2013;88(5):331–8.

34. Rytter D, Christensen JH, Bech BH, et al. The effect of maternal fish oil supplementation during the last trimester of pregnancy on blood pressure, heart rate and heart rate variability in the 19-year-old offspring. Br J Nutr. 2012;108(8):1475–83.

35. Rytter D, Bech BH, Halldorsson T, et al. No association between the intake of marine n-3 PUFA during the second trimester of pregnancy and factors associated with cardiometabolic risk in the 20-year-old offspring. Br J Nutr. 2013;110(11):2037–46.

36. Olofsson SO, Bostrom P, Andersson L, et al. Lipid droplets as dynamic organelles connecting storage and efflux of lipids. Biochim Biophys Acta. 2009;1791(6):448–58.

37. Jensen CL, Prager TC, Zou Y, et al. Effects of maternal docosahexaenoic acid supplementation on visual function and growth of breast-fed term infants. Lipids. 1999;34(Suppl):S225.

38. Montgomery C, Speake BK, Cameron A, Sattar N, Weaver LT. Maternal docosahexaenoic acid supplementation and fetal accretion. Br J Nutr. Jul 2003;90(1):135–45.

39. Arenz S, Ruckerl R, Koletzko B, von Kries R. Breast-feeding and childhood obesity – a systematic review. Int J Obes Relat Metab Disord. 2004;28(10):1247–56.

40. Cunnane SC, Francescutti V, Brenna JT, Crawford MA. Breast-fed infants achieve a higher rate of brain and whole body docosahexaenoate accumulation than formula-fed infants not consuming dietary docosahexaenoate. Lipids. 2000;35(1):105–11.

41. Wilson AC, Forsyth JS, Greene SA, et al. Relation of infant diet to childhood health: seven year follow up of cohort of children in Dundee infant feeding study. BMJ. 1998;316(7124):21–5.

42. Taittonen L, Nuutinen M, Turtinen J, Uhari M. Prenatal and postnatal factors in predicting later blood pressure among children: cardiovascular risk in young Finns. Pediatr Res. 1996;40(4):627–32.

43. Singhal A, Cole TJ, Lucas A. Early nutrition in preterm infants and later blood pressure: two cohorts after randomised trials. Lancet. 2001;357(9254):413–9.

44. Pivik RT, Dykman RA, Jing H, Gilchrist JM, Badger TM. Early infant diet and the omega 3 fatty acid DHA: effects on resting cardiovascular activity and behavioral development during the first half-year of life. Dev Neuropsychol. 2009;34(2):139–58.

45. Larnkjaer A, Christensen JH, Michaelsen KF, Lauritzen L. Maternal fish oil supplementation during lactation does not affect blood pressure, pulse wave velocity, or heart rate variability in 2.5-y-old children. J Nutr. 2006; 136(6):1539–44.

46. Forsyth JS, Willatts P, Agostoni C, et al. Long chain polyunsaturated fatty acid supplementation in infant formula and blood pressure in later childhood: follow up of a randomised controlled trial. BMJ. 2003;326(7396):953.

47. Damsgaard CT, Schack-Nielsen L, Michaelsen KF, et al. Fish oil affects blood pressure and the plasma lipid profile in healthy Danish infants. J Nutr. 2006;136(1):94–9.

48. Greenberg JA, Bell SJ, Ausdal WV. Omega-3 fatty acid supplementation during pregnancy. Rev Obstet Gynecol. 2008;1(4):162–9.

49. Skilton MR, Ayer JG, Harmer JA, et al. Impaired fetal growth and arterial wall thickening: a randomized trial of omega-3 supplementation. Pediatrics. 2012;129(3):e698–703.

50. Skilton MR, Phang M. From the alpha to the omega-3: breaking the link between impaired fetal growth and adult cardiovascular disease. Nutrition. 2016;32:725.

Chapter 22
Maternal Folate, Methyl Donors, One-Carbon Metabolism, Vitamin B12 and Choline in Foetal Programming

Jean-Louis Guéant and Rosa-Maria Guéant-Rodriguez

Key Points

- The deficit in dietary methyl donors before and during pregnancy produces profound effects on child development and long-term health.
- The foetal programming of rat by deficiency in methyl donors produces manifestations of metabolic syndrome in liver and heart and altered neurodevelopment and neuroplasticity.
- Accumulating evidence shows that maternal status in methyl donor nutrients affects DNA methylation, in population studies.
- Low B12 in the first trimester of pregnancy predicts higher central obesity and higher insulin resistance at 6 years in the offspring, especially when associated with high maternal folate status.
- Association studies and interventional studies converge in showing an influence of maternal folate on cognitive performances of offspring.

Keywords Folate • Vitamin B12 • Epigenomics • Methylome • Birth weight • Metabolic syndrome • Cognition

Abbreviations

MTHFD1, MTHFD2	Methylenetetrahydrofolate dehydrogenase 1 and 2
1-CM	One-carbon metabolisms
AHCY	Adenosylhomocysteinase
BHMT	Betaine homocysteine methyltransferase
BMI	Body mass index
CBS	Cystathionine beta-synthase
CTH	Cystathionine gamma-lyase
DHFR	Dihydrofolate reductase
DMR	Differentially methylated region

J.-L. Guéant, MD, DSc (✉) • R.-M. Guéant-Rodriguez, MD, PhD
University Hospital Nancy and Inserm 954 Research Unity, N-GERE, (Nutrition-Genetics-Environmental Risks),
Institute of Medical Research (Pôle BMS), University of Lorraine, Vandoeuvre les Nancy, France
e-mail: Jean-Louis.Gueant@univ-lorraine.fr

© Springer International Publishing AG 2017
R. Rajendram et al. (eds.), *Diet, Nutrition, and Fetal Programming*,
Nutrition and Health, DOI 10.1007/978-3-319-60289-9_22

293

DOHaD	Developmental origins of health and disease
ER-α	Oestrogen receptor alpha
ERR-α	Oestrogen-related receptor alpha
EWAS	Epigenome wide association studies
HAT	Histone acetyltransferase
HDAC	Histone deacetylase
HDM	Histone demethylase
HIF-1α	Hypoxia-inducible factor
HMT	Histone methyltransferase
HNF-4	Hepatic nuclear factor 4
HOMA-IR	Homeostasis model assessment of insulin resistance
HSF1	Heat shock factor protein 1
IGF1	Insulin-like growth factor 1
IUGR	Intrauterine growth restriction
MDD	Methyl donor deficiency
MTHFD	Methylenetetrahydrofolate dehydrogenase
MTHFR	Methylenetetrahydrofolate reductase
MTR	Methionine synthase
NASH	Non-alcoholic steatohepatitis
PGC-1α	Peroxisome proliferator-activated receptor γ coactivator1α
PPAR-α	Peroxisome proliferator-activated receptor alpha
PRMT1	Protein arginine methyltransferase 1
SAH	S-adenosylhomocysteine
SAM	S-adenosylmethionine
SHMT	Serine hydroxymethyltransferase
SIRT	Sirtuins
TYMS	Thymidylate synthase

The developmental origins of health and disease (DOHaD) concept consider that the development events and the related environment influence during early life (at conception, and/or during foetal life, infancy and early childhood) can have a long-term impact on later health and disease risk. Consequences of negative gene-environment interactions for early health and development include increased risk of pregnancy complications such as intrauterine growth retardation and subsequent foetal programming outcomes such as obesity, increased insulin resistance and impaired cognitive development in children. These conditions are also known to predict later outcomes of age-related chronic diseases, such as outcomes of metabolic syndrome and cognitive decline, through programming mechanisms.

Experimental and human population studies have established links between the deficit in dietary methyl donors (MDD) involved in the one-carbon metabolism and foetal programming in early and later outcomes in the offspring. This review will be focused on the associations and underlying mechanisms of MDD foetal programming on outcomes of obesity and metabolic syndrome and cognition.

1-CM Participates in a Network of Pathways Related with Early Programming

1-CM plays a central role in the influence of metabolic and nutritional factors on DNA methylation and regulation of gene expression. This complex metabolic network is regulated by a number of genes and requires micronutrients such as folate, vitamins B12, B6, B2 among others to function correctly.

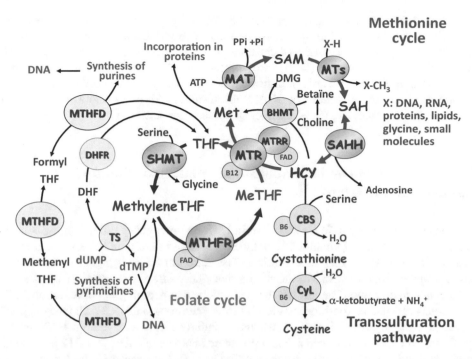

Fig. 22.1 One-carbon metabolism pathways and so-called dietary methyl donors that acts as precursors of methyl and other one-carbon radicals (*in yellow*). In the folate cycle monocarbons are used for synthesis of purines and thymidylate. In the methionine cycle, the methyl group provided by methyl-tetrahydrofolate is used in homocysteine remethylation to methionine. The transsulfuration of homocysteine is catalyzed by cystathionine beta-synthase and cystathionine gamma-lyase, two enzymes that are B6-dependent. *Abbreviations*. *THF* tetrahydrofolate, *MTHFD 1 and 2* methylene-tetrahydrofolate dehydrogenase 1 et 2, *MTHFR* methylene-tetrahydrofolate reductase, *SHMT1* "cytoplasmic serine hydroxymethyltransferase", *TYMS* thymidylate synthase, *DIIFR* dihydrofolate reductase, *MTR* methionine synthase, *SHMT* serine hydroxymethyltransferase, *BHMT* betaine homocysteine methyltransferase, *MAT* methionine adenosyl-transferase, *CBS* cystathionine beta-synthase, *CTH* cystathionine gamma-lyase, *AHCY* adenosylhomocysteinase (Figure adapted from Ref. [19])

Some of them, folate, vitamin B12 and choline are methyl donors, which are involved in the synthesis of the precursor of S-adenosylmethionine, the universal donor of methyl groups needed for DNA methylation (Fig. 22.1). Thus, dysregulation in any of the regulatory components (nutritional, metabolic or genetic determinants) of 1-CM can alter the epigenomic regulation of gene expression.

1-CM displays complex biochemical regulation and participates in a network of interconnected pathways necessary for the synthesis of purine nucleotides, thymidylate and amino acids. Cellular methionine originates from the remethylation pathway of homocysteine by methionine synthase, which uses vitamin B12 (methyl-cobalamin) as a cofactor. The deficit in folate and vitamin B12 leads to two metabolic consequences, the decreased synthesis of methionine and S-adenosylmethionine (SAM) and the accumulation of homocysteine. Choline is also a methyl donor for the synthesis of methionine in the liver. Coenzymes derived from vitamin B2 are cofactors of several enzymes of the 1-CM, including methylenetetrahydrofolate reductase (MTHFR), while B6-derived coenzymes are cofactors of the enzymes involved in the transsulfuration pathway of homocysteine, which produces cysteine and glutathione. Novel aspects of the association of 1-CM with diseases concern low vitamin B6. Vitamins B6 and B2 are involved in the formation of kynurenines, which are neuroactive metabolites with immunomodulatory effects.

Over the past two decades, many epidemiological and experimental studies have showed an association between homocysteine (homocysteine) and manifestations of foetal programming. The consequences of folate and vitamin B12 deficiency on the decreased cellular concentration of SAM, increased S-adenosylhomocysteine (SAH) and decrease of the SAM/SAH ratio illustrate their importance in maintaining the homeostasis of transmethylations. The decreased SAM/SAH ratio impairs the cell's ability to ensure methylation of DNA, RNA, histones and co-regulators of nuclear receptors, all of which play a key role in epigenetic and epigenomic mechanisms [1].

The Nutritional Status and Metabolism of Folate and Vitamin B12 in Pregnancy and In Utero Life

The prevalence of deficiency in folate and vitamin 12 during pregnancy differs among countries and continents. The prevalence of vitamin B12 deficiency is high in India. In Europe, the prevalence of vitamin B12 deficit is lower than that of folate. The deficit in folate is higher in Northern than in Southern European countries. In Northern America, the folate fortification of cereals has been introduced since nearly two decades, but there is a debate concerning possible harmful effects of the supplementation and/or food fortification by folic acid in case of B12 deficiency [2]. It is well established that dietary methyl donor nutrients, including folate and vitamin B12, are vital for embryo, foetal and early development. The imbalance in status of folate and B12 has been associated with increased risk of adverse pregnancy outcomes [3]. However the links between the 1-CM network, epigenetic processes and phenotype are not clear. Different components of the process from diet and 1-CM to DNA methylation have been shown to affect development from the earliest stages and also long-term health outcomes. However these components have largely been studied as separate entities.

Fertility is influenced by folate and vitamin B12 in both males and females. Folate deficiency is associated with altered spermatogenesis and impaired ovarian reserve [4]. Pre-implantation embryos express almost all enzymes that participate in one-carbon metabolism, and the role of exogenous folate on their development is still under debate [5, 6]. Folate is crucial for proper foetal development and its deficiency is associated with Down syndrome and neural crest-related birth defects through mechanisms that may involve DNA methylation [7]. The effect of folate supplementation throughout pregnancy remains controversial, compared to its well-established protective influence in the preconceptional period of life. A recent meta-analysis concluded that increased folate intake is associated with higher birth weight after the first trimester, but has no effect on length of gestation [8]. The mechanisms of vitamin B12 availability during the foetal life are complex. Intrinsic factor is the digestive transporter of dietary B12 that is needed for its absorption and transcobalamin the blood transporter that delivers vitamin B12 to tissues. There is a progressive decrease in holotranscobalamin and free transcobalamin in amniotic fluid and blood during pregnancy [9, 10] and a higher concentration in cord blood than in maternal blood [11]. However, in congenital transcobalamin deficiency, the foetus is not B12-deficient and develops normally to full term, suggesting alternate pathways of B12 delivery. Transcobalamin and intrinsic factor of amniotic fluid have mainly a foetal origin [9]. Vitamin B12 bound to intrinsic factor can be a foetal source of B12 in utero, through the amniotic fluid swallowed by the foetus [12]. There is some specificity of the 1-CM during the foetal life regarding the absence of transsulfuration activity and the unique metabolism of serine and glycine in the foetus (see for review Kalhan SC, *Mol Cell Endocrinol*, 2016) [13].

1-CM Markers and Methyl Donor Status Influence Foetal Programming Outcomes

Experimental Evidences (Fig. 22.2)

Rodents provide suitable models to investigate promoter and histone demethylations, with gene and tissue-specific effects [14, 15]. Maternal dietary supplementation of folate produces epigenetic effects in the progeny of the agouti mice model. A mutation designed Avy is caused by the retrotransposition of a CpG-containing intracisternal A particle (IAP) upstream of the transcription start site of the wild-type agouti gene. The locus displays epigenetic inheritance following maternal but not paternal transmission [16]. Maternal dietary supplementation with folic acid, vitamin B12, choline and betaine induces IAP methylation and shifts the phenotype distribution by increasing the proportion of coat colour. The offspring are also leaner, healthier and have a longer lifespan [17]. Reduced periconceptional supply of folate, vitamin B12 and methionine in sheep led to greater body fat, insulin resistance and hypertension and at the molecular level, to variation in epigenetic patterns [18]. The foetal programming of rat by deficiency in methyl donors, vitamin B12 and folate produces central manifestations of metabolic syndrome in liver and heart [19]. Deficiency in folate and vitamin B12 during gestation and lactation produces manifestations of foetal programming, with decreased birth weight, increased central fat mass, liver steatosis and cardiac hypertrophy, in pups from deficient rat mothers [20, 21]. These manifestations result from increased import of free fatty acids, impaired fatty acid β-oxidation and impaired energy metabolism in myocardium and liver. The underlying molecular mechanisms are linked to the decreased expression and activity of SIRT1 and PRMT1 and the subsequent hyperacetylation and hypomethylation of PGC1-α and epigenomic dysregulation of nuclear receptors, ER-α, PPARs, ERR-α and HNF-4. Interestingly, overnutrition produces similar effects with decreased expression and activity of SIRT1. The differential gene expression associated with DNA methylation is related to the outcomes of metabolic syndrome, including blood pressure. Some of these expression changes are involved in renin-angiotensin system and energy metabolism [22].

Epidemiological Facts

Over the past two decades, many epidemiological studies and meta-analyses have clearly demonstrated an association between markers of the 1-CM, including methyl donors and homocysteine, and birth weight and other manifestations of foetal programming [19].

Various studies in India and Nepal have reported an association between maternal vitamin B12 status during pregnancy and central obesity and insulin resistance in childhood. Indian babies have low weight but are fat (lean-fat phenotype), and there is a higher prevalence of mothers with low serum vitamin B12 and folate deficiency, compared to Europe [23]. Offspring birthweight is inversely related to maternal homocysteine concentration and *MTHFR* gene variant rs1801133 (formerly *677 C>T*) predicts higher homocysteine concentration and lower birth weight, in the Pune Maternal Nutrition Study and Parthenon Cohort Study of India [24]. Pune Maternal Nutrition Study shows also that low cobalamin in the first trimester of pregnancy predicts higher central obesity and higher insulin resistance at 6 years in the offspring, especially when associated with high maternal folate status [25]. A study in the rural district of Nepal confirmed that low pregnancy cobalamin status was associated with an increased risk of insulin resistance in the offspring by early school age [26]. In another cohort from India, maternal homocysteine at 30 gestational weeks was associated with higher post

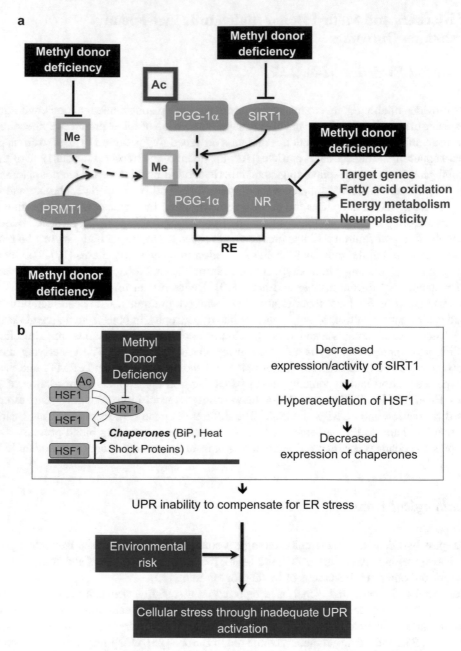

Fig. 22.2 (**a, b**) Methyl donor deficiency (MDD) foetal programming effects on nuclear receptor pathways. MDD decreases the expression of peroxisome proliferator-activated receptor alpha (PPARα), oestrogen-related receptor alpha (ERR-α) and hepatic nuclear factor 4 (HNF-4). It impairs the co-regulation of these nuclear receptors (NRs) by peroxisome proliferator-activated receptor gamma coactivator 1-alpha (PGC-1α), through its decreased methylation and/or increased acetylation. This imbalanced methylation/acetylation is the consequence of the decreased expression of arginine methyl-transferase PRMT1, the decreased cellular ratio of S-adenosylmethionine (SAM)/S-adenosylhomocysteine (SAH) that directly influences PRMT1 activity and the decreased expression of deacetylase sirtuin 1 (SIRT1); These mechanisms produce some of the effects of MDD foetal programming through altered expression of genes involved in energy metabolism, fatty oxidation, and neuroplasticity (Figure adapted from Ref. [19])

load glucose concentrations in the offspring at 5 and 9 years. Higher maternal folate status during the same period was associated with a higher degree of insulin resistance in the offspring [27]. A variant of adenosylmethionine decarboxylase was associated with childhood obesity, in another Indian study [28].

Epidemiological studies have also shown that 1-CM markers and methyl donor status during pregnancy influence the risk of small birth weight and of subsequent events related to foetal programming, in Europe and Western countries. Children born from mothers with homocysteine in the top quartile weighted less than the rest of the children [29]. Other studies have also reported an inverse association between maternal homocysteine and birth weight in the offspring [27, 30], while no association was found in a large study from Canada, a country in which folate fortification in cereals has been introduced 15 years ago [31]. Maternal erythrocyte folate concentration during pregnancy was also reported to be positively associated with birth weight [32, 33]. A meta-analysis confirmed the inverse association between homocysteine and birth weight and estimated the OR for small-for-gestational-age (SGA) at 1.25 for maternal homocysteine above the 90th percentile [34]. In contrast, a double-blinded randomized controlled trial of folic acid supplementation, taken over 14–36 gestational weeks in women who also received folic acid supplements in the first trimester prevented the gestational decline of folate observed at 36 gestational weeks in the placebo group, but had no significant impact on infant size at birth [35]. In a more recent study, maternal concentrations of B12, B6 and Hcy did not associate with birth weight, but they predicted the 3-year weight gain [36].

The influence of folate intake seems to have an influence on outcomes of metabolic syndrome in childhood, in Europe, despite contrasted results among populations. In a population-based cohort from South UK, folate intake estimated by questionnaire did not influence childhood body composition [37]. In contrast, it was associated with birth weight and insulin resistance in a French study of obese adolescents [38]. Contrasted results have been also found with a genetic determinant of folate metabolism, the *MTHFR 677C>T* polymorphism. This gene variant not associated with obesity and BMI, in three cohorts from the UK and Denmark, or with metabolic syndrome, in an Italian population study [39, 40]. In contrast, in France, Frelut et al. reported that *MTHFR 677C>T* was associated with low birth weight and high insulin resistance in morbidly obese adolescents [38]. A cohort study of 2819 mothers and their children showed that higher vitamin B 12 concentrations in mothers predicted higher childhood bone mass, whereas homocysteine concentrations were associated with lower childhood bone mass [41].

Methyl Donors and Environmental Factors Influence the Epigenome in Early Life

Experimental Facts

The epigenome appears to be particularly malleable during embryogenesis and in utero life and epigenetic changes that occur at this time may have roles in disease susceptibility after birth [42]. Epigenetic imprinting is influenced by maternal environmental exposure, including nutritional status. It has a permanent effect on the developing foetus and lifelong genome adaptation [43].

Epidemiological Facts During Pregnancy and Postnatal Life

Accumulating evidence shows that maternal status in methyl donor nutrients affects DNA methylation. Pregnancy choline intake is associated with increased methylation of genes that regulate the foetal hypothalmic-pituitary axis reactivity in cord blood and in placenta [44]. Inverse associations have been reported between maternal fasting plasma homocysteine and global methylation of cord *LINE-I* DNA [45]. DNA methylation was increased in 17-month-old infants of mothers that had used periconceptional folic acid at the recommended dose of 400 µg/d [46], a result, which was not found in the folate-repleted population from the Viva cohort in the USA, where food fortification with folic acid is widespread [47]. Recently maternal riboflavin and cysteine were shown to affect DNA methylation of metastable epialleles in the offspring [48]. The genetic determinants of 1-CM and folate status may also affects DNA methylation on offsprings. A study of mother-child pairs of Dutch national origin found an association between the maternal *MTHFR 677C>T* genotype and the epigenome of a selection of seven genes in newborns [49].

The methyl donor deficient diet influences the development and later health of offspring through altered expression of methylated region (DMR) and imprinted genes. A recent study of pregnant women, the Newborn Epigenetics Study found an association of maternal erythrocyte folate levels with DNA methylation changes of *MEG3* DMR and birth weight [50]. Another study estimated the associations between maternal vitamins B12, B6 (pyridoxal phosphate and 4-pyridoxic acid) and homocysteine concentrations with offspring DNA methylation of 4 DMRs involved in foetal growth, namely, *H19, MEG3, SGCE/PEG10* and *PLAGL1*. The most relevant result was the association of higher maternal PLP concentrations with offspring DNA methylation levels at the *MEG3* DMR [36]. Imprinted genes are organized in clusters and are expressed predominantly from only one of the parental alleles. In the *H19/IGF2* cluster, H19 encodes a non-coding RNA, while IGF2 influences embryonic development and foetal programming through expression of insulin-like growth factor 2 [51]. Igf2 is expressed almost exclusively from the paternal allele, and the tightly linked H19 from the maternal allele. The loss of imprinting for *H19* and *IGF2* has been observed in human blood cells [50]. Patients heterozygous for a *H19* polymorphism and presenting with high plasma homocysteine concentrations due to renal failure (60 µmol/L) display a bi-allelic expression for *H19* that correlates with decreased DNA methylation and which reverts to mono-allelic expression and increased Igf2 expression after treatment with Me-THF [52]. These results show therefore that the influence of folate on Igf2 expression is not limited to early development but extends to the postnatal period. Similar results have been obtained with periconception global undernutrition. For example, the Dutch famine was associated with reduced DNA methylation at the IGF2 locus in the offspring 60 years later [53].

Epigenome Wide Changes Influence Metabolism and Traits of Metabolic Syndrome in Later Life

Heritability estimates are between 30% and 70% for age-related conditions such as diabetes, Alzheimer's disease, obesity and hypertension. The crucial role of the epigenome in this scenario is only beginning to be evaluated as powerful methods to analyse the whole DNA methylome emerge [54].

Epigenome Influence on Metabolic Traits

Many interacting mechanisms and confounding factors participate in the links between DNA methylation, gene expression and metabotypes. Genetic variance in CpG sites or in their vicinity could influence DNA methylation. Previous GWAS with metabolic traits linked to disease outcomes have identified many so-called genetically influenced metabotypes (GIMs) [55], which have been shown to predict complex disorders. Associations between metabolic traits and DNA methylation may result from complex interactions in contrast to GIM, where a genetic variant may be directly causal for an association between a SNP and a phenotype. DNA methylation is an important gene-regulatory mechanism expected to play a prominent role in disease/outcome-related metabotypes. For instance, DNA methylation can influence C-glycosyl tryptophan, a metabolite, which is also associated with birth weight [56]. Few longitudinal studies have compared the respective influence of environment and 1-CM among life. Bjornsson et al. studied the time-dependent changes in global DNA methylation of a panel of 1505 CpG dinucleotides from 807 genes within 337 individuals from two separate populations of widely separated geographic locations [57]. The author found 8–10% of individuals in both populations showing changes greater than 20% over an 11- to 16-year span. The data suggested an age-related loss of normal epigenetic patterns, which is a potential mechanism for late onset of common human diseases. The familial clustering of methylation changes raised the possibility that methylation might be directly related to genes controlling 1-CM or DNA methyltransferase activity.

Epigenome Influence on Age-Related Outcomes of Metabolic Syndrome

DNA methylation is considered as a 'key' for understanding the molecular mechanisms of normal and premature ageing. However, very few epigenome wide association studies (EWAS) have been performed for evaluating the association between the DNA methylome and age-related outcomes and none of them have considered the dietary methyl donors and metabolic determinants of 1-CM in their study design. A recent EWAS with BMI in 479 individuals of European origin showed an association of increased BMI with increased methylation at the *HIF3A* locus in blood cells and in adipose tissue [58]. To date, most of the knowledge on the influence of the epigenome on metabolic syndrome outcomes is generated from experimental data and cannot be easily extrapolated to human situations. An increase in adipose tissue mass has been associated with elevated secretion of proinflammatory adipokines, such as TNF-α and leptin, whose expression is determined by the epigenetic status of the relevant genes [59]. A group of obese women who responded well to a calorie-restricted diet had a lower level of promoter methylation on the TNF-α and leptin genes [60], suggesting that methylation levels of these genes could be used as epigenetic biomarkers in predicting response to low-energy diets. Furthermore, a study of obese men showed differential DNA methylation levels in several CpGs located in the *ATP10A* and *CD44* genes depending on the weight-loss outcome [61]. Non-alcoholic fatty liver disease (NAFLD) is considered as a visceral manifestation of metabolic syndrome, which linearly correlates with all components of metabolic syndrome. In a study of liver biopsies from NAFLD patients, methylation of PGC1-α promoter, a co-regulator involved in energy metabolism was linked to HOMA-IR and plasma fasting insulin levels [62]. Bell et al. explored the hypothesis that epigenetic changes contribute to the rate of ageing phenotype in a sample of middle-aged female twins [63]. They reported 490 genomic regions that were differentially methylated with chronological age and a differentially methylated region (DMR) associated with total cholesterol. None was associated with blood pressure.

Dietary Methyl Donors Influence the Effects of Toxic Dietary Factors on Epigenome

Toxic dietary factors can influence the epigenetic hallmarks related to folate status, in experimental studies. In mice, maternal exposure to bisphenol A, an oestrogenic xenobiotic, decreases DNA methylation in the retrotransposon upstream of the agouti gene and shifts coat colour distribution in the offspring. This effect is neutralized by maternal supplementation with folic acid, betaine and choline [64].

Fumonisins from corn- and maize-based diets are associated with growth retardation in exposed infants in Tanzania [65]. Part of the toxicity could be related to impaired folate metabolism and epigenetic alterations. Indeed, fumonisin FB1 inhibits folate receptor expression [66, 67] and methyl donor deficiency and fumonisin FB1 act synergistically on DNA instability through alteration of heterochromatin assembly [68].

1-CM Markers and Methyl Donor Status During Pregnancy and Lactation Influence Postnatal Neurodevelopment and Cognition Through Epigenomic Mechanisms

Experimental Facts (Figs. 22.2 and 22.3)

The deficiency of vitamin B12 and folate during pregnancy and postnatal life impairs the proper development of brain, in animal models. The increased homocysteine triggers oxidative stress and homocysteinylation of functional cargo proteins involved in the transport of neurotransmitters. Vitamin B12 and folate deficiency in dams during gestation and lactation produces deregulations of nuclear receptors in pups, a mechanism which is also observed in heart and liver. In particular, the imbalanced methylation/acetylation of PGC1-α disrupts the activation of ER-α with subsequent altered cerebellum neuroplasticity through impaired expression of synapsins [69]. In a N1E115 neuroblastoma cell model, the most discernible consequences of decreased cellular availability of vitamin B12 are reduced proliferation and accelerated differentiation through PP2A, NGF and TACE pathways and increased reticulum stress through decreased expression of deacetylase SIRT1 and greater acetylation of heat shock factor protein 1 (HSF1) [70, 71]. Folate deficit sensitizes H19-7 neuronal progenitors to differentiation-associated apoptosis, with increased expression of histone deacetylases (HDAC), leading to impaired differentiation, cell polarity, vesicular transport, synaptic plasticity and neurite outgrowth. Expression and phosphorylation at both Tyr705 and Ser727 of Stat3 are decreased in the brains of deprived foetuses and in differentiating progenitors. Vitamin shortage down regulates Stat3 signalling through miR-124 upregulation, leading to altered brain development [72].

Population Studies

Association studies and interventional studies converge in showing an influence of maternal folate on cognitive performances of offspring. In Europe, children from mothers with increase of homocysteine during pre-pregnancy and early pregnancy were more likely to score lower in IQ tests at 6 years of age than children with mothers whose homocysteine are in the low–normal range [73]. The children had normal plasma homocysteine at the time of the development tests and no correlation between homocysteine and their IQ scores. Folic acid supplement intake during early pregnancy was positively associated with neurodevelopment in 4-year-old children in Spain [73]. Maternal red cell folate at 14 weeks of pregnancy was inversely associated with hyperactivity in 8–9 year old children [73] and positively associated with foetal head growth. Late pregnancy folate status (but not vitamin B12) was positively associated with cognitive test scores in 9–10 year-old children in India [74]. Multivitamin supplementation from early pregnancy throughout 3 months post-partum was associated with improved IQ tests in 7–9 year old children from rural Nepal [75]. The same study observed no added benefit to their IQ when supplementing these children from 12 to 36 months of age [76]. In contrast, another study found no association between mid–late pregnancy folate status or homocysteine and

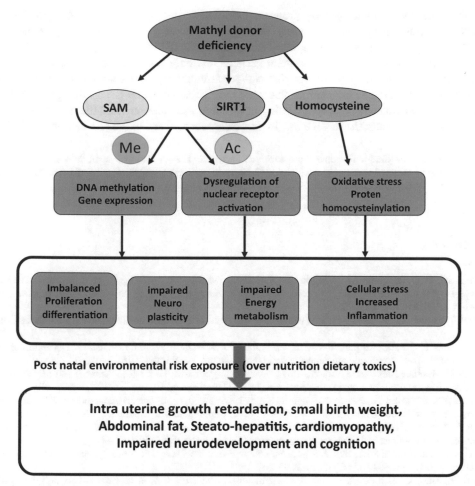

Fig. 22.3 Overview of the mechanisms observed in the dam-progeny rat model of MDD (methyl donor-deficient diet) foetal programming. MDD produces sequential events related to increased homocysteine and decreased SAM and sirtuin (SIRT)1 activity. Decreased production of S-adenosylmethionine and altered SIRT1 expression lead to epigenomic dysregulations, with methylome changes and disruption of nuclear receptor coactivation by imbalanced methylation/ acetylation of the coactivator PGC-1α. Homocysteine accumulation produces cellular stress and protein homocysteinylation. The consequences include reduced proliferation and sensitized progenitors to differentiation, impaired neuroplasticity and energy metabolism and increased cellular stress and inflammation. These consequences may trigger outcomes related to non-alcoholic steatohepatitis (NASH), cardiomyopathy and cognition in animals exposed to over nutrition or proinflammatory agents in later life

neurodevelopment in 5-year-old black American children of low socioeconomic status [77], while the maternal *MTHFR 677 T* variant allele was associated with lower developmental scores at 24 months of age in Mexican children [78].

In Conclusion

The deficit in dietary methyl donors before and during pregnancy produces profound effects on child development and long-term health. Childhood obesity and cognition development are growing concerns. There are now experimental evidences suggesting that this deficit in maternal micronutrient status create an environment that may program a child towards higher risk of disease in later life by influencing prenatal epigenomic profiles, leading to lifelong genome adaptation. However, the influence of epigenome in the underlying mechanisms of MDD foetal programming has received insufficient attention to date. Common gene variants and epigenome are key determinants of early development and health outcomes that predict and/or participate in the development and progression of chronic ageing diseases. The correlations that have been observed so far are encouraging for the prospects of further integrated analyses associating epigenome wide analyses and the metabolic and nutritional factors that influence the methylome, in particular those related to the one-carbon metabolism.

Acknowledgements Institutional grants were received from the French national institute for medical research (Inserm), the French national agency for research (ANR Nutrivigene project) and the Region of Lorraine (France). The authors declare no competing financial interests.

References

1. Gueant JL, Caillerez-Fofou M, Battaglia-Hsu S, Alberto JM, Freund JN, Dulluc I, et al. Molecular and cellular effects of vitamin B12 in brain, myocardium and liver through its role as co-factor of methionine synthase. Biochimie. 2013;95(5):1033–40.
2. Selhub J, Rosenberg IH. Excessive folic acid intake and relation to adverse health outcome. Biochimie. 2016;126: 71–8.
3. Sole-Navais P, Cavalle-Busquets P, Fernandez-Ballart JD, Murphy MM. Early pregnancy B vitamin status, one carbon metabolism, pregnancy outcome and child development. Biochimie. 2016;126:91–6.
4. Forges T, Monnier-Barbarino P, Alberto JM, Gueant-Rodriguez RM, Daval JL, Gueant JL. Impact of folate and homocysteine metabolism on human reproductive health. Hum Reprod Update. 2007;13(3):225–38.
5. Kwong WY, Adamiak SJ, Gwynn A, Singh R, Sinclair KD. Endogenous folates and single-carbon metabolism in the ovarian follicle, oocyte and pre-implantation embryo. Reproduction. 2010;139(4):705–15.
6. Ikeda S, Koyama H, Sugimoto M, Kume S. Roles of one-carbon metabolism in preimplantation period – effects on short-term development and long-term programming. J Reprod Dev. 2012;58(1):38–43.
7. Kim KC, Friso S, Choi SW. DNA methylation, an epigenetic mechanism connecting folate to healthy embryonic development and aging. J Nutr Biochem. 2009;20(12):917–26.
8. Fekete K, Berti C, Trovato M, Lohner S, Dullemeijer C, Souverein OW, et al. Effect of folate intake on health outcomes in pregnancy: a systematic review and meta-analysis on birth weight, placental weight and length of gestation. Nutr J. 2012;11:75.
9. Gueant JL, Hambaba L, Vidailhet M, Schaefer C, Wahlstedt V, Nicolas JP. Concentration and physicochemical characterisation of unsaturated cobalamin binding proteins in amniotic fluid. Clin Chim Acta. 1989;181(2):151–61.
10. Greibe E, Andreasen BH, Lildballe DL, Morkbak AL, Hvas AM, Nexo E. Uptake of cobalamin and markers of cobalamin status: a longitudinal study of healthy pregnant women. Clin Chem Lab Med. 2011;49(11):1877–82.
11. Amarin ZO, Obeidat AZ. Effect of folic acid fortification on the incidence of neural tube defects. Paediatr Perinat Epidemiol. 2010;24(4):349–51.
12. Aimone-Gastin I, Gueant JL, Plenat F, Muhale F, Maury F, Djalali M, et al. Assimilation of [57Co]-labeled cobalamin in human fetal gastrointestinal xenografts into nude mice. Pediatr Res. 1999;45(6):860–6.
13. Kalhan SC. One carbon metabolism in pregnancy: impact on maternal, fetal and neonatal health. Mol Cell Endocrinol. 2016;435:48–60.
14. McCabe DC, Caudill MA. DNA methylation, genomic silencing, and links to nutrition and cancer. Nutr Rev. 2005;63(6 Pt 1):183–95.
15. Ghoshal K, Li X, Datta J, Bai S, Pogribny I, Pogribny M, et al. A folate- and methyl-deficient diet alters the expression of DNA methyltransferases and methyl CpG binding proteins involved in epigenetic gene silencing in livers of F344 rats. J Nutr. 2006;136(6):1522–7.
16. Wolff GL, Kodell RL, Moore SR, Cooney CA. Maternal epigenetics and methyl supplements affect agouti gene expression in Avy/a mice. FASEB J. 1998;12(11):949–57.
17. Waterland RA, Jirtle RL. Transposable elements: targets for early nutritional effects on epigenetic gene regulation. Mol Cell Biol. 2003;23(15):5293–300.
18. Sinclair KD, Allegrucci C, Singh R, Gardner DS, Sebastian S, Bispham J, et al. DNA methylation, insulin resistance, and blood pressure in offspring determined by maternal periconceptional B vitamin and methionine status. Proc Natl Acad Sci U S A. 2007;104(49):19351–6.

19. Gueant JL, Namour F, Gueant-Rodriguez RM, Daval JL. Folate and fetal programming: a play in epigenomics? Trends Endocrinol Metab. 2013;24(6):279–89.
20. Garcia MM, Guéant-Rodriguez RM, Pooya S, Brachet P, Alberto JM, Jeannesson E, et al. Methyl donor deficiency induces cardiomyopathy through altered methylation/acetylation of PGC-1α by PRMT1 and SIRT1. J Pathol. 2011;225(3):324–35.
21. Pooya S, Blaise S, Moreno Garcia M, Giudicelli J, Alberto JM, Gueant-Rodriguez RM, et al. Methyl donor deficiency impairs fatty acid oxidation through PGC-1alpha hypomethylation and decreased ER-alpha, ERR-alpha, and HNF-4al(6)pha in the rat liver. J Hepatol. 2012;57(2):344–51.
22. Chen G, Broseus J, Hergalant S, Donnart A, Chevalier C, Bolanos-Jimenez F, et al. Identification of master genes involved in liver key functions through transcriptomics and epigenomics of methyl donor deficiency in rat: relevance to nonalcoholic liver disease. Mol Nutr Food Res. 2015;59(2):293–302.
23. Yajnik CS, Deshmukh US. Fetal programming: maternal nutrition and role of one-carbon metabolism. Rev Endocr Metab Disord. 2012;13(2):121–7.
24. Yajnik CS, Chandak GR, Joglekar C, Katre P, Bhat DS, Singh SN, et al. Maternal homocysteine in pregnancy and offspring birthweight: epidemiological associations and Mendelian randomization analysis. Int J Epidemiol. 2014;43(5):1487–97.
25. Yajnik CS, Deshpande SS, Jackson AA, Refsum H, Rao S, Fisher DJ, et al. Vitamin B12 and folate concentrations during pregnancy and insulin resistance in the offspring: the Pune maternal nutrition study. Diabetologia. 2008;51(1):29–38.
26. Stewart CP, Christian P, Schulze KJ, Arguello M, Leclerq SC, Khatry SK, et al. Low maternal vitamin B-12 status is associated with offspring insulin resistance regardless of antenatal micronutrient supplementation in rural Nepal. J Nutr. 2011;141(10):1912–7.
27. Krishnaveni GV, Veena SR, Karat SC, Yajnik CS, Fall CH. Association between maternal folate concentrations during pregnancy and insulin resistance in Indian children. Diabetologia. 2014;57(1):110–21.
28. Tabassum R, Jaiswal A, Chauhan G, Dwivedi OP, Ghosh S, Marwaha RK, et al. Genetic variant of AMD1 is associated with obesity in urban Indian children. PLoS One. 2012;7(4):e33162.
29. Murphy MM, Scott JM, Arija V, Molloy AM, Fernandez-Ballart JD. Maternal homocysteine before conception and throughout pregnancy predicts fetal homocysteine and birth weight. Clin Chem. 2004;50(8):1406–12.
30. Onalan R, Onalan G, Gunenc Z, Karabulut E. Combining 2nd-trimester maternal serum homocysteine levels and uterine artery Doppler for prediction of preeclampsia and isolated intrauterine growth restriction. Gynecol Obstet Investig. 2006;61(3):142–8.
31. Dodds L, Fell DB, Dooley KC, Armson BA, Allen AC, Nassar BA, et al. Effect of homocysteine concentration in early pregnancy on gestational hypertensive disorders and other pregnancy outcomes. Clin Chem. 2008;54(2):326–34.
32. Rao L, Puschner B, Prolla TA. Gene expression profiling of low selenium status in the mouse intestine: transcriptional activation of genes linked to DNA damage, cell cycle control and oxidative stress. J Nutr. 2001;131(12):3175–81.
33. Relton CL, Pearce MS, Parker L. The influence of erythrocyte folate and serum vitamin B12 status on birth weight. Br J Nutr. 2005;93(5):593–9.
34. Hogeveen M, Blom HJ, den Heijer M. Maternal homocysteine and small-for-gestational-age offspring: systematic review and meta-analysis. Am J Clin Nutr. 2012;95(1):130–6.
35. McNulty B, McNulty H, Marshall B, Ward M, Molloy AM, Scott JM, et al. Impact of continuing folic acid after the first trimester of pregnancy: findings of a randomized trial of folic acid supplementation in the second and third trimesters. Am J Clin Nutr. 2013;98(1):92–8.
36. McCullough LE, Miller EE, Mendez MA, Murtha AP, Murphy SK, Hoyo C. Maternal B vitamins: effects on offspring weight and DNA methylation at genomically imprinted domains. Clin Epigenetics. 2016;8:8.
37. Lewis SJ, Leary S, Davey Smith G, Ness A. Body composition at age 9 years, maternal folate intake during pregnancy and methyltetrahydrofolate reductase (MTHFR) C677T genotype. Br J Nutr. 2009;102(4):493–6.
38. Frelut ML, Nicolas JP, Guilland JC, de Courcy GP. Methylenetetrahydrofolate reductase 677 C->T polymorphism: a link between birth weight and insulin resistance in obese adolescents. Int J Pediatr Obes. 2011;6(2-2):e312–7.
39. Lewis SJ, Lawlor DA, Nordestgaard BG, Tybjaerg-Hansen A, Ebrahim S, Zacho J, et al. The methylenetetrahydrofolate reductase C677T genotype and the risk of obesity in three large population-based cohorts. Eur J Endocrinol. 2008;159(1):35–40.
40. Russo GT, Di Benedetto A, Alessi E, Ientile R, Antico A, Nicocia G, et al. Mild hyperhomocysteinemia and the common C677T polymorphism of methylene tetrahydrofolate reductase gene are not associated with the metabolic syndrome in type 2 diabetes. J Endocrinol Investig. 2006;29(3):201–7.
41. Heppe DH, Medina-Gomez C, Hofman A, Franco OH, Rivadeneira F, Jaddoe VW. Maternal first-trimester diet and childhood bone mass: the Generation R Study. Am J Clin Nutr. 2013;98(1):224–32.
42. Mill J, Heijmans BT. From promises to practical strategies in epigenetic epidemiology. Nat Rev Genet. 2013; 14(8):585–94.
43. Szyf M. DNA methylation, the early-life social environment and behavioral disorders. J Neurodev Disord. 2011;3(3):238–49.

44. Jiang X, Bar HY, Yan J, Jones S, Brannon PM, West AA, et al. A higher maternal choline intake among third-trimester pregnant women lowers placental and circulating concentrations of the antiangiogenic factor fms-like tyrosine kinase-1 (sFLT1). FASEB J. 2013;27(3):1245–53.

45. Fryer AA, Nafee TM, Ismail KM, Carroll WD, Emes RD, Farrell WE. LINE-1 DNA methylation is inversely correlated with cord plasma homocysteine in man: a preliminary study. Epigenetics. 2009;4(6):394–8.

46. Steegers-Theunissen RP, Obermann-Borst SA, Kremer D, Lindemans J, Siebel C, Steegers EA, et al. Periconceptional maternal folic acid use of 400 microg per day is related to increased methylation of the IGF2 gene in the very young child. PLoS One. 2009;4(11):e7845.

47. Boeke CE, Baccarelli A, Kleinman KP, Burris HH, Litonjua AA, Rifas-Shiman SL, et al. Gestational intake of methyl donors and global LINE-1 DNA methylation in maternal and cord blood: prospective results from a folate-replete population. Epigenetics. 2012;7(3):253–60.

48. Dominguez-Salas P, Moore SE, Baker MS, Bergen AW, Cox SE, Dyer RA, et al. Maternal nutrition at conception modulates DNA methylation of human metastable epialleles. Nat Commun. 2014;5:3746.

49. van Mil NH, Bouwland-Both MI, Stolk L, Verbiest MM, Hofman A, Jaddoe VW, et al. Determinants of maternal pregnancy one-carbon metabolism and newborn human DNA methylation profiles. Reproduction. 2014;148(6):581–92.

50. Hoyo C, Murtha AP, Schildkraut JM, Jirtle RL, Demark-Wahnefried W, Forman MR, et al. Methylation variation at IGF2 differentially methylated regions and maternal folic acid use before and during pregnancy. Epigenetics. 2011;6(7):928–36.

51. Ideraabdullah FY, Vigneau S, Bartolomei MS. Genomic imprinting mechanisms in mammals. Mutat Res. 2008; 647(1-2):77–85.

52. Ingrosso D, Cimmino A, Perna AF, Masella L, De Santo NG, De Bonis ML, et al. Folate treatment and unbalanced methylation and changes of allelic expression induced by hyperhomocysteinaemia in patients with uraemia. Lancet. 2003;361(9370):1693–9.

53. Heijmans BT, Tobi EW, Stein AD, Putter H, Blauw GJ, Susser ES, et al. Persistent epigenetic differences associated with prenatal exposure to famine in humans. Proc Natl Acad Sci U S A. 2008;105(44):17046–9.

54. Rakyan VK, Down TA, Balding DJ, Beck S. Epigenome-wide association studies for common human diseases. Nat Rev Genet. 2011;12(8):529–41.

55. Suhre K, Gieger C. Genetic variation in metabolic phenotypes: study designs and applications. Nat Rev Genet. 2012;13(11):759–69.

56. Menni C, Kastenmuller G, Petersen AK, Bell JT, Psatha M, Tsai PC, et al. Metabolomic markers reveal novel pathways of ageing and early development in human populations. Int J Epidemiol. 2013;42(4):1111–9.

57. Bjornsson HT, Sigurdsson MI, Fallin MD, Irizarry RA, Aspelund T, Cui H, et al. Intra-individual change over time in DNA methylation with familial clustering. JAMA. 2008;299(24):2877–83.

58. Dick KJ, Nelson CP, Tsaprouni L, Sandling JK, Aissi D, Wahl S, et al. DNA methylation and body-mass index: a genome-wide analysis. Lancet. 2014;383(9933):1990–8.

59. Hermsdorff HH, Puchau B, Zulet MA, Martinez JA. Association of body fat distribution with proinflammatory gene expression in peripheral blood mononuclear cells from young adult subjects. OMICS. 2010;14(3):297–307.

60. Cordero P, Campion J, Milagro FI, Goyenechea E, Steemburgo T, Javierre BM, et al. Leptin and TNF-alpha promoter methylation levels measured by MSP could predict the response to a low-calorie diet. J Physiol Biochem. 2011;67(3):463–70.

61. Milagro FI, Campion J, Cordero P, Goyenechea E, Gomez-Uriz AM, Abete I, et al. A dual epigenomic approach for the search of obesity biomarkers: DNA methylation in relation to diet-induced weight loss. FASEB J. 2011; 25(4):1378–89.

62. Sookoian S, Rosselli MS, Gemma C, Burgueno AL, Fernandez Gianotti T, Castano GO, et al. Epigenetic regulation of insulin resistance in nonalcoholic fatty liver disease: impact of liver methylation of the peroxisome proliferator-activated receptor gamma coactivator 1alpha promoter. Hepatology. 2010;52(6):1992–2000.

63. Bell JT, Tsai PC, Yang TP, Pidsley R, Nisbet J, Glass D, et al. Epigenome-wide scans identify differentially methylated regions for age and age-related phenotypes in a healthy ageing population. PLoS Genet. 2012;8(4):e1002629.

64. Dolinoy DC, Huang D, Jirtle RL. Maternal nutrient supplementation counteracts bisphenol A-induced DNA hypomethylation in early development. Proc Natl Acad Sci U S A. 2007;104(32):13056–61.

65. Kimanya ME, De Meulenaer B, Roberfroid D, Lachat C, Kolsteren P. Fumonisin exposure through maize in complementary foods is inversely associated with linear growth of infants in Tanzania. Mol Nutr Food Res. 2010;54(11):1659–67.

66. Chango A, Nour AA, Bousserouel S, Eveillard D, Anton PM, Gueant JL. Time course gene expression in the one-carbon metabolism network using HepG2 cell line grown in folate-deficient medium. J Nutr Biochem. 2009;20(4):312–20.

67. Abdel Nour AM, Ringot D, Gueant JL, Chango A. Folate receptor and human reduced folate carrier expression in HepG2 cell line exposed to fumonisin B1 and folate deficiency. Carcinogenesis. 2007;28(11):2291–7.

68. Pellanda H, Forges T, Bressenot A, Chango A, Bronowicki JP, Gueant JL, et al. Fumonisin FB1 treatment acts synergistically with methyl donor deficiency during rat pregnancy to produce alterations of H3- and H4-histone methylation patterns in fetuses. Mol Nutr Food Res. 2012;56(6):976–85.
69. Pourie G, Martin N, Bossenmeyer-Pourie C, Akchiche N, Gueant-Rodriguez RM, Geoffroy A, et al. Folate- and vitamin B12-deficient diet during gestation and lactation alters cerebellar synapsin expression via impaired influence of estrogen nuclear receptor alpha. FASEB J. 2015;29(9):3713–25.
70. Battaglia-Hsu SF, Akchiche N, Noel N, Alberto JM, Jeannesson E, Orozco-Barrios CE, et al. Vitamin B12 deficiency reduces proliferation and promotes differentiation of neuroblastoma cells and up-regulates PP2A, proNGF, and TACE. Proc Natl Acad Sci U S A. 2009;106(51):21930–5.
71. Ghemrawi R, Pooya S, Lorentz S, Gauchotte G, Arnold C, Gueant JL, et al. Decreased vitamin B12 availability induces ER stress through impaired SIRT1-deacetylation of HSF1. Cell Death Dis. 2013;4:e553.
72. Kerek R, Geoffroy A, Bison A, Martin N, Akchiche N, Pourie G, et al. Early methyl donor deficiency may induce persistent brain defects by reducing Stat3 signaling targeted by miR-124. Cell Death Dis. 2013;4:e755.
73. Julvez J, Fortuny J, Mendez M, Torrent M, Ribas-Fito N, Sunyer J. Maternal use of folic acid supplements during pregnancy and four-year-old neurodevelopment in a population-based birth cohort. Paediatr Perinat Epidemiol. 2009;23(3):199–206.
74. Veena SR, Krishnaveni GV, Srinivasan K, Wills AK, Muthayya S, Kurpad AV, et al. Higher maternal plasma folate but not vitamin B-12 concentrations during pregnancy are associated with better cognitive function scores in 9- to 10- year-old children in South India. J Nutr. 2010;140(5):1014–22.
75. Christian P, Murray-Kolb LE, Khatry SK, Katz J, Schaefer BA, Cole PM, et al. Prenatal micronutrient supplementation and intellectual and motor function in early school-aged children in Nepal. JAMA. 2010;304(24):2716–23.
76. Christian P, Morgan ME, Murray-Kolb L, LeClerq SC, Khatry SK, Schaefer B, et al. Preschool iron-folic acid and zinc supplementation in children exposed to iron-folic acid in utero confers no added cognitive benefit in early school-age. J Nutr. 2011;141(11):2042–8.
77. Tamura T, Goldenberg RL, Chapman VR, Johnston KE, Ramey SL, Nelson KG. Folate status of mothers during pregnancy and mental and psychomotor development of their children at five years of age. Pediatrics. 2005;116(3):703–8.
78. Pilsner JR, Hu H, Wright RO, Kordas K, Ettinger AS, Sanchez BN, et al. Maternal MTHFR genotype and haplotype predict deficits in early cognitive development in a lead-exposed birth cohort in Mexico City. Am J Clin Nutr. 2010;92(1):226–34.

Chapter 23
Maternal Taurine Supplementation Prevents Misprogramming

Edith Arany

Key Points

- This chapter focuses on animal and human studies related to the role of taurine (Tau) in glucose and lipid metabolism.
- Maternal diabetes and maternal dietary deficiencies influences fetal development and increases the risks of developing glucose intolerance, insulin resistance, obesity and hypertension in the offspring in adulthood.
- Tau is a sulfur amino acid that plays an important part in multiple cellular functions related to osmoregulation, energy storage, anti-oxidation, cytoprotection and absorption of intestinal fat.
- Maternal dietary intake is the main source of fetal Tau and is transported from the mother to fetus through the placenta by Tau transporters (TauT). The fetus during development lacks the enzyme cysteine-dioxygenase (CDO) and cannot synthesize Tau from methionine and cysteine.
- The absence or deficiency of Tau during intrauterine life alters fetal and pancreatic development predisposing the offspring to T2D in adulthood.
- Tau supplementation to dams with diabetes or exposed to protein restricted diets reverted the damage to the endocrine pancreas in the fetus, rescuing the offspring from developing disease later in life.

Keywords Taurine • Maternal taurine deficiency • Fetal taurine deficiency • DOHAD • Type 1 diabetes (T1D) and Type 2 diabetes (T2D) • Obesity

Abbreviations

α	Alpha cells
ATP	Adenosine triphosphate
Akt	Protein kinase B
β	Beta cells
BMI	Body mass index
[Ca2+] i	Intracellular Ca 2+ concentration

E. Arany, MD, PhD (✉)
Schulich School of Medicine and Dentistry, Department of Pathology and Laboratory Medicine, Lawson Health Research Institute & the Children Health Institute, University of Western Ontario, London, ON, Canada N6A 4V2
e-mail: earany@uwo.ca

© Springer International Publishing AG 2017
R. Rajendram et al. (eds.), *Diet, Nutrition, and Fetal Programming*,
Nutrition and Health, DOI 10.1007/978-3-319-60289-9_23

CDO	Cysteine dioxygenase
CHOL	Cholesterol
C57 Bl/6J	Black inbred laboratory mice
C-peptide	Connecting peptide (A and B insulin chain)
C	Control
CYP7A1	Cholesterol-7-hydrolase
δ	Delta cells
DNA	Deoxyribonucleic acid
DM	Diabetes mellitus
Flk-1	Receptor for vascular endothelial growth factor
HbA1C	Glycosylated hemoglobin
HF	High Fat
HOMA	Homeostatic model of assessment index
HPLC	High-performance liquid chromatography
IUGR	Intrauterine growth restriction
IGF-II	Insulin-like growth factor-II
IR	Insulin receptor
KKAy mice	Genetically obese diabetic mice
LP	Low protein
LP1	Low protein diet during gestation and lactation
LP2	Low protein diet all life
LDL	Low-density lipoprotein
NOD	Non-obese diabetic
OLEFT	Otsuka Long Evans Tokushima Fatty rats
Pdx-1	Pancreatic and duodenal homeobox 1
PGC-1α	Peroxisome proliferator-activated receptor gamma coactivator 1-alpha
pp.	Pancreatic polypeptide
PPAR-α	Peroxisome proliferator-activated receptor alpha
PPAR-Y	Peroxisome proliferator-activated receptor gamma
RNA	Ribonucleic acid
RIA	Radioimmunoassay
SST	Somatostatin
STB	Syncytiotrophoblast
T1D	Type 1 diabetes
T2D	Type 2 diabetes
TAU	Taurine
TauT	Taurine transporters
TG	Triglycerides
UCP	Uncoupling protein 2
VLDL	Very low density lipoprotein
WAT	White adipose tissue

Introduction

What Is Taurine?

In 1838, Demarcay extracted an amino-acid from the bile of the ox (*Bos Taurus*) [1] that he called Taurine (Tau). This sulfur containing amino-acid was often called "non-essential" as it differs from most amino-acids in that it is not metabolized or incorporated into proteins and remains free in the intracellular fluid.

Since 1968, studies showed that Tau has a significant array of physiological functions associated with the conjugation of bile acids, cellular osmoregulation, and energy storage, absorption of intestinal fat, glucose metabolism, anti-oxidation, and cytoprotective effects during cell development and survival.

Tau is undoubtedly considered one of the most important substances in the body. It is synthesized from ingested methionine and cysteine and oxidized in the presence of pyridoxal 5'-phosphate (as a cofactor) by the rate limiting enzyme cysteine–dioxygenase (CDO) in the liver [2]. At a cellular level Tau plays a crucial role in cell membrane stabilization, osmoregulation and detoxification [3]. It has the ability to modulate Ca^2+ binding in a variety of tissues and to phosphorylate proteins. Tau serves as a regulator of mitochondrial protein synthesis by enhancing the electron transport chain activity and protecting the mitochondria against excessive superoxide generation.

High concentrations of Tau are found in tissues with high oxidative activity and may prevent leakage of the reactive compounds formed in the mitochondrial environment. Tau indirectly acts as an antioxidant by providing sufficient pH buffering in the mitochondrial matrix [4].

In most vertebrates, plasma Tau concentrations are lower than 1 mM and its intracellular concentration ranges from 10 to 50 mM. All these values are usually altered by diet, disease and aging [5].

In humans, Tau is the most abundant amino acid found in the developing brain, skeletal muscle, liver, spinal cord, retina, pancreas, heart, white blood cells and platelets.

Epidemiological studies showed that communities that consume diets enriched with meat and seafood have lower risks of developing metabolic diseases such as obesity, diabetes, dyslipidemia, and hypertension [6].

It is important to note that lacto-ovo- vegetarian diets lack Tau, and who follow these diets have very low levels of Tau in plasma and tissues. Children raised in strictly vegetarian diets, have an increased incidence in childhood disease [7]. Multiple studies have shown that all these conditions can be reversed altering the diets by including meat and seafood products or by the administration of Tau [8] as a supplement.

The concept that Tau is a 'conditionally essential' amino acid arose from studies showing that in chronic conditions of reduced intake, increased need, or reduced conservation, the body loses its ability to maintain the required Tau pools necessary for its normal function.

Taurine in Development

The β-amino-acid taurine (2-aminoethanesulfonic acid), although not a constituent of proteins, is essential for fetal growth and organogenesis [9]. Tau cannot be synthesized by the fetus as the enzyme required for its synthesis is absent during development in human fetal tissues [10]. Fetal Tau is mainly provided by maternal dietary intake and is the most abundant free amino acid present in the human placenta [11]. The fetal requirements of Tau are met by its uptake from the maternal blood by the Tau transporter (TauT) present on the syncytiotrophoblast (STB) microvillus plasma membrane. In the STB, the activity of the TauT is critical to achieve a high intracellular Tau concentration to maintain a gradient that favours Tau efflux towards the fetus, where it is readily used in organ development [12].

Intrauterine restricted babies (IUGR) exposed to maternal dietary deficiencies have lower plasma Tau concentrations compared with normal pregnancies supporting its importance for fetal growth [13].

Tau is also present in human milk [14]. Babies that are not breast feed are Tau deficient. Currently, all infant milk formula is supplemented with Tau to compensate these babies Tau insufficiency. Tau is crucial for the absorption of fat. This addition to milk formula was enough to improve the absorption of fat and to maintain plasma and urine concentrations of Tau to values found in breast fed children [15].

Tau Regulation in Adults

The balance of Tau concentration in tissues and circulation is regulated by the liver and the kidney. Tau deficiency is rare in adults. In Tau-restricted diets, Tau is conserved by reducing its urinary excretion and enhancing reabsorption.

Patients with Gaucher's disease, retinitis pigmentosa [16], receiving long- term Tau-free parenteral nutrition [14] or poorly controlled diabetes mellitus (DM) [17] have very low plasma levels of Tau.

Tau concentration is mainly regulated by the taurine transporter (TauT) which is widely expressed and distributed in most tissues. It transports Tau from the extracellular space into cells to help maintain a high intracellular content. Alterations in Tau tissue content are associated with the reduction of TauT leading to cardiopathy with cardiac atrophy, accelerated skeletal muscle senescence and altered metabolic response to exercise [18].

Programming the Pancreas in Utero

In humans and rodents, the endocrine pancreas, or islets of Langherhans, comprises 2–3% of the total pancreatic volume and plays a vital function in maintaining nutritional homeostasis. The islets develop from ductal-like cells in the embryo, fetus, and neonate which further form primitive islets in the mesenchyme adjacent to the ducts. Final differentiation into the different cell types such as insulin-expressing (β), glucagon (α), somatostatin (δ), and pancreatic polypeptide (pp) cells occurs by the expression of a cascade of transcription factors, such as the master regulator *Pdx*-1 [19], and by the actions of local peptide growth factors within the surrounding mesenchyme [20] (Fig. 23.1).

In humans the third trimester is essential to pancreatic development as it undergoes a remodeling process to enable its response to nutrients at birth [21]. In the rat 2–3 days before birth β-cells duplicate in number by replication, cell recruitment, and maturation of undifferentiated β-cell precursors [22]. This process continues throughout neonatal life and declines at weaning. Simultaneously, during this period a remodeling process occurs with the absence of IGFs [23] (which are known to act as

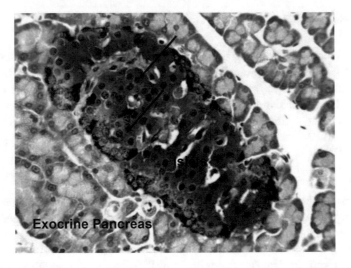

Fig. 23.1 Representative microphotograph of a rat pancreas section. The exocrine and endocrine pancreas is labelled. The *arrows* in the endocrine pancreas show two different cells types. The *brown* cells in the mantle of the islets correspond to glucagon (α) cells and the red cells in the core to insulin (β) cells

survival factors) where a transient wave of apoptosis at day 14 occurs after a rise in neogenesis at day 10 to conserve beta cell mass. This process by which part of the β-cell population with low glucose responsiveness for insulin release is replaced by cells with acute glucose stimulated insulin release takes place to give rise to a β-cell population that will be better adapted to control glucose metabolism in adult life [23].

Islets are also surrounded by a rich network of capillaries to allow nutrient and growth factor delivery, as well as accurate glucose sensing and dispersion of hormones into the systemic circulation [24]. Inadequate islet vasculature results in reduced insulin secretion and glucose intolerance [25]. The signaling mechanism between vasculature and islet cells involves the vascular endothelial growth factor-A (VEGF-A) and a deficiency in its expression can result in β-cell loss.

David Barker and Charles N. Hales after extensive epidemiological studies coined the term "fetal programming" in 2001 [26], suggesting that poor nutrition or altered delivery of nutrients during fetal development impairs the offspring long-term. More so, the timing of the nutritional challenges in early, mid or late gestation will have different effects on organogenesis and could increase the risk to disease later in life [27].

Multiple animal models have been utilized trying to extrapolate these results to humans, to understand and explore the mechanisms of these "in utero" effects on the development of disease. All models of IUGR result in impairment of placental development and function which leads to a reduction of nutrient availability and oxygen to the fetus and are associated with a reduction in fetal growth [28].

Rodents were exposed to different types of dietary manipulations at different windows of development such as calorie restriction (50% calorie reduction), protein restriction (LP 8% vs C 20% protein diets) or over nutrition given (high fat diets).

Maternal protein restriction or low protein diet (LP) is an extensively studied rodent model of intrauterine growth restriction. Our laboratory explored the effects of this LP diet (8% protein restriction and otherwise isocalorific) during gestation on pancreas development and our results showed that the offspring had a reduced pancreatic weight at birth, diminished islet size and β-cell mass with decreased insulin content and pancreatic vascularity. This reduced β-cell mass was paralleled by a diminished rate of β cell replication and an increased developmental apoptosis. The slow recovery of β-mass was due to an increased length in the cell cycle kinetics with an extended G1phase [29]. Maternal and fetal plasma glucose levels were not altered by maternal protein restriction; however, plasma amino acid profiles were perturbed, and plasma concentration of Tau and its synthesis were decreased in both the mother and fetus [30].

These LP diets given at critical windows of development during gestation (first week, second week and third week) had different effects on the morphometric analysis of the endocrine pancreas followed by an altered postnatal glucose metabolism, with set phenotypes showing the same sexual dimorphisms as in humans [27].

The administration of LP diet during early gestation reflected primarily an influence on pancreatic embryogenesis and endocrine progenitor cells. The nutritional insult in mid-gestation represented a change in islet formation, which begins around day E12, while in late gestation, the LP diet influenced β-cell mass and maturation. These studies showed that the LP diet nutritional insult in early, middle or late gestation results in a relative deficiency of beta cell mass following birth due to the failure to develop larger islets. Females were particularly susceptible in mid-gestation and males in late gestation [27].

When nutritional restriction was extended into weaning, our laboratory showed that the effects were irreversible contributing to glucose intolerance later in life. We observed for the first time that at 130 days of age, LP offspring of both sexes showed signs of impaired glucose tolerance and the mechanisms by which this deterioration occurred was different in males than in females. Specifically, males exhibited decreased insulin sensitivity as calculated by the homeostatic model assessment (HOMA) index, while females exhibited a significant reduction in mean pancreatic islet number, islet size and beta cell mass. In LP males, basal insulin levels were twofold higher and Akt phosphorylation in response to insulin was reduced in adipose and skeletal muscle at 130 days of age when compared

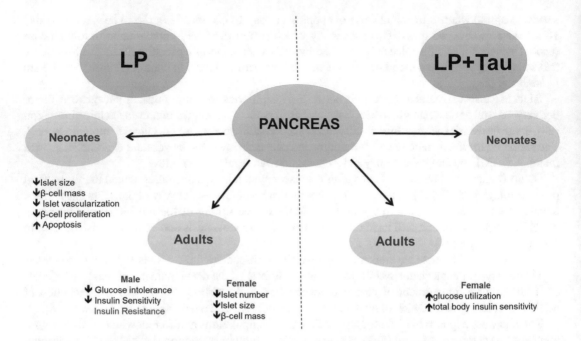

Fig. 23.2 Diagram outlining the effects of low protein diets (LP) and LP supplemented with taurine (Tau) during pregnancy and lactation on neonatal and adult offspring. On the *left*, the LP diet alone alters β-cell function and number in the offspring with impaired glucose homeostasis. On the *right*, the addition of Tau to the diet (LP+Tau) restored β-cell morphology and function preventing glucose intolerance in adulthood. Sexual differences are noted

to control-fed animals. Hence, females became relatively more insulin deficient while males were more insulin resistant. It also suggests that there is a sexual difference in the mechanism by which these alterations occur that may be related to hormonal changes. LP males had reduction of plasma testosterone levels along with a significant increase in visceral adiposity relative to their body weight at 130 days [31]. These gender-specific findings are consistent with observations in humans that showed that men are more insulin resistant than women [32]. In LP-fed males, the two major classic peripheral insulin-responsive tissues, muscle and adipose, displayed a diminished response to insulin resulting in decreased disposal of excess circulating glucose and fatty acids. Increased body fat mass, visceral fat mass and an adverse lipid profile are all observed in the human metabolic syndrome which is characterized by decreased insulin sensitivity whereby the degree of insulin resistance is related to the percentage of total body fat mass [33]. Collectively, all of these factors contributed to the onset of glucose intolerance in later life (Fig. 23.2).

It has been suggested that postnatal catch-up growth due to changes to the diet like the increase of calories or the proportion of the components of the diet such as the increase of proteins, carbohydrates or fat at birth, following fetal growth restriction may increase the predisposition to diseases such as type 2 (T2D) diabetes and hypertension [34].

A theory has been proposed to explain these results through the predictive adaptive response [35] which states that the fetus is constantly interpreting the environment created by the maternal milieu and placental function and predicts the environment into which it is likely to be born. However, this can be detrimental when inadequate or excessive nutrients are present following birth protein deprivation.

In order to further understand the effects of LP diets on offspring we performed the gold standard hyperinsulinemic–euglycemic clamp and hyperglycemic clamp to assess insulin sensitivity and β-cell function. Two groups were compared, one was given the LP diet during gestation and lactation (LP1) and another group kept the LP diet all life (LP2). These clamp studies showed that LP2 had better glucose metabolism than the LP1. In males, LP2 exposure had a tendency to increase hepatic insulin sensitivity and increase C-peptide levels in response to glucose during the hyperglycemic clamp and had improved β-cell function compared to the LP1 [36].

These results confirmed the adaptive response theory, showing that dietary changes at birth or weaning have detrimental effects on the offspring and when the environment is maintained throughout life the offspring thrives better. It also followed the observations seen in humans, where fetal growth restriction and catch up growth impacts insulin action and glucose metabolism in adulthood [37].

Role of Taurine Regulating the Endocrine Pancreas

Tau is localized mainly in the α (glucagon) and in some δ (Somatostatin) cells in the endocrine pancreas, whereas it is absent in β (insulin) cells [38]. This presence of Tau in the islets raised a lot of interest in the last decades into understanding its cellular and physiological role.

In 1996, Cherif et al. showed that Tau controls insulin secretion and appears to be age-dependent. In adults Tau reduces insulin secretion whereas in the fetus, Tau stimulates the insulin release induced by the secretagogues, leucine and arginine [39].

In fetal islets of dams exposed to a protein restricted diet (LP), the addition of Tau to the media did not stimulate insulin secretion. Interestingly, the addition of Tau to the maternal LP diet restored insulin secretion in the fetal islets to normal values and increased the expression of genes involved in β-cell proliferation, indicating the importance of Tau during fetal pancreas development [40].

Tau has been shown to be severely reduced in both maternal and fetal plasma as well as in fetal islets during maternal protein restriction [30]. Measuring Tau levels by HPLC we found that they were significantly lower ($P < 0.001$) at day 1 after birth in LP offspring compared to those of control-treated mothers. At 130 days there were no differences in Tau levels between the two groups [36].

When Tau was added to the LP diet (LP+Tau) during gestation and lactation, the loss of β-cell mass was prevented in the offspring probably by an increase of IGF-II expression [41] that was also translated to an increased number of cells positive for IGF-II in the islets. Previously, we showed that IGF-II acts as a survival factor in islet cells [23] stimulating DNA synthesis and protecting β-cells from apoptosis [42, 43]. In this LP+Tau group, Tau may induce IGF-II to promote the increase of β-cell proliferation and reduce apoptosis, thus normalizing islet size in these offspring.

In rodents, the islets are a richly vascularized tissue, where the blood supply arrives from a highly specialized network of microvessels arranged as a local intra-islet portal system [44] through which blood flows from the central core of β-cells to the cell mantle. Previous studies have shown that vascular islet blood vessel development was very sensitive to the lack of protein availability in utero. LP fetuses had a marked reduction in the islet blood vessel density [45]. When the LP diet was fed until adult age, there was a 65% decrease in the islet blood flow [30].

We demonstrated that Tau restored the expression and presence of VEGF in the islets by increasing the number of VEGF-positive cells in LP-fed pups at all ages. VEGF receptor Flk-1 was also increased in islet cells stating that Tau has an important role during fetal vascular and endocrine system development [46] (Fig. 23.2).

Tau has been recently implicated in the regulation of mitochondrial function through various actions, such as modulation of mitochondrial transfer RNA, buffer action and calcium movement [47, 48], supporting the idea that Tau might play an important role in energy production. Microarray analysis of the pancreas revealed that one of the pathways most affected by fetal protein malnutrition was cellular respiration as genes encoded for the TCA (tricarboxylic acid cycle) and mitochondrial proteins were affected. Furthermore, those islets were unable to enhance their ATP (adenosine triphosphate) production when stimulated with glucose. Maternal LP+Tau normalized the expression of all the altered genes and ATP production [49]. This was supported by another study where Tau increased the amount of ATP in UCP2 (uncoupling protein2) -overexpressing β-cells, probably by both increasing mitochondrial Ca++ influx through the Ca++ uniporter, and the ATP:ADP ratio and restoring glucose-stimulated insulin secretion [48].

Whether this beneficial effect of Tau was sustained until adulthood was not clearly understood. A study demonstrated that maternal Tau supplementation restored insulin response to a glucose challenge in 11-week-old female offspring of LP-fed dams, but Tau supplementation to control animals had detrimental effects including weak glucose intolerance [50].

Additionally, another study has demonstrated that the addition of Tau to a similar model of maternal protein restriction used by us (gestation and lactation) restored both β- cell mass and insulin secretory responses to glucose load in male offspring at 20 weeks of age, possibly by its protective role in maintaining mitochondrial morphology and function in β-cells and expression of the mtDNA-encoded COX I (mitochondrial DNA-cyclooxygenase 1) gene in islet cells [51].

Using the hyperinsulinemic–euglycemic clamp and hyperglycemic clamp we demonstrated that in both genders, maternal Tau supplementation improves glucose metabolism in adult LP offspring. In males, Tau supplementation tended to improve hepatic insulin sensitivity and increase body insulin sensitivity above that of the controls and completely restored β-cell function. Similar results were previously reported but unlike that study, we did not observe the effect of Tau on first-phase insulin secretion. In females, Tau improved glucose utilization and overall insulin sensitivity.

Role of Taurine and Diabetes

Type 1 diabetes (T1D) results from insulin deficiency due to the autoimmune-mediated destruction of the insulin producing pancreatic islet β-cells (insulitis). This inflammatory response arises from incompletely understood interactions between *β* cells, the immune system, and the environment in genetically susceptible individuals [52].

Tau levels are reduced in both plasma and platelets in patients with T1D [17] and type 2 diabetes (T2D) [53]. The reduction in Tau could be explained by the renal complications of these conditions due to impaired renal reabsorption or enhanced urinary clearance and fractional excretion in addition to a possible decrease in the net intestinal absorption [54].

In clinical studies the use of Tau to improve glucose metabolism in diabetic patients is not clear. A clinical trial conducted in a group of T1D patients treated with insulin and oral supplementation of Tau twice a day, at a dose of 0.5 g over 30 days improved carbohydrate metabolism and decreased triglycerides [55]. Although these results were promising, the number of patients studied was very small to have a power analysis. Another study showed that long-term Tau administration once a day, at a dose of 1.5 g per day for 90 days did not modify glucose metabolism in IDDM patients making Tau effects in humans arguable [17].

Currently, there are no accepted recommendations for daily taurine intake.

In an additional study conducted on T2D patients, Tau showed similar results to the previous. In this case HbA1C levels between patients and placebo did not change [56].

As mentioned before the average daily taurine intake in man is between 80 and 1000 mg, originating mainly from products of animal origin and can vary depending on the diet [57].

In animal models Tau reduces oxidative stress induced by hyperglycaemia [58], attenuates the age related increase of oxidative damage, decreases carbonyl group production [59], suggesting a role as a glycation scavenger. In diabetes, the depletion of Tau enhances the formation of glycosylated proteins and this overload of detoxification mechanisms [60] could promote the accumulation of reactive carbonyl and advanced glycosylation end products [61]. Therefore, dietary addition of Tau could reduce glycosylated hemoglobin levels.

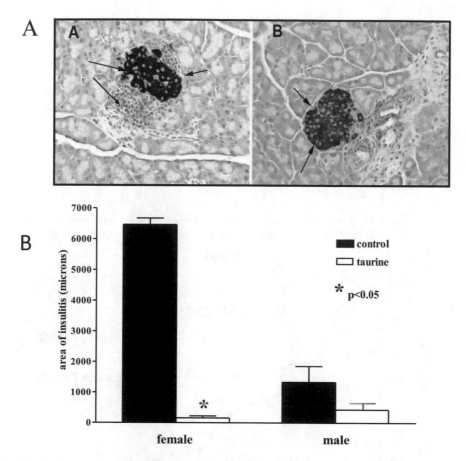

Fig. 23.3 Effects of taurine on insulitis. (**a**) Immuno-histochemical localization of insulin within islets (*arrows*) from control (*left*) or taurine-supplemented (*right*) female NOD mice at 8 weeks of age. Peri-insulitis is seen in the control animal (*arrow*), but is absent in the taurine treated one. Magnification bar 10 μm. (**b**) Area of insulitis. (mean ± SEM) in female or male control (*black bars*) or taurine-treated (*white bars*) mice. Values are from 12 animals for each group. *$p < 0.001$ vs control mice (Figure taken from Arany et al. [63], with permission)

Tau also regulates the immune response [62] and has anti-inflammatory properties [63]. Previous data from our laboratory showed that Tau given during gestation to NOD mice (a mouse model of T1D) resulted in increased in β-cell DNA synthesis, increased islet area, and reduced apoptosis in both sexes along with an elevated number of islet cells containing immune reactive IGF-II in mice at 14 days after birth, and prior to any evidence of insulitis [64] .

In the NOD female, peri-insulitis is first found at around 4–5 weeks after birth and affects 70–90% of islets by 9–10 weeks [65]. At 8 weeks, Tau supplemented female mice had a 90% reduction in the mean area of insulitis per islet suggesting that the immune infiltration within the islets was impaired (Fig. 23.3). This could imply that recognition of the beta cell auto-antigens by macrophages or dendritic cells were reduced, leading to diminished T cell recruitment or action. Tau is abundant in neutrophils and Tau- chloramines, reducing inflammation and the number of inflammatory cells [66] (Fig. 23.4). Tau has no effect on males at the same age. Although the onset of diabetes was delayed for both females and males, only 1 in 5 females developed diabetes after 1 year showing that short term Tau exposure during fetal life had a long term consequence, either in β-cell responsiveness to autoimmune attack or in autoimmune inter-cellular communication [64] (Fig. 23.5).

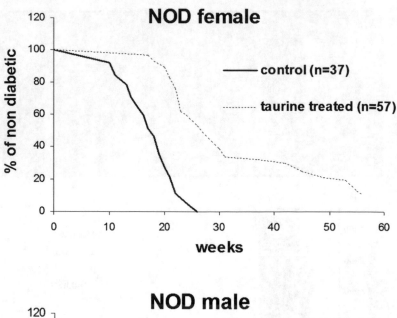

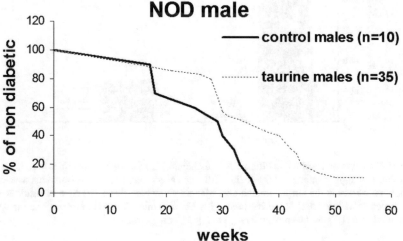

Fig. 23.4 Proposed mechanisms of taurine on the onset of TD1 in NOD female mice. The effects of the Tau during gestation and lactation were sustained reducing insulitis and maintaining β-cell mass

Tau supplementation from birth in NOD mice increased glucose tolerance in adult females and improved islet insulin release due to a better [Ca 2+] i response to glucose stimulus. However, no changes in pancreatic islet morphology were seen in either gender. In vitro, islets exposed to Tau showed a protective action against cytokine- induced β-cell secretory dysfunction [67].

In Otsuka Long Evans Tokushima Fatty (OLETF) rats, Tau acted as an antioxidant to attenuate islet fibrosis, which is important in the progression of pancreatic beta cell failure induced by oxidative stress in T2DM [68]. Metabolomics studies of sulfur amino acids [69] conducted in Zucker diabetic fatty (ZDF) rats showed a reduction of methionine and its metabolites (homocysteine, cysteine) in the liver suggesting that this deficiency contributed to a reduction of Tau synthesis and led to insulin resistance and development of T2D seen in this model.

Tau is concentrated mainly in the α and δ-cells [38] in the endocrine pancreas and may indicate that this amino acid could regulate glucagon secretion. Leptin-deficient obese (ob) mice given Tau showed a reduction in insulin and glucagon hypersecretion, and ameliorated β-cell responsiveness to δ-cells

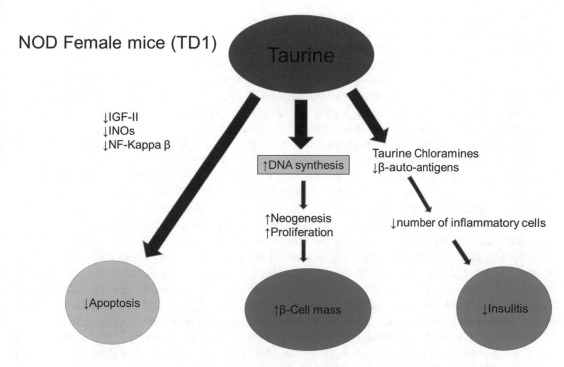

Fig. 23.5 Survival of NOD female and male mice with or without diabetes with increasing age (in weeks). Control (NOD-early onset diabetes). (*dark*), (*n* = 37–40). Taurine supplemented (NOD- late onset of diabetes). (*light*), *n* = (45–51) animals (*p* < 0.001). (Wilcoxon test). Kaplan–Meier survival plots (Figure modified from Arany et al. [63], with permission)

in islets. It also decreased islet hypertrophy, increased δ-cell mass, regulated Ca2+ handling in β and α-cells, and modified the expression of transcription factors and genes that participate in islet cell differentiation and function. This data suggested that Tau may prevent glucagon and insulin compensatory hyper- secretion in obesity and T2D, by maintenance of somatostatin (SST) paracrine interactions in the endocrine pancreas [70].

Another mechanism has been postulated by which this amino-acid may improve glucose control in diabetic conditions [71–73] by its interaction with the insulin receptor [74] through stimulation of the insulin signaling pathway by the activation of Akt in different insulin target tissues [75–78] increasing glucose uptake in muscle and liver [79].

Taurine and Obesity

Tau plasma levels are lower in obese subjects [80, 81] as compared with their non-obese counterparts [82] and in diet-induced and congenital animal models of obesity [82]. It has been demonstrated in Swiss mice that the addition of Tau to High fat (HF) diets after weaning prevented β-cell morpho-functional alterations after 6 months of treatment [83]. Similar diet given over 8 weeks to Sprague–Dawley rats at weaning, resulted in higher serum adiponectin levels and reduced total serum cholesterol (TC) level compared to the HF group [84]. It is important to point out that adiponectin increases fatty acid combustion and energy consumption in muscle and liver. Through these mechanisms, adiponectin contributes to improve insulin-induced signal transduction, and hence insulin sensitivity [85].

Tau reduced body weight (BW) and abdominal fat pads in genetically (Kondo spontaneous mild T2D obese) KKAy mice. Meanwhile in OLETF (obese T2D) rats, it did not significantly reduce BW but they had an improved insulin sensitivity, reductions in serum lipid, leptin and glucose concentrations with no changes in adiponectin [86]. Tau prevents the elevation of LDL and very LDL (VLDL) cholesterol in diet-induced hyper-lipidemic animals. Several studies showed that the cholesterol-lowering effect of Tau was associated with the stimulation of cholesterol catabolism into bile acids. In fact, the expression and activity of hepatic cholesterol 7-hydroxylase (CYP7A1), a rate-limiting enzyme of bile acid synthesis, was increased by Tau treatment [87].

Tau synthesis has been shown to change during the process of differentiation and hypertrophy of the adipocytes [75]. The decrease of Tau plasma levels was associated with a decrease in the expression of cysteine dioxygenase (CDO), a rate-limiting enzyme in the liver [2]. Recently it was reported that CDO mRNA was also expressed in white adipose tissue (WAT) [88]. Primary cell culture of adipocytes isolated from parametrial WAT of C57BL/6J incubated in KRHA buffer at 37 C showed that Tau concentration increased gradually suggesting that adipocytes secrete taurine. To further examine whether CDO is involved in Tau secretion in adipocytes, CDO was overexpressed in 3T3-L1 cells by means of a retroviral vector, and Tau and cysteine concentrations were measured in culture media. The level of Tau secreted into culture media for 3 d was increased significantly by CDO overexpression in comparison with the control level. In contrast, the level of used cysteine, which is the substrate of CDO for synthesis of Tau, was decreased significantly. These results suggest that CDO increases the synthesis of taurine from cysteine and that Tau is secreted from adipocytes [82].

On the other hand, "in vivo" high-fat diet-induced obese mice had decreased CDO expression in WAT and had decreased plasma Tau concentration. Similar results were seen in KKAy mice, a model of genetically obese diabetic mice in which a slight decrease in plasma Tau concentration was accompanied by a 50% reduction of CDO mRNA level in WAT [82]. When Tau was supplemented to these KKAy mice an up-regulation of PGC-1α, PPARγ, and PPARα and their target genes leading to increased energy expenditure, including fatty acid β-oxidation, was observed in WAT suggesting its role in preventing obesity [82].

In human studies Tau content was significantly lower in a healthy obese population (48 μmol/l) with a body mass index (BMI) of 30 and in patients with diabetes (32 μmol/l) with a (BMI) of 28 and compared to age- and sex-matched non-obese control subjects (85 μmol/l) with a BMI of 25 [89, 90].

Although the mechanisms by which Tau ameliorates obesity are at present unclear, these observations indicate that metabolic dysfunctions such as obesity and diabetes may be an effect of Tau deficiency.

In overweight men with a genetic predisposition for T2D the daily administration of 1.5 g Tau for 8 weeks had no effect on insulin secretion, insulin sensitivity, or blood lipid levels suggesting that at that dosage dietary Tau may enough to prevent T2D development [91]. However, oral Tau improved insulin sensitivity in overweight non-diabetic men [92].

Obese women given 3 g/day Tau for 8 weeks in combination with nutritional counseling were able to increase adiponectin levels and decrease markers of inflammation (high-sensitivity C-reactive protein) and lipid peroxidation (TBARS) [80].

Conclusions

Tau is an essential amino acid that can be synthesized in the liver and in WAT and is present in the plasma and tissues of humans and in multiple species of animals after birth. It is deficient in the fetal plasma when maternal daily requirements are low as a consequence of dietary deficiencies or by maternal diabetes. Multiple studies showed that Tau is also deficient in animal models of obesity, T1D and T2D. This shortage of Tau alters glucose metabolism, reduces insulin sensitivity, β- cell number and function. All these effects were reverted by the administration of Tau.

In humans Tau was reduced in both plasma and platelets in T1D and T2D and in obese subjects. The addition of Tau to the diet did not show the same results than in rodents. Although some studies showed some partial benefits on glucose and lipid metabolisms the results were controversial, mostly by the reduced number of subjects tested. Further clinical studies are needed to prove Tau effects as a lipid and glucose regulator in metabolic diseases and as a putative regulator of obesity.

References

1. Demarcay H. Ueber die natur der galle. AmPharm. 1838;27:270–91.
2. Stipanuk MH, Bagley PJ, Hou YC, Bella DL, Banks MF, Hirschberger L. Hepatic regulationof cysteine utilization for taurine synthesis. Taurine in health and disease. In: Huxtable RJ, Michak D, editors. Advances in experimental medicine and biology. New York: Plenum Press; 1994.
3. Schaffer S, Takahashi K, Azuma J. Role of osmoregulation in the actions of taurine. Amino Acids. 2000;19:527–46.
4. Jong CJ, Azuma J, Schaffer S. Mechanism underlying the antioxidant activity of taurine: prevention of mitochondrial oxidant production. Amino Acids. 2012;42:2223–32.
5. Lambert IH. Regulation of the cellular content of the organic Osmolyte taurine in mammalian cells. Neurochem Res. 2004;29(1):27–63.
6. Yamori Y, Taguchi T, Mori H, Mori M. Low cardiovascular risks in the middle aged males and females excreting greater 24-hour urinary taurine and magnesium in 41 WHO-CARDIAC study populations in the world. J Biomed Sci. 2010;17(Suppl 1(Suppl 1)):S21.
7. Shinwell ED, Gorodischer R. Totally vegetarian diets and infant nutrition. Pediatrics. 1982;70:582–6.
8. Geggel H, Ament M. Nutritional requirement for taurine in patients receiving long-term parenteral nutrition. N Engl J Med. 1985;312(May 1982):142–6.
9. Sturman JA. Taurine in development. J Nutr. 1988;118(10):1169–76. doi:10.1016/0024-3205(77)90420-9.
10. Gaull G, Sturman J, Räihä N. Development of mammalian sulfur metabolism: absence of cystathionase in human fetal tissues. Pediatr Res. 1972;6(6):538–47.
11. Philipps AF, Holzman IR, Teng C, Battaglia FC. Tissue concentrations of free amino acids in term human placentas. Am J Obstet Gynecol. 1978;131(8):881–7.
12. Norberg S, Powell TL, Jansson T. Intrauterine growth restriction is associated with a reduced activity of placental taurine transporters. Pediatr Res. 1998;44(2):233–8.
13. Economides DL, Nicolaides KH, Gahl WA, Bernardini I, Evans MI. Plasma amino acids in appropriate- and small-for-gestational-age fetuses. Am J Obstet Gynecol. 1989;161(5):1219–27.
14. Sturman JA, Chesney RW. Taurine in pediatric nutrition. Pediatr Clin N Am. 1995;42(4):879–97.
15. Rassin D, Gaull G, Järvenpää A, Räihä N. Feeding the low-birth-weight infant:II. Effects of taurine and cholesterol supplementation on amino acids and cholesterol. Pediatrics. 1983;71(2):179–86.
16. Vom Dahl S, Mönnighoff I, Häussinger D. Decrease of plasma taurine in Gaucher disease and its sustained correction during enzyme replacement therapy. Amino Acids. 2000;19(3–4):585–92.
17. Franconi F, Bennardini F, Mattana A, et al. Plasma and platelet taurine are reduced in subjects with insulin-dependent diabetes mellitus: effects of taurine supplementation. Am J Clin Nutr. 1995;61(5):1115–9.
18. Ito T, Oishi S, Takai M, et al. Cardiac and skeletal muscle abnormality in taurine transporter-knockout mice. J Biomed Sci. 2010;17(Suppl 1(Suppl 1)):S20.
19. Fernandes A, King LC, Guz Y, Stein R, Wright CV, Teitelman G. Differentiation of new insulin-producing cells is induced by injury in adult pancreatic islets. Endocrinology. 1997;138(4):1750–62.
20. Scharfmann R. Control of early development of the pancreas in rodents and humans: implications of signals from the mesenchyme. Diabetologia. 2000;43:1083–92.
21. Piper K, Brickwood S, Turnpenny LW, et al. Beta cell differentiation during early human pancreas development. J Endocrinol. 2004;181(1):11–23.
22. Kaung HL. Growth dynamics of pancreatic islet cell populations during fetal and neonatal development of the rat. Dev Dyn. 1994;200(2):163–75.
23. Petrik J, Arany E, McDonald TJ, Hill D. Apoptosis in the pancreatic islet cells of the neonatal rat is associated with the reduced expression of insulin-like growth factor II that may act as a survival factor. Endocrinology. 1998;139:2994–3004.
24. Lammert E, Cleaver OMD. Role of endothelial cells in early pancreas and liver development. Mech Dev. 2003; 120:59–64.
25. Brissova M, Shostak A, Shiota M, et al. Pancreatic islet production of vascular endothelial growth factor-A is essential for islet vascularization, revascularization, and function. Diabetes. 2006;55(11):2974–85.

26. Hales CN, Barker DJP. The thrifty phenotype hypothesis: type 2 diabetes. Br Med Bull. 2001;60(1):5–20.
27. Chamson-Reig A, Thyssen SM, Arany E, Hill DJ. Altered pancreatic morphology in the offspring of pregnant rats given reduced dietary protein is time and gender specific. J Endocrinol. 2006;191(1):83–92.
28. Morrison JL. Sheep models of intrauterine growth restriction: fetal adaptations and consequences. Clin Exp Pharmacol Physiol. 2008;35(7):730–43.
29. Petrik J, Reusens B, Arany E, Remacle C, Coelho C, Hoet JJ Hill, D. A low protein diet alters the balance of islet cell replication and apoptosis in the fetal and neonatal rat and is associated with a reduced pancreatic expression of insulin-like growth factor-II. Endocrinology. 1999;140(10):4861–73.
30. Reusens BDS, Snoek A, Bennis-Taleb N, Remacle C, Hoett J. Long-term consequences of diabetes and its complications may have a fetal origin: experimental and epidemiological evidence. In: Cowett RM, editor. Diabetes, Nestle: Workshop Series, vol. 25. New York: Raven Press; 1995. p. 187–8.
31. Chamson-Reig A, Thyssen SM, Hill DJ, Arany E. Exposure of the pregnant rat to low protein diet causes impaired glucose homeostasis in the young adult offspring by different mechanisms in males and females. Exp Biol Med. 2009;234(12):1425–36.
32. Shi H, Priya S, Senthil D. Sex differences in obesity-related glucose intolerance and insulin resistance. Glucose Toler. 2012:37–66.
33. Miyazaki Y, DeFronzo RA. Visceral fat dominant distribution in male type 2 diabetic patients is closely related to hepatic insulin resistance, irrespective of body type. Cardiovasc Diabetol. 2009;8:44–53.
34. Barker DJ, Forsen T, Eriksson JG, Osmond C. Growth and living conditions in childhood and hypertension in adult life: a longitudinal study. J Hypertens. 2002;20(10):1951–6.
35. Gluckman PD, Hanson MA. The consequences of being born small – An adaptive perspective. Hormone Res. 2006;65:5–14.
36. Tang C, Marchand K, Lam L, et al. Maternal taurine supplementation in rats partially prevents the adverse effects of early-life protein deprivation on β-cell function and insulin sensitivity. Reproduction. 2013;145(6):609–20.
37. Hales CN. Fetal and infant growth and impaired glucose tolerance in adulthood: the "thrifty phenotype" hypothesis revisited. Acta Paediatr Suppl. 1997;422(7):73–7.
38. Bustamante J, Lobo MV, Alonso FJ, et al. An osmotic-sensitive taurine pool is localized in rat pancreatic islet cells containing glucagon and somatostatin. Am J Physiol Endocrinol Metab. 2001;281:E1275–85.
39. Cherif H, Reusens B, Dahri S, Remacle C, Hoet JJ. Stimulatory effects of taurine on insulin secretion by fetal rat islets cultured in vitro. J Endocrinol. 1996;151(3):501–6.
40. Cherif H, Reusens B, Ahn MT, Hoet JJ, Remacle C. Effects of taurine on the insulin secretion of rat fetal islets from dams fed a low-protein diet. J Endocrinol. 1998;159(2):341–8.
41. Boujendar S, Reusens B, Merezak S, et al. Taurine supplementation to a low protein diet during foetal and early postnatal life restores a normal proliferation and apoptosis of rat pancreatic islets. Diabetologia. 2002;45(6):856–66.
42. Hogg J, Hill DJHV. The ontogeny of insulin-like growth factor (IGF) and IGF binding protein gene expression in the rat pancreas. Diabetes. 1994;36:465–71.
43. Hill DJ, Petrik J, Arany E, McDonald TJ, Delovitch TL. Insulin-like growth factors prevent cytokine-mediated cell death in isolated islets of Langerhans from pre-diabetic non-obese diabetic mice. J Endocrinol. 1999;161(1):153–65.
44. Bonner-Weir S, Orci L. New perspectives on the microvasculature of the islets of Langerhans in the rat. Diabetes. 1982;31(10):883–9.
45. Snoeck A, Remacle C, Reusens B, Hoet JJ. Effect of a low protein diet during pregnancy on the fetal rat endocrine pancreas. Biol Neonate. 1990;57(2):107–18.
46. Boujendar S, Arany E, Hill D, Remacle C, Reusens B. Taurine supplementation of a low protein diet fed to rat dams normalizes the vascularization of the fetal endocrine pancreas. J Nutr. 2003;133(9):2820–5.
47. Hansen SH, Andersen ML, Cornett C, Gradinaru R, Grunnet N. A role for taurine in mitochondrial function. J Biomed Sci. 2010;17(Suppl 1(Suppl 1)):S23.
48. Han J, Bae JH, Kim S-Y, et al. Taurine increases glucose sensity of UCP2-overexpressing beta-cells by ameliorating mitochondrial metabolism. Am J Physiol Endocrinol Metab. 2004;287:E1008–18.
49. Reusens B, Sparre T, Kalbe L, et al. The intrauterine metabolic environment modulates the gene expression pattern in fetal rat islets: prevention by maternal taurine supplementation. Diabetologia. 2008;51(5):836–45.
50. Merezak S, Reusens B, Renard A, et al. Effect of maternal low-protein diet and taurine on the vulnerability of adult Wistar rat islets to cytokines. Diabetologia. 2004;47(4):669–75.
51. Lee YY, Lee H-J, Lee S-S, et al. Taurine supplementation restored the changes in pancreatic islet mitochondria in the fetal protein-malnourished rat. Br J Nutr. 2011;106(08):1198–206.
52. Rabinowe SL, Eisenbarth GS. Type I diabetes mellitus. A chronic autoimmune disease. N Engl J Med. 1986;31:1360–8.
53. De Luca G, Calpona PR, Caponetti A, et al. Taurine and osmoregulation: platelet taurine content, uptake, and release in type 2 diabetic patients. Metabolism. 2001;50(1):60–4.
54. Merheb M, Daher RT, Nasrallah M, Sabra R, Ziyadeh FNBK. Taurine intestinal absorption and renal excretion test in diabetic patients: a pilot study. Diabetes Care. 2007;30:2652–4.

55. Elizarova EPNL. First experiments in taurine administration for diabetes mellitus. The effect on erythrocyte membranes. Adv Exp Med Biol. 1996;403:583–8.
56. Chauncey KB, Tenner TE Jr, Lombardini JB, Jones BG, Brooks ML, Warner RD, et al. The effect of taurine supplementation on patients with type 2 diabetes mellitus. Adv Exp Med Biol. 2003;526:91–6.
57. Hayes KCSJ. Taurine in metabolism. Annu Rev Nutr. 1981;1:401–25. (Annu Rev Nutr. 1981;1:401–25. Taurine in metabolism. Hayes KC, Sturman JA).
58. Haber CA, Lam TKT, Yu Z, et al. N-acetylcysteine and taurine prevent hyperglycemia-induced insulin resistance in vivo: possible role of oxidative stress. Am J Physiol Endocrinol Metab. 2003;285(4):E744–53.
59. Eppler B, Dawson R. Dietary taurine manipulations in aged male Fischer 344 rat tissue: taurine concentration, taurine biosynthesis, and oxidative markers. Biochem Pharmacol. 2001;62(1):29–39.
60. Baynes JW, Thorpe SR. Role of oxidative stress in diabetic complications: a new perspective on an old paradigm. Diabetes. 1999;48(1):1–9.
61. Hansen SH. The role of taurine in diabetes and the development of diabetic complications. Diabetes Metab Res Rev. 2001;17(5):330–46.
62. Grimble RF. The effects of Sulphur amino-acids intake on immune function in humans. J Nutr. 2006;36(6):1160S–665S.
63. Marcinkiewicz J, Kontny E. Taurine and inflammatory diseases. Amino Acids. 2014;46(1):7–20.
64. Arany E, Strutt B, Romanus P, Remacle C, Reusens B, Hill DJ. Taurine supplement in early life altered islet morphology, decreased insulitis and delayed the onset of diabetes in non-obese diabetic mice. Diabetologia. 2004;47(10):1831–7.
65. Pozzilli P, Signore A, Williams AJ, Beales PE. NOD mouse colonies around the world – recent facts and figures. Immunol Today. 1993;14(5):193–6.
66. Marcinkiewicz J, Nowak B, Grabowska A, Bobek M, Petrovska L, Chain B. Regulation of murine dendritic cell functions in vitro by taurine chloramine, a major product of the neutrophil myeloperoxidase-halide system. Immunology. 1999;98(3):371–8.
67. Ribeiro RA, Santos-Silva J, Vettorazzi JF, Borghi Cotrim B, Boschero AC, Magalhães CE. Taurine supplementation enhances insulin secretion without altering islet morphology in non-obese diabetic mice. Adv Exp Med Biol. 2015;803:353–70.
68. Lee YY, Lee H-JHK, Lee S-S, et al. Taurine supplementation restored the changes in pancreatic islet mitochondria in the fetal protein-malnourished rat. Br J Nutr. 2011;106(08):1198–206.
69. Kwak HC, Kim Y-M, Oh SJ, Kim SK. Sulfur amino acid metabolism in Zucker diabetic fatty rats. Biochem Pharmacol. 2015;96(3):256–66.
70. Santos-Silva JC, Ribeiro RA, Vettorazzi JF, et al. Taurine supplementation ameliorates glucose homeostasis, prevents insulin and glucagon hypersecretion, and controls α, β, and δ-cell masses in genetic obese mice. Amino Acids. 2015;47(8):1533–48.
71. Kim KS, Oh DH, Kim JY, et al. Taurine ameliorates hyperglycemia and dyslipidemia by reducing insulin resistance and leptin level in Otsuka long-Evans Tokushima fatty (OLETF) rats with long-term diabetes. Exp Mol Med. 2012;44(11):665–73.
72. Batista TM, da Silva PMR, Amaral AG, Ribeiro RA, Boschero AC, Carneiro EM. Taurine supplementation restores insulin secretion and reduces ER stress markers in protein-malnourished mice. Adv Exp Med Biol. 2013;776:129–39.
73. Vettorazzi JF, Ribeiro RA, Santos-Silva JC, Borck PC, Batista TM, Nardelli TR, Boschero AC, Carneiro E. Taurine supplementation increases K channel protein content, improving Ca handling and insulin secretion in islets from malnourished mice fed on a high-fat diet. Amino Acids. 2014;46(9):2123–36.
74. Maturo J, Kulakowski EC. Taurine binding to the purified insulin receptor. Biochem Pharmacol. 1988;37(19):3755–60.
75. Batista TM, Ribeiro RA, da Silva PMR, Camargo RL, Lollo PCB, Boschero AC, Carneiro EM. Taurine supplementation improves liver glucose control in normal protein and malnourished mice fed a high-fat diet. Mol Nutr Food Res. 2013;57:423–34.
76. Baek YY, Cho DH, Choe J, et al. Extracellular taurine induces angiogenesis by activating ERK-, Akt-, and FAK-dependent signal pathways. Eur J Pharmacol. 2012;674(2–3):188–99.
77. Das J, Sil PC. Taurine ameliorates alloxan-induced diabetic renal injury, oxidative stress-related signaling pathways and apoptosis in rats. Amino Acids. 2012;43(4):1509–23.
78. Ribeiro RA, Santos-Silva JC, Vettorazzi JF, et al. Taurine supplementation prevents morpho-physiological alterations in high-fat diet mice pancreatic β-cells. Amino Acids. 2012;43(4):1791–801.
79. Kulakowski EC, Maturo J. Hypoglycemic properties of taurine: not mediated by enhanced insulin release. Biochem Pharmacol. 1984;33(18):2835–8.
80. Rosa FT, Freitas EC, Deminice R, Jordao AA, Marchini J. Oxidative stress and inflammation in obesity after taurine supplementation: a double-blind, placebo-controlled study. Eur J Nutr. 2014;53:823–30.
81. Lee MY, Cheong SH, Chang KJ, Choi MJKS. Effect of the obesity index on plasma taurine levels in Korean female adolescents. Adv Exp Med Biol. 2003;526:285–90.
82. Tsuboyama-Kasaoka N, Shozawa C, Sano K, et al. Taurine (2-Aminoethanesulfonic acid) deficiency creates a vicious circle promoting obesity. Endocrinology. 2006;147(7):3276–84.

83. Ribeiro RA, Santos-Silva JC, Vettorazzi JF, et al. Taurine supplementation prevents morpho-physiological alterations in high-fat diet mice pancreatic β-cells. Amino Acids. 2012;43:1791–801.
84. You JS, Zhao X, Kim SH, Chang KJ. Positive correlation between serum taurine and adiponectin levels in high-fat diet-induced obesity rats. Adv Exp Med Biol. 2013;776:105–11.
85. Yamauchi T, Kamon J, Waki H, et al. The fat-derived hormone adiponectin reverses insulin resistance associated with both lipoatrophy and obesity. Nat Med. 2001;7(8):941–6.
86. Nakaya Y, Minami A, Harada N, Sakamoto S, Niwa Y, Ohnaka M. Taurine improves insulin sensitivity in the Otsuka Long-Evans Tokushima fatty rat, a model of spontaneous type 2 diabetes. Am J Clin Nutr. 2000;71(1):54–8.
87. Yokogoshi H, Oda H. Dietary taurine enhances cholesterol degradation and reduces serum and liver cholesterol concentrations in rats fed a high-cholesterol diet. Amino Acids. 2002;23(4):433–9.
88. Ide T, Kushiro M, Takahashi Y, Shinohara K, Cha S. mRNA expression of enzymes involved in taurine biosynthesis in rat adipose tissues. Metabolism. 2002;51(9):1191–7.
89. Jeevanandam M, Ramias L, Schiller WR. Altered plasma free amino acid levels in obese traumatized man. Metabolism. 1991;40(4):385–90.
90. Zhang M, Bi LF, Fang JH, et al. Beneficial effects of taurine on serum lipids in overweight or obese non-diabetic subjects. Amino Acids. 2004;26:267–71.
91. Brøns C, Spohr C, Storgaard H, Dyerberg J. Vaag a. Effect of taurine treatment on insulin secretion and action, and on serum lipid levels in overweight men with a genetic predisposition for type II diabetes mellitus. Eur J Clin Nutr. 2004;58:1239–47.
92. Xiao C, Giacca A, Lewis GF. Oral taurine but not N-acetylcysteine ameliorates NEFA-induced impairment in insulin sensitivity and beta cell function in obese and overweight, non-diabetic men. Diabetologia. 2008;51(1):139–46.

Chapter 24
Fetal Programming: Maternal Diets, Tryptophan, and Postnatal Development

Giuseppe Musumeci, Paola Castrogiovanni, Francesca Maria Trovato, Marta Anna Szychlinska, and Rosa Imbesi

Key Points

- Nutrient reduction, deprivation, or imbalance before implantation could result in somatic hypoevolutism at birth and alterations in endocrine and metabolic functions in postnatal life.
- Maternal malnutrition can cause alterations in both growth and maturation of specific developing brain regions and secretion of hormones such as GH, TRH, PRL, and gonadotropins.
- Maternal malnutrition exerts a suppressive effect on the immune response of both mother and fetus, with inevitable repercussions on the development of the immune system.
- Maternal malnutrition can affect the proliferation of myogenic precursors reducing the number of muscle fibers, especially in the fetal stage.
- Maternal malnutrition can affect future reproductive maturation with possible consequent impaired fertility and quality of gametes.
- The abnormal intake (in defect or excess) of tryptophan in the maternal diet, during pregnancy, has effects on different body areas of the progeny and on reproductive function.

Keywords Malnutrition • Postnatal development • Fetal programming • Tryptophan • Brain • Myogenesis • Fibrogenesis • Adipogenesis • Gametogenesis

Abbreviations

BMI   Body mass index
DOHaD   Developmental Origins of Health and Disease
DTH   Delayed-type hypersensitivity
GH   Growth hormone

G. Musumeci, PhD (✉) • P. Castrogiovanni, PhD • M.A. Szychlinska, PhD • R. Imbesi, MD
Department of Biomedical and Biotechnological Sciences, Human Anatomy and Histology Section,
School of Medicine, University of Catania, Catania, Italy
e-mail: g.musumeci@unict.it

F.M. Trovato, MD
Department of Clinical and Experimental Medicine, Internal Medicine Division, School of Medicine,
University of Catania, Catania, Italy

© Springer International Publishing AG 2017   325
R. Rajendram et al. (eds.), *Diet, Nutrition, and Fetal Programming*,
Nutrition and Health, DOI 10.1007/978-3-319-60289-9_24

HIV	Human immunodeficiency virus
IGF	Insulin-like growth factor
IHD	Ischaemic heart disease
IL-2	Interleukin-2
IUGR	Intrauterine growth restriction
NTDs	Neural tube defects
PMS	Premenstrual syndrome
PRL	Prolactin
T_3	Triiodothyronine
T_4	Tetraiodothyronine
TSH	Thyroid-stimulating hormone

Introduction

A lifelong healthy and varied diet is important, and, particularly during pregnancy, the mother's diet should provide energy and nutrients to both herself and fetus' growth and for future lactation. The nutritional status of the mother at conception is a key factor for development and fetal growth, so a healthy, balanced diet is essential, both before and during pregnancy. Moreover, in the last 10–15 years, much evidence has emerged linking nutrition during fetal life to the potential risk of disease in adulthood. According to the so-called "Barker hypothesis," chronic diseases in adulthood would be a result of the "fetal programming," through which any stimulus or insult during embryonic development would have a permanent effect on the structure and physiology of the human body. Experimental observations clearly indicate that the preimplantation phase is the period of the greatest vulnerability for the future embryo in relation to several endogenous and/or exogenous factors, including nutritional ones [1]. Nutrient reduction, deprivation, or imbalance before implantation could result in somatic hypoevolutism at birth [2], alterations in endocrine and metabolic functions in the postnatal life [3], and, often, impaired maturation of the reproductive system [4]. From clinical, epidemiological, and experimental observations, both in vivo and in vitro, several nutrients seem to influence the regular course of pregnancy and the embryo-fetal development in different animal species, including humans (Fig. 24.1). In fact, experimental results in mice have shown that undernutrition in pregnancy significantly reduces the number of puppies, increases the resorption of fetuses, and increases neonatal mortality [5]; in sheep, it retards intrauterine development of the fetus [6]; in rats, it reduces the weight of puppies at birth [4]. With regard to the human species, evaluating the specific influence of different nutrients on prenatal development is difficult, since a severe maternal undernutrition, with a reduction in caloric intake, will trigger a proportional increase in catabolic activity of the maternal tissues that cause the release in blood and then in maternal-fetal circulation of many aminoacids, vitamins, and minerals that will balance the deficit "diet" of the fetus. Considering selective deficiency of essential micronutrients during the embryo-fetal development, some malformation syndromes, such as congenital defects of the neural tube, are known to be a result of such deficits (Table 24.1) [7]. The intrauterine environment seems to "program" the developing fetus to be able to deal with a postnatal environment similar to the intrauterine one ("predictive adaptive response"). If the postnatal environment is discordant with the intrauterine one, diseases could establish. People undergoing a rapid transition from undernutrition in the early years of life to overnutrition in later years are more exposed to type 2 diabetes and other chronic diseases in their lifetime.

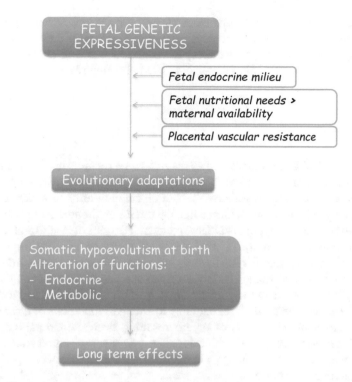

Fig. 24.1 Diagram of interrelations between fetal development and the long-term effects on the body

Table 24.1 Advantages of micronutrients supplementation

Reduction in incidence of NTDs and neonatal malformations	Folic acid
	Polyvitamins
	Zinc
Reduction in preterm birth incidence	Folic acid
	Polyvitamins
	Zinc
Reduction in low birth weight incidence	Folic acid
	Polyvitamins
	Zinc
Reduction in incidence of PMS	Calcium
Reduction in gestosis incidence	Calcium
	Vitamin C
	Vitamin E
Improved bone mineral composition in the newborn	Calcium
Reduction in maternal mortality	Vitamin A
	β-carotene
Reduction in fetal mortality	Polyvitamins
Higher levels of immune cells in HIV-positive pregnant women	Polyvitamins

The mother is the source of all molecular elements that allow a regular development and growth of the embryo until birth; therefore nutrition plays a key role, both before and during pregnancy. In the following paragraphs, we will analyze some aspects of the influence of maternal nutrition on "fetal programming" and any consequent alterations of a maternal malnutrition.

Fetal Programming

Over the past 20 years, epidemiological studies have shown a relationship between the early growth of the individual and the risk of diseases such as type 2 diabetes, cardiovascular disease, and metabolic syndrome. Studies on monozygotic twins, both on children of undernourished mothers and on animal models, have provided strong evidence that the uterine environment plays an important role in mediating this relationship. The hypothesis "Developmental Origins of Health and Disease" (DOHaD) suggests that environmental conditions during fetal and early postnatal development influence the health and ability of an individual for the lifetime, with permanent effects on growth, structure, and metabolism. This concept is nowadays widely accepted and is called "programming." Nevertheless, the mechanisms by which events of the prenatal life may affect cell function and then the metabolism of an organism after several years are just beginning to emerge. Alterations of these mechanisms may induce permanent structural alterations of organs resulting from suboptimal concentrations of an important factor during a critical period of development, persistent structural and/or metabolic alterations due to epigenetic changes leading to alterations in gene expression, and permanent effects on cellular aging regulation. The phenomenon known as "fetal programming" (Table 24.2) implies that nutritional and/or hormonal changes in the embryofetal microenvironment may affect the fetal genomic expression and exert permanent effects on a wide range of physiological processes [8]. Over 20 years ago, Hales and Barker proposed the hypothesis of the thrifty phenotype [9], according to which nonoptimal conditions of nutrition in uterus permanently alter the structure of organs of the fetus, which also adapts its metabolism to ensure its own survival. This is possible through the "saving" of some organs, in particular the brain, to the detriment of others, such as the heart, pancreas,

Table 24.2 Fetal programming in tissues and organs

Bone	Bone mineral composition
Liver	Metabolism of cholesterol
	Fibrinogen synthesis
	Factor VII synthesis
Kidney	Renin-angiotensin system activation
Musculoskeletal apparatus	Glycolysis
	Insulin resistance
Immune system	Autoimmunity of thyroid
Respiratory apparatus	Lung volume
Cardiovascular apparatus	Endothelial function
	Vascular compliance
	Left ventricle thickness
Endocrine system	Glucose metabolism
	GH-IGF1 axis
	Hypothalamic-pituitary-adrenocortical axis
	Hypothalamic-pituitary-gonadal axis

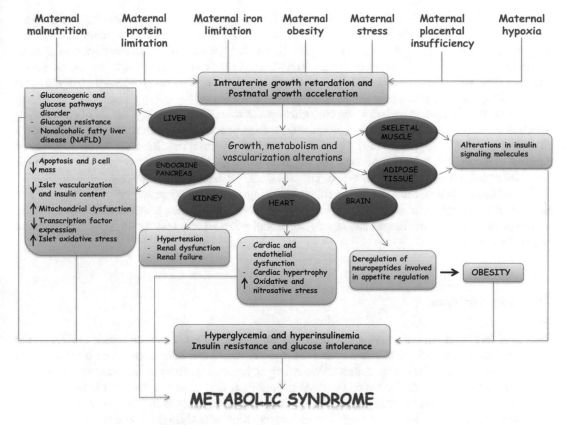

Fig. 24.2 Hypothesis of the thrifty phenotype

kidney, and skeletal muscle (Fig. 24.2). This hypothesis was the result of suggestive epidemiological studies by Barker et al. [10] and Hales et al. [11] that showed how individuals with a lower weight at birth and at 1 year of age had a higher mortality rate by ischemic heart disease (IHD) [10], a higher incidence of diabetes type 2, and abnormal glucose tolerance [11] – effects that are amplified by an inadequate postnatal nutrition. The DOHaD hypothesis includes several critical time windows, including preconception, fetal, and early postnatal periods, during which it is possible to establish the "fetal programming." Actually, the first time window should be considered puberty, since sexual reproduction begins long before fertilization. Indeed, the prerequisite for fertilization is the existence of the germline and the subsequent gametogenesis, which will be completed at puberty onset. So, for a good outcome of the fetal programming, an optimal nutrition is crucial not only during pregnancy but also in adult life from puberty.

Alterations in nutrient intake during prenatal life may be responsible not only for structural changes in organs but also for the onset of postnatal endocrine-metabolic disorders such as insulin resistance, type 2 diabetes, obesity, and puberty disorders [3]. It must also be taken into account that a general or selective deficiency in essential nutrients is not the sole cause of potential congenital malformative deficits. Indeed, many important endocrine and paracrine factors are involved in the growth and differentiation of embryonic tissues. Among them, insulin and insulin-like growth factors (IGFs) play a crucial role, not only during development but also during postnatal life. In fact, these molecules are considered, as amply demonstrated in animals, the most potent regulators of cell proliferation, apoptosis, oogenesis, embryogenesis, and ovarian secretion [12]. During intrauterine life, IGFs, in particular IGF-1 and IGF-2 to a certain extent, play an important role in regulating the nutrient metabolism (especially in the later stages of gestation), while in the immediately neonatal period, they promote and control the use of energy for growth and for the definitive differentiation of tissues, especially musculoskeletal and nervous ones, and the progressive adaptation to the extrauterine environment [13]. IGFs perform essential functions such as increasing protein synthesis and, at the same time, limiting their catabolism.

Lastly, it is important to underline the emerging area of research concerning the role of epigenetics, which is broadly defined as "heritable modifications in gene function which cannot be explained by changes in the DNA sequence" [14]. Epigenetic alterations in utero may have the ability to program diseases in adulthood. Scientific research has begun to investigate if epigenetic changes through nutritional interventions can affect the health of an individual, for example, in old age.

Given the vastness of the topic, in the following paragraphs, only some aspects of "fetal programming" will be analyzed, including the importance of mother's diet during pregnancy and its effects on the development of certain tissues and organs of particular importance and the possible consequences on postnatal life.

Immune Response

Results of recent researches confirm that maternal-fetal malnutrition exerts a suppressive effect on the immune response of both mother and fetus [15]. Indeed, nutritional imbalances, both deficiency and excess, can have inevitable repercussions on the emerging immune system and its development throughout life [15]. The pathways by which maternal malnutrition may influence the fetal immune system include alterations to the hypothalamus/pituitary axis, limited nutrients availability for embryonic and fetal development, and altered transfer of immunity from mother to child (placental transfer and breast milk transfer) [15]. Undernutrition, in fact, induces a significant hypertrophy of lymphoid organs, and overnutrition, especially if characterized by the abundance of fat, may have a suppressive effect on the immune response [15]. Maternal malnutrition is a serious risk even during postnatal life and childhood, when the child no longer enjoys the, albeit precarious, maternal protection [16]. Malnutrition during weaning and in early childhood can affect important aspects of the whole postnatal life such as somatic growth and protection against infectious diseases [15]. Primary and secondary lymphoid organs (e.g., gut-associated lymphoid tissue) undergo rapid expansion during the late fetal and early neonatal periods, during which time they may be uniquely sensitive to nutritional insults [15]. Moreover, the gastrointestinal immune system mainly develops through the relationship with bacteria [17]. The development of bacterial flora begins at birth and continues, especially in human, with a precise temporal series of bacterial strains that change depending on the nutritional steps of the baby, from breastfeeding to weaning [18]. Furthermore, the bacterial flora intervenes directly on the digestive function and for this reason acts as an indirect supplier of nutrients to the gastrointestinal tract [17], with subsequent effects on the development of the gut immune system of the child [16] (Table 24.3).

Pre- and Postnatal Brain Development

The development of the brain depends on complex processes of interaction between genetic and environmental factors. Among the environmental factors, nutrition, from conception to adulthood, is particularly important for the role of nutrients in specific metabolic pathways, so that a diet lacking in essential nutrients during the pre- and postnatal development may be responsible for permanent brain alterations [19]. From the 24th week of pregnancy until the early stages of postnatal life, the brain is

Table 24.3 Immunity in pregnancy and micronutrients supplementation

Stop to UV-induced immunosuppression	β-carotene
Better NK cells function	
Better response to DTH skin test	Vitamin C
Better response to DTH skin test	Vitamin E
Reduction in levels of IGF-2	
Increase in IL-2 levels	
Improvement in immune response to hepatitis B	
Vaccination	
Proliferation of immune cells	
Control in T-helper cells number	Polyvitamins
Better response to DTH skin test	
Reduction in infectious disease morbidity	
Antibody levels increase in influenza vaccination	

particularly vulnerable to adequate nutrition, given the strong neuronal proliferation and myelination that characterize neuronal development [20]. Among the fundamental nutrients, tryptophan, folate, and B vitamins are of particular relevance. Folate and B vitamins have a specific role in C1 metabolism and particularly in the production of S-adenosylmethionine, a methyl donor also necessary for the production of neurotransmitters; moreover folate and B vitamins are essential in the processes of transcription, nucleotide synthesis, and methylation.

An optimal supply of folate is essential during pregnancy. In pregnant women, given the increased folate request for rapid cell proliferation in the uterus and placenta tissues and for the fetus growth, there is a decrease in concentration of folate of about 50%, compared to the norm. From this comes the need for folic acid integration during pregnancy, thanks to its protective role against possible neural tube defects [21, 22], especially in the closing stages (21–28 days after conception). This has led to recommendations, worldwide, on the consumption of 400 µg of folic acid daily, from conception to the end of the first trimester of pregnancy [23]. Scientific data, even if not entirely consistent, suggest that the concentration of folate during pregnancy can affect the neurological development and behavior of offspring. Indeed, according to some studies, the low concentration of maternal folate is linked to increased inattention, hyperactivity problems, and emotional problems in the progeny [24], considerations that deserve further investigation. Few studies, however, have investigated the status of maternal folate after the recommended period, in the second and third trimester of pregnancy, to determine if the effect of folate is specific for some stages of pregnancy or if extended to the whole gestational period.

The B vitamins are necessary for essential metabolic pathways of the brain, being crucial for a healthy brain development and maintenance throughout life [25]. Also the B vitamins appear to have direct roles on neuronal development through their involvement in the C1 metabolism, and their effects on cognitive health may be independent or mediated by nutrient-nutrient and/or gene-nutrient interactions. Given the importance of C1 metabolism in a wide range of processes, it is not surprising that its possible perturbations can have strong effects on both brain development and brain aging. In a recent clinical study, performed in patients with mild cognitive impairment, there was evidence that the integration, for a period of 2 years, with folic acid and vitamins B6 and B12 reduced their cognitive decline; in addition, in these patients a brain atrophy reduction of about 30% was observed by magnetic resonance imaging [26].

Tryptophan is an essential amino acid that must be taken with food since it cannot be synthesized by the body. It is the precursor of serotonin, a neurotransmitter synthesized by serotonergic neurons of the central nervous system and by enterochromaffin cells, that is involved in the regulation of several body functions. The literature widely shows the link between dietary tryptophan and serotonin production, so the abnormal intake (in defect or excess) of tryptophan in the maternal diet, during pregnancy, has effects on different body areas of the progeny. For example, it is highlighted that the strong decrease of serotonin, caused by a maternal diet deficient in tryptophan, causes alterations of both growth and maturation of specific developing brain regions [13] and secretion of hormones such as GH, TRH, PRL, and gonadotropins [27, 28]. In contrast, the excess of serotonin in the CNS can cause alterations, hindering the normal differentiation of the serotonergic neurons of the raphe nuclei of the brainstem and preventing the serotonergic processes from reaching the hypothalamus [29], with a consequent reduction in the production of GH by the pituitary gland [30] and, therefore, of IGF-1 by the liver [16, 31].

Improving knowledge about potential epigenetic mechanisms, during pregnancy and postnatal life, will provide information on important links between folate, B vitamins, tryptophan, and status of brain health.

Pre- and Postnatal Myogenesis, Fibrogenesis, and Adipogenesis

Myogenesis, adipogenesis, and fibrogenesis are mechanisms directly involved in fetal and neonatal development of skeletal muscle [32], since skeletal muscle, fat, and connective tissues originate from mesenchymal stem cells. The commitment of these cells to myogenic, adipogenic, or fibrogenic lines can be considered a competitive process, and it is "due" to numerous inductive regulators. As a result of the controlled distribution of nutrients during embryonic and fetal development, skeletal muscle and adipose tissue, compared to brain and heart, have a lower priority, making the development of the skeletal muscle and adipose tissue particularly vulnerable to maternal nutritional deficiency [33]. The critical period for development of skeletal muscle, connective, and adipose tissues is mainly the fetal stage; therefore, just in this stage, the maternal undernutrition affects the proliferation of myogenic precursors reducing the number of muscle fibers. Instead, maternal nutrition has relatively minor effects on the development of skeletal muscle during the embryonic stage, since only a very small number of muscle fibers are formed during this stage. Even maternal overnutrition influences fetal development of skeletal muscle, intensifying intramuscular adipogenesis and fibrogenesis. Normally, during fetal development of skeletal muscle, a small portion of progenitor cells differentiate into adipocytes generating intramuscular fat; maternal overnutrition increases the expression of markers of adipogenesis in fetal skeletal muscle, at half gestation, compromising myogenesis in favor of adipogenesis which leads to a further increase of intramuscular fat, an event also associated with insulin resistance in skeletal muscle caused by paracrine effect of intramuscular adipocytes [34]. In addition to myofibrils and adipocytes, mesodermal progenitor cells can also differentiate into fibroblasts, which give rise to the connective tissue of endomysium, perimysium, and epimysium in fetal skeletal muscle during late gestation [32]. Maternal overnutrition increases the production of collagen and reticulation of the skeletal muscle, heart, and large intestine of fetus, suggesting an important role of maternal nutrition also in fetal fibrogenesis. The switching induced by overnutrition, from myogenesis to fibrogenesis, leads to impairment of muscle function, including the oxidative capacity. In addition, the attenuation of myogenesis reduces the number of muscle fibers, exerting permanent negative effects on muscle strength. To be considered, finally, that during the aging process, there is a progressive loss of muscle mass, accompanied by an increase in adiposity and fibrosis with consequent decrease in structural integrity and functional capacity of muscle; therefore the proper differentiation of mesenchymal stem cells during fetal development is crucial for the individual's health over the long term [27, 32, 34].

An altered tryptophan intake in the mother's diet during pregnancy has an indirect effect on the regular development of skeletal muscle. In fact, as mentioned in the previous paragraph, a deficiency or an excess of this aminoacid causes hyposerotonemia or hyperserotonemia that, although with different pathways, induces alterations in the normal brain development with functional defects on the hypothalamus/pituitary axis resulting in lack of hormones such as GH, TSH, T3, and T4. These deficiencies are associated with low body weight and alterations in the normal development of muscle tissue [27, 35, 36]. In particular, the reduced production of GH by the pituitary gland [30] will induce a deficient production of IGF-1 by the liver [16, 31], and it is known that low levels of IGF-1 have negative consequences on the differentiation of muscle and bone tissue and, therefore, on the body growth [16, 31]. In addition, recent experimental data show that in pregnant rats, even the hyperserotonemia, induced in experimental conditions, causes alterations in the offspring such as lower body mass index (BMI) and a lower rate of survival [30, 37].

Ultimately, the mechanisms behind the observed changes in fetal skeletal muscle, in cases of maternal malnutrition, remain largely unknown. In addition to the alteration of inductive regulators, it is likely that microRNAs are involved in myogenesis and adipogenesis regulation, although further studies are needed. Furthermore, it is thought that epigenetic changes, such as DNA methylation, may modify the cell line commitment during muscle and adipose tissue fetal development.

Pre- and Postnatal Gametogenesis and Reproductive Function

The DOHaD hypothesis led to the identification of new goals of fetal programming, in particular the effects on future reproductive function. Germ cells, during their differentiation, undergo intense epigenetic modifications, even though the critical times for the action of epigenetic markers are different between males and females. Males are probably more sensitive during fetal life, as, in male germ cells, DNA methylation is reacquired during the proliferation of spermatogonia (fetal life). In contrast, the female gametes may be more sensitive to epigenetic disturbance during folliculogenesis, as DNA methylation occurs during the growth and maturation of oocytes (adult life) [38]. In addition, malnutrition during folliculogenesis, which is a phase characterized by active angiogenesis and protein synthesis, results in a deficient oocyte quality. Because gametogenesis begins and takes place mostly during pregnancy, the status of maternal nutrition can influence the future reproductive maturation with possible consequent impaired fertility and quality of gametes, thus creating a transgenerational effect [39]. Increasingly, the literature provides a growing amount of information on the consequences of nutritional deficiencies in parental germ cells, even before the ovum is fertilized [40]. Recently, it was shown that the DNA damage of spermatocytes in the adult, as a result of micronutrient deficiencies, can significantly increase the risk of congenital malformations in the offspring and even carcinogenesis [16]. Infertility in the progeny can be induced by a variety of mechanisms, such as oxidative stress and epigenetic changes [41]. Actually, epidemiological studies on maternal nutrition and its effects on fertility of the offspring are rare, and the existing data are generally focused on the long-term effects of low birth weight due to maternal malnutrition. In fetuses with intrauterine growth restriction (IUGR) and in babies born dead, a compromised development of gonads was observed [42]. Cryptorchidism is common in children born with IUGR and has been associated with lower sperm counts in adulthood [43]. An early onset of puberty was observed in girls whose mothers had a high BMI during pregnancy [44]. The high maternal BMI seems to determine a negative effect on the concentration of inhibin B and seminal plasma quality on male children, indicative of a decreased function of Sertoli cells [45]. Although these data need further confirmation, an interaction between inadequate maternal nutrition (excess or reduced nutritional intake, imbalance in micronutrients, alcohol intake) and reproductive maturation in progeny has been demonstrated in most of the studies. For example, it is well known that exposure to alcohol in utero influences the development of the fetus causing cognitive, neuropsychological, and behavioral problems in the progeny [46], but it also seems that maternal consumption of alcohol during pregnancy impairs the development of Sertoli cells and is associated with decreased sperm in sons [47]. In addition, there was an increased risk of cryptorchidism in boys who have undergone prenatal alcohol exposure [48].

In the context of maternal malnutrition, a maternal diet deficient in tryptophan has an effect even on reproductive function. Studies conducted on the offspring of rats fed with diet free of tryptophan, from the first day of pregnancy, showed a sex-dependent effect on the reproductive system: females showed a normal onset of puberty; on the contrary males showed neither testicular descensus nor spermatogenesis. The effects were, however, less marked if mothers were fed with a diet free of tryptophan from the 14th day of pregnancy [4].

Conclusion

As discussed in the sections of this chapter, the DOHaD hypothesis is supported by both epidemiological evidence, correlating newborn size, growth and child nutrition with status of adult health, and animal experiments, showing that maternal under- and overnutrition during pregnancy lead to anomalies in metabolism and body composition in adulthood. Nowadays, it is believed that a "programming" in the early stages of life could be important in the etiology of diseases such as obesity, type 2 diabetes and cardiovascular disease, suggesting, therefore, that these common diseases can be prevented through optimal development of both fetus and newborn.

Fetal nutrition is influenced by diet and by the size and composition of the mother's body. In humans, strong evidence that maternal nutrition programs the risk for disease in the progeny is currently limited, although it seems to indicate the accumulation of oxidative stress and the consequent rapid cell aging as major molecular mechanisms (Fig. 24.3). Several studies support the idea that maternal antioxidant therapy can reverse some of the deleterious effects of oxidative stress suffered in

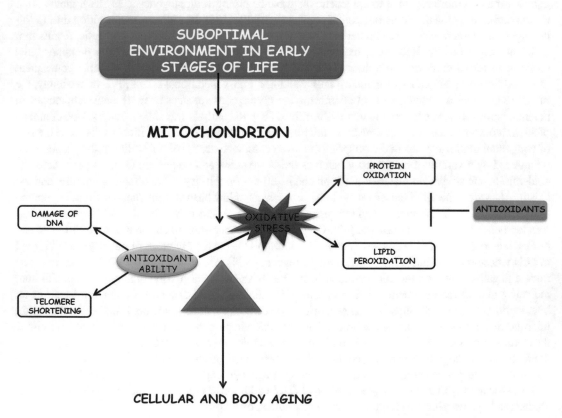

Fig. 24.3 Oxidative stress as a basic mechanism of the programming development and of aging

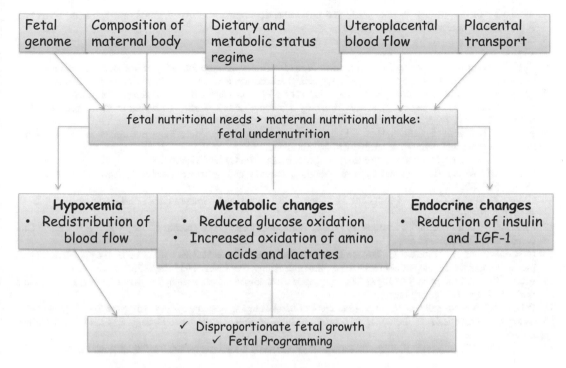

Fig. 24.4 Diagram explaining the maternal control of development and embryo-fetal programming

the early stages of prenatal life. Nevertheless, studies both in animals and humans [49, 50] show that a proper assessment can be possible only in postnatal life, and, therefore, further studies need to deal with the potential beneficial effects of postnatal supplementation with antioxidants. Other data on specific nutritional interventions, derived from the follow-up of children born after nutritional interventions during pregnancy, do not always agree even if they show beneficial effects on vascular function, lipid concentrations, glucose tolerance, and insulin resistance.

What has been observed clinically in humans has been confirmed in animal experiments, and this allows the use of new knowledge to reduce the onset of many diseases. Therefore, it is necessary to know both the factors that determine fetal growth and the conditions that limit the maternal-fetal supply of nutrients and oxygen to the fetus (Fig. 24.4). So much has already been done, but more studies need to understand how the fetus adapts to a limited supply of nutrients from the mother, how these adaptations can influence structure and physiology of the body, and which are the molecular mechanisms by which nutrients and hormones can alter gene expression. We believe that to improve the outcomes of pregnancy, promote growth and healthy child development, reduce the risk of chronic diseases, and slow down the metabolic decline associated with aging, it is necessary to develop dietary strategies to optimize nutrition, not only during pregnancy but already when this is programmed, by assuming adequate micronutrients and complementary foods, never forgetting the importance of breastfeeding.

References

1. Minkin MJ. Embryonic development and pregnancy test sensitivity: the importance of earlier pregnancy detection. Women's Health (Lond Engl). 2009;5(6):659–67.
2. Triunfo S, Lanzone A. Impact of maternal under nutrition on obstetric outcomes. J Endocrinol Investig. 2015;38(1): 31–8.
3. Reusens B, Ozanne SE, Remacle C. Fetal determinants of type 2 dyabetes. Curr Drug Targets. 2007;8(8):935–41.

4. Imbesi R, Castrogiovanni P. Embryonic and post natal development in experimental tryptophan deprived rats. A preliminary study. J Mol Histol. 2008;39(5):487–98.

5. Gabory A, Attig L, Junien C. Developmental programming and epigenetics. Am J Clin Nutr. 2011;94(6 Suppl): 1943S–52S.

6. Ford SP, Long NM. Evidence for similar changes in offspring phenotype following either maternal undernutrition or overnutrition: potential impact on fetal epigenetic mechanisms. Reprod Fertil Dev. 2011;24(1):105–11.

7. Simpson JL, Bailey LB, Pietrzik K, Shane B, Holzgreve W. Micronutrients and women of reproductive potential: required dietary intake and consequences of dietary deficiency or excess. Part II – itamin D, vitamin A, iron, zinc, iodine, essential fatty acids. J Matern Fetal Neonatal Med. 2011;24(1):1–24.

8. El Hajj N, Schneider E, Lehnen, Haaf T. Epigenetics and consequences of an adverse nutritional and diabetic intrauterine environment. Reproduction. 2014;148(6):R111–20.

9. Hales CN, Barker DJ. The thrifty phenotype hypothesis. Br Med Bull. 2001;60:5–20.

10. Barker DJ, Winter PD, Osmond C, et al. Weight in infancy and death from ischaemic heart disease. Lancet. 1989;2:577–80.

11. Hales CN, Barker DJ, Clark PMS, et al. Fetal and infant growth and impaired glucose tolerance at age 64. BMJ. 1991;303:1019–22.

12. Maki RG. Small is beautiful: insulin-like growth factors and their role in growth, development, and cancer. J Clin Oncol. 2010;28(33):4985–95.

13. Castrogiovanni P, Musumeci G, Trovato FM, Avola R, Magro G, Imbesi R. Effects of high-tryptophan diet on pre- and postnatal development in rats: a morphological study. Eur J Nutr. 2014;53(1):297–308.

14. Russo VEA, Martienssen RA, Riggs AD. Epigenetic mechanisms of gene regulation. Cold Springs Harbor: Cold Springs Harbor Laboratory Press; 1996.

15. Palmer AC. Nutritionally mediated programming of the developing immune system. Adv Nutr. 2011;2(5):377–95.

16. Strzepa A, Szczepanik M. Influence of natural gut flora on immune response. Postepy Hig Med Dosw Online. 2013;67:908–20.

17. MacDonald TT, Pettersson S. Bacterial regulation of intestinal immune responses. Inflamm Bowel Dis. 2000;6(2): 116–22.

18. Madan JC, Farzan SF, Hibberd PL, Karagas MR. Normal neonatal microbiome variation in relation to environmental factors, infection and allergy. Curr Opin Pediatr. 2012;24(6):753–9.

19. Anjos T, Altmäe S, Emmett P, et al. Nutrition and neurodevelopment in children: focus on NUTRIMENTHE Project. Eur J Nutr. 2013;52:1825–42.

20. Isaacs EB. Neuroimaging, a new tool for investigating the effects of early diet on cognitive and brain development. Front Hum Neurosci. 2013;7:445.

21. Czeizel AE, Dudás I. Prevention of the first occurrence of neural-tube defects by periconceptional vitamin supplementation. N Engl J Med. 1992;327:1832–5.

22. MRC Vitamin Study Research Group. Prevention of neural tube defects: results of the Medical Research Council Vitamin Study. Lancet. 1991;339:131–7.

23. Centers for Disease Control Prevention. Recommendations for the use of folic acid to reduce the number of cases of spina bifida and other neural tube defects. Morb Mortal Wkly Rep. 1992;41:1–8.

24. Pentieva K, McGarel C, McNulty B, et al. Effect of folic acid supplementation during pregnancy on growth and cognitive development of the offspring: a pilot followup investigation of children of FASSTT study participants. Proc Nutr Soc. 2012;71:E139.

25. van de Rest O, van Hooijdonk LWA, Doets E, et al. B vitamins and n-3 fatty acids for brain development and function: review of human studies. Ann Nutr Metab. 2012;60:272–92.

26. Smith AD, Smith SM, de Jager CA, et al. Homocysteine-lowering by B vitamins slows the rate of accelerated brain atrophy in mild cognitive impairment: a randomized controlled trial. PLoS One. 2010;5:e12244.

27. Imbesi R, D'Agata V, Musumeci G, Castrogiovanni P. Skeletal muscle: from development to function. Clin Ter. 2014;165:47–56.

28. Yoshimura M, Hagimoto M, Matsuura T, Ohkubo J, Ohno M, Maruyama T, et al. Effects of food deprivation on the hypothalamic feeding-regulating peptides gene expressions in serotonin depleted rats. J Physiol Sci. 2014;64:97–104.

29. Whitaker-Azmitia PM. Behavioral and cellular consequences of increasing serotonergic activity during brain development: a role in autism? Int J Dev Neurosci. 2005;23(1):75–83.

30. Hranilovic D, Blažević S, Ivica N, Cicin-Sain L, Oreskovic D. The effects of the perinatal treatment with 5-hydroxytryptophan or tranylcypromine on the peripheral and central serotonin homeostasis in adult rats. Neurochem Int. 2011;59(2):202–7.

31. Duan C. Nutritional and developmental regulation of insulin-like growth factors in fish. J Nutr. 1998;128:306S–14S.

32. Musumeci G, Castrogiovanni P, Coleman R, Szychlinska MA, Salvatorelli L, Parenti R, Magro G, Imbesi R. Somitogenesis: from somite to skeletal muscle. Acta Histochem. 2015;117(4–5):313–28.

33. Zhu MJ, Ford SP, Means WJ, Hess BW, Nathanielsz PW, Du M. Maternal nutrient restriction affects properties of skeletal muscle in offspring. J Physiol. 2006;575:241–50.
34. Trovato FM, Imbesi R, Conway N, Castrogiovanni P. Morphological and functional aspects of human skeletal muscle. J Funct Morphol Kinesiol. 2016;1(3):289–302.
35. Musumeci G, Imbesi R, Trovato FM, Szychlinska MA, Aiello FC, Buffa P, Castrogiovanni P. Importance of serotonin (5-HT) and its precursor l-tryptophan for homeostasis and function of skeletal muscle in rats. A morphological and endocrinological study. Acta Histochem. 2015;117(3):267–74.
36. Ruan Z, Yang Y, Wen Y, Zhou Y, Fu X, Ding S, et al. Metabolomic analysis of amino acid and fat metabolism in rats with l-tryptophan supplementation. Amino Acids. 2014;46:2681–91.
37. Musumeci G, Loreto C, Trovato FM, Giunta S, Imbesi R, Castrogiovanni P. Serotonin (5HT) expression in rat pups treated with high-tryptophan diet during fetal and early postnatal development. Acta Histochem. 2014; 116(2):335–43.
38. Bourc'his D, Proudhon C. Sexual dimorphism in parental imprint ontogeny and contribution to embryonic development. Mol Cell Endocrinol. 2008;282:87–94.
39. Sharpe RM, Franks S. Environment, lifestyle and infertility–an inter-generational issue. Nat Cell Biol. 2002; 4(Suppl):s33–40.
40. Kauffman AS, Bojkowska K, Rissman EF. Critical periods of susceptibility to short-term energy challenge during pregnancy: impact on fertility and offspring development. Physiol Behav. 2010;99(1):100–8.
41. Cetin I, Berti C, Calabrese S. Role of micronutrients in the periconceptional period. Hum Reprod Update. 2010;16:80–95.
42. de Bruin JP, Dorland M, Bruinse HW, Spliet W, Nikkels PG, Te Velde ER. Fetal growth retardation as a cause of impaired ovarian development. Early Hum Dev. 1998;51:39–46.
43. Boisen KA, Main KM, Rajpert-De Meyts E, Skakkebaek NE. Are male reproductive disorders a common entity? The testicular dysgenesis syndrome. Ann N Y Acad Sci. 2001;948:90–9.
44. Keim SA, Branum AM, Klebanoff MA, Zemel BS. Maternal body mass index and daughters' age at menarche. Epidemiology. 2009;20:677–81.
45. Toulis KA, Iliadou PK, Venetis CA, Tsametis C, Tarlatzis BC, Papadimas I, et al. Inhibin B and anti-Mullerian hormone as markers of persistent spermatogenesis in men with non-obstructive azoospermia: a meta-analysis of diagnostic accuracy studies. Hum Reprod Update. 2010;16:713–24.
46. Ornoy A, Ergaz Z. Alcohol abuse in pregnant women: effects on the fetus and newborn, mode of action and maternal treatment. Int J Environ Res Public Health. 2010;7:364–79.
47. Ramlau-Hansen CH, Toft G, Jensen MS, Strandberg-Larsen K, Hansen ML, Olsen J. Maternal alcohol consumption during pregnancy and semen quality in the male offspring: two decades of follow-up. Hum Reprod. 2010;25:2340–5.
48. Damgaard IN, Jensen TK, Petersen JH, Skakkebaek NE, Toppari J, Main KM. Cryptorchidism and maternal alcohol consumption during pregnancy. Environ Health Perspect. 2007;115:272–7.
49. Curhan GC, Willet WC, Rimm EB, et al. Birth weight and adult hypertension, diabetes mellitus and obesity in US men. Circulation. 1996;15:3246–50.
50. Mi J, Law C, Zhang KL, et al. Effects of infant birthweight and maternal body mass index in pregnancy on components of the insulin resistance syndrome in China. Ann Intern Med. 2000;132(4):253–60.

Chapter 25
Intrauterine Programming and Effects of Caffeine

Zhexiao Jiao, Hao Kou, Dan Xu, Hanwen Luo, and Hui Wang

Key Points

- Caffeine ingestion during pregnancy is a common phenomenon.
- Growing evidences indicate that prenatal caffeine ingestion can induce developmental toxicity.
- Developmental toxicity induced by prenatal caffeine ingestion is related to the susceptibility to adult metabolic diseases.
- Prenatal caffeine ingestion can significantly increase maternal blood corticosterone level and open the placental glucocorticoid barrier, thereby leading to overexposure of foetus to the maternal glucocorticoids.
- Excessive glucocorticoids and caffeine can exert powerful effects on the epigenome to influence the expression of important developmental genes, thereby leading to intrauterine programming alteration of the hypothalamic–pituitary–adrenal (HPA) axis and glucocorticoids-insulin-like growth factor 1 (GCs-IGF1) axis.
- We have proposed the common mechanisms of increased susceptibility to metabolic diseases in IUGR offspring, which is mechanism about 'two programming' and 'two hit' mediated by the overexposure to maternal glucocorticoids.

Keywords Caffeine • Developmental toxicity • Hypothalamic–pituitary–adrenal axis • Intrauterine programming • Epigenetic modifications • Metabolic diseases

Abbreviations

11β-HSD	11β-hydroxysteroid dehydrogenase
BMCCs	Bone mesenchymal stem cells
CRH	Corticotropin-releasing hormone
DNMT	DNA methyltransferase
DOHaD	Developmental Origins of Health and Disease

Z. Jiao, PhD • H. Kou, PhD • D. Xu, PhD • H. Luo, MD • H. Wang, PhD (✉)
Department of Pharmacology, Basic Medical School, Wuhan University, Wuhan, China
e-mail: wanghui19@whu.edu.cn

© Springer International Publishing AG 2017
R. Rajendram et al. (eds.), *Diet, Nutrition, and Fetal Programming*,
Nutrition and Health, DOI 10.1007/978-3-319-60289-9_25

GCs-IGF1   Glucocorticoids-insulin-like growth factor 1
GR   Glucocorticoid receptor
Hdac   Histone deacetylases
HPA   Hypothalamic–pituitary–adrenal
IUGR   Intrauterine growth retardation
MAPK   Mitogen-activated protein kinase
MR   Mineralocorticoid receptor
MS   Metabolic syndrome
NAFLD   Non-alcoholic fatty liver disease
NO   Nitric oxide
P450scc   P450 cholesterol side-chain cleavage enzyme
RAS   Renin–angiotensin system
SF-1   Steroidogenic factor 1
SR-BI   Scavenger receptor BI
SREBP1   Sterol-regulatory element-binding protein 1
StAR   Steroidogenic acute regulatory protein

Introduction

Intrauterine growth retardation (IUGR) is defined by a developing foetus weighing 10% or two standard deviations less than the mean body weight of normal foetuses at the same gestational age [1]. IUGR is the most common type of developmental toxicity and refers to the poor growth of a foetus while in the mother's uterus during pregnancy. The global incidence of IUGR is approximately 2.75–15.53% [2]. Recent epidemiological studies have revealed that IUGR can induce foetal distress, neonatal asphyxia, and perinatal death. Furthermore, IUGR offspring after birth are more likely to exhibit delayed physical and intellectual development and increased susceptibility to adult metabolic diseases [3–5]. Thus, the incidence of some adult diseases is influenced by the uterine environment, in addition to genetic and postnatal factors.

Caffeine (1,3,7-trimethylxanthine) is a methylxanthine alkaloid that is widely present in coffee, tea, soft drinks, foods, and some drugs [6]. Many previous studies have reported that caffeine ingestion can enhance mood and alertness, awareness, attention, and reaction time [7]. Owing to their excitation action on the central nervous system and beneficial effects on the cardiovascular system, caffeinated beverages are frequently consumed by different segments of society. According to statistical data from the WTO in 2009, the world's total export of caffeinated products totals 65 billion dollars per year. Furthermore, caffeine has gradually replaced theophylline as the drug of first choice for apnea of prematurity in clinical applications [8, 9]. Caffeine ingestion during pregnancy is a common phenomenon. It was reported that the intake of caffeine per capita in America is 2.64 mg/kg/day and that the mean caffeine exposure of women during pregnancy is 1.76 mg/kg/day [10].

As one of the most widely consumed products, caffeine has been extensively studied to evaluate its safety on human health. Following the introduction of the concept 'developmental origins of health and disease (DOHaD)' in the 1980s, research began on the adverse effect of prenatal caffeine exposure on adult metabolic diseases, although some epidemiological data demonstrated that adult caffeine intake can prevent and reduce the effects of the metabolic syndrome (MS) [7]. Realising the potential negative effects of caffeine, the US Food and Drug Administration set guidelines for the daily intake of caffeine for pregnant women in the 1980s. Moreover, epidemiological studies and animal experiments have indicated that prenatal caffeine ingestion leads to reproductive and developmental toxicities [11–13], and prenatal caffeine ingestion may be the developmental inducer of various adult metabolic diseases in offspring [14, 15]. Recent animal experiments in our laboratory have demonstrated that caffeine ingestion during pregnancy can induce IUGR and increase the susceptibility to adult metabolic diseases, such as non-alcoholic fatty liver disease (NAFLD). Based on the above-mentioned experiments, we have proposed a hypothesis regarding the alteration of hypothalamic–pituitary–adrenal (HPA) axis-associated neuroendocrine metabolic programming, of which the core mechanism is the alteration of the programming of glucocorticoid-insulin-like growth factor 1 (GC-IGF1) [16, 17]. This article reviews the current progress in understanding the developmental toxicity and intrauterine programming mechanism of the foetal origin of metabolic disease induced by prenatal caffeine ingestion.

Developmental Toxicity Induced by Caffeine

Developmental toxicity is defined as adverse structural or functional alterations caused by an environmental insult before and after birth, including short-term and long-term adverse effects [18]. The typical short-term effects include spontaneous abortion, congenital malformation, and IUGR; the typical long-term effects include intellectual and physical development retardation and increased susceptibility to adult metabolic diseases [3–5].

Adverse Pregnancy Outcomes Induced by Caffeine Exposure

Previous studies have suggested that prenatal caffeine ingestion is correlated with various developmental toxicities, including spontaneous abortion [13, 19–22], congenital malformation [23, 24], and IUGR [25, 26].

As a typical developmental toxicity, IUGR was discussed with regard to its correlation with prenatal caffeine ingestion in a previous review [6] that included 26 epidemiological surveys from different periods (before the year 2000 and 2000–2010). Among the reports before 2000, six reports indicated that prenatal caffeine ingestion was associated with IUGR, and three reports did not indicate a correlation. For the period from 2000 to 2010, the results of six reports were negative for the correlation between prenatal caffeine ingestion and IUGR, and 11 studies obtained an ambiguous correlation owing to serious deficiencies (effects of confounders such as nicotine or alcohol) in these studies. As mentioned above, the correlation between prenatal caffeine ingestion and IUGR remains controversial. Different doses of caffeine ingested, clinically insignificant magnitudes of IUGR, and other confounding factors (e.g. age and health condition of the pregnant women) may be possible reasons for the conflicting results. Therefore, animal experiments are necessary to validate the developmental toxicities induced by prenatal caffeine ingestion.

Previous studies in animal models have identified that foetal mortality has a dose-dependent relationship with prenatal caffeine ingestion, and the congenital malformation ratio was shown to increase in a group that received a high dose of caffeine [27]. Multiple studies support the same conclusion [28, 29]. Moreover, the ratios of stillbirth, IUGR, and osteodysplasty were shown to be markedly increased in a high-dose caffeine exposure group [30]. Prenatal caffeine ingestion can also reduce the birth weight of male rhesus macaques [31]. Recently, a series of animal experiments by our laboratory also indicated that prenatal caffeine ingestion during the second and third trimesters reduced the body weight and height of the foetus and increased the IUGR rate in dose-dependent manners [17, 26, 32]. Therefore, caffeine can induce developmental toxicities and is a definite inducer of IUGR (animal studies on caffeine developmental toxicity are listed in Table 25.1).

Table 25.1 Examples of developmental toxicities caused by caffeine exposure

Study	Developmental toxicities induced by caffeine
Collins et al. (1982)	Increasing the congenital malformation ratio
Ikeda et al. (1982)	
Smith et al. (1987)	
Gilbert and Rice (1991)	Reducing the birth weight of male offspring
Nehlig and Debry (1994)	Increasing the ratios of stillbirth, IUGR, and osteodysplasty
Liu et al. (2012)	Reducing the body weight and height of the foetus, increasing the IUGR rate
Xu et al. (2012)	

Increased Susceptibility to Adult Metabolic Diseases in Offspring

MS is an aggregation of a number of symptoms (including hypertension and hyperglycaemia dyslipidaemia), and its pathophysiological basis is insulin resistance. It can induce various metabolic diseases, such as NAFLD, diabetes, and cardiac–cerebral vascular disease. Recently, clinical studies have identified that an adverse intrauterine environment can increase the incidence of various metabolic diseases [33–49], indicating that MS may originate from intrauterine development. Separated from other symptoms, hypercholesterolemia is also the pathogenic basis and diagnosis target of MS [50]. Persistent dyslipidaemia in IUGR rats, resulting from an adverse intrauterine environment, can increase the susceptibility to MS in adulthood [51–54], indicating that hypercholesterolemia may have an intrauterine origin.

Some epidemiological studies have revealed that caffeine ingestion in adolescence can increase the susceptibility to MS [55, 56]. In addition, caffeine ingestion in infancy can induce insulin resistance in female rats [57]. However, epidemiological evidence that indicates a correlation between prenatal caffeine exposure and adult metabolic diseases is rare. Animal experiments by our laboratory revealed that prenatal caffeine ingestion could induce neuroendocrine metabolic programming alterations in offspring following the glucocorticoid-associated alteration of peripheral glucose and lipid metabolic pathways [17, 58], which presented as low blood glucose and high blood lipid levels under low activity of the HPA axis, and high blood glucose and low blood lipid levels under high activity of the HPA axis. As a result, this disorder of peripheral glucose and lipid metabolic function can increase the susceptibility to MS in offspring [16, 26]. Meanwhile, prenatal caffeine ingestion can induce changes in pancreatic development and lead to diabetic symptoms (high blood glucose and low blood insulin levels) after high-fat diet feeding [59]. Moreover, prenatal caffeine ingestion can damage the ultrastructure of foetal hepatocytes and alter the programming of lipid synthesis and output, presenting as enhanced lipogenesis in female offspring and reduced lipid output in male offspring, when fed a high-fat diet, catch-up growth appears in adult offspring, with increased lipid synthesis and reduced output, thereby aggravating hepatic lipid accumulation and causing NAFLD [16]. It has been shown that prenatal caffeine ingestion can increase the susceptibility to hypercholesterolaemia [26]. Cholesterol metabolism in foetal cartilage is also affected by prenatal caffeine exposure, resulting in an accumulation of cholesterol in articular cartilage and increased susceptibility to adult osteoarthritis [60]. Glomerulosclerosis, the vital mechanism of hypertension, can be induced by prenatal caffeine ingestion [61]. In conclusion, caffeine ingestion in developmental stages (gestation and adolescence) can increase the susceptibility to multiple adult metabolic diseases.

Damage Mechanisms and Influencing Factors of Caffeine Development Toxicity

Because of its high lipid solubility, caffeine can be rapidly absorbed from the mother's gastrointestinal tract and distributed to foetal tissues by passing through multiple tissue barriers (such as the placental barrier and the blood-brain barrier) [62]. Therefore, prenatal caffeine ingestion can act directly and indirectly on the matrix and the placenta and ultimately affect foetal development.

Effects on the Mother

In pregnant women, the peak plasma caffeine concentration is reached between 30 and 60 min after absorption from the gastrointestinal tract [63]. The biological half-life ($t_{1/2}$) of caffeine varies widely among individuals, and it depends on multiple factors such as age, gender, liver enzyme function level (related to caffeine metabolism), and pregnancy. The $t_{1/2}$ of caffeine is approximately 2–6 h in healthy adults, and it increases to 18 h in the third trimester [14]. The activity of CYP1A2 (primary enzyme for caffeine metabolism) decreases during pregnancy, which may make the $t_{1/2}$ longer in pregnant women and induce the cumulative effects of caffeine [64].

The HPA axis is an important component of the endocrine system. As the terminal effector organ of the HPA axis, the adrenal gland is responsible for synthesising glucocorticoids and plays an important role in growth and development [65]. Steroidogenic acute regulatory protein (StAR) and P450 cholesterol side-chain cleavage enzyme (P450scc) are vital rate-limiting enzymes in adrenal steroidogenesis [66–68]. It has been reported that the alteration of the maternal glucocorticoid level may be an important endocrine mechanism of foetal developmental toxicity [65, 69]. Previously, we have shown that that prenatal caffeine ingestion can significantly increase the maternal blood corticosterone level [70]. Further findings from an in vitro study indicate that caffeine can promote the expression of StAR and increase the rate of steroid hormone synthesis [71]. As discussed later in this review, the level of maternal glucocorticoids, resulting from prenatal caffeine ingestion, is considered the cause of increased susceptibility to adult metabolic diseases in offspring.

Effects on the Placenta

The placenta is an important organ responsible for material exchange between the foetus and the mother. Moreover, the endocrine function of the placenta plays an important role in foetal development [72]. Placental lesions are the most common cause of IUGR and are primarily caused by the increased apoptosis and the decreased proliferation of trophoblast cells [73]. Bax (pro-apoptotic) and Bcl-2 (anti-apoptotic) are two genes closely related to apoptosis, and the balance between their expressions is crucial for maintaining the normal function of the placenta [74]. p53 is a widely expressed tumour suppressor gene in placental trophoblast cells and can accelerate apoptosis through up-regulating the expression of Bax and downregulating the expression of Bcl-2 [75]. Our laboratory found that prenatal caffeine ingestion could increase the expression of p53 and Bax while decreasing the expression of Bcl-2, which is consistent with Nomura's result [76]. It was suggested that caffeine could accelerate apoptosis in placental trophoblast cells by increasing the expression of p53 [25]. A recent study showed that prenatal caffeine ingestion could decrease leptin expression in placental trophoblast cells, which increased the expression of p53 in the placenta [77]. It was reported that many factors such as inhibition of adenosine receptors, disorder of the rein-angiotensin system (RAS), oxidative damage by nitric oxide (NO), and CYP1A1 are involved in placental damage caused by caffeine [78].

Effects on the Foetus

The 11β-hydroxysteroid dehydrogenase system (11β-HSDs) includes two dehydrogenases (11β-HSD1 and 11β-HSD2) with glucocorticoid metabolic function. 11β-HSD1 activates glucocorticoids by reduction, whereas 11β-HSD2 inactivates glucocorticoids by oxidation [79]. A previous study confirmed that caffeine could inhibit the expression of 11β-HSD2 in primary hippocampal neurons of foetal rats, as well as increase the expression of 11β-HSD1 and glucocorticoid receptor (GR) [17]. In addition, it was found that caffeine might decrease the expression of 11β-HSD2 by increasing promoter methylation. As a result, the concentration of glucocorticoids in the foetal hippocampus increases, leading to the excessive activation of GR and a toxic effect on the hippocampus, thereby causing high stress sensitivity of the HPA axis in offspring.

Caffeine Ingestion and Foetal Programming of Metabolic Diseases

An increasing number of studies have shown that the alteration of offspring endocrine and metabolic programming caused by an adverse intrauterine environment [80], especially inhibition of the development of the HPA axis (with high postnatal stress susceptibility), may be the potential mechanism of the intrauterine origin of MS [81, 82]. Based on numerous systematic studies by our laboratory [16, 17, 26, 32, 70, 83, 84], the mechanism of intrauterine neuroendocrine metabolic programming of increased susceptibility to adult diseases in offspring caused by prenatal caffeine ingestion was recently proposed. It suggested that foetal overexposure to maternal glucocorticoids caused by prenatal caffeine ingestion could alter the intrauterine programming of the HPA axis and GC-IGF1 axis in offspring, which results in the postnatal dysfunction of the HPA axis and the functional alteration of glucocorticoid-associated glucolipid metabolism and the increased susceptibility to multiple adult metabolic diseases. Postnatal chronic stimulations (such as overnutrition and high mental stress) could accelerate the alteration of neuroendocrine metabolic programming, thereby inducing a variety of metabolic diseases.

Maternal Glucocorticoids and the Placental Barrier

Under physiological conditions, maternal glucocorticoids are involved in early foetal growth and development, and the intrauterine glucocorticoid level is the key factor involved in adjusting foetal tissue formation and functional maturation. However, exposure to high glucocorticoid levels could cause foetal dysplasia [65]. During pregnancy, the endogenous maternal cortisol concentration is five to ten times higher than that in the foetal compartment. The concentration gradient is maintained by the placental glucocorticoid barrier [85], and 11β-HSDs are involved in the regulation of this placental glucocorticoid barrier (Fig. 25.1). It has been proven that 11β-HSD1 [17] and 11β-HSD2 are expressed in the placenta [86]. Previous reports show that a variety of adverse intrauterine environments (such as hypoxia, ischemia, and stress in pregnant woman) can downregulate the expression of 11β-HSD2 in

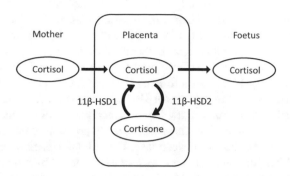

Fig. 25.1 The placental glucocorticoid barrier. 11β-HSD1/11β-HSD2 can catalyse an oxidation-reduction reaction, which results in the reciprocal transformation between active cortisol and inactive cortisone. 11β-HSD2, acting as glucocorticoid barrier, is expressed abundantly in the placenta during pregnancy

the placenta and then destroy the placental glucocorticoid barrier, resulting in the overexposure of the foetus to the maternal glucocorticoids [87–89]. A study by our laboratory [17] showed that caffeine exposure during pregnancy could enhance the corticosterone levels in maternal and foetal blood and could up-regulate placental 11β-HSD1 and downregulate placental 11β-HSD2. A study by Yang et al. showed that caffeine could directly downregulate 11β-HSD2 [90]. These results reveal that caffeine exposure during pregnancy can increase the level of maternal blood glucocorticoids and open the placental glucocorticoid barrier by the action of 11β-HSDs, thereby leading to overexposure of the foetus to maternal glucocorticoids.

Foetal Programming of Metabolic Diseases Caused by Excessive Glucocorticoids

Excessive Glucocorticoids and Programming of the HPA Axis

The HPA axis is an important neuroendocrine axis responsible for systemic stress response, and is a vital vulnerable target during the intrauterine period [91]. Glucocorticoid exposure during pregnancy could cause postnatal functional abnormalities in the neuroendocrine system in offspring, and the permanent alteration of the endocrine system has a significant long-term impact on physical health [92]. Programming alterations of the HPA axis are most likely to be responsible for the intrauterine origin of MS [93]. Previous studies showed that low basal activity and high stress sensitivity of the HPA axis in IUGR offspring may have resulted from caffeine exposure during pregnancy [17, 26]. These results indicate that intrauterine programming alterations of the HPA axis induced by prenatal caffeine ingestion may be the major mechanism for the increased susceptibility to adult metabolic diseases.

In rats, caffeine ingestion during pregnancy induces low-functional programming alterations of the HPA axis in the offspring [26]. Animal experiments found that after caffeine ingestion during pregnancy, the expression of corticotropin-releasing hormone (CRH) was reduced in the foetal hypothalamus and StAR and P450scc as well as the synthesis of endogenous corticosterone were significantly decreased. The activity of the HPA axis in these offspring rats reflected a low basal activity after weaning [26]. To date, no other laboratory has reported an underlying mechanism for the low-functional programming alteration of the HPA axis caused by caffeine ingestion during pregnancy. It is known that there are specific binding sites for steroidogenic factor 1 (SF-1) in all of the promoter regions of the adrenal steroid synthetase system, including StAR, P450scc, 3β-HSD, P450c21, and P450c11, indicating that SF-1 is one of the most important transcriptional factors in the regulation of steroid synthetase expression [94–96]. Studies have shown that both DNA methylation and histone acetylation can affect the expression of SF-1 [97, 98]. One study found that caffeine up-regulates the expression of StAR in foetal adrenal cortical cells and then increases the synthetic rate of cortisol [71], indicating that caffeine has a direct excitatory effect on adrenal steroid synthesis function. However, it was found through animal experiments [17] that foetal overexposure to maternal gluco-corticoids reduced the expression of foetal adrenal SF-1 and the steroid synthetase system. Furthermore, the total rate of DNA methylation was increased, and the acetylation of histone H3K9 and H3K14 was decreased in the promoter region of SF-1; meanwhile, the expression of the DNA methyltransferases (Dnmt1 and Dnmt3a/3b) and the histone deacetylases (Hdac1 and Hdac2) increased. Thus, the altera-tions of epigenetic modifications and the expression of SF-1 caused by high maternal glucocorticoid levels may be the main reasons for the reduced expression and function of the steroidal synthetase system, instead of a direct effect of caffeine. A recent study found that caffeine exposure during preg-nancy could also reduce the expression of the foetal adrenal scavenger receptor BI (SR-BI) gene by increasing the DNA methylation level. SR-BI had a direct effect on the influx of blood cholesterol to the adrenal gland; thus, reduced SR-BI expression could reduce steroidogenesis function [99].

The activity of the HPA axis in adult offspring rats with prenatal caffeine exposure showed a high stress sensitivity and gender difference after a fortnight ice-water swimming test [26]. It is known that the hippocampus is the negative feedback regulating centre of the HPA axis, where cortical receptors (CRs), including mineralocorticoid receptor (MR) and GR, are expressed. Both MR and GR can bind to glucocorticoids. In addition to participating in the control of the HPA axis, MR can protect hippo-campal neurons, whereas excessive activation of GR can induce neuronal damage [100]. Therefore, a decrease in the expression ratio of MR and GR reflects the damage level of hippocampal neurons to some degree [101]. Caffeine exposure in pregnancy increases the hippocampal expression of GR and 11β-HSD1 [17], and the excessive activation of GR could injure the neurons. The expression ratio of MR and GR was shown to dramatically decrease when chronic stress was experienced after birth; therefore, chronic stress further aggravated the damage to the hippocampal neurons, thereby reducing the negative feedback adjustment ability of the hippocampus to the HPA axis. As a result, the HPA axis presented high stress sensitivity. The adrenal gland is the end-organ of the HPA axis, and our laboratory recently found [102] that in the case of prenatal caffeine ingestion, the reduction of adrenal steroid synthetic function is related to the inhibition of the IGF1 signalling pathway caused by the activation of the local 11β-HSDs/CR system. The function alteration of the adrenal gland could persist until after birth, characterised by mild accelerated growth with a normal diet and moderate to severe accelerated growth with a high-fat diet; both scenarios were associated with the inhibition of the IGF1 signalling pathway caused by activation of the local 11β-HSDs/CR system. A gender difference was also found.

Excessive Glucocorticoids and Programming of the IGF1 Signalling Pathway

IGF1 is a type of polypeptide hormone mainly synthesised by the liver, and it participates in the pro-liferation, differentiation, and metabolism of multiple cells and tissues [103–105]. After binding to its receptor (IGF1R), IGF1 phosphorylates MEK/ERK and activates mitogen-activated protein kinase (MAPK) to promote cell proliferation and resist cell apoptosis; on the other hand, it can phosphorylate PI3K/Akt and regulate cell glucolipid metabolism via transcriptional factors such as sterol-regulatory element-binding protein 1 (SREBP1). In the early development of the foetus, IGF1 is mainly synthe-sised by the liver, whereas multiple tissues establish autocrine and paracrine of IGF1 at post-conceptual ages [106–108]. Therefore, the synthesis of IGF1 by the liver during the intrauterine period directly plays a decisive role in birth weight, organic structure, and functional development of the foetus [103, 105, 107]. It has been shown that the blood IGF1 level is reduced in IUGR foetuses [109, 110], and the accelerated growth after birth is always accompanied by an increase in the IGF1 level [111, 112].

It is postulated that the alteration of the IGF1 pathway in the liver is the main reason for IUGR caused by an adverse environment during pregnancy and the principal factor in catch-up growth when there is sufficient nutrition after birth.

Research has shown that the glucocorticoid level regulates the expression of IGF1 in multiple tissues and cells [113], specifically the increased secretion of IGF1 under low glucocorticoid levels and inhibition of the secretion of IGF1 under high glucocorticoid levels [114, 115]. The hepatic IGF1 pathway in foetal rats exposed to prenatal caffeine ingestion is suppressed by high maternal glucocorticoid levels, which manifests as phenotypic variations such as hyperglycaemia and lipid lowering [32]. The low activity of the HPA axis in IUGR offspring resulting from caffeine ingestion during pregnancy can last until after birth; the hepatic IGF1 signalling pathway is enhanced under low levels of glucocorticoids, and rat offspring shows the phenotypic changes of hypoglycaemia and hyperlipidaemia [16, 26] and a more obvious catch-up growth on a high-fat diet [16, 116]. The risk for MS was shown to increase in offspring that underwent adverse intrauterine development and catch-up growth in early life [117].

IGF1 plays a vital role in skeletal development. IGF1 in circulation and bone tissues is important for the processes of proliferation, differentiation, and apoptosis of bone mesenchymal stem cells (BMSCs), chondrocytes, and osteoblasts [118–120]. High maternal glucocorticoid levels caused by caffeine ingestion during pregnancy were shown to significantly reduce the expression of the relevant genes in the IGF1 signalling pathway in foetal long epiphyseal cartilage, resulting in a reduction in cartilage extracellular matrix synthesis [84]. In addition, overexposure to glucocorticoids results in reduced cartilage differentiation, decreased cartilage cell proliferation, decreased matrix synthesis, and the attenuation of articular cartilage. The responsible mechanism could be the decreased expression of the IGF1 pathway in the epiphyseal cartilage of foetal rats caused by high maternal glucocorticoid levels [121].

Mechanism of Foetal-Originated Metabolic Disease Induced by Prenatal Caffeine Ingestion

To date, a complete and systematic theory for the intrauterine programming mechanisms of foetal-originated metabolic disease caused by an adverse intrauterine environment is lacking. In the last 5 years, our laboratory has utilised an IUGR rat model produced by caffeine ingestion in pregnancy to investigate the intrauterine mechanisms of foetal-originated metabolic diseases, such as foetal NAFLD, diabetes, glomerulosclerosis, and osteoarthritis. Based on the research results, we have proposed the common mechanisms for the increased susceptibility to metabolic diseases in IUGR offspring, which is a mechanism involving 'two programming' types and a 'two-hit' scenario mediated by the overexposure to maternal glucocorticoids (Fig. 25.2):

'The first programming' is permanent alteration of various specific organ functions (such as the reduction of adrenal steroid synthetic function and the enhancement of liver lipid de novo synthesis function), and it is relevant to 'the thrifty phenotype' and abnormal epigenetic modifications. This programming can last until afterbirth and even adulthood. 'The second programming' is the GC-IGF1 axis programming in various foetal tissues, which can induce a low IGF1 level in utero and high IGF1 level after birth, thereby causing IUGR and catch-up growth after birth in the case of nutritional sufficiency. It is the foundation of the structural and functional compensation of multiple organs in IUGR offspring after birth. These two types of programming interact with each other and finally result in the alteration of the general glucolipid metabolism and the increased disease susceptibility of multiple organs. The 'the second hit' refers to a postnatal unhealthy lifestyle (such as chronic stress and high-fat diet), which can accelerate or aggravate the occurrence of metabolic diseases in the offspring.

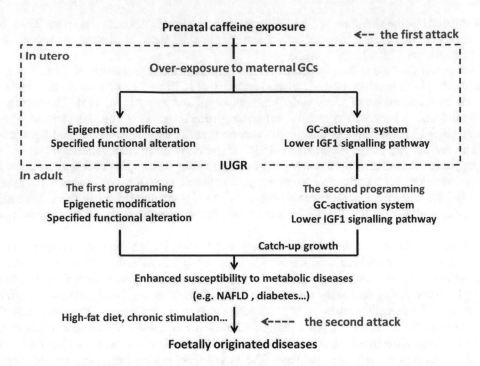

Fig. 25.2 Mechanisms of increased susceptibility to metabolic diseases induced by prenatal caffeine exposure

Conclusion

With the increased consumption of caffeinated foods and beverages, safety issues related to caffeine have attracted much attention. Although some studies have revealed that prenatal caffeine exposure could induce reproductive and developmental toxicities, the mechanism of the toxicities induced by caffeine remains unclear. As discussed in this review, overexposure of the foetus to maternal gluco-corticoids resulting from prenatal caffeine ingestion can induce alterations in intrauterine neuroendo-crine metabolic programming and abnormal functional development of various organs. This aberrant developmental trajectory has a long-term effect on glucose and lipid metabolism, which may contrib-ute to the increased susceptibility to various metabolic diseases. Along with the advancement of mod-ern medical science, researchers will improve the understanding of caffeine-induced effects on women and children. Exploring the underlying mechanism of developmental toxicity induced by caffeine intake will help to prevent potential adverse effects. Meanwhile, future studies may deepen our knowl-edge of the developmental origins of adult metabolic diseases and provide the theoretical foundation for the early prevention and treatment of metabolic diseases.

References

1. Silveira VM, Horta BL. Birth weight and metabolic syndrome in adults: meta-analysis. Rev Saude Publica. 2008;42(1):10–8.
2. Skarsgard ED, Amii LA, Dimmitt RA, Sakamoto G, Brindle ME, Moss RL. Fetal therapy with rhIGF-1 in a rabbit model of intrauterine growth retardation. J Surg Res. 2001;99(1):142–6.
3. Szostak-Wegierek D, Szamotulska K. Fetal development and risk of cardiovascular diseases and diabetes type 2 in adult life. Med Wieku Rozwoj. 2011;15(3):203–15.

4. Sohi G, Revesz A, Hardy DB. Permanent implications of intrauterine growth restriction on cholesterol homeostasis. Semin Reprod Med. 2011;29(3):246–56.
5. Desai M, Gayle D, Babu J, Ross MG. The timing of nutrient restriction during rat pregnancy/lactation alters metabolic syndrome phenotype. Am J Obstet Gynecol. 2007;196(6):555.e1–7.
6. Brent RL, Christian MS, Diener RM. Evaluation of the reproductive and developmental risks of caffeine. Birth Defects Res B Dev Reprod Toxicol. 2011;92(2):152–87.
7. Heckman MA, Weil J, Gonzalez de Mejia E. Caffeine (1, 3, 7-trimethylxanthine) in foods: a comprehensive review on consumption, functionality, safety, and regulatory matters. J Food Sci. 2010;75(3):R77–87.
8. Aranda JV, Beharry K, Valencia GB, Natarajan G, Davis J. Caffeine impact on neonatal morbidities. J Matern-Fetal Neonatal Med. 2010;23(Suppl 3):20–3.
9. Picone S, Bedetta M, Paolillo P. Caffeine citrate: when and for how long. A literature review. J Matern-Fetal Neonatal Med. 2012;25(Suppl 3):11–4.
10. Frary CD, Johnson RK, Wang MQ. Food sources and intakes of caffeine in the diets of persons in the United States. J Am Diet Assoc. 2005;105(1):110–3.
11. Kuczkowski KM. Caffeine in pregnancy: a cause for concern? Ann Fr Anesth Reanim. 2009;28(6):605–7.
12. Fortier I, Marcoux S, Beaulac-Baillargeon L. Relation of caffeine intake during pregnancy to intrauterine growth retardation and preterm birth. Am J Epidemiol. 1993;137(9):931–40.
13. Weng X, Odouli R, Li DK. Maternal caffeine consumption during pregnancy and the risk of miscarriage: a prospective cohort study. Am J Obstet Gynecol. 2008;198(3):279.e1–8.
14. Bakker R, Steegers EA, Obradov A, Raat H, Hofman A, Jaddoe VW. Maternal caffeine intake from coffee and tea, fetal growth, and the risks of adverse birth outcomes: the Generation R Study. Am J Clin Nutr. 2010;91(6):1691–8.
15. Momoi N, Tinney JP, Liu LJ, et al. Modest maternal caffeine exposure affects developing embryonic cardiovascular function and growth. Am J Physiol Heart Circ Physiol. 2008;294(5):H2248–56.
16. Wang L, Shen L, Ping J, et al. Intrauterine metabolic programming alteration increased susceptibility to nonalcoholic adult fatty liver disease in prenatal caffeine-exposed rat offspring. Toxicol Lett. 2014;224(3):311–8.
17. Xu D, Zhang B, Liang G, et al. Caffeine-induced activated glucocorticoid metabolism in the hippocampus causes hypothalamic-pituitary-adrenal axis inhibition in fetal rats. PLoS One. 2012;7(9):e44497.
18. Setzer RW, Lau C, Mole ML, Copeland MF, Rogers JM, Kavlock RJ. Toward a biologically based dose-response model for developmental toxicity of 5-fluorouracil in the rat: a mathematical construct. Toxicol Sci. 2001;59(1):49–58.
19. Giannelli M, Doyle P, Roman E, Pelerin M, Hermon C. The effect of caffeine consumption and nausea on the risk of miscarriage. Paediatr Perinat Epidemiol. 2003;17(4):316–23.
20. George L, Granath F, Johansson AL, Olander B, Cnattingius S. Risks of repeated miscarriage. Paediatr Perinat Epidemiol. 2006;20(2):119–26.
21. Greenwood DC, Alwan N, Boylan S, et al. Caffeine intake during pregnancy, late miscarriage and stillbirth. Eur J Epidemiol. 2010;25(4):275–80.
22. Cnattingius S, Signorello LB, Anneren G, et al. Caffeine intake and the risk of first-trimester spontaneous abortion. N Engl J Med. 2000;343(25):1839–45.
23. Schmidt RJ, Romitti PA, Burns TL, et al. Maternal caffeine consumption and risk of neural tube defects. Birth Defects Res A Clin Mol Teratol. 2009;85(11):879–89.
24. Collier SA, Browne ML, Rasmussen SA, Honein MA, National Birth Defects Prevention S. Maternal caffeine intake during pregnancy and orofacial clefts. Birth Defects Res A Clin Mol Teratol. 2009;85(10):842–9.
25. Huang J, Zhou S, Ping J, et al. Role of p53-dependent placental apoptosis in the reproductive and developmental toxicities of caffeine in rodents. Clin Exp Pharmacol Physiol. 2012;39(4):357–63.
26. Xu D, Wu Y, Liu F, et al. A hypothalamic-pituitary-adrenal axis-associated neuroendocrine metabolic programmed alteration in offspring rats of IUGR induced by prenatal caffeine ingestion. Toxicol Appl Pharmacol. 2012;264(3):395–403.
27. Collins T, Welsh J, Black T, Ruggles D. Teratogenic potential of caffeine in rats. Paper presented at: alternative dietary practices and nutritional abuses in pregnancy. Proceedings of a workshop. Washington, DC: National Academy Press; 1982.
28. Ikeda GJ, Sapienza PP, McGinnis ML, Bragg LE, Walsh JJ, Collins TF. Blood levels of caffeine and results of fetal examination after oral administration of caffeine to pregnant rats. J Appl Toxicol: JAT. 1982;2(6):307–14.
29. Smith SE, McElhatton PR, Sullivan FM. Effects of administering caffeine to pregnant rats either as a single daily dose or as divided doses four times a day. Food Chem Toxicol. 1987;25(2):125–33.
30. Nehlig A, Debry G. Consequences on the newborn of chronic maternal consumption of coffee during gestation and lactation: a review. J Am Coll Nutr. 1994;13(1):6–21.
31. Gilbert SG, Rice DC. Somatic development of the infant monkey following in utero exposure to caffeine. Fundam Appl Toxicol. 1991;17(3):454–65.

32. Liu Y, Xu D, Feng J, et al. Fetal rat metabonome alteration by prenatal caffeine ingestion probably due to the increased circulatory glucocorticoid level and altered peripheral glucose and lipid metabolic pathways. Toxicol Appl Pharmacol. 2012;262(2):205–16.

33. Nobili V, Marcellini M, Marchesini G, et al. Intrauterine growth retardation, insulin resistance, and nonalcoholic fatty liver disease in children. Diabetes Care. 2007;30(10):2638–40.

34. Zandi-Nejad K, Luyckx VA, Brenner BM. Adult hypertension and kidney disease: the role of fetal programming. Hypertension. 2006;47(3):502–8.

35. Barker DJ. In utero programming of chronic disease. Clin Sci. 1998;95(2):115–28.

36. Gamborg M, Byberg L, Rasmussen F, et al. Birth weight and systolic blood pressure in adolescence and adulthood: meta-regression analysis of sex- and age-specific results from 20 Nordic studies. Am J Epidemiol. 2007;166(6):634–45.

37. Primatesta P, Falaschetti E, Poulter NR. Birth weight and blood pressure in childhood: results from the Health Survey for England. Hypertension. 2005;45(1):75–9.

38. Leon DA, Koupil I, Mann V, et al. Fetal, developmental, and parental influences on childhood systolic blood pressure in 600 sib pairs: the Uppsala Family study. Circulation. 2005;112(22):3478–85.

39. Hemachandra AH, Klebanoff MA, Furth SL. Racial disparities in the association between birth weight in the term infant and blood pressure at age 7 years: results from the collaborative perinatal project. J Am Soc Nephrol. 2006;17(9):2576–81.

40. Cruickshank JK, Mzayek F, Liu L, et al. Origins of the "black/white" difference in blood pressure: roles of birth weight, postnatal growth, early blood pressure, and adolescent body size: the Bogalusa heart study. Circulation. 2005;111(15):1932–7.

41. Iliadou A, Cnattingius S, Lichtenstein P. Low birthweight and type 2 diabetes: a study on 11 162 Swedish twins. Int J Epidemiol. 2004;33(5):948–53; discussion 953–4.

42. Hales CN, Barker DJ, Clark PM, et al. Fetal and infant growth and impaired glucose tolerance at age 64. BMJ. 1991;303(6809):1019–22.

43. Veenendaal MV, Painter RC, de Rooij SR, et al. Transgenerational effects of prenatal exposure to the 1944–45 Dutch famine. BJOG. 2013;120(5):548–53.

44. Painter RC, Osmond C, Gluckman P, Hanson M, Phillips DI, Roseboom TJ. Transgenerational effects of prenatal exposure to the Dutch famine on neonatal adiposity and health in later life. BJOG. 2008;115(10):1243–9.

45. Dennison EM, Syddall HE, Sayer AA, Gilbody HJ, Cooper C. Birth weight and weight at 1 year are independent determinants of bone mass in the seventh decade: the Hertfordshire cohort study. Pediatr Res. 2005;57(4):582–6.

46. Cooper C, Harvey N, Javaid K, Hanson M, Dennison E. Growth and bone development. Nestle Nutr Work Ser Paediatr Program. 2008;61:53–68.

47. Antoniades L, MacGregor AJ, Andrew T, Spector TD. Association of birth weight with osteoporosis and osteoarthritis in adult twins. Rheumatology. 2003;42(6):791–6.

48. Barker DJ, Gluckman PD, Godfrey KM, Harding JE, Owens JA, Robinson JS. Fetal nutrition and cardiovascular disease in adult life. Lancet. 1993;341(8850):938–41.

49. Barker DJ. The fetal and infant origins of adult disease. BMJ. 1990;301(6761):1111.

50. Mathieu P, Pibarot P, Despres JP. Metabolic syndrome: the danger signal in atherosclerosis. Vasc Health Risk Manag. 2006;2(3):285–302.

51. Pecks U, Brieger M, Schiessl B, et al. Maternal and fetal cord blood lipids in intrauterine growth restriction. J Perinat Med. 2012;40(3):287–96.

52. Sohi G, Marchand K, Revesz A, Arany E, Hardy DB. Maternal protein restriction elevates cholesterol in adult rat offspring due to repressive changes in histone modifications at the cholesterol 7alpha-hydroxylase promoter. Mol Endocrinol. 2011;25(5):785–98.

53. Rueda-Clausen CF, Dolinsky VW, Morton JS, Proctor SD, Dyck JR, Davidge ST. Hypoxia-induced intrauterine growth restriction increases the susceptibility of rats to high-fat diet-induced metabolic syndrome. Diabetes. 2011;60(2):507–16.

54. Drake AJ, Raubenheimer PJ, Kerrigan D, McInnes KJ, Seckl JR, Walker BR. Prenatal dexamethasone programs expression of genes in liver and adipose tissue and increased hepatic lipid accumulation but not obesity on a high-fat diet. Endocrinology. 2010;151(4):1581–7.

55. Hino A, Adachi H, Enomoto M, et al. Habitual coffee but not green tea consumption is inversely associated with metabolic syndrome: an epidemiological study in a general Japanese population. Diabetes Res Clin Pract. 2007;76(3):383–9.

56. Dhingra R, Sullivan L, Jacques PF, et al. Soft drink consumption and risk of developing cardiometabolic risk factors and the metabolic syndrome in middle-aged adults in the community. Circulation. 2007;116(5):480–8.

57. Ji Z, Chen B, Ni Q, Kou H, Guo Y, Wang H. Influence of long-term caffeine exposure on neuroendocrine metabolic function of infant rats. J Wuhan Univ. 2014;35(1):93–7.

58. Liu L, Liu F, Kou H, et al. Prenatal nicotine exposure induced a hypothalamic-pituitary-adrenal axis-associated neuroendocrine metabolic programmed alteration in intrauterine growth retardation offspring rats. Toxicol Lett. 2012;214(3):307–13.

59. Zhou J, Kou H, Guo Y, Zhang L, Wang H. Prenatal caffeine exposure induces abnormal glucose metabolism and insulin resistance in adult male offspring rats with high-fat diet and chronic stress. Chin J Pharmacol Toxicol. 2015;1(29):8.
60. Luo H, Li J, Cao H, et al. Prenatal caffeine exposure induces a poor quality of articular cartilage in male adult offspring rats via cholesterol accumulation in cartilage. Sci Rep. 2015;5:17746.
61. Ao Y, Sun Z, Hu S, et al. Low functional programming of renal AT2R mediates the developmental origin of glomerulosclerosis in adult offspring induced by prenatal caffeine exposure. Toxicol Appl Pharmacol. 2015;287(2): 128–38.
62. Miners JO, Birkett DJ. The use of caffeine as a metabolic probe for human drug metabolizing enzymes. Gen Pharmacol. 1996;27(2):245–9.
63. Newton R, Broughton LJ, Lind MJ, Morrison PJ, Rogers HJ, Bradbrook ID. Plasma and salivary pharmacokinetics of caffeine in man. Eur J Clin Pharmacol. 1981;21(1):45–52.
64. Tsutsumi K, Kotegawa T, Matsuki S, et al. The effect of pregnancy on cytochrome P4501A2, xanthine oxidase, and N-acetyltransferase activities in humans. Clin Pharmacol Ther. 2001;70(2):121–5.
65. Fowden AL, Li J, Forhead AJ. Glucocorticoids and the preparation for life after birth: are there long-term consequences of the life insurance? Proc Nutr Soc. 1998;57(1):113–22.
66. Bose HS, Lingappa VR, Miller WL. Rapid regulation of steroidogenesis by mitochondrial protein import. Nature. 2002;417(6884):87–91.
67. Manna PR, Stocco DM. Regulation of the steroidogenic acute regulatory protein expression: functional and physiological consequences. Curr Drug Targets Immune Endocr Metab Disord. 2005;5(1):93–108.
68. Manna PR, Dyson MT, Stocco DM. Regulation of the steroidogenic acute regulatory protein gene expression: present and future perspectives. Mol Hum Reprod. 2009;15(6):321–33.
69. Andrews MH, Matthews SG. Regulation of glucocorticoid receptor mRNA and heat shock protein 70 mRNA in the developing sheep brain. Brain Res. 2000;878(1–2):174–82.
70. Kou H, Liu Y, Liang G, et al. Maternal glucocorticoid elevation and associated blood metabonome changes might be involved in metabolic programming of intrauterine growth retardation in rats exposed to caffeine prenatally. Toxicol Appl Pharmacol. 2014;275(2):79–87.
71. Ping J, Lei YY, Liu L, Wang TT, Feng YH, Wang H. Inheritable stimulatory effects of caffeine on steroidogenic acute regulatory protein expression and cortisol production in human adrenocortical cells. Chem Biol Interact. 2012;195(1):68–75.
72. Salafia CM, Charles AK, Maas EM. Placenta and fetal growth restriction. Clin Obstet Gynecol. 2006;49(2):236–56.
73. Cox P, Marton T. Pathological assessment of intrauterine growth restriction. Best Pract Res Clin Obstet Gynaecol. 2009;23(6):751–64.
74. Cobellis L, De Falco M, Torella M, et al. Modulation of Bax expression in physiological and pathological human placentas throughout pregnancy. In Vivo. 2007;21(5):777–83.
75. Qiao S, Nagasaka T, Harada T, Nakashima N. p53, Bax and Bcl-2 expression, and apoptosis in gestational trophoblast of complete hydatidiform mole. Placenta. 1998;19(5–6):361–9.
76. Nomura K, Saito S, Ide K, et al. Caffeine suppresses the expression of the Bcl-2 mRNA in BeWo cell culture and rat placenta. J Nutr Biochem. 2004;15(6):342–9.
77. Wu YM, Luo HW, Kou H, et al. Prenatal caffeine exposure induced a lower level of fetal blood leptin mainly via placental mechanism. Toxicol Appl Pharmacol. 2015;289(1):109–16.
78. Zhou S, Huang J, Bao C, Ping J, Wang H. Review of research on mechanism of IUGR induced by prenatal caffeine exposure. Chin J Pharmacol Toxicol. 2010;24(4):4.
79. Chapman K, Holmes M, Seckl J. 11beta-hydroxysteroid dehydrogenases: intracellular gate-keepers of tissue glucocorticoid action. Physiol Rev. 2013;93(3):1139–206.
80. Fowden AL, Giussani DA, Forhead AJ. Endocrine and metabolic programming during intrauterine development. Early Hum Dev. 2005;81(9):723–34.
81. Xita N, Tsatsoulis A. Fetal origins of the metabolic syndrome. Ann N Y Acad Sci. 2010;1205:148–55.
82. Kanaka-Gantenbein C. Fetal origins of adult diabetes. Ann N Y Acad Sci. 2010;1205:99–105.
83. Ping J, Wang JF, Liu L, et al. Prenatal caffeine ingestion induces aberrant DNA methylation and histone acetylation of steroidogenic factor 1 and inhibits fetal adrenal steroidogenesis. Toxicology. 2014;321:53–61.
84. Tan Y, Liu J, Deng Y, et al. Caffeine-induced fetal rat over-exposure to maternal glucocorticoid and histone methylation of liver IGF-1 might cause skeletal growth retardation. Toxicol Lett. 2012;214(3):279–87.
85. Hodyl NA, Stark MJ, Butler M, Clifton VL. Placental P-glycoprotein is unaffected by timing of antenatal glucocorticoid therapy but reduced in SGA preterm infants. Placenta. 2013;34(4):325–30.
86. Stewart PM, Whorwood CB. 11 beta-Hydroxysteroid dehydrogenase activity and corticosteroid hormone action. Steroids. 1994;59(2):90–5.
87. Wadhwa PD, Culhane JF, Rauh V, Barve SS. Stress and preterm birth: neuroendocrine, immune/inflammatory, and vascular mechanisms. Matern Child Health J. 2001;5(2):119–25.

88. McTernan CL, Draper N, Nicholson H, et al. Reduced placental 11beta-hydroxysteroid dehydrogenase type 2 mRNA levels in human pregnancies complicated by intrauterine growth restriction: an analysis of possible mechanisms. J Clin Endocrinol Metab. 2001;86(10):4979–83.

89. Lesage J, Blondeau B, Grino M, Breant B, Dupouy JP. Maternal undernutrition during late gestation induces fetal overexposure to glucocorticoids and intrauterine growth retardation, and disturbs the hypothalamo-pituitary adrenal axis in the newborn rat. Endocrinology. 2001;142(5):1692–702.

90. Sharmin S, Guan H, Williams AS, Yang K. Caffeine reduces 11beta-hydroxysteroid dehydrogenase type 2 expression in human trophoblast cells through the adenosine A(2B) receptor. PLoS One. 2012;7(6):e38082.

91. Xiong F, Zhang L. Role of the hypothalamic-pituitary-adrenal axis in developmental programming of health and disease. Front Neuroendocrinol. 2013;34(1):27–46.

92. Matthews SG, Owen D, Kalabis G, et al. Fetal glucocorticoid exposure and hypothalamo-pituitary-adrenal (HPA) function after birth. Endocr Res. 2004;30(4):827–36.

93. Reynolds RM. Corticosteroid-mediated programming and the pathogenesis of obesity and diabetes. J Steroid Biochem Mol Biol. 2010;122(1–3):3–9.

94. Lavoie HA, King SR. Transcriptional regulation of steroidogenic genes: STARD1, CYP11A1 and HSD3B. Exp Biol Med. 2009;234(8):880–907.

95. Morohashi K, Honda S, Inomata Y, Handa H, Omura T. A common trans-acting factor, Ad4-binding protein, to the promoters of steroidogenic P-450s. J Biol Chem. 1992;267(25):17913–9.

96. Parker KL, Rice DA, Lala DS, et al. Steroidogenic factor 1: an essential mediator of endocrine development. Recent Prog Horm Res. 2002;57:19–36.

97. Xue Q, Lin Z, Yin P, et al. Transcriptional activation of steroidogenic factor-1 by hypomethylation of the 5′ CpG island in endometriosis. J Clin Endocrinol Metab. 2007;92(8):3261–7.

98. Jacob AL, Lund J, Martinez P, Hedin L. Acetylation of steroidogenic factor 1 protein regulates its transcriptional activity and recruits the coactivator GCN5. J Biol Chem. 2001;276(40):37659–64.

99. Wu DM, He Z, Ma LP, Wang LL, Ping J, Wang H. Increased DNA methylation of scavenger receptor class B type I contributes to inhibitory effects of prenatal caffeine ingestion on cholesterol uptake and steroidogenesis in fetal adrenals. Toxicol Appl Pharmacol. 2015;285(2):89–97.

100. de Quervain DJ, Aerni A, Schelling G, Roozendaal B. Glucocorticoids and the regulation of memory in health and disease. Front Neuroendocrinol. 2009;30(3):358–70.

101. Zhe D, Fang H, Yuxiu S. Expressions of hippocampal mineralocorticoid receptor (MR) and glucocorticoid receptor (GR) in the single-prolonged stress-rats. Acta Histochem Cytochem. 2008;41(4):89–95.

102. He Z, Zhu C, Huang H, et al. Prenatal caffeine exposure-induced adrenal developmental abnormality in male offspring rats and its possible intrauterine programming mechanisms. Toxicol Res. 2016;5(2):388–98.

103. Netchine I, Azzi S, Houang M, et al. Partial primary deficiency of insulin-like growth factor (IGF)-I activity associated with IGF1 mutation demonstrates its critical role in growth and brain development. J Clin Endocrinol Metab. 2009;94(10):3913–21.

104. Randhawa R, Cohen P. The role of the insulin-like growth factor system in prenatal growth. Mol Genet Metab. 2005;86(1–2):84–90.

105. Roberts CT, Owens JA, Sferruzzi-Perri AN. Distinct actions of insulin-like growth factors (IGFs) on placental development and fetal growth: lessons from mice and guinea pigs. Placenta. 2008;29(Suppl A):S42–7.

106. Laviola L, Natalicchio A, Perrini S, Giorgino F. Abnormalities of IGF-I signaling in the pathogenesis of diseases of the bone, brain, and fetoplacental unit in humans. Am J Physiol Endocrinol Metab. 2008;295(5):E991–9.

107. Agrogiannis GD, Sifakis S, Patsouris ES, Konstantinidou AE. Insulin-like growth factors in embryonic and fetal growth and skeletal development (review). Mol Med Rep. 2014;10(2):579–84.

108. Netchine I, Azzi S, Le Bouc Y, Savage MO. IGF1 molecular anomalies demonstrate its critical role in fetal, postnatal growth and brain development. Best Pract Res Clin Endocrinol Metab. 2011;25(1):181–90.

109. Kenyon C. A conserved regulatory system for aging. Cell. 2001;105(2):165–8.

110. Gicquel C, Le Bouc Y. Hormonal regulation of fetal growth. Horm Res. 2006;65(Suppl 3):28–33.

111. Kamei H, Ding Y, Kajimura S, Wells M, Chiang P, Duan C. Role of IGF signaling in catch-up growth and accelerated temporal development in zebrafish embryos in response to oxygen availability. Development. 2011;138(4):777–86.

112. Fall CH, Pandit AN, Law CM, et al. Size at birth and plasma insulin-like growth factor-1 concentrations. Arch Dis Child. 1995;73(4):287–93.

113. Binoux M, Lassarre C, Hardouin N. Somatomedin production by rat liver in organ culture. III. Studies on the release of insulin-like growth factor and its carrier protein measured by radioligand assays. Effects of growth hormone, insulin and cortisol. Acta Endocrinol. 1982;99(3):422–30.

114. Inder WJ, Jang C, Obeyesekere VR, Alford FP. Dexamethasone administration inhibits skeletal muscle expression of the androgen receptor and IGF-1 – implications for steroid-induced myopathy. Clin Endocrinol. 2010;73(1):126–32.

115. Robson H, Siebler T, Shalet SM, Williams GR. Interactions between GH, IGF-I, glucocorticoids, and thyroid hormones during skeletal growth. Pediatr Res. 2002;52(2):137–47.
116. Li J, Luo H, Wu Y, et al. Gender-specific increase in susceptibility to metabolic syndrome of offspring rats after prenatal caffeine exposure with post-weaning high-fat diet. Toxicol Appl Pharmacol. 2015;284(3):345–53.
117. Jaquet D, Gaboriau A, Czernichow P, Levy-Marchal C. Insulin resistance early in adulthood in subjects born with intrauterine growth retardation. J Clin Endocrinol Metab. 2000;85(4):1401–6.
118. Woods KA, Camacho-Hubner C, Savage MO, Clark AJ. Intrauterine growth retardation and postnatal growth failure associated with deletion of the insulin-like growth factor I gene. N Engl J Med. 1996;335(18):1363–7.
119. Perrini S, Natalicchio A, Laviola L, et al. Abnormalities of insulin-like growth factor-I signaling and impaired cell proliferation in osteoblasts from subjects with osteoporosis. Endocrinology. 2008;149(3):1302–13.
120. Xian L, Wu X, Pang L, et al. Matrix IGF-1 maintains bone mass by activation of mTOR in mesenchymal stem cells. Nat Med. 2012;18(7):1095–101.
121. Fernandez-Cancio M, Esteban C, Carrascosa A, Toran N, Andaluz P, Audi L. IGF-I and not IGF-II expression is regulated by glucocorticoids in human fetal epiphyseal chondrocytes. Growth Horm IGF Res. 2008;18(6):497–505.

Part V
International Aspects and Policies

Chapter 26
Famines, Pregnancy and Effect on the Adults

Matthew Edwards

Key Points

- Maternal starvation during pregnancy causes lifelong effects on offspring.
- Metabolic syndrome is one such effect initially attributed to selection of a thrifty genotype, although this hypothesis has since been discredited.
- The cause of subsequent adult problems is attributed to foetal programming (the Barker hypothesis).
- Foetal programming is thought to involve changes in imprinting or other epigenetic patterns but might also involve non-coding RNA.
- These patterns might persist through to adult life and even to subsequent generations.
- Theories about transgenerational transmission of information resulting from environmental exposures have reawakened Lamarckian explanations for transmission of epigenotypes.
- It might be too early to completely put the thrifty genotype hypothesis to rest, until databases for whole genome sequencing are available for cases exposed to maternal starvation as foetuses and controls.
- A theory is presented for new germ line and/or somatic mosaicism as an effect of high rates of cell division in the early embryo and selection, in adverse intrauterine environments, of cell lines or tissues with favourable mutations or inherited polymorphisms.
- This Darwinian process of variation and selection could be analogous to the prolific accumulation of mutations and cell clones in embryonic lymphocyte precursors.

Keywords Foetus • Maternal malnutrition • Metabolic syndrome • Foetal programming • Somatic mosaicism • Whole genome sequencing • Thrifty genotype hypothesis • Phenotype

Abbreviations

CpG   Cytosine-guanosine dinucleotide sequence
DNA   Deoxyribonucleic acid
H19   Gene for a long non-coding RNA molecule in the Prader-Willi/Angelman syndrome differentially imprinted region

M. Edwards, MD, FRACP, FCCMG, FACMG (✉)
Department of Paediatrics, School of Medicine, Western Sydney University,
Penrith, NSW, Australia
e-mail: matthew.edwards@westernsydney.edu.au; matt.edwards@mac.com

© Springer International Publishing AG 2017
R. Rajendram et al. (eds.), *Diet, Nutrition, and Fetal Programming*,
Nutrition and Health, DOI 10.1007/978-3-319-60289-9_26

HDL	Plasma high-density lipoprotein
IAP	Intracisternal A particle, a retrotransposon in the agouti gene of a strain of mice
IGF1	Insulin-like growth factor 1
IUGR	Intrauterine (foetal) growth retardation
IVF	In vitro fertilisation
kJ	Kilojoules
MECP2	Gene for methyl-CpG-binding protein 2
miRNA	Micro-inhibitory RNA
mRNAs	Messenger RNA molecules
P12A	Substitution of arginine for proline at amino acid residue 12 (P12A) in the PPARγ protein, a genetic polymorphism
PPARs	Peroxisome proliferator-activated receptors
RNA	Ribonucleic acid
siRNA	Small interfering RNA, or short interfering RNA, or silencing RNA
UBE3A	Ubiquitin protein ligase E3A gene

Introduction

The metabolic syndrome has been identified in adults who were exposed in utero to maternal starvation or intrauterine growth retardation [1], followed by more plentiful nutrition and/or a period of rapid growth. Although its manifestations are not appreciated until adulthood, it has been attributed to the lifelong effects of foetal programming [2]. Foetal programming is currently considered to be an adaptation by which foetuses tailor their growth and development to the current nutritional conditions. That adaptation might in many situations even be passed on to subsequent generations and might not be appropriate to different subsequent prevailing environmental conditions. The mechanism of foetal programming might be multifactorial and complex. It could involve genetic imprinting, which includes deacetylation and methylation of histones; methylation of CpG sequences in DNA; altered relationships between genomic DNA, nucleosomes and the nuclear matrix; or other molecular mechanisms including non-coding RNA. Imprinting of gene tns off their expression was first described in genes largely associated with foetal growth in placental mammals. One of a pair of alleles for a gene promoting or inhibiting foetal growth was turned off or imprinted depending on the sex of the parent from which it was inherited [3].

Famines causing widespread starvation of women during pregnancy have been "natural" experiments that enabled the comparison of diseases in exposed humans with siblings or other controls born after unexposed pregnancies. Variation in individual degree of starvation, postnatal extent of starvation or confounding factors such as family history, socio-economic status, maternal health, age or parity, other exposures such as epidemics and the long time between exposure and adult assessment could be avoided or ameliorated by the study of large populations, of those with records of universal starvation and poverty and where individual health records of birth weight, gestational age, fertility, infant mortality and adult morbidity and mortality were available. Theories attempting to explain foetal programming included the thrifty genotype hypothesis which argued that deprived environments selected genes for thriftiness which were poorly suited to subsequent times of plenty [4]. If this was the case, evolutionary bottlenecks due to famine plus or minus migration should have selected genes for thriftiness in the entire population so that everyone should now have inherited these [5]. Conditions like metabolic syndrome have appeared very rapidly in some populations and reduced in frequency a generation or so later, a process that is too fast to be explained solely by classic theories of germ line evolutionary selection [6, 7]. These have added support to the foetal origins or Barker hypothesis that foetal programming did not necessarily alter genomic DNA but probably involved epigenetic mechanisms: a "thrifty phenotype". A subsequent "drifty" phenotype theory argues that there is a real increase in the frequency of genes for obesity due to genetic drift, allowed by relaxation of selection against an obese phenotype [5]. A period of rapid growth might be more important in relation to metabolic programming, so no measured IUGR need be present [8]. Metabolic syndrome was not observed after a Russian famine where maternal malnutrition had been long-standing, and there was no postnatal improvement in nutrition and catch-up growth spurt [9].

There is evidence that metabolic syndrome is influenced by certain gene sequences [10]. Foetal insulin phenotype determined by glucokinase mutations has been shown to affect both birth weight and the later development of type 2 diabetes [11]. The question as to whether the process is entirely explained by epigenetic processes or is additionally associated with changes in somatic or constitutional genomic sequence might be answered with current advances in genomic sequencing and bioinformatics technology. These will enable the detection or exclusion of genomic changes, including those in intergenic non-coding RNA sequences, in different tissues of populations with and without metabolic syndrome or other adult diseases attributed to foetal programming.

Epidemiological Studies

These have been reviewed recently [12]:

- Norwegian research in the 1970s [13] identified an association between poverty during adolescence and later onset of coronary heart disease and a correlation between infant mortality, a surrogate of poverty and later male adult mortality from any disease, from cerebrovascular disease and from arteriosclerotic heart disease. There was a less marked but still significant correlation between total infant mortality in 1896–1925 and arteriosclerotic heart disease in 1964–1967 in adult females. At later dates when the standard of living throughout Norway had improved to "upper middle class" levels, the correlation had disappeared. There was a strong correlation between infant mortality and later adult development of lung cancer. These correlations were interpreted to relate to nutrition during adolescence, although authors considered the possibility of cigarette smoking as a confounding factor. As conditions are likely to have been similar when the subjects were adolescents and when they were in utero, it is also possible that maternal malnutrition could have contributed to this association.
- An association between low birth weight and development of coronary heart disease and type 2 diabetes in adults was identified in the United Kingdom in the 1980–1990s, leading to the thrifty phenotype hypothesis [2].
- A remote valley of Overkalix in northern Sweden was isolated by winter snow and steep mountains in the nineteenth to early twentieth century. People exposed to famine as preadolescent boys [14], for whom contemporary parish and municipal registers recorded dates of birth and harvest results, were found to have grandchildren who were more likely to die of heart disease or diabetes.
- The Dutch famine or Hunger Winter of 1944–1945, when occupied cities were blockaded for several months to prevent food deliveries or migration, was preceded and followed by normal nutrition. Food rations were limited to an average of 1600–3200 kJ per day from December 1944 to April 1945. Physical and mental health of adults have been analysed in a number of studies indicating worse outcomes for congenital abnormalities [15], obesity [16], metabolic syndrome [8], schizophrenia and unemployment in people whose birth dates and locations indicated exposure to maternal starvation at different stages of development in utero during the famine. Although genal intelligence was not affected in army conscripts [17], specific impairments of adult cognitive ability were noted in the sixth decade [18], most markedly in those exposed to maternal malnutrition early in the pregnancy. Malnutrition at any stage of pregnancy was associated with glucose intolerance

and reduced head circumference [8, 18]. Starvation restricted to the last trimester was associated with reduced foetal and postnatal growth but not with adult metabolic syndrome. Starvation in mid-pregnancy was associated with microalbuminuria in adults, and exposure in the first trimester was followed by metabolic syndrome in adults [8].

- The "Great Leap Forward," which involved a famine, starvation, limited ability to migrate away from the starved region within China and detailed follow-up records of the population kept by the regime [19].
- The Avon Longitudinal Study of Pregnancy and Childhood in the United Kingdom. This showed that men who had been malnourished in mid-childhood and exposed to deprivation, measured by early age of commencement of cigarette smoking, had larger sons but did not have larger daughters. The grandsons of men exposed to starvation in preadolescence had higher mortality but not their granddaughters. After paternal grandmothers were exposed to malnutrition, their granddaughters had increased mortality but not their grandsons. This was attributed to epigenetic changes, possibly involving miRNA [12].
- A large proportion of the adult Pima people in Arizona and the population of Nauru have had a very high prevalence of metabolic syndrome after introduction of a western diet [20, 21]. In subsequent generations exposed to higher-energy diet, the incidence of metabolic syndrome has dropped in Nauru, although it still remains high [22]. The drop in incidence was attributed initially to the loss of genes from the population that predisposed to diabetes [20] but could have been influenced by improvement of nutrition during pregnancy [6] or to changes in the proportion of people of different ages in the population.
- A large analysis of population studies in Central America, sub-Saharan Africa and South and Southeast Asia showed a range of poorer outcomes of mental, educational and physical health in adults after they were subjected to maternal malnutrition during pregnancy [23]. Metabolic syndrome was not as prevalent in these populations, which was an interesting difference to what was found in more wealthy countries.

Molecular Studies

Disturbances of imprinting have been implicated in foetal programming, and in a number of common diseases including metabolic syndrome and cancer. Imprinting in most genomic sites is reversible, being reset in the zygote according to the sex of the parent, but this can depend on an intact imprinting centre near the imprinted region of a chromosome. If an imprinting centre is deleted or inactivated, the imprint will not be reset when passed to offspring, as occurs in familial Angelman syndrome [24], and the disease can be passed on by unaffected parents to subsequent generations. Imprinting is limited to some chromosomal segments, its extent within a tissue can vary normally with age, and its distribution within different tissues of the body can be limited. Imprinting is possibly responsible for the long-term activation and deactivation of interacting sets of genes during development and aging. Loss of imprinting with age has been implicated in the aetiology of many neoplasms, in which genes promoting growth are released from methylation [25]. Mosaic imprinting where only a proportion of body cells have an imprinting abnormality has been identified in Beckwith-Wiedemann syndrome [26]. For some genes, it is normal for imprinting to occur in some tissues but not in others: the *UBE3A* gene involved in Angelman syndrome is an example of this [27]. Inheritance of Prader-Willi or Angelman syndrome can be caused by mutations in their imprinting centre that prevent the normal erasure an resetting of imprinting pattern that occurs in gametogenesis and parent-of-origin imprinting during embryogenesis. Imprinting changes of the X or Y chromosomes have been postulated to contribute to foetal programming [12].

The peroxisome proliferator-activated receptor alpha (PPARα) which increased the numbers of peroxisomes in hepatocytes was identified as the target of hypolipidaemic fibrate drugs. The PPARs are nuclear receptors which, as transcription factors activated by lipids and other ligands and cofactors, bind regulatory sequences within many target genes to influence diverse cellular processes. They have been implicated in the pathophysiology of metabolic syndrome and have a wide range of other effects [28]. While initial research on the PPARα isoform involved fatty acid catabolism, it also influences inflammation and atherogenesis and promotes cyclic AMP response element binding in the nucleus of hippocampal neurons, influencing neuronal plasticity, synapse formation and memory [29]. The gamma-isoform (PPARγ) has an important role in the development and function of white and brown fat and in a wide variety of immunological processes. It is the target of the thiazolidinedione drugs in treatment of type 2 diabetes to increase adipogenesis in adipose tissue, reduce adipogenesis in the muscle and liver and stimulate the release of adiponectin from adipose tissue, increasing sensitivity to insulin. PPARδ is activated during fasting to increase fatty acid oxidation in mitochondria, thermogenesis and energy consumption. It also affects inflammatory processes, wound healing and myelination. A recent review summarised research into ligands being developed to stimulate PPARδ activity in metabolic syndrome, increasing HDL levels, reducing plasma triglycerides and a range of pro-inflammatory and atherogenic mediators [28]. The protean actions of PPAR genes suggest they are important contributors to the expression of metabolic syndrome and might be relevant in the study of the effects of intrauterine malnutrition. A polymorphism affecting as many as 23% of people in some ethnic groups, a substitution of arginine for proline at amino acid residue 12 (P12A) in the PPARγ protein, increases susceptibility to type 2 diabetes, while mutations in the segment of the PPARγ gene that encodes the lipid ligand-binding domain are associated with polycystic ovary syndrome and severe manifestations of metabolic syndrome. There appears to be an interaction between birth weight, which could reflect intrauterine nutrition, the P12A polymorphism and the development of insulin resistance and hyperinsulinaemia in adults [30].

The wide variety of functions and expression patterns of genes involved in response to starvation and the metabolic syndrome, such as adiponectin, leptin and many others, will be relevant to the development of associated inflammatory, immune and neoplastic complications in virtually every system. Female, but not male, rats exposed in utero to maternal starvation and treated after birth with pharmacological doses of leptin were protected from the effects of maternal starvation and did not develop signs of the metabolic syndrome [31]. Specific abnormalities including raised levels of pro-inflammatory molecules and reduced expression of genes coding for antigen-presenting molecules developed in male rats treated with leptin after birth to normally nourished mothers.

In a mouse model, the agouti gene codes for a paracrine melanocortin receptor antagonist synthesised in hair follicle cells. Polymorphisms in the gene result in different patterns and colours of hair pigmentation. Maternal nutrition and early environmental influences alter the methylation of an intracisternal A particle (IAP) [32] retrotransposon within the agouti gene [33–35]. If the IAP is not methylated, it acts as an ectopic promoter, and yellow agouti protein, which is normally expressed only in hair cells, is expressed widely within the body, causing metabolic syndrome and carcinogenesis. Exposure of the moth to folate or phytoestrogens that promote methylation of the gene [36] or to environmental compounds that reduce methylation such as bisphenol A [37] modifies the development of metabolic syndrome in offspring. Variable levels of agouti expression are observed in isogenic mice, attributable to different levels of methylation of the gene. It is significant that 45% of the human genome consists of transposons, and about 3% consists of retrotransposons [38]. Stochastic alteration of methylation and other epigenetic processes by variation in maternal nutrition and subsequent environmental influences could also affect the expression of a wide range of genes in the adult human.

If epigenetic changes are inherited across multiple generations, there is limited molecular evidence to explain how a Lamarckian process like this happens. Treatment of embryonic mice by feeding endocrine disruptors to the mothers caused persistent changes in methylation and transcription in animals that were exposed as embryos, but they were not transmitted to the next generation [39]. This would suggest either that epigenetic changes are not passed to subsequent generations, or if they are, some process other than methylation or altered transcription must be involved. Without evidence of persistent change in methylation in subsequent generations, some protein, histone, chromatin, RNA or other molecular memory could substitute for an epigenetic mark [40] that results in the persistence or reappearance of an ancestral epigenetic pattern, but the mechanism is presently unknown. Expression of microRNAs can persist for prolonged periods and multiple generations [41], but the mechanism for their persistence is unexplained, unless they promote their own transcription in addition to altering the expression of other genes. Whole genome sequencing of well-characterised case and control populations will possibly enable testing of a hypothesis that the effects of ancestral starvation on adult offspring involve somatic and/or germline genomic modifications, i.e. a "thrifty genotype".

Behaviour is likely to be significantly affected by starvation, or at least the circumstances causing the starvation. The behaviour of the mother can alter the epigenotype of rat pups [42]. Maternal anxiety, likely to be increased if there is maternal starvation, has been associated with altered methylation of the imprinted IGF1 and H19 loci in newborn babies [43]. The incidence of schizophrenia was increased in the adult offspring of mothers starved in the Dutch Hunger Winter [44] and the Great Leap Forward [19].

Maternal malnutrition in various animal models was associated with raised glucocorticoid levels and hypertension in offspring [45]. This was also shown to occur if the mother was treated with corticosteroids as a surrogate for the stress of starvation and was postulated to reset foetal hypothalamic-pituitary-adrenal activity [46, 47]. Epidemiological studies of humans have shown a relationship between birth weight, reflecting intrauterine nutrition, and adult levels of cortisol and blood pressure [48].

Possibilities for Future Research

The questions that need to be answered about effects in the adult of foetal starvation include:

- How can it be prevented? If intrauterine starvation is unavoidable, how can normal health be maintained?
- What molecular mechanisms affecting the health of adults, and possibly their descendants, might enable prevention or treatment of adult effects after unavoidable maternal and/or foetal starvation. Does maternal malnutrition just alter the foetal epigenome, or does it involve genomic sequence alterations? Specific treatments might be different in each case. Does foetal starvation result in selection of certain genes and loss from the population, or from the individual cells making up the embryo, of other gene sequences through early embryonic or cell deaths?
- If as seems likely, the effects are multifactorial, what are the major ones that might be amenable to treatment? The *MECP2* mutation in Rett syndrome causes multiple disturbances of methylation and gene expression. Addressing a specific treatable target, IGF1 signalling holds promise in an animal model of Rett syndrome [49] and might inform the management of common complex problems like the metabolic syndrome. Genomic or epigenetic changes, even if they are heritable, might be managed with drugs that amplify or inactivate specific mRNAs or other means of regulating gene expression.

Infection/Colonisation

The relationship between symbiotic or pathogenic/saprophytic organisms and humans is of potential importance as it involves the transfer of organisms largely between mother and child [50], so a large proportion of the genes inherited by a child from its mother are actually in the bacteria colonising the baby's formerly sterile epithelia. There is a détente between microorganisms and the human host, possibly mediated by micro-inhibitory RNA (miRNA) and other regulators of gene expression, including methylation and histone deacetylation. The population of s-biotic bacteria in the gut might be altered in the mother if she is malnourished and possibly in the respiratory epithelium and skin of the child if the level or type of nutrition changes. This mechanism might contribute to the different effects during adulthood of intrauterine malnutrition, where the mother might also have been mal-nourished with altered gut flora and postnatal malnutrition. It might partially explain different patterns of "inherited" disease seen after starvation of the mother during her pregnancy versus starvation of the father during his adolescence [12]. Metabolic syndrome and other mortality from common diseases of multifactorial origin are common in many indigenous adult populations, but there are also high rates of childhood bacterial infection [51], dental disease and malnutrition. Chronic bacterial infection due to dental, periodontal and respiratory disease is associated, possibly causally, with a number of adult diseases, so studies of maternal malnutrition can be complicated by coexistent socioeconomic factors (and an emerging repertoire of known genetic factors) that predispose to chronic infection.

Genomic Mutations, Epigenesis vs Mutation in Genes Involved in Methylation or RNA Regulation

Metabolic syndrome has been attributed to changes in the epigenotype, caused by environmental influences during intrauterine or later development and altering the phenotype of metabolic syndrome within congenic strains of laboratory animals or human identical twins. These experimental groups were formerly thought to consist of individuals that were genetically identical. It seemed reasonable then to conclude that if epigenetic differences were caused by experimental manipulation in congenic strains of animals, or if they were associated in discordant monozygotic human twins with alterations in prenatal or postnatal environment, there would be no need to look for alterations in genomic DNA that could have caused or be associated with epigenetic changes. The spontaneously hypertensive rat is a congenic strain inbred for many generations but is still heterozygous at every 2.5×10^{-5} nucleo-tides on whole genome sequencing [52], which would be in keeping with estimates of new mutation in other species. There might have been pre-existing discordance for imprinting in human twins regardless of their environmental differences. One of monozygotic twins, having less access to pla-cental nutrition, can have IUGR and adult-onset metabolic syndrome, while the other twin, with higher birth weight, has a lower risk of metabolic syndrome [53]. Beckwith-Wiedemann syndrome is associated with abnormal foetal growth and somatic mosaicism for an imprinting defect of chromo-some 11 or other less common mechanisms [54]. Mosaicism refers to a mixture of cells containing the genotype present at conception and a population with a new mutation or perhaps a new imprinting pattern. It is more frequent in one of monozygotic twins [55, 56]. A number of conditions have been found to be discordant in monozygotic twins [57–59], including epigenetic differences that seem to develop with age [60], suggesting either that disease-causing mutations or imprinting abnormalities can occur after conception of these twins or even that monozygotic twinning might be caused somehow by mosaicism for mutations [57] or imprinting patterns.

Metabolic effects that are not passed on to future generations might be due to somatic mutations that do not involve the germ line, and this might be related to the timing of the intrauterine stimulus. Human monozygotic twins, besides having different epigenotypes [61], can have significant differ-ences in DNA sequence, including copy number variations caused by postzygotic mutations [62], occurring after the conception of the embryo. A growing list of patients is reported with subclinical and often unsuspected or mild expression of disease because of dilution of its effects by mosaicism, or nonpenetrance because the mosaicism spared the cell line usually involved in pathogenesis, but was only detected in an accessible tissue like blood [63]. To date no whole genome sequencing study has compared adult somatic and germ line sequences in metabolic syndrome with controls or compared genome sequences in different tissues of the same subject [61, 64]. This potentially applies to animals thought to be congenic.

Although famines have enabled "natural experiments" involving humans, conclusions from epidemiological research have been limited by the possibility of biased ascertainment, where the group actually analysed is relatively small and unrepresentative of the exposed population, especially if subjects might preferentially participate because they have health problems. Genetic selection by famine has been dismissed because of rapid changes in disease prevalence. Any decrease in birth rate was attributed to reduction of fertility. Genotype is however a plausible influence on fertility during famine [10]. The birth rate dropped at the same time as an increase in mortality in China during the starvation associated with their Great Leap Forward [19]. A similar phenomenon was observed in the number of young people eligible for conscription, who were conceived during the Dutch famine [15]. It was concluded that a rebound increase in birth rates following relief of the famine negated any selective effect of the famine [5]. Famine has been thought to affect conception but embryonic survival has not been considered or mentioned in earlier research [10, 65]. Fertility might be noticeably affected if conception of a genetically "fit" embryo was delayed until after the very early loss of genetically "unfit" one(s). In multiple pregnancies in animals, the death of a foetus might not influence litter size because of selective death of foetuses [66]. In about 10% of human twin pregnancies, one of the twins is known to have vanished during the pregnancy [57]. The smaller twin might have died in utero but for postzygotic mutation(s) predisposing to a thrifty genotype in some of the cells of the conceptus, that later founded a surviving embryo, and later development of metabolic syndrome. Past epidemiological studies of humans were unlikely to have detected early foetal loss, because this could masquerade as a late or irregular menstrual cycle or as infertility. Mortality and fertility data were usually collected retrospectively and were limited to records of live births or foetal mortality in advanced pregnancy, and comparisons might have been influenced by social class [7].

With whole genome sequencing, especially of single cells or single cell types, it will become possible to test a hypothesis that reduction in birth rate might have been due to very early mortality of embryos, or genetic selection of cells within embryos, in addition to, or rather than reduced conception [10, 67]. The embryo implanting into the decidua relies on residual energy stores of the ovum and surrounding cells, and metabolic processes determined by maternal RNA and proteins, and on absorption of nutrients from the uterine decidua [68]. The implanting embryo is surrounded by dendritic cells which influence immunological tolerance [69]. Maternal malnutrition, obesity, autoimmune or vascular diseases might affect the behaviour of these cells, as shown in other tissues [70, 71]. Selection pressure must be high at the best of times in the early intrauterine environment when only 30–40% of ovulations result in clinically recognisable pregnancy, and 30% of conceptions survive to live birth [72]. After pregnancy is confirmed by ultrasound at 6 weeks, between 4.2% and 12.7% of pregnancies are miscarried [73]. There is high rate of embryonic loss after aneuploid embryos conceived by IVF are excluded by laboratory screening [74]. As most embryo implantations fail, foetal and/or intrauterine factors that alter the success of implantation could have significant effects on birth rates, or if birth rates are unchanged, on genotype frequencies [10] in surviving embryos or in the case of somatic mosaicism, in cells within surviving embryos. This could lead to physiological and pathological changes in adulthood. A plausible hypothesis is that the decidua around the embryo would be less hospitable in malnourished mothers or in those with pathology contributing to later placental insufficiency, such as the metabolic syndrome itself. Entire embryos, or cells within embryos (see below), might be selected for survival by genotypes most suited to the intrauterine environment. It is estimated that the average baby has 50–100 new mutations [75]. Evidence for the concept of foetal loss and its relationship with epigenetic inheritance, leading to the loss of certain genotypes in offspring, has been available since heterozygous yellow agouti mice were interbred [66, 76]. In women who are starved, or those whose pregnancy is complicated by placental insufficiency and/or intrauterine growth retardation, the selective pressure would be higher. Among the new mutations likely to be present in a newborn animal, some could be found that confer a selective advantage in some intrauterine conditions, e.g. starvation or placental insufficiency, but are unfavourable in later times of rapid growth or high caloric intake. Maternal starvation could thus be a driver of somatic mutation and possibly also of selection of cells with mutations favourable to the current environment. Selection of cells within the embryo, or of total embryos based on their epigenotype, could be enabled by mutation or other mechanisms. Looking for missing polymorphism genotypes, present in parents, affected children and their unexposed siblings, but lost and undetectable in embryos lost too early to be sampled, might assist the search for genetic contributors to metabolic syndrome in adults [67].

Somatic Mosaicism

There is opportunity for selection within organs of cells with somatic mutations, as by age 15 years the average human is predicted to have 10^{-7}–10^{-6} mutations per nucleotide per somatic cell [75], which could equate to 100–1000 mutations per non-replicating diploid cell and 1000–10,000 per replicating cell. Non-replicating adult cells can also accumulate genomic mutations which could also affect function, epigenotype and phenotype [75]. If the mutation affected genes for double stranded siRNA, it might be possible for these to act in a paracrine or endocrine manner. The germ line in a 15 year old adolescent would have 10–1000 mutations [75]. Although conceived by IVF and therefore cultured in vitro, a very high proportion of human embryos from healthy parents have somatic mosaicism for copy number variations [77]. To these, can be added an unknown frequency of smaller insertion, deletion and point mutations in protein-coding and regulatory genomic sequences in cells within embryos, implying that there is a significant opportunity for selection of cells within each embryo and that the body of each adult is the product of a complex evolutionary process just within their own life span. Attribution of differences in phenotype and methylation patterns to postnatal environmental differences and metabolic programming might be refined when it becomes possible to compare whole genome sequences of different tissues in different types of monozygotic twins [62] or congenic strains of laboratory animals. Acknowledgment of this possibility is starting to appear in recent publications including fascinating new research into childhood obesity [78].

Reverse Transcription?

It has been shown that germ cells take up small RNA molecules to alter chromatin structure and affect gene expression for many generations in worms [41]. A similar process has occurred following ancestral starvation. Double-stranded RNA coming from somatic tissue mutations might even alter the genomic sequence [79] by a process involving reverse transcription, or analogous to it, and be passed on to the next generation in the genomic DNA. This would involve an epigenetic process but its fixation in subsequent generations might involve genomic DNA changes in addition to, or rather than, a Lamarckian mechanism. These might only be detectable with whole genomic sequencing research involving multiple generations including one exposed to starvation, controls, descendants and multiple tissue types, not just bloods.

Conclusions

There is no molecular evidence that epigenetic changes caused by starvation or other environmental influences are part of an ordered predictable (or programmed) response. The targets of drugs or xenobiotics that influence DNA methylation appear to be nonspecific [37]. As with other Darwinian selection processes, the environmental influence could cause random and nonspecific stochastic effects on individual cells within the organism. Somatic and germ cells with favourable epigenotypes and/or genotypes could then be selected on the basis of their ability to survive and proliferate in the developing organism in the prevailing environmental circumstances. An orderly process of imprinting occurs in human development so that genes are appropriately silenced and activated depending on the age of the organism and the tissue type. There seems to be little dispute that this can be explained by the interaction of cells with each other within the organism, coordinated by genomic sequences and their products including proteins and coding or non-coding regulatory RNAs. By the same reasoning, it is plausible that environmental conditions within an organism, such as maternal starvation, could select germ cells and somatic cells with genotypes that promote certain patterns of imprinting, which might then be transmitted to subsequent generations of body cells to adulthood in humans and even to descendants. There are political incentives and bias in ethics committees in favour of funding and adopting epigenetic theories to reinforce the idea that everyone is born with equal potential and that ancestral deprivation or discrimination against groups has molecular transgenerational effects. This might be the case: at present it is easy to find research funded and published in influential journals on single-cell genome-wide methylome study and transcriptome sequencing of single cells [80]. There are strong incentives to publish positive findings on transgenerational epigenetics, but it is harder to publish negative studies [81]. It remains to be seen whether it is as feasible to obtain funding for, and acceptance by ethics committees of, whole *genome* sequencing of single cells or single tissues in people of different ages exposed in utero to starvation or other environmental insults and suitable controls. Until that happens, the thrifty genotype hypothesis needs to be kept on the list of possible mechanisms for adult disease after maternal malnutrition.

A modification of the thrifty genotype theory could begin by asking how postzygotic mutation could be thought of as an adaptive process? Arguments against genetic selection occurring within short periods of history mention the long generation time of humans. But there is a very short time between the generations of cells that form a human embryo. For example, an enormous somatic variation of point mutations and somatic recombinations in genes for antibodies occurs in a relatively short period of development, resulting in different people having a repertoire of lymphocytes which can synthesise antibodies to virtually all of millions of possible foreign complex molecules, to most of which they will never be exposed. How can different people each happen to have a set of antibodies that recognise identical foreign molecules, if this occurs by a random process independent of any vertical (parental inheritance) or horizontal transmission of information between people (at least until they infect each other with a transmissible disease)? It has been universally accepted that this is enabled by the enormous random genetic *mutation or variation* with each division of embryonic lymphocytes, in association with *selection*, within the thymus against lymphocytes which recognise self-antigens, and in favour of those which recognise foreign molecules introduced into the body, i.e. a Darwinian process of evolution within each of us as we develop. If this is the case, there could be a similar process of selection within every embryo's body (including possibly their germ line) for the rapidly dividing cell that is most suited to the local environment, whether it be in a starving mother or one offering a poor intrauterine environment due to her own manifest or incipient metabolic syndrome. That process of genomic variation and selection could indeed be mediated by changes in methylation or gene expression that are being detected by current research. It might be detectable if involving mosaic genomic variation, when single cells or tissues can be sequenced and compared between databases of subjects exposed to maternal malnutrition and controls.

References

1. Barker DJ, Hales CN, Fall CH, Osmond C, Phipps K, Clark PM. Type 2 (non-insulin-dependent) diabetes mellitus, hypertension and hyperlipidaemia (syndrome X): relation to reduced fetal growth. Diabetologia. 1993;36(1):62–7.
2. Hales CN, Barker DJ. Type 2 (non-insulin-dependent) diabetes mellitus: the thrifty phenotype hypothesis. Diabetologia. 1992;35(7):595–601.

3. Constancia M, Hemberger M, Hughes J, Dean W, Ferguson-Smith A, Fundele R, et al. Placental-specific IGF-II is a major modulator of placental and fetal growth. Nature. 2002;417(6892):945–8.
4. Neel JV. Diabetes mellitus: a "thrifty" genotype rendered detrimental by "progress"? Am J Hum Genet. 1962;14:353–62.
5. Speakman JR. Thrifty genes for obesity, an attractive but flawed idea, and an alternative perspective: the 'drifty gene' hypothesis. Int J Obes. 2008;32(11):1611–7.
6. Stoger R. The thrifty epigenotype: an acquired and heritable predisposition for obesity and diabetes? BioEssays. 2008;30(2):156–66.
7. Hart N. Famine, maternal nutrition and infant mortality: a re-examination of the Dutch hunger winter. Popul Stud (Camb). 1993;47(1):27–46.
8. Roseboom T, de Rooij S, Painter R. The Dutch famine and its long-term consequences for adult health. Early Hum Dev. 2006;82(8):485–91.
9. Stanner SA, Yudkin JS. Fetal programming and the Leningrad Siege study. Twin Res. 2001;4(5):287–92.
10. Prentice AM, Hennig BJ, Fulford AJ. Evolutionary origins of the obesity epidemic: natural selection of thrifty genes or genetic drift following predation release? Int J Obes. 2008;32(11):1607–10.
11. Hattersley AT, Beards F, Ballantyne E, Appleton M, Harvey R, Ellard S. Mutations in the glucokinase gene of the fetus result in reduced birth weight. Nat Genet. 1998;19(3):268–70.
12. Pembrey M, Saffery R, Bygren LO, Carstensen J, Edvinsson S, Faresjo T, et al. Human transgenerational responses to early-life experience: potential impact on development, health and biomedical research. J Med Genet. 2014;51(9):590–5.
13. Forsdahl A. Are poor living conditions in childhood and adolescence an important risk factor for arteriosclerotic heart disease? Br J Prev Soc Med. 1977;31(2):91–5.
14. Kaati G, Bygren LO, Edvinsson S. Cardiovascular and diabetes mortality determined by nutrition during parents' and grandparents' slow growth period. Eur J Hum Genet. 2002;10(11):682–8.
15. Stein Z. Famine and human development: the Dutch hunger winter of 1944–45. Oxford: Oxford University Press; 1975.
16. Ravelli GP, Stein ZA, Susser MW. Obesity in young men after famine exposure in utero and early infancy. N Engl J Med. 1976;295(7):349–53.
17. Stein Z, Susser M, Saenger G, Marolla F. Nutrition and mental performance. Prenatal exposure to the Dutch famine of 1944–1945 seems not related to mental performance at age 19. Science. 1972;178(4062):708–13.
18. de Rooij SR, Wouters H, Yonker JE, Painter RC, Roseboom TJ. Prenatal undernutrition and cognitive function in late adulthood. Proc Natl Acad Sci U S A. 2010;107(39):16881–6.
19. St Clair D, Xu M, Wang P, Yu Y, Fang Y, Zhang F, et al. Rates of adult schizophrenia following prenatal exposure to the Chinese famine of 1959–1961. JAMA. 2005;294(5):557–62.
20. Dowse GK, Zimmet PZ, Finch CF, Collins VR. Decline in incidence of epidemic glucose intolerance in Nauruans: implications for the "thrifty genotype". Am J Epidemiol. 1991;133(11):1093–104.
21. Diamond J. The double puzzle of diabetes. Nature. 2003;423(6940):599–602.
22. Khambalia A, Phongsavan P, Smith BJ, Keke K, Dan L, Fitzhardinge A, et al. Prevalence and risk factors of diabetes and impaired fasting glucose in Nauru. BMC Public Health. 2011;11:719.
23. Victora CG, Adair L, Fall C, Hallal PC, Martorell R, Richter L, et al. Maternal and child undernutrition: consequences for adult health and human capital. Lancet. 2008;371(9609):340–57.
24. Lewis MW, Brant JO, Kramer JM, Moss JI, Yang TP, Hansen PJ, et al. Angelman syndrome imprinting center encodes a transcriptional promoter. Proc Natl Acad Sci. 2015;112(22):6871–5.
25. Jones PA, Laird PW. Cancer epigenetics comes of age. Nat Genet. 1999;21(2):163–7.
26. Weksberg R, Shuman C, Beckwith JB. Beckwith-Wiedemann syndrome. Eur J Hum Genet. 2010;18(1):8–14.
27. Albrecht U, Sutcliffe JS, Cattanach BM, Beechey CV, Armstrong D, Eichele G, et al. Imprinted expression of the murine Angelman syndrome gene, Ube3a, in hippocampal and Purkinje neurons. Nat Genet. 1997;17(1):75–8.
28. Ahmadian M, Suh JM, Hah N, Liddle C, Atkins AR, Downes M, et al. PPARgamma signaling and metabolism: the good, the bad and the future. Nat Med. 2013;19(5):557–66.
29. Roy A, Jana M, Corbett GT, Ramaswamy S, Kordower JH, Gonzalez FJ, et al. Regulation of cyclic AMP response element binding and hippocampal plasticity-related genes by peroxisome proliferator-activated receptor alpha. Cell Rep. 2013;4(4):724–37.
30. Eriksson JG, Lindi V, Uusitupa M, Forsen TJ, Laakso M, Osmond C, et al. The effects of the Pro12Ala polymorphism of the peroxisome proliferator-activated receptor-gamma2 gene on insulin sensitivity and insulin metabolism interact with size at birth. Diabetes. 2002;51(7):2321–4.
31. Ellis PJ, Morris TJ, Skinner BM, Sargent CA, Vickers MH, Gluckman PD, et al. Thrifty metabolic programming in rats is induced by both maternal undernutrition and postnatal leptin treatment, but masked in the presence of both: implications for models of developmental programming. BMC Genomics. 2014;15:49.
32. Bernhard W. The detection and study of tumor viruses with the electron microscope. Cancer Res. 1960;20:712–27.
33. Dolinoy DC. The agouti mouse model: an epigenetic biosensor for nutritional and environmental alterations on the fetal epigenome. Nutr Rev. 2008;66(Suppl 1):S7–11.

34. Miller MW, Duhl DM, Vrieling H, Cordes SP, Ollmann MM, Winkes BM, et al. Cloning of the mouse agouti gene predicts a secreted protein ubiquitously expressed in mice carrying the lethal yellow mutation. Genes Dev. 1993;7(3):454–67.
35. Bultman SJ, Michaud EJ, Woychik RP. Molecular characterization of the mouse agouti locus. Cell. 1992;71(7):1195–204.
36. Dolinoy DC, Weidman JR, Waterland RA, Jirtle RL. Maternal genistein alters coat color and protects Avy mouse offspring from obesity by modifying the fetal epigenome. Environ Health Perspect. 2006;114(4):567–72.
37. Dolinoy DC, Huang D, Jirtle RL. Maternal nutrient supplementation counteracts bisphenol A-induced DNA hypomethylation in early development. Proc Natl Acad Sci U S A. 2007;104(32):13056–61.
38. Lander ES, Linton LM, Birren B, Nusbaum C, Zody MC, Baldwin J, et al. Initial sequencing and analysis of the human genome. Nature. 2001;409(6822):860–921.
39. Iqbal K, Tran DA, Li AX, Warden C, Bai AY, Singh P, et al. Deleterious effects of endocrine disruptors are corrected in the mammalian germline by epigenome reprogramming. Genome Biol. 2015;16(1):1–24.
40. Radford EJ, Ito M, Shi H, Corish JA, Yamazawa K, Isganaitis E, et al. In utero effects. In utero undernourishment perturbs the adult sperm methylome and intergenerational metabolism. Science. 2014;345(6198):1255903.
41. Devanapally S, Ravikumar S, Jose AM. Double-stranded RNA made in *C. elegans* neurons can enter the germline and cause transgenerational gene silencing. Proc Natl Acad Sci U S A. 2015;112(7):2133–8.
42. Weaver IC, Cervoni N, Champagne FA, D'Alessio AC, Sharma S, Seckl JR, et al. Epigenetic programming by maternal behavior. Nat Neurosci. 2004;7(8):847–54.
43. Mansell T, Novakovic B, Meyer B, Rzehak P, Vuillermin P, Ponsonby AL, et al. The effects of maternal anxiety during pregnancy on IGF2/H19 methylation in cord blood. Transl Psychiatry. 2016;6:e765.
44. Hulshoff Pol HE, Hoek HW, Susser E, Brown AS, Dingemans A, Schnack HG, et al. Prenatal exposure to famine and brain morphology in schizophrenia. Am J Psychiatry. 2000;157(7):1170–2.
45. Bloomfield FH, Oliver MH, Giannoulias CD, Gluckman PD, Harding JE, Challis JR. Brief undernutrition in late-gestation sheep programs the hypothalamic-pituitary-adrenal axis in adult offspring. Endocrinology. 2003;144(7):2933–40.
46. Levitt NS, Lindsay RS, Holmes MC, Seckl JR. Dexamethasone in the last week of pregnancy attenuates hippocampal glucocorticoid receptor gene expression and elevates blood pressure in the adult offspring in the rat. Neuroendocrinology. 1996;64(6):412–8.
47. Dodic M, May CN, Wintour EM, Coghlan JP. An early prenatal exposure to excess glucocorticoid leads to hypertensive offspring in sheep. Clin Sci (Lond). 1998;94(2):149–55.
48. Phillips DI, Barker DJ, Fall CH, Seckl JR, Whorwood CB, Wood PJ, et al. Elevated plasma cortisol concentrations: a link between low birth weight and the insulin resistance syndrome? J Clin Endocrinol Metab. 1998;83(3):757–60.
49. Castro J, Garcia RI, Kwok S, Banerjee A, Petravicz J, Woodson J, et al. Functional recovery with recombinant human IGF1 treatment in a mouse model of Rett syndrome. Proc Natl Acad Sci. 2014;111(27):9941–6.
50. Negri I, Jablonka E. Editorial: epigenetics as a deep intimate dialogue between host and symbionts. Front Genet. 2016;7:7.
51. Janu EK, Annabattula BI, Kumariah S, Zajaczkowska M, Whitehall JS, Edwards MJ, et al. Paediatric hospitalisations for lower respiratory tract infections in Mount Isa. Med J Aust. 2014;200(10):591–4.
52. Atanur SS, Birol I, Guryev V, Hirst M, Hummel O, Morrissey C, et al. The genome sequence of the spontaneously hypertensive rat: analysis and functional significance. Genome Res. 2010;20(6):791–803.
53. Poulsen P, Vaag AA, Kyvik KO, Moller Jensen D, Beck-Nielsen H. Low birth weight is associated with NIDDM in discordant monozygotic and dizygotic twin pairs. Diabetologia. 1997;40(4):439–46.
54. Zollino M, Orteschi D, Marangi G, De Crescenzo A, Pecile V, Riccio A, et al. A case of Beckwith-Wiedemann syndrome caused by a cryptic 11p15 deletion encompassing the centromeric imprinted domain of the BWS locus. J Med Genet. 2010;47(6):429–32.
55. Bose B, Wilkie RA, Madlom M, Forsyth JS, Faed MJ. Wiedemann-Beckwith syndrome in one of monozygotic twins. Arch Dis Child. 1985;60(12):1191–2.
56. Bo S, Cavallo-Perin P, Scaglione L, Ciccone G, Pagano G. Low birthweight and metabolic abnormalities in twins with increased susceptibility to type 2 diabetes mellitus. Diabet Med. 2000;17(5):365–70.
57. Hall JG. Twinning: mechanisms and genetic implications. Curr Opin Genet Dev. 1996;6(3):343–7.
58. Hall JG. Twins and twinning. Am J Med Genet. 1996;61(3):202–4.
59. Hall JG, Lopez-Rangel E. Embryologic development and monozygotic twinning. Acta Genet Med Gemellol. 1996;45(1–2):53–7.
60. Fraga MF, Ballestar E, Paz MF, Ropero S, Setien F, Ballestar ML, et al. Epigenetic differences arise during the lifetime of monozygotic twins. Proc Natl Acad Sci U S A. 2005;102(30):10604–9.
61. Martin GM. Epigenetic drift in aging identical twins. Proc Natl Acad Sci U S A. 2005;102(30):10413–4.
62. Czyz W, Morahan JM, Ebers GC, Ramagopalan SV. Genetic, environmental and stochastic factors in monozygotic twin discordance with a focus on epigenetic differences. BMC Med. 2012;10:93.

63. Erickson RP. Somatic gene mutation and human disease other than cancer: an update. Mutat Res. 2010;705(2):96–106.
64. Frank SA. Evolution in health and medicine Sackler colloquium: somatic evolutionary genomics: mutations during development cause highly variable genetic mosaicism with risk of cancer and neurodegeneration. Proc Natl Acad Sci U S A. 2010;107(Suppl 1):1725–30.
65. Prentice A. Surviving famine. Survival: survival of the human race. Cambridge: Cambridge University Press; 2007. p. 146–7.
66. Castle WE, Little CC. On a modified Mendelian ratio among yellow mice. Science. 1910;32(833):868–70.
67. Edwards MJ. Genetic selection of embryos that later develop the metabolic syndrome. Med Hypotheses. 2012;78(5):621–5.
68. Deanesly R. Termination of early pregnancy in rats after ovariectomy is due to immediate collapse of the progesterone-dependent decidua. J Reprod Fertil. 1973;35(1):183–6.
69. Kammerer U, Schoppet M, McLellan AD, Kapp M, Huppertz HI, Kampgen E, et al. Human decidua contains potent immunostimulatory CD83(+) dendritic cells. Am J Pathol. 2000;157(1):159–69.
70. Rocha VZ, Libby P. Obesity, inflammation, and atherosclerosis. Nat Rev Cardiol. 2009;6(6):399–409.
71. Chandra RK. Nutrition and immunology: from the clinic to cellular biology and back again. Proc Nutr Soc. 1999;58(3):681–3.
72. Macklon NS, Geraedts JP, Fauser BC. Conception to ongoing pregnancy: the 'black box' of early pregnancy loss. Hum Reprod Update. 2002;8(4):333–43.
73. Hill LM, Guzick D, Fries J, Hixson J. Fetal loss rate after ultrasonically documented cardiac activity between 6 and 14 weeks, menstrual age. J Clin Ultrasound. 1991;19(4):221–3.
74. Staessen C, Verpoest W, Donoso P, Haentjens P, Van der Elst J, Liebaers I, et al. Preimplantation genetic screening does not improve delivery rate in women under the age of 36 following single-embryo transfer. Hum Reprod. 2008;23(12):2818–25.
75. Lynch M. Rate, molecular spectrum, and consequences of human mutation. Proc Natl Acad Sci. 2010;107(3):961–8.
76. Cuenot L. Sur quelques anomalies apparentes des proportions Mendeliennes. Arch Zool Exp Gen. 1908;9:7–15.
77. Voet T, Vanneste E, Vermeesch JR. The human cleavage stage embryo is a cradle of chromosomal rearrangements. Cytogenet Genome Res. 2011;133(2–4):160–8.
78. Dalgaard K, Landgraf K, Heyne S, Lempradl A, Longinotto J, Gossens K, et al. Trim28 haploinsufficiency triggers bi-stable epigenetic obesity. Cell. 2016;164(3):353–64.
79. Steele EJ. Commentary: past, present, and future of epigenetics applied to livestock breeding – hard versus soft Lamarckian inheritance mechanisms. Front Genet. 2016;7:29.
80. Angermueller C, Clark SJ, Lee HJ, Macaulay IC, Teng MJ, Hu TX, et al. Parallel single-cell sequencing links transcriptional and epigenetic heterogencity. Nat Meth. 2016;13(3):229–32.
81. Whitelaw E. Disputing Lamarckian epigenetic inheritance in mammals. Genome Biol. 2015;16:60.

Chapter 27
Maternal Malnutrition, Foetal Programming, Outcomes and Strategies in India

Poornima Prabhakaran and Prabhakaran Dorairaj

Key Points

- Maternal nutrition has direct consequences for foetal well-being, both in the form of immediate effects and long-term impacts.
- India faces a dual burden of undernutrition and overnutrition, with adolescent girls and women in the childbearing age group, both in rural and urban areas affected.
- Maternal nutrition is a modifiable factor, and research in India has established the role of supplemental maternal nutrition on birth weight of the offspring.
- Both macro- and micronutrients are shown to impact birth outcomes.
- Early nutrition has influence on birth weight, childhood morbidity and long-term disease risk.
- Postnatal growth patterns and lifestyle factors, including diet and physical activity patterns, play a synergistic role on later life disease risk.
- Research in India has shown the need to adopt a life-course approach to deal with chronic disease.

Keywords Maternal nutrition • Foetal programming • Critical period • Risk factors • Policy

Abbreviations

APCAPS	Andhra Pradesh Children and Parents Study
BMI	Body mass index
DLHS	District level household and facility survey
DOHaD	Developmental Origins of Health and Disease
ICDS	Integrated Child Development Scheme
INR	Indian national rupee

P. Prabhakaran, MBBS, MSc(Epidemiology), PhD(Social Medicine) (✉)
Associate Professor and Senior Research Scientist, Chronic Disease Epidemiology and Fellow,
Centre for Environmental Health, Public Health Foundation of India, Gurgaon, Haryana, India
e-mail: poornima.prabhakaran@phfi.org

P. Dorairaj, MD, DM(Cardiology), MSc, FRCP, FNASc
Professor, Chronic Disease Epidemiology and Vice-President, Research & Policy, Public Health foundation of India, Gurgaon, Haryana, India

© Springer International Publishing AG 2017
R. Rajendram et al. (eds.), *Diet, Nutrition, and Fetal Programming*,
Nutrition and Health, DOI 10.1007/978-3-319-60289-9_27

IQ   Intelligence quotient
LBW   Low birth weight
MMA   Methylmalonic acid
MRI   Magnetic resonance imaging
NDBC   New Delhi Birth Cohort
NFHS   National Family Health Survey
NIN   National Institute of Nutrition

Background

Nutrition of a mother through her lifetime has significant impact on the health and well-being of her offspring. Appropriate nutrition, in particular during adolescence, pregnancy and lactation, affects the growth and development of the foetus, thereby translating into healthy statistics for birth outcomes, childhood health and long-term health and economic benefits [1]. Nutritional programmes around the world have rightly focussed on women and mothers during pregnancy, with many countries recognising the importance of appropriate maternal nutrition as a strategy to reduce increasing maternal, infant and neonatal morbidity and mortality rates.

Overview on Nutritional Status of Indian Women

India, a lower middle-income country, is host to a huge population of poorly nourished women. According to the National Family Health Survey (NFHS 2005–2006), the prevalence of undernourished women, based on a body mass index (BMI) less than 18.5 kg/m^2, was 36.5%; nearly half of these (15.8%) had a BMI less than 17 kg/m^2, pointing to the widespread prevalence of moderate to severe undernutrition. The prevalence of anaemia among women in their childbearing years, aged 15–49 years, ranges from 32.7% in the state of Kerala to 76.3% in West Bengal (Source: District Level Household and Facility Survey). This exemplifies the wide variation across states in India. Among adolescent girls alone, 15–18 years of age, nearly 35% have a BMI less than 18.5 kg/m^2 in Kerala, while the figure in Rajasthan is nearly 60%; anaemia levels vary from 35% in Kerala to almost double this prevalence among adolescents in Bihar [2].

On the other end of the spectrum of malnourishment, overweight and obesity levels among Indian women have also shown a steady rise. According to the National Family Health Survey 3 (2005–2006), the overall prevalence of overweight women aged 15–49 years was 13%, with about 3% falling in the obese category (BMI greater than 30 kg/m^2). What is even more discouraging is the fact that this double burden of malnutrition is not restricted to a particular socio-economic stratum. With rapid urbanisation, increasing migration from rural to urban locations for work opportunities and the accompanying changes in lifestyle and dietary practices, the socio-economic reversal of risk factors for lifestyle disorders is evident across rural and urban populations [3] (Figs. 27.1 and 27.2).

The prevalence of malnutrition among women in India is clearly linked to their educational status. NFHS-3 data shows no education associated with twice the levels of undernutrition and 12 or more years of education associated with three times higher level of overweight/obesity.

Maternal Nutritional Status and Foetal Programming

Early life factors, including the nutritional status of mothers, impact the intrauterine milieu and have ramifications for the foetus through intergenerational effects [4]. Poor nutritional and environmental influences during critical stages of development cause permanent changes in structure, physiology

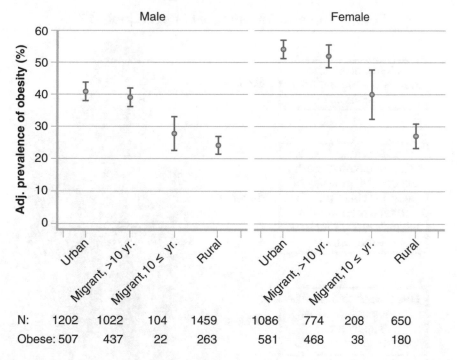

Fig. 27.1 Prevalence of obesity across migration/residence status (Source: *PLOS Medicine* 2010 Ebrahim et al.)

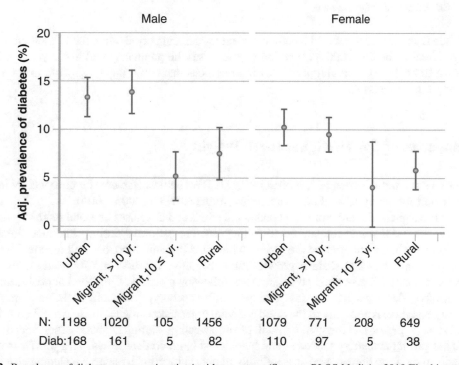

Fig. 27.2 Prevalence of diabetes across migration/residence status (Source: *PLOS Medicine* 2010 Ebrahim et al.)

and metabolism of the growing embryo and foetus (Fig. 27.3). This "foetal programming" paradigm proposed by Prof. David Barker triggered a whole school of research on the Developmental Origins of Health and Disease (DOHaD) [5, 6]. Poor intrauterine nutrition (including those resulting from maternal hyperglycaemic states) and development impact birth weight, and abnormal birth weight has been shown to have long-term consequences.

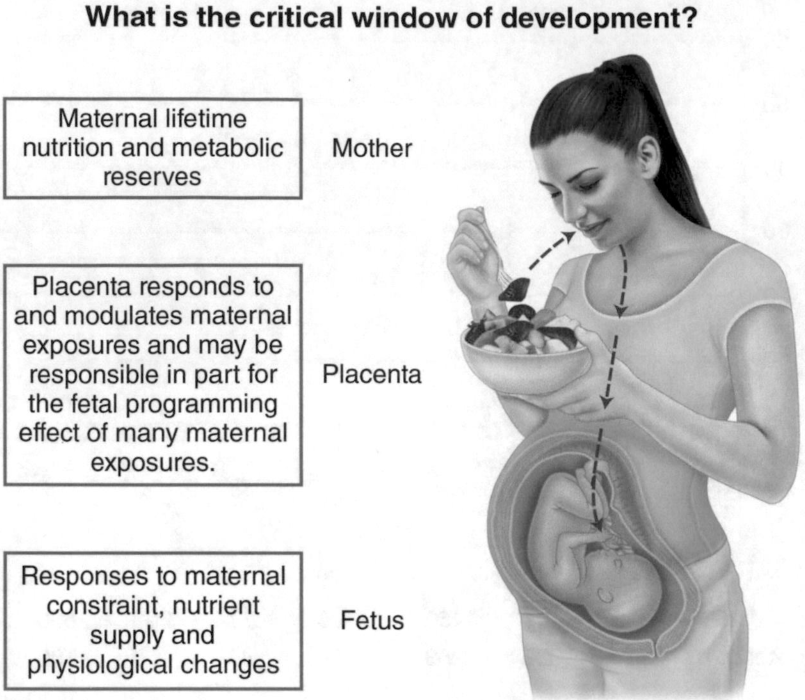

What is the critical window of development?

Maternal lifetime nutrition and metabolic reserves — Mother

Placenta responds to and modulates maternal exposures and may be responsible in part for the fetal programming effect of many maternal exposures. — Placenta

Responses to maternal constraint, nutrient supply and physiological changes — Fetus

Fig. 27.3 Critical period of development

Evidence from around the world has focussed on the critical period when foetal programming has long-term effects. The first 1000 days which encompasses the pregnancy and first 2 years of life has been shown to be the most crucial period for interventions that could impact short-term survival and reduce long-term effects [7].

Consequences of Lower/Higher Birth Weight

India faces a substantial burden of low birth weight (LBW) babies. Babies with birth weight less than 2500 g account for nearly 30% of births according to the NFHS 3 (2005–2006).

Low birth weight babies are prone to neonatal infections and this raises neonatal morbidity and mortality; those that survive into infancy could follow different pathways during childhood. Infants and children that remain undernourished are prone to impaired immune functions and recurrent infections and have poor muscular and skeletal growth, lower cognitive function and IQ resulting in reduced schooling and poor adult economic potential. Also, following a period of impaired nourishment during critical periods of development, foetuses develop a "thrifty phenotype" whereby a "defence" mechanism comes into play; there is a sparing of the brain and vital organs, downregulation of overall growth, muscular and skeletal tissues and increased growth of simple energy-storing adipose tissue, reduced insulin sensitivity, a pro-inflammatory tendency and heightened basal cortisol levels. This translates to long-term effects in the form of increased susceptibility to unhealthy growth patterns including an early adiposity rebound, overweight and obesity, increased cardiometabolic risk factors such as impaired glucose tolerance, lipid abnormalities and high blood pressure [8, 9]. Research in the mid-1980s following the Barker hypothesis showed an inverse relation between low birth weight and later risk of coronary heart disease [10, 11]. The studies, largely based in the UK and other western populations, established an

Summary and framework

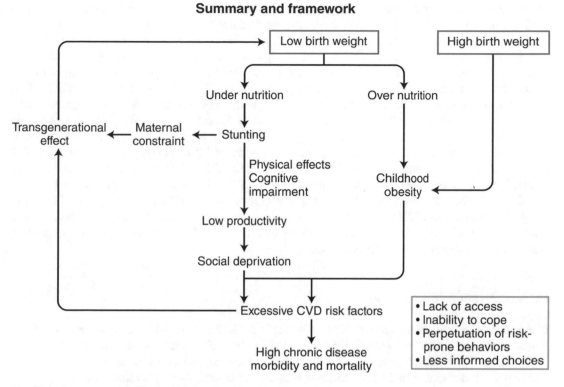

Fig. 27.4 Consequences of low and high birth weight

association between lower birth weight and later elevated risk of non-communicable diseases, in particular type 2 diabetes and cardiovascular disease [12, 13]. Higher birth weight, a consequence of maternal overnutrition and hyperglycaemic states, is a precursor for childhood overweight and obesity. The following figure (Fig. 27.4) provides a summary of the consequences of low and high birth weight.

India

Studies in India have long contributed to the evidence base on maternal malnutrition, foetal programming and long-term outcomes.

Maternal Nutrition Studies

Hyderabad Nutrition Trial

Nearly four decades ago, India's policy response to the dire situation of childhood malnutrition – the Integrated Child Development Services (ICDS) scheme – was launched by the Government of India on October 2, 1975 [14]. While its central focus was the improvement of nutritional status of pregnant and lactating women and children less than 6 years of age, it also included complementary programmes for early childhood education, health, hygiene and nutrition education for the mothers and delivery of other national programmes (immunisation, anaemia control and basic health care) from the ICDS centres. As the programme saw stepwise expansion in the 1980s and 1990s, the National Institute of Nutrition (NIN) in Hyderabad, Andhra Pradesh state, in Southern India conducted an impact evaluation trial to study the effect of nutritional supplementation in pregnancy on the birth weight of the offspring. A controlled, cluster randomised trial of the nutrition supplementation of pregnant mothers was carried out between 1987 and 1990. Mothers in 15 intervention villages received a nutritional supplement of a locally made preparation "upma" that provided 2.09 MJ and 20–25 g protein to mothers and about 1.25 MJ and 8–10 g protein to children up to 6 years of age, while no supplement was provided to the mothers and children in 14 control villages. All children born between January 1, 1987, and December 31, 1990, in the study villages ($N = 4338$) formed a birth cohort within the trial groups. Mean birth weight recorded within 48 h of delivery and available in 2964 (68%) newborns was higher in the 15 intervention villages (2655(SD 430) g) than that in control villages (2594(SD430) g); the mean difference was 61 g (95% CI 18–104), $p = 0.007$. Incidence of low birth weight was higher (34.3%) in control than in intervention villages (31.3%). The incidence of low birth weight was also lower (27%) in infants born to mothers who consumed supplements at least 3 days in a week compared to those who did so occasionally (36.3%) [15]. Maternal nutritional supplementation had a small but definite impact on birth weight.

Pune Maternal Nutrition Study

The contributory role of maternal nutritional status in the low birth weight scenario was again established in the Pune Maternal Nutrition Study [16].Women in six villages near Pune in the southern Indian state of Maharashtra were studied through pregnancy and assessed for nutrition and physical and metabolic activity, with detailed studies using foetal ultrasound and postnatal growth. The mothers in this study had an average BMI of 18.1 kg/m², while babies weighed 2.7 kg on an average. However, compared to Caucasian babies (average birth weight of 3.5 kg), these babies were thinner by ponderal index (24.1 kg/m³ versus 28.2 kg/m³). However, both subcutaneous and visceral fats were higher in MRI studies in the Indian babies compared to their Caucasian counterparts. This added to the evidence from earlier studies by the Pune team that had established for the first time – the "thin-fat" hypothesis. This posited that Indians had greater levels of fat at lower levels of BMI, and type 2 diabetes in Indian adults was shown to occur at a younger age, in individuals with lower levels of BMI but greater central adiposity, measured by waist-hip ratio [17, 18].The PMNS established that such pathways are established quite early in life.

Maternal Macro- Versus Micronutrients

Further, studies in PMNS mothers established the critical role of micronutrients rather than macronutrients in the diet. Birth size was directly related to a higher intake of green leafy vegetables, fruit and milk. The mothers had high levels of vitamin B12 deficiency (nearly 70%), with 90% of these women showing high methylmalonic acid (MMA) levels (≥ 0.26 μmol/L) – a specific indicator of vitamin B 12 deficiency. The low B12 levels, rather than folate levels, were associated with prevalence of high homocysteine levels (30%). Higher maternal total homocysteine levels predicted lower birth weight for gestational age [20].The role of 1-C metabolism that involves the donation and regeneration of 1-C groups, including the methyl group, has since been widely debated [21]. Maternal nutrition should provide an adequate supply of methyl donors such as folate, vitamin B12, betaine, methionine and choline – all important nutrients essential for optimal foetal organogenesis, growth and development [22]. The Pune work has shown the association of these maternal micronutrients in predicting birth weight, body composition, insulin resistance and cognitive function of the offspring of PMNS mothers [23, 24].

Pune Intervention Study

An ongoing randomised controlled trial – Pune Intervention Study that involves adolescent males and females receiving a daily supplement for at least 3 years or until their first delivery – seeks to test the role of pre-conception nutrition. The micronutrient supplement composition based on the United Nations Multiple Micronutrient Preparation (UNIMAP) formulation [25] provides approximately one recommended dietary allowance (RDA) of 15 vitamins and minerals. The findings from this study will add to the evidence base for appropriate nutrients even from adolescence to have optimal foetal growth and birth outcomes.

Mumbai SARAS Kids Study

A similar intervention study among women in an urban Mumbai (Maharashtra state, India) slum provided micronutrient-rich foods in the form of a snack made from green leafy vegetables, fruit and milk, before and throughout pregnancy. The study enrolled 6513 women, 2067 babies were born, and the birth weight in the intervention group was greater by 26 g ($p = 0.20$), with a slightly greater difference of 48 g ($p = 0.05$) if women started the supplement >3 months before conception. The study interestingly found a significant interaction with maternal BMI; there was no effect on newborn weight in mothers in the lowest BMI category (<18.6 kg/m^2) compared to those born to mothers in the higher BMI categories (BMI>18.6 kg/m^2) [26].The children in this cohort are currently being followed for assessment of cardiometabolic risk factors and cognitive function.

Longitudinal Studies

Studies of a prospective nature established in India have provided a rich repository of data to evaluate the Barker hypothesis.

Retrospective Studies

Mysore Birth Cohort

A retrospective hospital records-based study in Holdsworth Memorial Hospital in Mysore, Karnataka state, in South India [27] corroborated the low birth weight-later NCD risk evidence base in an Indian setting. Men and women, born between 1934 and 1954, were retraced using their hospital records several years later. Those with the lowest birth weights, shorter birth lengths and smaller head circumferences had a higher prevalence of coronary heart disease, when assessed between 40 and 70 years [28] (Fig. 27.5). The relation of offspring coronary heart disease to lower maternal weights was also shown, again pointing to the importance of adequate nourishment of pregnant mothers and the consequent cyclical intergenerational effects. Those in the lowest birth weight categories in this cohort were also prone to higher levels of insulin resistance [29] (Fig. 27.6).

Hyderabad Nutrition Trial Follow-Up

The children born within the Hyderabad Nutrition Trial mentioned earlier were retraced at adolescence and assessed for cardiovascular risk factors. Among 1165 adolescents 11–15 years of age, offspring of mothers within the intervention group were taller and had a lower level of insulin resistance and

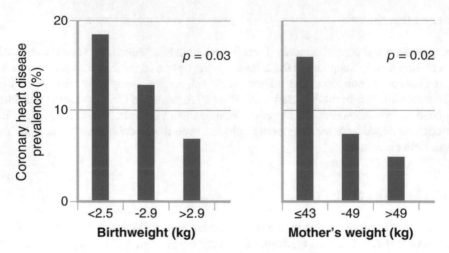

Fig. 27.5 Prevalence (%) of coronary heart disease in men and women aged >45 years in Mysore, India

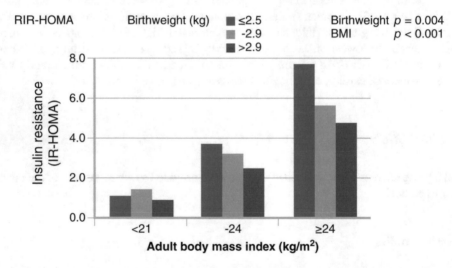

Fig. 27.6 Relative insulin resistance (HOMA) – men born in HMH, Mysore, South India 1934–1954 (*n* = 266)

vascular function assessed by augmentation index. This was early pragmatic evidence that better early life nutrition apparently translated into both improved birth weight and improved cardiovascular risk profile at adolescence [30].

Prospective Studies

New Delhi Birth Cohort (NDBC)

Two longitudinal studies were established in India in 1969 in New Delhi (North India) and Vellore (South India) to study the long-term outcomes of pregnancy in these semiurban/urban populations. In the post-Barker research environment of the 1980s, these birth cohorts served as the ideal populations to test the hypothesis in a developing country setting, with particular emphasis on early childhood and adult outcomes.

A geographically defined area in an urban community in South Delhi (12 km² area) was selected. All families living there between December 1, 1969, and November 30, 1972, were identified. Among a population of nearly 120,000, there were 20,755 married women of reproductive age (13–49 years) who were assessed every other month (±3 days) at home in order to record menstrual dates. Women who became pregnant were seen by a health visitor every 2 months (±3 days) initially and on alternate days from the 37th week of gestation. There were 9169 pregnancies resulting in 8181 live births (8030 singletons and 151 from twin pairs), 202 stillbirths and 867 abortions. Trained personnel recorded the weight and length/height and head circumference of the babies within 72 h of birth and then at the ages of 3, 6, 9 and 12 months (±7 days) and 6 monthly intervals (+15 days) thereafter until 20 years of age. The NDBC saw intermittent phases of revival and data collection. While the initial phases saw the collection of anthropometric data on the birth cohort from birth until 20 years of age, the revival in 1995 of the cohort of young adults (26–32 years) added to the repository, data on cardiometabolic disorders.

Studies in the New Delhi birth cohort were therefore the first to use comprehensive growth data from birth through childhood to exemplify that those born small, having accelerated childhood growth and crossing over earlier into higher centiles of BMI categories, were those most prone to adult cardiometabolic disorders [31] Early age at adiposity rebound (the age at which BMI starts to rise) was clearly shown to be a risk factor for later disease. The detailed anthropometric measurements provided data to establish growth patterns using BMI. When assessed as young adults, those who were small at birth and in infancy and showed rapid childhood weight gain had greatest propensity to develop impaired fasting glucose (Fig. 27.7), dyslipidaemia, higher blood pressure and features of the metabolic syndrome compared to the average cohort growth rate [32].

This cohort also showed how the rapid nutritional and epidemiological transitions in India can translate into an escalation of risk factors for chronic disease over a very short period of time [33]. The prevalence rates of high blood pressure and impaired fasting glucose levels showed significant increases over a period of 6 years in this adult cohort. Additional research contributed to the evidence base on the associations between early life factors and later disease risk patterns, including impaired fasting glucose, dyslipidaemia, hypertension, obesity and impaired bone metabolism [34–36]. This New Delhi cohort has under follow-up children in the next generation with new studies focusing on mental health, pulmonary and cardiac function of the adults and growth and development of their children in relation to intergenerational influences.

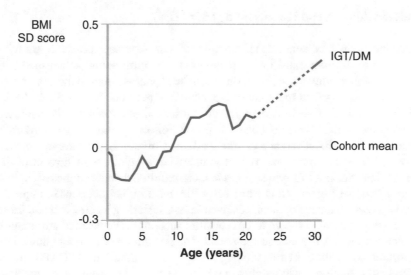

Fig. 27.7 New Delhi: childhood BMI of men and women who developed diabetes or prediabetes, 230 out of 1518, aged 30 years

Vellore Birth Cohort

The original study sample was based on a population census carried out in defined areas of Vellore town and adjoining rural villages in Southern India, representing different socio-economic strata. All married non-pregnant women of childbearing potential in the study areas were identified, and 20,626 women (rural 11,628; urban 8998) were recruited. If found pregnant, the woman was enrolled in a pregnancy follow-up, and on delivery, birth measurements were recorded and an infancy follow-up commenced. Thus, this birth cohort is defined as all children born to these women during the period, 1969–1973.The average BMI of pre-pregnant mothers was 18.6 and 19.4 kg/m² in rural and urban areas, respectively. There were 10,670 single live-born babies (rural 6260; urban 4410), and 4092 had complete birth and parental measurements [37]. All the babies were examined and measured at birth with monthly follow-up up to the first 3 months and thereafter every 3 months up to 1 year. Infant height and weight measurements were made only up to 3 months, while head and chest circumferences, breastfeeding pattern, morbidity and mortality were recorded at each of the follow-ups.

Women who were themselves small at birth had nearly three times the risk of delivering low birth babies [38]. Glucose intolerance, insulin resistance and other cardiometabolic risk factors, including blood pressure and lipid abnormalities, were studied in relation to parental size, neonatal size and childhood growth [39]. These findings added to the evidence base in India testing the Barker hypothesis.

The Pune Children's Study

The Pune Children's study in 1991 showed that children with lower birth weight were more insulin resistant at 4 years of age [40]; at 8 years, the same children were heavier and had the highest levels of cardiovascular risk factors [41]. This again points to the dual role of lower birth weight and factors in the postnatal life that perpetuates the chronic disease risk.

Life-Course Studies in India

Andhra Pradesh Children and Parents Study (APCAPS)

The Hyderabad Nutrition Trial cohort is an exemplar of a life-course approach to studying the evolution of cardiovascular risk in a transitioning population. The birth cohort established within the trial was followed up as young adults. Studies during these later phases enrolled the cohort members, their parents and siblings to establish the Andhra Pradesh Children and Parents Study (APCAPS) [42]. Living within a transitioning socio-economic and nutritional environment, the adolescent children who had earlier shown better cardiovascular risk profile following early maternal nutritional supplementation seemed to lose the advantage as young adults. Children in the intervention villages of the earlier trial showed similar, if not worse, risk as compared to the children in the control sites (personal communication). The diet and lifestyle changes in these children that accompanied rapid urbanisation were important causative factors. Thus while early life nutrition is important in improving the birth weight and early growth and development, postnatal factors including healthy diet and lifestyle patterns across the life course were also shown to be crucial in sustaining the accrued advantage of early life nutrition supplementation. A life-course approach to the prevention of non-communicable diseases is therefore important, particularly in transitioning countries like India. The APCAPS cohort provided a classical example of changing lifestyles affecting later life health status within a generation that faced rapid social and environmental change within a span of a decade. Thus earlier evidence from another study – Indian Migration study – which showed the trends across rural-migrant-urban populations to steadily adopt the diet and lifestyle behaviours of the adoptive place of residence, moving to consumption of more energy-dense foods and sedentary behaviour, was further confirmed [3].

The above overview of Indian studies emphasises the role of adequate maternal macro- and micro-nutrients from adolescence to adulthood, pregnancy and lactation to ensure optimal nourishment and growth and development of the foetus. Early maternal nutrition together with postnatal factors including diet, physical activity and socio-economic influences across the life course has a synergistic role in the development of chronic diseases and their risk factors.

Strategies for prevention should therefore be cognisant of the need to include action and policies that encompass the entire spectrum of nutrition-sensitive and nutrition-specific interventions, disease prevention and health promotion strategies. India has taken initial steps in this direction, and below is an outline of the broader domains of action over the last few years.

Strategies for Nutrition Policies to Address Malnutrition India

In an environment where poverty exists among plenty, and undernutrition coexists with over-nourishment, India's dual burden of malnutrition requires adequate and appropriate policies to be in place. These should ideally straddle multiple sectors from agriculture, food production, procurement and distribution, food subsidies, water, sanitation and hygiene measures, apart from the health and development sectors of women and child ministries. India has initiated a number of programmes and policies to deal with its burden of malnutrition.

The previously mentioned *Integrated Child Development Scheme (ICDS)* was a flagship programme established in 1975 by the Government of India and was envisaged to achieve universal coverage. As with all such mammoth nationwide exercises, this programme too saw multiple hurdles including the effective roll-out, gaps in uptake and utilisation and barriers in 100% coverage across the delivery centres. Nevertheless, the ICDS programme has remained as one of the most effective of national programmes in reaching out to the remotest of regions to deliver its objectives, achieving nearly 100% coverage across the country over the years. Apart from nutritional supplements, early child care, growth and development monitoring and other programmes including anaemia control and immunisation were simultaneously delivered through the core delivery centres – the anganwadis. "Anganwadi" literally means a courtyard and functions as the centre for delivery of the nutrition and education components of the ICDS programme. It functions through the deployment of a team comprising a locally appointed woman as the teacher aided in her tasks by a helper, both being provided incentives for their targeted delivery of services to pregnant, lactating women and children below 6 years of age.

The *National Nutrition Policy of 1993* was a first in placing nutrition in the context of development. However undernutrition was a major focus of this programme and obesity remained conspicuously out of its ambit.

The *National Food Security Bill 2013* has as its objective *"to provide for food and nutritional security in human life cycle approach, by ensuring access to adequate quantity of quality food at affordable prices to people to live a life with dignity"*.

Under the provisions of the bill, beneficiaries of the public distribution system were entitled to 5 kg (11 lb) per person per month of cereals at prices ranging from rice at 3 INR (4.8¢ US) per kg to wheat at 2 INR (3.2¢ US) per kg and coarse grains (millet) at 1INR (1.6¢ US) per kg. Pregnant and lactating women and certain categories of children are eligible for free meals.

There are several other programmes and policy initiatives in India to combat undernutrition, and these are summarised in the table below (Table 27.1).

On policies to tackle, the overweight and obesity burden, taxation on sugar-sweetened beverages and policies for food labelling and modification of processed foods have been advocated. The use of

Table 27.1 Programmes and policy initiatives in India for nutrition

Policies	Strategic documents/reports
National Nutrition Policy, 1993	National Plan of Action for Children, 2005
National Health Policy, MoHFW (2002)	Report of the Working Group on Integrating Nutrition with Health(11th Five Year Plan, 2007–2012)
Policy on Infant and Young Child Feeding (2004)	5-Year strategic Plan (2011–2016), (Towards a New Dawn) Ministry of Women and Child Development (MoWCD)
Policy on Control of Anemia, MoHFW (2004)	Working Group on Food and Nutrition Security, Planning Commission, 2006
Policy on Micronutrient Vitamin A, MoHFW	Recommendations for a Reformed and Strengthened ICDS, National Advisory Council (NAC)
Guidelines for Administration of Zinc Supplements (Diarrhea Management, 2007)	Draft Policy Note on Nutrition and Health, submitted to MoHFW, 2007
National Iodine Deficiency Disorder Control Program (1992)	ICDS and Nutrition in the 11th 5-Year Plan
Operational Guidelines on Facility-based Management of Children with Severe Acute Malnutrition (SAM) (2011)	Report of the Inter-Ministerial group on ICDS Restructuring 2011
Operational Framework for Weekly Iron-Folic Acid (WIFS) tablets to Adolescent Girls (2011)	Report of the Working Group on Nutrition for the XIIth 5-Year Plan(2012–2017)
Provision of supplementary feeding to pregnant and lactating children and children <6 (ICDS)	India Health Report: Nutrition 2015

Source: Health Communication Division, Public Health Foundation of India
ICDS Integrated Child Development Scheme, *MoHFW* Ministry of Health and Family Welfare, *NAC* National Advisory Committee, *MoWCD* Ministry of Women and Child Development

added salt to cooked meals is a social custom in many parts of India that is not readily amenable to change. Policies on dietary restriction of salt and salt restriction in processed foods are therefore fraught with regulatory hurdles and are yet to be rolled out effectively. On the other hand, fortification of salt with iodine in the light of iodine deficiency disorders was welcomed and effectively implemented some years ago.

Conclusions

Maternal malnutrition is predominantly affecting transitioning societies like India, with a dual burden of undernutrition and overnutrition evident across all socio-economic strata.

Overall, the Indian scenario is an exemplar of a transitioning population faced with a dual burden of under- and overnutrition, and the policymakers need a holistic approach across multisectoral domains to combat the problems resulting from maternal malnutrition, foetal programming and later life adverse health outcomes, particularly non-communicable diseases.

References

1. Victora CG, Adair L, Fall C, Hallal PC, Martorell R, Richter L, et al. Maternal and child undernutrition: consequences for adult health and human capital. Lancet [Internet]. 2008;371(9609):340–57. [cited 2013 Dec 11].
2. India Health Report-Nutrition-2015. http://www.transformnutrition.org/india-health-report-on-nutrition-2015/.
3. Ebrahim S, Kinra S, Bowen L, Andersen E, Ben-Shlomo Y, Lyngdoh T, et al. The effect of rural-to-urban migration on obesity and diabetes in India: a cross-sectional study. PLoS Med [Internet]. 2010;7(4):e1000268. [cited 2013 Dec 28].

4. Fall C. Maternal nutrition: effects on health in the next generation. Indian J Med Res [Internet]. 2009;130(5):593–9. [cited 2013 Dec 28].
5. Barker DJ, Fall CH. Fetal and infant origins of cardiovascular disease. Arch Dis Child [Internet]. 1993;68(6):797–9.l. [cited 2016 Apr 14].
6. Fall CHD. Fetal programming and the risk of noncommunicable disease. Indian J Pediatr [Internet]. 2013;80(Suppl 1(0 1)):S13–20. [cited 2016 Jun 9].
7. Why 1000 days. http://thousanddays.org/the-issue/why-1000-days/.
8. Gluckman PD, Hanson MA, Beedle AS. Early life events and their consequences for later disease: a life history and evolutionary perspective. Am J Hum Biol [Internet]. 2007;19(1):1–19. [cited 2016 Jul 7].
9. Wells JCK. The thrifty phenotype as an adaptive maternal effect. Biol Rev Camb Philos Soc. 2007;82:143–72.
10. Martyn CN, Barker DJ, Osmond C. Mothers' pelvic size, fetal growth, and death from stroke and coronary heart disease in men in the UK. Lancet [Internet]. 1996;348(9037):1264–8. [cited 2013 Dec 28].
11. Barker DJ. Fetal origins of cardiovascular disease. Ann Med [Internet]. 1999;31(Suppl 1):3–6. [cited 2013 Dec 13].
12. Hales CN, Barker DJ. The thrifty phenotype hypothesis. Br Med Bull [Internet]. 2001;60:5–20. [cited 2016 Jul 7].
13. Law CM, de Swiet M, Osmond C, Fayers PM, Barker DJ, Cruddas AM, et al. Initiation of hypertension in utero and its amplification throughout life. BMJ [Internet]. 1993;306(6869):24–7. [cited 2016 Jul 7].
14. Integrated Child Development Services. http://icds-wcd.nic.in/icds/.
15. Annual Reports -National Institute of Nutrition. http://ninindia.org/annualreports.htm.
16. Rao S, Yajnik CS, Kanade A, Fall CH, Margetts BM, Jackson AA, et al. Intake of micronutrient-rich foods in rural Indian mothers is associated with the size of their babies at birth: Pune Maternal Nutrition Study. J Nutr [Internet]. 2001;131(4):1217–24. [cited 2016 Mar 11].
17. Shelgikar KM, Hockaday TD, Yajnik CS. Central rather than generalized obesity is related to hyperglycaemia in Asian Indian subjects. Diabet Med [Internet]. 1991;8(8):712–7. [cited 2016 Jul 7].
18. Yajnik CS. The lifecycle effects of nutrition and body size on adult adiposity, diabetes and cardiovascular disease. Obes Rev [Internet]. 2002;3(3):217–24. [cited 2013 Dec 28].
19. Yajnik CS, Fall CHD, Coyaji KJ, Hirve SS, Rao S, Barker DJP, et al. Neonatal anthropometry: the thin-fat Indian baby. The Pune Maternal Nutrition Study. Int J Obes Relat Metab Disord [Internet]. 2003;27(2):173–80. [cited 2013 Dec 28].
20. Yajnik CS, Frcp M, Deshpande Msc SS, Panchanadikar Phd AV, Naik Phd SS, Deshpande Msc JA, et al. Maternal total homocysteine concentration and neonatal size in India. Asia Pac J Clin Nutr. 2005;14(2):179–81.
21. Yajnik CS, Deshmukh US. Fetal programming: maternal nutrition and role of one-carbon metabolism. Rev Endocr Metab Disord [Internet]. 2012;13(2):121–7. [cited 2016 Jul 7].
22. Dominguez-Salas P, Cox SE, Prentice AM, Hennig BJ, Moore SE. Maternal nutritional status, C(1) metabolism and offspring DNA methylation: a review of current evidence in human subjects. Proc Nutr Soc [Internet]. 2012;71(1):154–65. [cited 2016 Jul 7].
23. Yajnik CS, Deshpande SS, Jackson AA, Refsum H, Rao S, Fisher DJ, et al. Vitamin B12 and folate concentrations during pregnancy and insulin resistance in the offspring: the Pune Maternal Nutrition Study. Diabetologia [Internet]. 2008;51(1):29–38. [cited 2016 Mar 8].
24. Bhate V, Deshpande S, Bhat D, Joshi N, Ladkat R, Watve S, et al. Vitamin B12 status of pregnant Indian women and cognitive function in their 9-year-old children. Food Nutr Bull. 2008;29(4):249–54.
25. Margetts BM, Fall CHD, Ronsmans C, Allen LH, Fisher DJ, Maternal Micronutrient Supplementation Study Group. Multiple micronutrient supplementation during pregnancy in low-income countries: review of methods and characteristics of studies included in the meta-analyses. Food Nutr Bull [Internet]. 2009;30(4 Suppl):S517–26. [cited 2016 Jul 7].
26. Potdar RD, Sahariah SA, Gandhi M, Kehoe SH, Brown N, Sane H, et al. Improving women's diet quality preconceptionally and during gestation: effects on birth weight and prevalence of low birth weight – a randomized controlled efficacy trial in India (Mumbai Maternal Nutrition Project). Am J Clin Nutr [Internet]. 2014;100(5):1257–68. [cited 2016 Apr 14].
27. Krishna M, Kalyanaraman K, Veena SR, Krishanveni GV, Karat SC, Cox V, et al. Cohort profile: the 1934–66 Mysore birth records cohort in South India. Int J Epidemiol. 2015;44(6):1833–41.
28. Stein CE, Fall CH, Kumaran K, Osmond C, Cox V, Barker DJ. Fetal growth and coronary heart disease in south India. Lancet. 1996;348(9037):1269–73.
29. Fall CHD, Stein CE, Kumaran K, Cox V, Osmond C, Barker DJP, et al. Size at birth, maternal weight, and type 2 diabetes in South India. Diabet Med. 1998;15(3):220–7.
30. Kinra S, Rameshwar Sarma KV, Ghafoorunissa MVVR, Ravikumar R, Mohan V, et al. Effect of integration of supplemental nutrition with public health programmes in pregnancy and early childhood on cardiovascular risk in rural Indian adolescents: long term follow-up of Hyderabad nutrition trial. BMJ [Internet]. 2008;337:a605. [cited 2013 Dec 28].
31. Bhargava SK, Sachdev HS, Fall CHD, Osmond C, Lakshmy R, Barker DJP, et al. Relation of serial changes in childhood body-mass index to impaired glucose tolerance in young adulthood. N Engl J Med [Internet]. 2004;350(9):865–75. [cited 2013 Dec 28].

32. Sachdev HPS, Osmond C, Fall CHD, Lakshmy R, Ramji S, Dey Biswas SK, et al. Predicting adult metabolic syndrome from childhood body mass index: follow-up of the New Delhi birth cohort. Arch Dis Child. 2009;94:768–74.

33. Huffman MD, Prabhakaran D, Osmond C, Fall CHD, Tandon N, Lakshmy R, et al. Incidence of cardiovascular risk factors in an Indian urban cohort results from the New Delhi birth cohort. J Am Coll Cardiol [Internet]. 2011;57(17):1765–74. [cited 2013 Dec 28].

34. Khalil A, Huffman MD, Prabhakaran D, Osmond C, Fall CHD, Tandon N, et al. Predictors of carotid intima-media thickness and carotid plaque in young Indian adults: the New Delhi birth cohort. Int J Cardiol [Internet]. 2013;167(4):1322–8. [cited 2013 Dec 28].

35. Tandon N, Fall CHD, Osmond C, Sachdev HPS, Prabhakaran D, Ramakrishnan L, et al. Growth from birth to adulthood and peak bone mass and density data from the New Delhi birth cohort. Osteoporos Int [Internet]. 2012;23(10):2447–59. [cited 2014 Apr 15].

36. Lakshmy R, Fall CH, Sachdev HS, Osmond C, Prabhakaran D, Biswas SD, et al. Childhood body mass index and adult pro-inflammatory and pro-thrombotic risk factors: data from the New Delhi birth cohort. Int J Epidemiol. 2011;40:102–11.

37. Antonisamy B, Raghupathy P, Christopher S, Richard J, Rao PSS, Barker DJP, et al. Cohort profile: the 1969–73 Vellore birth cohort study in South India. Int J Epidemiol [Internet]. 2009;38(3):663–9. [cited 2016 Feb 29].

38. Agnihotri B, Antonisamy B, Priya G, Fall CHD, Raghupathy P. Trends in human birth weight across two successive generations. Indian J Pediatr [Internet]. 2008;75(2):111–7. [cited 2013 Dec 28].

39. Raghupathy P, Antonisamy B, Geethanjali FS, Saperia J, Leary SD, Priya G, et al. Glucose tolerance, insulin resistance and insulin secretion in young south Indian adults: relationships to parental size, neonatal size and childhood body mass index. Diabetes Res Clin Pract [Internet]. 2010;87(2):283–92. [cited 2013 Dec 28].

40. Yajnik CS, Fall CH, Vaidya U, Pandit AN, Bavdekar A, Bhat DS, et al. Fetal growth and glucose and insulin metabolism in four-year-old Indian children. Diabet Med [Internet]. 1995;12(4):330–6. [cited 2013 Dec 28].

41. Bavdekar A, Yajnik CS, Fall CH, Bapat S, Pandit AN, Deshpande V, et al. Insulin resistance syndrome in 8-year-old Indian children: small at birth, big at 8 years, or both? Diabetes [Internet]. 1999;48(12):2422–9. [cited 2013 Dec 28].

42. Kinra S, Radha Krishna KV, Kuper H, Rameshwar Sarma KV, Prabhakaran P, Gupta V, et al. Cohort profile: Andhra Pradesh Children and Parents Study (APCAPS). Int J Epidemiol. 2014;43(5):1417–24.

Chapter 28
Maternal Nutritional Factors Dictating Birth Weights: African Perspectives

Baba Usman Ahmadu

Key Points

- Baby's birthweight (BW) in Africa is influenced by maternal stature, weight, composition and metabolism, all of which are determined by maternal nutrition.
- Maternal food security in Nigeria and Africa at large can easily be evaluated by the use of simple indicator known as Household Dietary Diversity Score (HDDS), built on 12 food groups namely: (a) Cereals, (b) Roots or tubers, (c) Vegetables, (d) Fruits, (e) Meat, poultry and offal, (f) Eggs, (g) Fish or shellfish, (h) Beans, peas, lentils, or nuts, (i) Cheese, yoghurt, milk, or other milk products, (j) Oil, fat, or butter, (k) Sugar or honey and (l) Other foods.
- Many international bodies monitor food availability in Africa. They include Food and Agriculture Organization, International Association for Food Protection, International Food Information Council, World Resources Institute and World Food Programme etc.
- Physical environment, political economy, cultural and religious values determine maternal food consumption and ultimately baby's BW in Africa.
- The weight of a baby to an extent depend on foetal supply line. Starved and stunted mothers mostly found in Africa have both macro and micronutrient deficiencies and are more likely to have small babies with low birth weight (LBW).
- Embryonic mass is characterized by inner and outer cell mass both are dependent on maternal nutrition. Therefore, maternal under nutrition widely seen in Africa is associated with reduce embryonic cell density leading to LBW. Adequate maternal nutrition improves fetal growth velocity to normal range of BW. Maternal obesity (high caloric/energy intake) can further increase foetal

B.U. Ahmadu (MBBS, MHPM, FMCPaed) (✉)
Fellow National Postgraduate Medical College Nigeria, Paediatrics (FMCPaed). Member Paediatric Association of Nigeria (PAN), Member Medical and Dental Consultant Association of Nigeria (MDCAN), Member Nigerian Medical Association (NMA). Paediatrician and Visiting Paediatrician at Federal Medical Centre Yola, Abubakar Tafawa Balewa Teaching Hospital Bauchi and Federal Medical Centre Jalingo. Chair, Co-Chair and Member of Committees, Yola, Adamawa State, Nigeria
e-mail: ahmadu4u2003@yahoo.com

© Springer International Publishing AG 2017
R. Rajendram et al. (eds.), *Diet, Nutrition, and Fetal Programming*,
Nutrition and Health, DOI 10.1007/978-3-319-60289-9_28

growth trajectory producing big (macrosomic) babies. The later trend has been observed in emerging African cities like Lagos, Nigeria, Soweto, South-Africa, Gaborone, Botswana etcetera.

- Traditionally, the African society gets its food through hunting activity, gathering and farming. Now, food pattern in Africa runs two major parallels. Urbanization has favored the consumption of high caloric/energy food. Consequences being maternal obesity and macrosomic babies. Food insecurity has led to consumption of food low in calories, thus, favoring under nutrition and LBW.
- High energy food generates high levels of amino acid, pyruvate and lactate for energy to support foetal growth. This is complimented by glucose supply from high sugars. Maternal under nutrition from starvation majorly seen in sub-Saharan Africa results in slowing down of fetal growth trajectory all through pregnancy resulting to a LBW child.
- Financial security is essential to ensure regular supply of food varieties. Household food security in Africa depends chiefly on family income greatly under pressure by food price inflation. Therefore, low-income earners suffer food shortages more than rich households. Mothers found in the low-income category are more vulnerable to LBW delivery.

Keywords Maternal nutrition • Babies' birthweight • African perspectives • Food security • Acculturation • Urbanization • Starvation • Obesity • Anthropology

Abbreviations

BW   Birthweight
HDDS   Household dietary diversity score
HFIAP   Household food insecurity access prevalence
HFIAS   Household food insecurity access scale
ICESCR   International covenant on economic, social and cultural rights
LBW   Low birthweight
MAHFP   Months of adequate household food provision indicator

Introduction

Food is any edible substance basically of plant or animal origin, which contains essential nutrients like carbohydrates, fats, proteins, vitamins, minerals and water. The essence of food in an individual is to provide nutrition, health, energy and to sustain life and growth. Adequate diet is an individual right as enshrined in the International Covenant on Economic, Social and Cultural Rights (ICESCR) [1], which recognized the right to adequate food, the right to be free from hunger and the right to adequate standard of living. Nutrition is the science that interprets the interaction of nutrients and other substances found in food in relation to maintenance, growth, reproduction and health of an individual [2–5]. Nutrients in food are grouped into mainly two categories. One, macronutrients such as fats, proteins and carbohydrates [2–5]. Two, micronutrients such as minerals and vitamins [2–5]. Macronutrient is food required in large quantity, micronutrient on the other hand is food required in small amount. Furthermore, food also contains water and dietary fiber. BW is influenced by many maternal factors interacting with foetal programming sequence. Maternal factors like age, parity are less significant compared to maternal body size (stature), weight, composition and metabolism, all representing mothers' nutritional experience [6]. Babies weighing >3.99 kg are classified as macrosomia, those weighing 2.5–3.99 kg are normal and those <2.5 kg are termed low birth-weight (LBW).

Food Security and Its Evaluation

Food security defined as access to adequate nutritious food that meet dietary needs and preferences for active healthy life is unfortunately being challenged by many factors, poverty being foremost in Africa [2–5, 7]. One-third of the world undernourished is found in Africa. Sufficient, safe and variety of food supply could prevent starvation or obesity, thus, preventing LBW or foetal macrosomia. Out of the four commonly used measures of household food security namely: Household Food Insecurity Access Scale (HFIAS), Household Food Insecurity Access Prevalence (HFIAP), Household Dietary Diversity Score (HDDS) and Months of Adequate Household Food Provision Indicator (MAHFP), HDDS score is more meaningful and nutritionally relevant model widely adopted by African countries [3, 8–10]. It shows the diversity of both macro and micronutrients as well as other food substance an individual eats that amount to adequate nutrition. HDDS is designed on 12 simple food groups namely: (a) Cereals, (b) Roots or tubers, (c) Vegetables, (d) Fruits, (e) Meat, poultry and offal, (f) Eggs, (g) Fish or shellfish, (h) Beans, peas, lentils, or nuts, (i) Cheese, yoghurt, milk, or other milk products, (j) Oil, fat, or butter, (k) Sugar or honey and (l) Other foods. These food varieties are easily accessible in most African states.

Stakeholders Involved in Quality and Safety of Food

Several bodies control and monitor food safety and security in Africa and the world at large. They include Food and Agriculture Organization, International Association for Food Protection, International Food Information Council, World Resources Institute, World Food Programme etc [2, 7, 11] Cereals like guinea corn, millet, maize, wheat, rice etcetera provide most of the staple food in Africa [2–5, 7]. Legumes such as beans, soya beans couple with vegetables, fruits and nuts compliment the cereals. Meat, fish, dairy and their products are consumed mostly by a minute affluent African families [2–4, 7]. Other foods consumed which are not of animal or plant source include things like edible fungi [12], mushrooms for instance. Ambient bacteria [13] are used in the preparation of fermented foods like pap, leavened bread, alcoholic drinks and yogurt among others [2–4, 7, 12, 13]. Salt, baking soda, potash, cream of tartar are few among endless list of food additives used to preserve or chemically alter food ingredient in Africa.

Factors Affecting Maternal Nutrition and Birthweight in Africa

Differences in geopolitical environs, economies, cultural and religious ideology in Africa have underpinned maternal food consumption patterns and might, as well determine BW of babies [3, 4, 7]. The environment of Southern African countries and some Central and West African states are highly productive for agriculture, with favorable soils and rainfall patterns suitable for adequate maternal nutrition that might yield babies with normal range of BW. Saharan and sub-Saharan countries of Africa by contrast are located in semi-arid desert environment which could produce maternal under-nutrition and LBW babies. Most African political economy are un-stable with a negative impact on both maternal nutrition and BW of babies. Some cultures in Africa forbid children consuming meat, others consume it in an unhealthy manner, some serve best portion of food to the father of the house before attending to mother and child, which in most cases feed in groups. Some only permit food considered as halal (food gotten through legal and lawful means). Consumption of nutritious food like vegetables and fish in some African states was partly motivated by cultural philosophies of eating such food with starchy staple. Low consumption of fish in some African communities was not because fish is not available or affordable, but rather people who eat fish are affiliated to inferior cultural groups. Many of these food preferences, food taboos, eating neutral food like beverage and miscellaneous ones like mushroom are purely based on ethno-cultural, socio-religious affiliations that often lead to maternal under-nutrition or obesity, resulting to LBW or macrosomic babies.

Embryology of Maternal Nutrition and Birthweight of Babies

The weight of a baby strongly depend on nutrients and oxygen supply it receives from the mother, otherwise, called foetal supply line [5, 6]. Foetus is undernourished having LBW when its demand for nutrients exceeds supply, as it is the case with starved mothers or placental failure or from excess demand of nutrients by a rapidly growing foetus. Placental failure in Africa is majorly caused by infections like placental malaria, HIV which damages the placenta thereby impeding the flow of nutrient in mother-infant pair. Mothers who are starved have LBW (acute malnutrition) and are most prone to having small babies with LBW [4–6, 14]. Chronic under nutrition also influences BW through its effect on maternal stature, independent of body weight [6, 15]. Short stature may be associated with LBW, whereas, tallness may lead to appropriate BW. Both acute and chronic maternal under nutrition are also linked to deficiencies in specific nutrients like vitamins A, C, D, folate, iron and zinc resulting to a LBW baby [6].

Prior to implantation, the embryo comprised of two types of cell mass, the inner cell mass which will metamorphosed to foetus and the outer cell mass which becomes the placenta [6, 16]. The density of cells in these two cell masses are widely determined by mothers' nutrition [16]. Therefore, maternal under nutrition at the time of conception leads to paucity of cells in the inner and outer cell mass. Aftermath being LBW, atrophied placenta, reduced postnatal growth and altered organ/body weight ratios. Adequate maternal nutrition will raise fetal growth velocity to normal BW limits [6]. Maternal obesity from high caloric/energy consumption can further shoot the foetal growth trajectory producing macrosomic babies.

African Perspective of Maternal Nutrition and Babies' Birthweight

African families by tradition secure food through farming, hunting and gathering. The food is high in carbohydrate and fibre, low in fat, protein and sugar [3, 4, 7]. This is so because cornmeal, rice and other starchy carbohydrates form the basis of most African dishes taking alongside vegetables and fruits [17–20]. Meat, fish, poultry and dairy products are seldom consumed because of poverty amidst large family size. Examples of African dishes are Luhya and Nshima cuisines consumed mostly in Kenya, Ugali or Posho consumed in other parts of East Africa, Sadza in Zimbabwe and Pap in South Africa, Fufu in West Africa; meat, cuscus, olives and dates in North Africa [17–20]. African food is diverse and full of flavor for instance hot spices, chili peppers and peanut sauces are favorites in West Africa [19]. All over Africa, no meal is complete without a starchy component [17–20]. Table 28.1 represents food components of which most African cuisines are made off [17, 18]. The food component are of low to medium calorie with only few exceptions per serving. When mothers eat these food mix rightly, they will maintain normal weight together with their babies.

Currently, most food requirements of the world is highly processed and supplied by food industry, these foods are high in fat, protein and sugar, low in carbohydrate and fibre [3, 4, 7]. Diet play a significant role in mothers' health. The quantity and quality of food eaten are determined by multiple interacting variables. These are media advertisement, time constraint, access to retail outlets and markets, access to cooking, refrigeration and storage facilities. Imbalances between consumed foods results in either starvation and wasting (under nutrition) or obesity (over nutrition). Africa has a growing concern about the paradoxical expansion of both hunger and obesity culminating into LBW or macrosomic deliveries. Meal formats in Africa is presently undergoing evolution, which implies a shift from a local traditional diets containing required energy value to a potentially dense caloric food because of development and urbanization on one hand [3, 5]. On the other hand, low-income, inadequate information from illiteracy, poverty, food insecurity, inadequate government policies and escalation of conflict, war, insurgency and

Table 28.1 Food and energy consumption of a traditional African meal

Food item[a]	Energy in Cal per 100 g (3.5 oz.) serving	Remarks
Cereals	135–310	Low–medium Cal
Vegetables	8–130	Very low-low Cal
Fruits	10–235	Low–medium Cal
Pepper	16	Very low Cal
Peanut sauce	581	High Cal
Food item[b]		
Meat and meat product	150–400	Low-high Cal
Fish and fish product (sea food)	90–490	Low-high Cal
Dairy and dairy products	80–440	Low-high Cal

Cal calorie
[a]Food item often consumed
[b]Food item seldom consumed

famine among others had led to low caloric/energy intake with rising cases of maternal under nutrition and LBW babies [2, 3, 5]. Pinstrup-Anderson described Africa's hunger problems as a triple burden of malnutrition, where hunger, micronutrient deficiencies and obesity co-exist [21].

Transition to Urbanization in Africa

Urbanization in African societies had led to individuals squatting in camps and in informal houses with poor sanitation and sewage disposal. No portable water supply, epileptic electricity and inadequate utilities. Meals have to be cooked on kerosene stoves or with fire wood. Individuals are separated from their families, which calls for adjustment of people to new surroundings. People work longer hours far away from home as such patronize fast foods, which are more available, affordable and contain energy as high as 3470 kcal/capita/day [5, 6, 17–20, 22]. Lifestyle changes are that of increased sedentary lifestyle, high alcohol intake and a change in dietary patterns. A more of European diet (fast food) high in energy, containing more salt, high saturated fat and fat soluble vitamins A, D, E and likes, high protein and sugar is consumed [5, 7, 17–20]. Consumption of fibre, vitamins and minerals are low because less fruits and vegetables are eaten [5, 7, 17–20]. Mothers on this kind of diet are often obese with a tendency of giving birth to macrosomic babies. The dense protein and fats provides high levels of amino acid, pyruvate and lactate for energy and to maintain foetal growth during first trimester of pregnancy; which might be complimented by glucose supply from high sugars [5, 20]. Similar pattern with a preferential switch to glucose supplying most of the energy for foetal growth is seen during second and third trimester of pregnancy [6, 20]. Table 28.2 lists some fast food, alcoholic beverage as well as their energy content [17, 18].

Human Catastrophe, Starvation and Financial Security

Escalation of human catastrophe [2], particularly, insurgency in Africa has led to many internally displaced people whose families are deprived of food. Ultimately leading to starvation with a devastating and widespread effect on maternal health and LBW deliveries. Food deprivation is regarded as a deficit need in Maslow's hierarchy of needs. Maternal under nutrition results in immediate slowing of fetal growth all through pregnancy giving rise to a LBW child. Financial security is essential to

Table 28.2 Caloric density of fast food, beverages, refined sugar, fruit and vegetable of emerging African cities

Food item[a]	Caloric density per serving	Remarks
FF, Biscuit digestives	480–562 Cal	High calorie
FF, Cheese, Ice creams	180–550 Cal	Medium-high calorie
FF, Sandwich	523 Cal	High calorie
FF, Cakes, Hamburger	375–576 Cal	High calorie
FF, Hotdog, Pancake, Taco	460–5711 Cal	High calorie
Alcoholic beverages	97–245 Cal	Low-medium calorie
Fats and Sugars	400–900 Cal	Medium-high calorie
Carbonated beverages	120–500 Cal	Low-high calorie
Food item[b]		
Fruits and vegetables	8–581 Cal	Very low-high calorie

NB: Standard conversion factors used for energy value of macronutrients: 4 kcal/g of protein, 9 kcal/g of fat, 4 kcal/g of carbohydrate and 7 kcal/g of alcohol [20]
FF Fast food, *Cal* Calorie
[a]Food item consumed often
[b]Food item seldom consumed

Table 28.3 Maternal food preferences occasioned by poverty and food insecurity in Africa

Food item[a]	Caloric density per serving	Remarks
Macaroni	95 Cal	Low calorie
Noodles	70 Cal	Low calorie
Plain porridge	55 Cal	Low calorie
Bread	220 Cal	Low-medium calorie
Spaghetti	101 Cal	Low calorie
Rice	140 Cal	Low calorie
Fruit and vegetable	8–130 Cal	Low calorie
Oils	900 Cal	High calorie
Table sugar	400 Cal	Medium-high calorie
Food item[b]		
Meat, fish and poultry	50–500 Cal	Low-high calorie
Milk and dairy product	38–600 Cal	Low-high calorie
Beverages	124–500 Cal	Low-high calorie

Cal calorie
[a]Frequently consumed food
[b]Less frequently consumed food

ensure regular supply of food choices macro and micronutrient for consumption. Household food security in Africa depends principally on household income that is greatly affected by food price inflation. Low-income households suffer food shortages more than rich ones. Because of poverty, poor homes depend more on low calorie cereals for a staple food producing less than 2500 kcal/capita/day [5, 6, 17, 18, 20, 22], as shown in Table 28.3. Mothers found in this category are more vulnerable to LBW delivery. Therefore, political will, enriching economic policies, maternal nutrition education etcetera must be revamped and strengthened to mitigate food insecurity, avert food crisis situation due to hunger and starvation. Disaster, conflict and refugee problems must be managed effectively and efficiently. This can be done via national emergency response squad or a task force committee mandated to coordinate food supply and other stuffs to the affected to prevent starvation and its dire effect on foetal weight.

Conclusions

The influence of maternal nutrition on BW of a child cannot be overemphasized. Maternal nutrition in Africa is a bit complex because of events and global acculturation. Originally the traditional African diet which is low in fat and protein, high in unrefined carbohydrates, vegetables, legumes, nuts and fruit has undergone a shift. Urbanization has led to a choice of a high energy/caloric food that has increased level of refined carbohydrate, high fat and salt. Such food also has high sugar examples are sweets, soft drinks, biscuits, cakes and chocolates. Anthropological values had led to maternal deprivation of some important food stuff with negative impact on both maternal-infant pair. Human disasters, poor government policies and diseases had worsened poverty levels and heightened starvation in parts of Africa. These are responsible for maternal consumption of low energy/caloric diet. Whereas, mothers feeding on high energy/caloric food are likely going to give birth to babies with normal BW or macrosomia; those on low energy/caloric diet could end up with LBW babies.

References

1. Health and Human Rights. International covenant on economic, social and cultural rights. www.ohchr.org.
2. Food and Agriculture Organization of the United Nations Rome. Addressing food insecurity in protracted crises. The state of food insecurity in the world; 2010.
3. Alexander FL, Liam R. Food, place, and culture in urban Africa: comparative consumption in Gaborone and Blantyre. J Hung Environ Nutr. 2014;9(2):256–79.
4. Pretorius S, Sliwa K. Perspectives and perceptions on the consumption of a healthy diet in Soweto, an urban African community in South Africa. SAHeart. 2011;8:178–83.
5. Talat JH, Khushnaseeb Ibrahim S, Ejaz A, et al. Maternal factors affecting birth weight of uncomplicated pregnancy. JPMA. 1991;41:164–7.
6. David JPB. The malnourished baby and infant. Br Med Bull. 2001;60:69–88.
7. Drimie S, Faber M, Vearey J, et al. Dietary diversity of formal and informal residents in Johannesburg, South Africa. BMC Public Health. 2013;13:911–1000.
8. Frayne B, Pendleton W, Crush J, et al. The state of urban food insecurity in Southern Africa. Vol No. 2: African Food Security Urban Network (AFSUN); 2010.
9. Coates J, Swindale A, Bilinsky P. Household food insecurity access Scale (HFIAS) for measurement of food access: indicator guide (v.3). Washington, DC: Food and Nutrition Technical Assistance Project, Academy for Educational Development; 2007.
10. Swindale A, Bilinsky P. Household dietary diversity score (HDDS) for measurement of household food access: indicator guide. Washington, DC: Food and Nutrition Technical Assistance Project; 2006.
11. Gillespie S, McLachlan M, Shrimpton R. Combatting malnutrition: time to act. Washington, DC: World Bank; 2003.
12. Guillamón E, García-Lafuente A, Lozano M, et al. Edible mushrooms: role in the prevention of cardiovascular diseases. Fitoterapia. 2010;81(7):715–23.
13. Cavalieri D, McGovern PE, Hartl DL, et al. Evidence for S. cerevisiae fermentation in ancient wine. J Mol Evol. 2003;57(Suppl 1):S226–32.
14. Naeye RL, Blanc W, Paul C. Effects of maternal nutrition on the human fetus. Pediatrics. 1973;52:494–503.
15. Cawley RH, McKeown T, Record RG. Parental stature and birth weight. Ann Hum Genet. 1954;6:448–56.
16. Walker SK, Hartwich KM, Seamark RF. The production of unusually large offspring following embryo manipulation: concepts and challenges. Theriogenology. 1996;45:111–20.
17. Food Calories List. www.weightlossforall.com.
18. USDA National Nutrient Database for Standard Reference, Release 20. Energy content of selected foods per common measure, sorted alphabetically.
19. The BS, Cookbook A. Diane and Leo Dillon (illust). New York: Carol Publishing Group; 1993.
20. Donald R, Lesley B, Debbie B. Food and nutrient availability in South African households: development of a nationally representative database. Health and development research group and the burden of disease research unit technical report, 2002.

21. Pinstrup-Andersen P. The African food system and human health and nutrition: a conceptual and empirical overview. In: Pinstrup-Andersen P, editor. The African food system and its interaction with human health and nutrition. Ithaca: Cornell University Press; 2010. p. 1–13.
22. Lechtig A, Klein RE, Dobbing J, editors. Maternal nutrition in pregnancy – eating for two? London: Academic Press; 1981. p. 131–74.

Chapter 29
Maternal Nutrition in Ireland: Issues of Public Health Concern

John M. Kearney and Elizabeth J. O'Sullivan

Key Points

- The prevalence of obesity is increasing in Ireland, and maternal obesity is a major public health concern. Interventions to promote a healthy weight during pregnancy may need to begin in the pre-conception period.
- The majority of Irish women gain more weight than is recommended during pregnancy. Although one dietary intervention to reduce excessive gestational weight gain has been successful, whether this also improves infant outcomes is unclear.
- The Irish Health Service Executive does not recommend universal screening for gestational diabetes mellitus; only those with pre-specified risk factors are screened. Prevalence of gestational diabetes in Ireland may depend on geographic location; the west of Ireland may be a particular "pocket" with high prevalence.
- Since the 1980s Ireland has had a policy of voluntary fortification with folic acid. Recent increases in incidence rates for NTDs and research suggesting that a significant proportion of women in Ireland have sub-optimal folate status indicate the need to adopt a policy of mandatory fortification.
- A supplement of 400 μg folic acid/daily is recommended periconceptionally but adherence is less than 45% and in decline suggesting more proactive national strategies to communicate its importance periconceptionally for reducing NTD risk.
- Strategies aimed at ensuring optimal intakes are required to improve intakes and status of vitamin D in pregnancy based on current research involving pregnancy-specific requirements and fortification scenarios based on national dietary survey data.
- As alcohol usage both before and during the first trimester of pregnancy in the Irish population is so prevalent, health professionals have an important role in advocating total abstinence from alcohol during pregnancy.

Keywords Perinatal nutrition • Folic acid • Vitamin D • Supplementation • Alcohol usage • Obesity • Gestational weight gain • Gestational diabetes

J.M. Kearney, BSc (Ag), PgDip, PhD (✉) • E.J. O'Sullivan, BA, BSc, PgDip, PhD
Dublin Institute of Technology (DIT), School of Biological Sciences, Dublin, Ireland
e-mail: john.kearney@dit.ie

© Springer International Publishing AG 2017
R. Rajendram et al. (eds.), *Diet, Nutrition, and Fetal Programming*,
Nutrition and Health, DOI 10.1007/978-3-319-60289-9_29

Abbreviations

25(OH)D	25 – hydroxyvitamin D
Atlantic-DIP	Atlantic diabetes in pregnancy
BMI	Body mass index
DHA	Docosahexaenoic acid
EFSA	European Food Safety Authority
EPA	Eicosapentaenoic acid
FSAI	Food Safety Authority of Ireland
GDM	Gestational diabetes mellitus
GUI	Growing up in Ireland
GWG	Gestational weight gain
HSE	Health Services Executive
IADPSG	International Association of Diabetes and Pregnancy Study Groups
ICGP	Irish College of General Practitioners
IOM	Institute of Medicine
IUNA	Irish Universities Nutrition Alliance
LC-PUFA	Long chain polyunsaturated fatty acids
NANS	National adult nutrition survey
NTD	Neural tube defect
OGTT	Oral glucose tolerance test
PRAMS	Pregnancy Risk Assessment Monitoring System
RDA	Recommended daily allowance
RNI	Reference nutrient intake
ROLO	Randomized cOntrol trial of LOw glycaemic index diet to prevent macrosomia in euglycemic women
SCOPE	Screening for Pregnancy Endpoints
SLAN	Survey on lifestyle and attitudes to nutrition
US	United States
WHO	World Health Organization

Introduction

Nutrition before and during pregnancy not only effects fetal growth and development but also the risk of chronic diseases for the infant in adulthood [1]. Nutrient availability for the fetus is influenced by maternal body composition, nutritional stores, diet, as well as the ability of the placenta to transfer nutrients. This chapter aims to explore maternal nutrition in Ireland in terms of outcomes, research and strategies to address a number of the key nutritional issues of concern: pre-pregnancy weight status, gestational weight gain, gestational diabetes, periconceptional nutrition and macro- and micro-nutrient intakes in pregnancy with an emphasis on those nutrients of particular concern in the Irish population (Fig. 29.1). A substantial amount of research has been conducted in the area of maternal nutrition and fetal outcomes in the Republic of Ireland (or Éire, in the Irish language). Nutrition-related issues in the perinatal period fall under two broad problem areas: excessive caloric intakes and inappropriate nutrient intakes. This chapter will examine these two areas of nutritional concern in the Irish context, in each case outlining the extent of the problem and the underlying nutritional causes. In addition, the strategies, policies and clinical guidelines to tackle these nutrition-related concerns will be outlined.

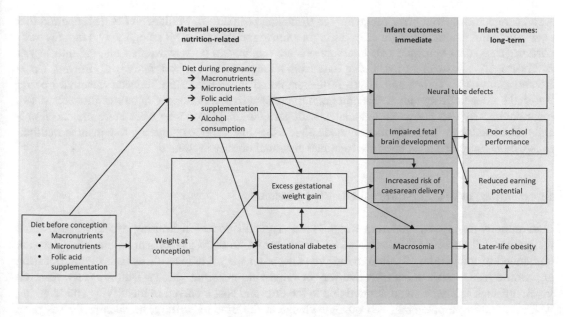

Fig. 29.1 Conceptual framework for issues of concern relating to maternal nutrition in Ireland

Problems Associated with Excessive Caloric Intake

Pre-conception Weight/Maternal Obesity

Ireland is on track to be the most obese nation in Europe by 2030 [2]. The diverse range of health problems for the mother-infant dyad that maternal obesity poses makes maternal weight a major public health nutrition problem in Ireland. Among other things, obesity increases the risk of gestational diabetes, pre-eclampsia, delivery by caesarean section, infant admission to the neonatal unit, infant hypoglycemia, and macrosomia (birthweight ≥4 kg). Delivering by caesarean section and infant admission to the neonatal unit are associated with significant costs to the Irish health service [3], making maternal obesity an issue of both public health *and* economic importance.

Despite the known adverse outcomes associated with obesity, there is no national surveillance system for monitoring weight among Irish women of child-bearing age. Based on data from ~1000 women recruited through the Coombe Women and Infants University Hospital, Fattah and colleagues [4] observed that mean maternal weight was not different among mothers in their first trimester (up to 14 weeks) when grouped by gestational age; the authors concluded that changes in maternal weight during pregnancy occur after the first trimester. Thus, weight at first antenatal visit may be a reasonable proxy for pre-conception BMI among pregnant women in Ireland.

Using weight at first antenatal visit, the prevalence of maternal obesity in Ireland has been reported by different researchers to be 14% [5], 17% [6], 19% [4] and 25% [7]. Maternal obesity is particularly problematic among multigravid women in Ireland. Lynch and colleagues [7] reported that, while 25% of all women attending an antenatal clinic at a tertiary referral centre in the west of Ireland over a 3-year period (2001–2003) were obese, only 20% of primigravid women were obese compared with 29% of multigravid women. McKeating and colleagues [6] reported that prevalence of maternal obesity remained stable at ~17% over a 5-year period (2009–2013) and obesity rates increased with age, social disadvantage, and increased parity. Similarly, in a Dublin, Ireland-based study following maternal weight trajectories from early pregnancy to 9 months postpartum, Mullaney et al. [5] reported that over one in three normal-weight or overweight women moved up 1 BMI category by 4 months post-partum. Thus, they conclude that interventions are required to prevent women moving into higher BMI categories postpartum [5]. Using data from a large national cohort study (the Growing Up in Ireland study) [8], Turner and Layte further explored the relationship between maternal obesity 9 months after delivery and sociodemographic characteristics. Among mothers in this cohort [8], maternal obesity was positively associated with parity among those who were more socioeconomi-cally disadvantaged. These data combined suggest that interventions targeting low-income multipa-rous women might be most effective to reduce maternal obesity in Ireland.

Interventions to Reduce Maternal Obesity in Ireland

Interventions to improve maternal weight status typically focus on limiting excessive gestational weight gain (discussed in the next section). Given that ~47% of pregnancies in developed regions are unplanned or unintended [9], improving pre-conception weight among all women of child-bearing age would likely be the most effective way of improving maternal obesity. Unfortunately, research involving such interventions is limited due to the time and cost involved in identifying and targeting women planning a pregnancy. To our knowledge at the time of writing, no such study has been conducted, or is currently underway, in Ireland.

Policy and Clinical Practice Guidelines Around Management of Maternal Obesity

The Irish Health Service Executive (HSE), in conjunction with the Irish College of General Practitioners (ICGP), have published weight-management guidelines for before, during and after pregnancy [10]. These guidelines were produced to assist general practitioners and primary care staff to prevent, detect, and manage overweight and obesity. The HSE/ICGP recommend that clinicians encourage 5–10% weight loss among overweight women prior to conceiving [10]. The document also highlights that BMI should ideally be in the range 19.0–30.0 kg/m^2 before a woman commences assisted reproduction [10].

Clinical practice guidelines specifically aiming to improve the management of obese women before, during and after pregnancy have also been published by the Clinical Strategy and Programmes Directorate of the HSE in conjunction with the Institute of Obstetricians and Gynaecologists [11]. Similar to the HSE/ICGP guidelines, these clinical practice guidelines highlight the beneficial effects of losing weight prior to conception [11]; however, greater emphasis is placed on providing optimal care for the obese woman during pregnancy. The guidelines provide several nutrition-related recom-mendations, specifically that weight and height be measured at the first antenatal appointment and BMI should be calculated, women who are obese should be advised to take a high dose of folic acid periconceptionally, they should have an oral glucose tolerance test between 24 and 28 weeks' gesta-tion to screen for gestational diabetes mellitus, and they should be provided with extra support to help them initiate and continue breastfeeding [11].

Excessive Gestational Weight Gain

Gestational weight gain (GWG) is a concern because of the association between GWG and negative maternal outcomes (increased risk of caesarean delivery and postpartum weight retention) and nega-tive infant outcomes (increased risk of preterm birth and small- or large-for-gestational-age) [12].

Table 29.1   Institute of medicine gestational weight gain guidelines [12]

Pre-pregnancy BMI	Recommended gestational weight gain range (kg)
Underweight (<18.5 kg/m^2)	12.5–18.0
Normal-weight (18.5–24.9 kg/m^2)	11.5–16.0
Overweight (25–29.9 kg/m^2)	7–11.5
Obese (≥30 kg/m^2)	5–9

Table 29.2   Prevalence of excess gestational weight gain in Ireland as reported by independent researchers

Study authors (reference)	Year(s) of participant recruitment	Sample size	How total GWG was calculated	Excessive GWG by baseline BMI category Presented as the proportion of mothers within each BMI category in each study exceeding the GWG guidelines (%)			
				Underweight	Normal-weight	Overweight	Obese
Heery et al. [13]	2011	799	(Final weight available in pregnancy) – (self-reported pre-pregnancy weight)	42.9	57.8	81.1	62.7
Walsh et al. [14]	2007–2011	621	(Last recorded weight gain at greater than or equal to 37 weeks' gestation) – (measured weight at 1st antenatal visit)	–	21	61	54
O'Dwyer et al. [15]	2011	604	(Measured weight at 38 weeks' gestation) – (measured weight at 1st antenatal visit)	0	3.4	17.5	46.3

The Institute of Medicine (IOM) in the United States (US) developed guidelines for GWG in an American population. These guidelines were originally developed in 1990 and were updated in 2009 due to the increasing proportion of overweight and obesity among women of reproductive age in the US [12]. The IOM recommended weight-gain ranges for pregnant women are stratified by pre-pregnancy BMI (Table 29.1); the higher the pre-pregnancy BMI, the lower the recommended GWG. Although these guidelines are specific to a US population, no such guidelines exist for an Irish population so the US guidelines have been used by some researchers to report prevalence of excessive GWG in Ireland.

In Ireland, several researchers have explored GWG among cohorts of mothers recruited through maternity hospitals [13–15] (Table 29.2). Heery and colleagues [13] recruited a prospective cohort of pregnant women in their first trimester between March and May 2011 in The National Maternity Hospital, Dublin, Ireland. Using the difference between the last weight measured before delivery and self-reported pre-pregnancy weight, they reported the proportion of participants who exceeded the IOM guidelines within each BMI category [13]. Calculation of the proportion of mothers who exceeded the guidelines took the gestational age at the time the final weight was measured into account [13]. Among this sample of 799 women, 4.4% were underweight, 64.7% were normal-weight, 20.5% were overweight, and 10.4% were obese [13]. A total of 62.5% of pregnant women had excessive GWG, and this was most common among overweight women, 81.1% of whom exceeded the guidelines [13] (Table 29.2). A secondary analysis of data collected as part of a large randomised controlled trial conducted at The National Maternity Hospital [14] reported that while 43% of the total sample gained in excess of the IOM guidelines, 21% of normal-weight, 61% of overweight, and 54% of obese women gained above the guidelines (Table 29.2). Finally, among a sample of 604 pregnant women recruited from the Coombe Women and Infants University Hospital in 2011, O'Dwyer and colleagues [15] reported that 1.1% were underweight, 46.4% were normal-weight, 27.2% were overweight, and 25.3% were obese based on their 1st trimester weight. Excessive GWG was observed in 18.3% of the total sample, but was more prevalent among obese pregnant women, 46.3% of whom exceeded the GWG recommendation (Table 29.2) [15].

Excessive GWG may be particularly problematic among Irish mothers as data from the screening for pregnancy endpoints (SCOPE) study indicate that pregnant women in Cork, Ireland were at higher risk of gaining excess GWG than mothers in Adelaide, Australia and mothers in Auckland, New Zealand [16]. The authors of this multi-centre study [16], speculate that societal-cultural factors may explain the excessive GWG in Ireland as mothers may believe that "eating for two" is expected.

The higher proportion of mothers exceeding the GWG guidelines in the study conducted by Heery et al. [13] may be explained by their use of self-reported pre-pregnancy weight, which is often under-reported, as their baseline weight measurement. Despite this limitation and although the number of studies reporting GWG among Irish women is small, Irish women consistently gain more weight than the IOM guidelines, and this is more pronounced among overweight and obese mothers.

Interventions to Prevent Excessive Gestational Weight Gain in Ireland

Preventing excessive GWG was an a priori secondary outcome of the ROLO (Randomized cOntrol trial of LOw glycaemic index diet to prevent macrosomia in euglycemic women) study [17] conducted in The National Maternity Hospital in Dublin, Ireland. McGowan and colleagues reported that a group dietary education session with information about following a low glycaemic index diet before 22 weeks' gestation reduced energy intake and improved glycaemic index among participants in the intervention group [17]. Mothers in this trial who received the dietary intervention gained less weight during pregnancy and were less likely to exceed the IOM GWG guidelines [17], however, there was no difference in infant birthweight between the intervention and control group. A second randomized controlled trial of a lifestyle intervention supported by an app is currently underway at The National Maternity Hospital with the primary aim of reducing gestational diabetes [18]. Gestational weight gain is also a secondary outcome of this intervention; results are yet to be reported [18].

Although there has been a lot of interest in GWG and preventing excess GWG, a group of Irish authors are recommending that we switch focus from monitoring weight during pregnancy to providing advice about physical activity and improving nutritional intakes [19]. A recent prospective observational study by the same group reported no independent association between excess GWG and negative outcomes, but strong independent associations between maternal obesity and negative outcomes [15].

Policy and Clinical Guidelines

To our knowledge, no national policy or clinical guidelines for the management of GWG exist in Ireland. Though some clinicians measure maternal weight throughout pregnancy, it is not systematically measured at each antenatal visit in Ireland. According to the HSE and the Institute of Obstetricians and Gynaecologists "[a]t present, there is insufficient evidence to justify a repeat measurement of maternal weight in all pregnancies" [11]. However, the HSE recommends measurement of body weight at each antenatal visit for pregnancies complicated by gestational diabetes mellitus [20].

Gestational Diabetes Mellitus

Introduction and Prevalence

Gestational diabetes mellitus (GDM) is any form of diabetes or glucose intolerance with first onset during pregnancy [20]. GDM is associated with macrosomia, increased risk of injury to mother and/or baby during the birth, and increased risk of Caesarean section delivery. Table 29.3 provides the prevalence of GDM in the three maternity hospitals in Co. Dublin, Ireland. Together, these hospitals account for ~50% of all Irish births annually.

The Atlantic Diabetes in Pregnancy (Atlantic-DIP) study is a multicentre study established in 2005 involving five antenatal centres on the west coast of Ireland [21]. One of the primary aims of this study was to determine the prevalence of hyperglycaemia during pregnancy. The Atlantic-DIP group compared the prevalence of GDM using the standard criteria from the World Health Organization (WHO) to newer guidelines released by the International Association of Diabetes and Pregnancy Study Groups (IADPSG). All pregnant women who presented to five antenatal centres along the west coast of Ireland were offered screening for GDM at 24–28 weeks' gestation [21]. Of the 12,487 women who were offered the screening, 5500 completed the study; those who consented to participate were slightly older and more overweight than those who did not [21]. Using the new criteria, 12.4% of participants had GDM, compared with 9.4% when using the WHO criteria [21]. GDM, as defined by the IADPSG was associated with adverse maternal and neonatal outcomes; thus, the authors conclude that using the new diagnostic criteria could increase diagnosis of GDM and reduce the associated morbidity for the mother and infant [21]. However, they caution that identifying more women with GDM will place significant burden on the healthcare system.

Of note is the high prevalence of DGM in the Atlantic-DIP cohort. Regardless of the diagnostic criteria used; the proportion of mothers in the Atlantic-DIP study with GDM is higher than the proportions observed in the three Dublin, Ireland-based maternity hospitals (Table 29.3). It has been suggested that there may be "pockets of high prevalence" of GDM, and that the West of Ireland may be one of them, along with Finland and Sardinia [22].

Interventions to Reduce Incidence of Gestational Diabetes Mellitus in Ireland

Although the low glycaemic index dietary advice offered to mothers in the previously mentioned ROLO study [17] resulted in pregnant women in the intervention arm having less glucose intolerance, this intervention had no effect on overt GDM [23]. However, incidence of GDM in this cohort was very low, which would reduce the ability to detect a difference between study arms. A randomized controlled trial of a lifestyle intervention with the primary aim of reducing gestational diabetes is currently underway at The National Maternity Hospital [18].

Table 29.3 Prevalence of gestational diabetes among the patients of three large Dublin, Ireland maternity hospitals (2014)

Hospital	n (% of total live births)
The National Maternity Hospital	258 (2.6%)
The Rotunda Hospital	644 (6.1%)
The Coombe Women and Infants University Hospital	672 (7.3%)

Data obtained from the annual report published by each hospital

Policy and Clinical Guidelines

Universal screening for GDM is controversial; the HSE recommends selective screening for GDM among at-risk pregnant women between 24 and 28 weeks' gestation [20]. At-risk pregnant women (e.g. women who are obese, have a family history of diabetes or have had a previously unexplained perinatal death) are provided with a 75 g oral glucose tolerance test (OGTT) and GDM is diagnosed using the HAPO criteria [24]. The HSE also recommend that women with GDM be treated by a multidisciplinary team, have an increased frequency of hospital visits, and that they should be followed-up postpartum because they are at increased risk of developing Type 2 diabetes. This follow-up should consist of an OGTT at 6 weeks postpartum and yearly there after. Reports of a prospective observational cohort study comparing two models of care in the management of GDM in Ireland have been published this year [25]. This group of researchers compared lifestyle and dietary intervention followed by insulin therapy where necessary managed by a combined obstetric/endocrinology clinic with the same dietary and lifestyle intervention but a midwife-led clinic for glucose monitoring [25]. There were no differences in outcomes between the two models of care; thus, the authors conclude that a stratified model of care may represent a more cost-effective use of healthcare resources [25].

Problems Associated with Inappropriate Nutrient Intakes

Folate

A major public health issue related to maternal nutrition in Ireland is the elevated prevalence of infants born with Neural Tube Defects (NTDs). Along with the UK, Ireland has the highest rates in Europe. Owing to the absence of a comprehensive register of pregnancies affected by NTDs in Ireland, it is difficult to obtain reliable estimates of the current incidence of NTDs. Between 2009 and 2011 the incidence rate increased from 1.04/1000 births in 2009 to 1.17/1000 in 2011, on average 80 NTD births/year [26], a reverse in the trend from the previous decade showing a decline in NTDs.

In Ireland, folate can be obtained from the diet in three ways: natural sources of folate, e.g. leafy green vegetables; foods which are voluntarily fortified with folic acid and food supplements. The HSE, in conjunction with The Institute of Obstetricians and Gynaecologists, has published a clinical practice guideline on Nutrition in Pregnancy [27]. One of their key recommendations states that all women of reproductive age should be advised to take a daily supplement of 400 μg folic acid, or 4 mg if they have a history of NTDs or pre-existing diabetes mellitus, while for obese women it is 4 mg/day (Table 29.4, [27]). Taking folic acid before conception and during the very early stages of pregnancy can prevent up to 70% of NTDs. However, just 44% of Irish mothers comply with this recommendation pre-conception [28–30]. A decline in folic acid supplementation among 42,000 women booking for

Table 29.4 Recommendations for micronutrient supplementation in pregnancy in Ireland [27]

Micronutrient	All women	BMI ≥30 kg/m² obese
Folic acid	400 μg	4 mg
Vitamin B12	No pregnancy specific recommendation for supplementation	–
Vitamin D	5 μg	10 μg
Iodine	No pregnancy-specific national guideline for supplementation	–
Iron	Supplements only recommended for women with a low serum ferritin or those at risk of developing iron-deficiency anaemia	–
Calcium	No pregnancy-specific recommendation	–

antenatal care between 2009 and 2013 in a large maternity hospital in Ireland was seen, with the periconceptional folic acid supplementation rate were decreasing from 45.1% in 2009 to 43.1% in 2013 [29].

The women most likely to take folic acid were those who planned their pregnancy and were >30 years old, non-obese, Irish-born and employed professionally. Even lower rates of folic acid supplementation have been seen in the National Adult Nutrition Survey (NANS), which was carried out between 2008 and 2010 and which did not include pregnant women. Only 2% of women surveyed aged 18–35 years and 1% of women aged 36–50 years consumed the recommended 400 µg folic acid from food supplements [31].

The dietary patterns and associated folate intakes during pregnancy in a cohort of 398 healthy pregnant women were assessed using a food frequency questionnaire in each trimester of pregnancy [32]. Mean daily intakes of total folate were 272 µg/day in pregnancy. Furthermore, intakes of folate did not vary greatly across trimesters. Overall, only 2.1% were compliant with the RDA for folate from dietary sources alone (Table 29.5). Thus, it is clear that action is required to promote the supplementation of folic acid among women in Ireland and to consider other strategies for ensuring adequate folate status.

Table 29.5 Mean daily energy, macro and micronutrient intakes and % compliance to the current recommendations for pregnancy for the total sample and across the clusters during each trimester of pregnancy in Ireland

				Dietary pattern					
	All (n = 285)			Unhealthy (n = 124)		Health conscious (n = 161)		p^b	p^c
	R	Mean (SD)	%C	Mean (SD)	%C	Mean (SD)	%C		
Energy (MJ)	–	8.0 (1.7)	–	8.0 (1.9)	–	8.0 (1.5)	–	–	–
Protein (%TE)	10–15	16.7 (2.3)	23.0	15.9 (2.1)	**32.3**	17.3 (2.2)	**16.0**	<0.001	<0.001
CHO (%TE)	≥55	50.1 (4.9)	15.0	49.9 (5.2)	16.1	50.3 (4.7)	14.1	NS	NS
Total fat (%TE)	<30	36.1 (4.3)	8.0	37.1 (4.4)	6.5	35.4 (4.1)	9.2	0.001	NS
SFA (%TE)	<10	13.9 (2.4)	4.2	14.5 (2.3)	**1.6**	13.4 (2.3)	**6.1**	<0.001	0.058
PUFA (%TE)	5–10	5.7 (1.4)	68.2	11.9 (1.7)	71.8	11.1 (1.6)	65.4	NS	NS
MUFA (%TE)	≤10	11.4 (1.7)	21.0	5.9 (1.4)	**13.0**	5.6 (1.4)	**27.0**	<0.001	0.004
Fibre (g)	20	19.0 (5.4)	38.3	16.4 (4.8)	**15.3**	20.9 (4.9)	**55.8**	<0.001	<0.001
Vitamin A (RE µg)[a]	700	878.9 (426.4)	64.8	742.2 (344.3)	**48.4**	983.0 (453.7)	**77.3**	<0.001	<0.001
Vitamin C (mg)[a]	80	116.4 (67.8)	66.2	93.1 (66.5)	**51.6**	134.1 (63.4)	**77.3**	<0.001	<0.001
Vitamin D (µg)[a]	10	2.7 (1.7)	0.3	2.2 (1.3)	0.0	3.0 (1.8)	0.6	<0.001	NS
Vitamin B_{12} (µg)[a]	1.6	4.5 (1.8)	98.3	4.1 (1.5)	96.8	4.8 (1.9)	99.4	0.001	NS
Folate (µg)[a]	500	272.3 (90.7)	2.1	252.0 (97.5)	2.4	287.7 (82.2)	1.8	<0.001	NS
Calcium (mg)	1200	914.3 (265.7)	12.2	885.9 (291.0)	11.3	935.9 (243.4)	12.9	NS	NS
Iron (mg)	15	11.4 (3.0)	12.5	10.5 (2.7)	**7.3**	12.0 (3.2)	**16.6**	<0.001	0.018
Iodine (µg)	130	136.6 (51.0)	50.5	125.9 (48.5)	**41.1**	144.8 (51.4)	**57.7**	0.002	0.006
Sodium (mg)	2400	2702.5 (642.6)	31.7	2721.2 (674.7)	25.8	2688.3 (618.8)	36.2	NS	NS

Reproduced with permission from the authors [32]

%C, percentage of compliance; R, current Irish and European recommendations for pregnant women (acceptable macronutrient distribution range (AMDR) for macronutrients or the recommended dietary allowances (RDA) for micronutrients or the population target for dietary fibre and sodium)

[a] p value assessed using the Mann-Whitney U test

[b] p value assessing the difference in nutrient intake across the two clusters (one-way ANOVA)

[c] p value assessing the difference in level of compliance to the recommendations for pregnancy (χ^2 test)

Strategies to Increase Folic Acid Intakes

Voluntary fortification of food with folic acid, introduced in the early 1980s, has made a significant contribution to reducing the risk of NTD-affected pregnancies in Ireland. However, the approach has been shown to be less effective than mandatory fortification schemes in countries such as the US and Canada, where rates of NTDs dropped significantly following the introduction of mandatory fortification. Direct evidence in Ireland in support of mandatory fortification is provided by the work of Hopkins et al., involving an analyses of data from the cross-sectional NANS survey [33]. Hopkins and colleagues explored the relative impact of voluntary fortification and supplement use on dietary intakes and biomarker status of folate as measured by red blood cell folate in Irish adults. They found that the consumption of voluntarily fortified foods and/or supplement use was associated with significantly higher dietary intakes and biomarker status of folate in Irish adults. Of particular concern, however, was the fact that just 36% of women of childbearing age in Ireland have blood folate levels that are adequate for optimal protection against NTDs with as many as 20% of young women in Ireland not consuming folic acid at all being non-consumers of supplements or fortified food. Such findings provide the evidence base for the option of mandatory fortification of bread or flour in Ireland to provide about 150 μg of folic acid per day in women of childbearing age, which could reduce the prevalence of NTDs by approximately 30%, being proposed by the FSAI's scientific committee for food [34].

Vitamin D

Vitamin D and its active metabolite 25 –hydroxyvitamin D (25(OH)D) is required for optimal fetal bone development, fetal growth and has a potential role in normal glucose homeostasis while insufficient intakes may result in negative outcomes such as preeclampsia, low birth weight, and an increased incidence of autoimmune diseases [35]. There is a strong association between adequate maternal and neonatal serum levels and optimal bone health in childhood and later life. Deficiency of vitamin D can result in rickets in children and in a study conducted in 2006 in two major Dublin, Ireland paediatric hospitals, 20 cases of rickets in infants and toddlers were identified. In Ireland, due to its high latitude (53° North), sunlight intensity during the winter months is too low to stimulate synthesis of Vitamin D. Thus, dietary intake is required to maintain adequate vitamin D status. Vitamin D occurs naturally in very few foods: oil-rich fish, egg yolks, liver, meat and milk. Alternative dietary sources are fortified foods and nutritional supplements.

A number of cross-sectional dietary surveys have observed the average intake of vitamin D in Irish women of reproductive age (18–50 years) to be below recommended levels [31, 36]. Vitamin D status has been assessed in a sample of 1132 adults in the NANS whereby the influence of season and supplementation practice was also assessed across age- and gender-specific subgroups [37]. Vitamin D status as measured by serum 25(OH)D was influenced by both season and supplementation use. Moreover, while Vitamin D deficiency (<30 nmol/L) was only found in 6% of women, 42.2% of women aged 18–35 years and 38.3% of women aged 36–50 years had levels considered by the Institute of Medicine (<50 nmol/L) as being inadequate for health [37]. A recent study looked at the trends in vitamin D intakes and dietary sources of vitamin D in Irish adults in two nationally representative dietary surveys conducted in 1999 and 2009 [38]. This analysis also explored the contribution of fortified foods and nutritional supplements and examined the effect of potential vitamin D food-fortification scenarios on the distribution of vitamin D intakes in Irish adults using the 2011 IUNA food consumption survey data [31]. The percentage of Irish adults with inadequate intakes of Vitamin D exceeded 90% in all age groups between 18 and 50 and this high prevalence of Vitamin D inadequacy was also seen a decade later in 2009 [38]. This same study found that vitamin D supplementation among Irish adults aged 18–50 was just 18%. A considerably higher proportion of adults (>50%) in the 2009 survey consumed vitamin D–fortified foods, the majority of which were fat spreads and breakfast cereals.

Suboptimal vitamin D intakes [39] as well as low serum vitamin D status has also been reported in pregnancy [35, 40]. Vitamin D insufficiency (defined as serum 25(OH)D <50 nmol/L) was prevalent in Irish women throughout pregnancy. In particular, most women had vitamin D insufficiency during the extended winter period (October to March); with about 91% of women insufficient during the first trimester. Even between April and September about 41% of women still had insufficient vitamin D status. None of the pregnant women in this study were taking vitamin D-containing supplements [40]. The specific nutritional requirements for vitamin D to promote a healthy pregnancy have yet to be determined as the current suggested cut-offs for serum 25-hydroxyvitamin D concentrations representing vitamin D sufficiency/deficiency are based on evidence from non-pregnant adults. A recent Irish study involving a sample of 30 women looking at vitamin D status as gestation progresses reported a decrease in circulating total and free 25(OH)D concentrations as pregnancy advances suggestive of a higher requirement for vitamin D [41]. At 15 weeks' gestation, the proportion of women with serum 25(OH)D concentration <30 and 50 nmol/L was 10% and 63%, respectively, and this increased to 53% and 80%, respectively, at 36 weeks' gestation.

Clinical Practice Guidelines

The HSE Obesity and Pregnancy Clinical Practice Guidelines recommend that obese women take a 10 µg/day supplement of Vitamin D during pregnancy, double that of the general recommendation for non-obese pregnant women of 5 µg/day (Table 29.4) [27]. This level is considerably lower than the recommended level in the UK – 10 µg/day and the US – 15 µg/day and is currently being reviewed by an expert working group. In terms of clinical practice, health professionals and parents need to be made aware that vitamin D deficiency is prevalent in Ireland, particularly among dark-skinned infants and young children. A higher dose is recommended if there is a history of rickets in a sibling or a known maternal vitamin D deficiency.

Iron

Maternal iron deficiency has been associated with low birthweight and small-for-gestational age babies and poor weight and height gain during childhood. Iron requirements increase progressively after 25 weeks' gestation; thus, it is vital that maternal iron intake is sufficient throughout pregnancy to meet the increased requirement for fetal growth while maintaining adequate maternal stores. Dietary surveys in Ireland have found that a significant proportion of women of reproductive age are not meeting the daily requirement for iron [31, 36]. The mean intake in 2007 for women of all ages was 13.1 mg/day which decreased significantly with age [36]. Similarly, in a dietary intake study of pregnant women the majority were not reaching their daily requirements for iron intake during pregnancy [32] (Table 29.5). Currently the Irish recommendation for iron during pregnancy is 15 mg/day. In a secondary analysis of the ROLO study, Horan et al. observed that 54% of the cohort of pregnant Irish women were non-compliant in the first trimester. The 15 mg RNI was not achieved by 38% and 41% of women in the second and third trimesters, respectively [42].

Women suspected of iron deficiency should have a full blood count at booking and 28 weeks' gestation and, if possible, serum ferritin checked [27]. Iron supplementation is only recommended for women with a low serum ferritin or those deemed at risk of developing iron-deficiency anaemia. Appropriate use of supplementation and an iron-rich diet has the potential of reducing incidence of anaemia in pregnancy and subsequent adverse outcomes and therefore the threshold for iron supplementation in pregnancy should be low [27]. This is mainly due to the higher iron requirement during pregnancy, which becomes difficult to meet with dietary sources alone. Iron supplementation during pregnancy has an evident role in preventing maternal anaemia and the risk of preterm delivery associated with it. However, in Ireland routine iron supplementation for all women in pregnancy is not recommended. If, however, there is evidence of iron deficiency, the recommended treatment is oral iron supplementation. A recent study suggests that obesity may hamper transfer of iron to the foetus due to inflammation responses [43], therefore, in this instance iron supplementation should be followed according to health professional advice [44].

Long Chain Omega 3-PUFA (EPA and DHA)

While there are no pregnancy-specific recommendations for altering lipid intakes, there is a recommendation to ensure adequate intakes of long-chain omega-3 polyunsaturated fatty acids (LC-PUFA), specifically docosahexaenoic acid (DHA) and eicosapentaenoic acid (EPA). DHA is particularly important for the developing fetus being linked to improved retinal development and as an important component of brain tissue [45]. While a role for maternal supplementation remains inconclusive, maternal fish consumption has been positively associated in some studies with visual and cognitive function in the offspring [46].

The proportion of Irish women of reproductive age (18–50 years) consuming fish, specifically oily fish, has been reported to be low. A recent study [47] examining fat intakes in two national dietary surveys in 2001 and 2011 found lower mean intakes of EPA and DHA of 161 mg/day among younger women aged 18–35 years. While fish was the main contributor of EPA and DHA, 'nutritional supplements' were also major contributors. Among consumers, supplements contributed up to 55% of total EPA and DHA intake. While the use of n-3 supplements was higher in 2011 (12·5%) when compared to 2001 (7·5%), these levels of supplement usage are still low in terms of recommended intakes. The lowest compliance with the recommended adequate intake of $\geq$250 mg/d of 47% was seen for female non-supplement users aged 18–35 years. This has implications for adequate intakes of LC-PUFA for women of reproductive age and specifically in pregnancy. No data are available on DHA and EPA intakes during pregnancy in Ireland. However, intakes of LC-PUFA (including both omega-3 and omega-6 fatty acids) have been reported in a recent study of diet in pregnancy with 68.2% compliance with recommended intakes [32] (Table 29.5). Thus, given the beneficial role of these fatty acids during pregnancy where the European Food Safety Authority (EFSA) recommend increasing intakes of DHA by an additional 100–200 mg/day [48], such low intakes by younger women in Ireland may have implications in pregnancy for the long-term health of the fetus.

The EFSA recommend that all pregnant women should consume an additional 100–200 mg/day of DHA [48]. This is in addition to the requirement of 250 mg/week combined EPA and DHA. Such an increased intake can be achieved by consuming one to two portions of oil-rich fish per week [49]. While total maternal requirements for LC-PUFA during pregnancy are unknown, it has been estimated that pregnant women may need to consume as much as 300 mg/d to provide for the additional requirement owing to increased fetal accretion especially in the third trimester. In the Irish diet, the best food sources of DHA are oily fish including trout, salmon, mackerel, tuna and sardines [49]. However, given that that only 52.6% of Irish adults are consumers of fish and that consumption levels were higher among supplement users, this suggests that there is a significant segment of the Irish population who do not consume fish or fish oil supplements and with inadequate intakes of beneficial long-chain n-3 fatty acids. The relatively low fish consumption and supplementation usage of LC-PUFA by young women in Ireland highlights the need for increased awareness about the importance of omega-3 LC-PUFA in pregnancy and the potential adverse effects on the developing fetus and infant if dietary intake is inadequate.

Alcohol

Heavy alcohol consumption during pregnancy is associated with several adverse birth outcomes including preterm birth, low birth weight and negative cognitive and behavioural outcomes; sustained high consumption can result in fetal alcohol syndrome [50]. However, the effects of low-level alcohol exposure in utero are equivocal with some studies reporting no evidence of fetal harm, whilst others have indicated an increased risk of neurodevelopmental problems. Recently published research involving three different cohort studies: GUI (Growing Up in Ireland), SCOPE (Screening for Pregnancy Endpoints) and PRAMS (Pregnancy Risk Assessment Monitoring System) examined alcohol consumption patterns and their determinants in over 17,000 Irish women before and during the different trimesters of pregnancy [50]. Over 75% of Irish women were found to be consuming alcohol during their pregnancy and this high prevalence was seen across all social groups, highlighting the very low adherence to guidelines advising complete abstinence from alcohol during pregnancy (Table 29.6). Results from the SCOPE study indicate a higher prevalence of alcohol consumption among pre-pregnant Irish women (90%) when compared to the UK, New Zealand and Australia. Such a high prevalence of consumption continues into early pregnancy among Irish women with 82% consuming alcohol. With regard to binge drinking, according to the SCOPE study, 45% of Irish women were found to binge drink in the first trimester of their pregnancy with the rate of binge drinking falling to just 0.4% in the second trimester [50].

Results from all of these studies highlight the prevalence and social acceptability of this unhealthy behaviour during pregnancy. Socioeconomic status was not strongly related in this study and indeed this concurs with earlier studies [28, 51]. One retrospective cohort study investigated the prevalence, predictors and perinatal outcomes of periconceptional alcohol exposure and reported that 81% of the 61,241 women in the sample consumed alcohol during the periconceptional period [51]. Such high alcohol usage in Ireland has been reported in earlier studies [52, 53]. While assessing alcohol consumption during pregnancy may be problematic in that it is so susceptible to recall and reporting bias, given that these high rates have not declined over the past two decades, new policies and interventions are required to tackle the high prevalence of alcohol consumption both before and during pregnancy.

Current guidelines are that health professionals should continue to advise all pregnant women of the need to abstain from alcohol consumption in accordance with current national guidelines [54]. As alcohol is being consumed by such a high proportion of women in early pregnancy, albeit at low levels, this is occurring at a critical stage of pregnancy with regard to early development and growth of the fetus and represents a significant public health problem. As the evidence for harmful effects of low alcohol intakes in the later stages of pregnancy is lacking this may result in varying perceptions of risk by health professionals and a consequent lack of consistent advice for abstinence being given. More research is needed to determine the effectiveness of educational interventions in bringing about change in professional and maternal attitudes to alcohol drinking in pregnancy [55]. Unlike many other countries, such as the US, labels on alcohol products sold in Ireland do not include health warnings of consuming alcohol in pregnancy. Given the ambivalent attitude to alcohol usage in pregnancy in Ireland, this labelling policy may need to be considered.

Conclusion

In our exploration of the nutrition-related issues in the perinatal period in Ireland, we identified two broad problem areas: excessive caloric intakes and inappropriate nutrient intakes. Among the problems related to excessive caloric intake, maternal obesity is arguably the most important as this is also associated with excessive gestational weight gain and increased incidence of gestational diabetes.

Table 29.6 Prevalence of alcohol consumption in GUI (2008, 2009), SCOPE Ireland (2008–2011) and PRAMS Ireland (2012)

	GUI N = 10,953 N (%)	SCOPE Ireland N = 1766 N (%)	PRAMS N = 718 N (%)
Pre-pregnancy alcohol consumption	*Not recorded*	1586 (90)	545 (77)
Non-drinkers pre-pregnancy	*Not recorded*	180 (10)	173 (23)
Severity of consumption[a]			
1–2 units per week	*Not recorded*	287 (18)	168 (43)
3–7 units per week	*Not recorded*	602 (38)	96 (24)
8–14 units per week	*Not recorded*	451 (28)	73 (19)
>14 units per week	*Not recorded*	247 (16)	58 (15)
Median (Interquartile range (IQR))	*Not recorded*	6 (3, 11)	4 (1, 10)
Pre-pregnancy binging	*Not recorded*	1044 (59)	134 (24)
Any alcohol in pregnancy	2198 (20)	1444 (82)	325 (46)
Non-drinkers in pregnancy	8755 (80)	322 (18)	393 (54)
Binge [any in pregnancy]	*Not recorded*	795 (45)	23 (4)
First trimester alcohol consumption	1127 (11)	1415 (80)	211 (30)
Non-drinkers in first trimester	9826 (89)	351 (20)	507 (70)
Severity of consumption[a]			
1–2 units per week	572 (54)	424 (30)	142 (85)
3–7 units per week	332 (31)	600 (42)	11 (7)
8–14 units per week	117 (11)	266 (19)	8 (5)
>14 units per week	41 (4)	125 (9)	7 (4)
Median (IQR)	2 (2, 2)	4 (2, 7.5)	1 (1,2)
Binge first trimester (yes)	*Not recorded*	795 (45)	21 (3)
Second trimester alcohol consumption	1585 (15)	500 (29)	216 (31)
Non-drinkers in second trimester	9368 (85)	1266 (71)	502 (69)
Severity of consumption[a]			
1–2 units per week	1006 (76)	486 (98)	153 (91)
3–7 units per week	367 (25)	11 (2)	10 (6)
8–14 units per week	93 (6)	1 (0.2)	5 (3)
>14 units per week	23 (2)	0	1 (1)
Median (IQR)	1 (1, 2)	0.5 (0.3, 1.0)	1 (1,1)
Binge second trimester (yes)	*Not recorded*	7 (0.4)	4 (1)
Third trimester alcohol consumption	1559 (14)	*Not recorded*	225 (32)
Non-drinkers in third trimester	9394 (84)	*No recorded*	493 (68)
Severity of consumption[a]			
1–2 units per week	1016 (70)	*Not recorded*	161 (90)
3–7 units per week	341 (23)	*Not recorded*	13 (7)
8–14 units per week	78 (5)	*Not recorded*	4 (2)
>14 units per week	21 (1)	*Not recorded*	1 (1)
Median (IQR)	1 (1, 2)	*Not recorded*	1 (1,1)
Binge third trimester (yes)	*Not recorded*	*Not recorded*	6 (1)

[a]Note that severity of alcohol consumption only refers to women who consumed alcohol during pregnancy. Reproduced with permission from the publishers [50]

Given that many pregnancies are unplanned, interventions to reduce maternal obesity are likely to be more successful if implemented in the pre-pregnancy period. Thus, pre-conception health promotion interventions are likely warranted. Problems related to inappropriate nutrient intakes relate to the fact that diet during pregnancy is often sub-optimal and Ireland, like many other European countries, has a conservative approach to supplementation during pregnancy in contrast to North America. Health professionals in Ireland have a vital role to play towards ensuring optimal pregnancy outcomes in terms of fetal growth and development, particularly in terms of educating and advising women about alcohol intake during pregnancy.

References

1. Koletzko B, Brands B, Poston L, Godfrey K, Demmelmair H. Early nutrition programming of long-term health. Proc Nutr Soc. 2012;71(3):371–8.
2. Breda J, Jewell J, Webber L, Galea G. WHO projections in adults to 2030. 22nd European Congress on Obesity (ECO2015); May 6 2015; Prague, Czech Republic: Obes Facts; 2015. p. 18.
3. Gillespie P, Cullinan J, O'Neill C, Dunne F, Collaborators AD. Modeling the independent effects of gestational diabetes mellitus on maternity care and costs. Diabetes Care. 2013;36(5):1111–6.
4. Fattah C, Farah N, Barry SC, O'Connor N, Stuart B, Turner MJ. Maternal weight and body composition in the first trimester of pregnancy. Acta Obstet Gynecol Scand. 2010;89(7):952–5.
5. Mullaney L, O'Higgins AC, Cawley S, Daly N, McCartney D, Turner MJ. Maternal weight trajectories between early pregnancy and four and nine months postpartum. Public Health. 2016;135:144–6.
6. McKeating A, Maguire PJ, Daly N, Farren M, McMahon L, Turner MJ. Trends in maternal obesity in a large university hospital 2009–2013. Acta Obstet Gynecol Scand. 2015;94(9):969–75.
7. Lynch CM, Sexton DJ, Hession M, Morrison JJ. Obesity and mode of delivery in primigravid and multigravid women. Am J Perinatol. 2008;25(3):163–7.
8. Turner MJ, Layte R. Obesity levels in a national cohort of women 9 months after delivery. Am J Obstet Gynecol. 2013;209(2):124.e1–7.
9. Singh S, Sedgh G, Hussain R. Unintended pregnancy: worldwide levels, trends, and outcomes. Stud Fam Plan. 2010;41(4):241–50.
10. The Irish College of General Practitioners and The Health Service Executive. Healthy weight management guidelines before, during & after pregnancy: a quick reference guide for primary care staff. Dublin: Health Service Executive; 2013. https://www.icgp.ie/go/library/catalogue/item?spId=73ACFC19-4195-4F57-91E5F973ED955D72.
11. Health Service Executive, Institute of Obstetricians and Gynaecologists. Obesity and pregnancy: clinical practice guideline. 2013.
12. Rasmussen KM, Abrams B, Bodnar LM, Butte NF, Catalano PM, Maria Siega-Riz A. Recommendations for weight gain during pregnancy in the context of the obesity epidemic. Obstet Gynecol. 2010;116(5):1191–5.
13. Heery E, Kelleher CC, Wall PG, McAuliffe FM. Prediction of gestational weight gain – a biopsychosocial model. Public Health Nutr. 2015;18(08):1488–98.
14. Walsh JM, McGowan CA, Mahony RM, Foley ME, McAuliffe FM. Obstetric and metabolic implications of excessive gestational weight gain in pregnancy. Obesity. 2014;22(7):1594–600.
15. O'Dwyer V, O'Toole F, Darcy S, Farah N, Kennelly MM, Turner MJ. Maternal obesity and gestational weight gain. J Obstet Gynaecol. 2013;33(7):671–4.
16. Restall A, Taylor RS, Thompson JMD, Flower D, Dekker GA, Kenny LC, et al. Risk factors for excessive gestational weight gain in a healthy. Nulliparous Cohort J Obes. 2014;2014:9.
17. McGowan CA, Walsh JM, Byrne J, Curran S, McAuliffe FM. The influence of a low glycemic index dietary intervention on maternal dietary intake, glycemic index and gestational weight gain during pregnancy: a randomized controlled trial. Nutr J [Internet]. 2013. 2013;12(1):140.
18. Kennelly MA, Ainscough K, Lindsay K, Gibney E, Mc Carthy M, McAuliffe FM. Pregnancy, exercise and nutrition research study with smart phone app support (pears): study protocol of a randomized controlled trial. Contemp Clin Trials. 2016;46:92–9.
19. O'Higgins Amy C, Doolan A, Mullaney L, Daly N, McCartney D, Turner Michael J. The relationship between gestational weight gain and fetal growth: time to take stock? J Perinat Med. 2014;42(4):409–15.
20. Office of the Nursing & Midwifery Services Director. Guidelines for the management of pre-gestational and gestational diabetes mellitus from pre-conception to the postnatal period. In: Director OotNaMS, editor. Dublin: Health Service Executive; 2010. http://www.hse.ie/eng/services/publications/NursingMidwifery%20Services/onsdguidelinesgestationaldiabetes.pdf.
21. O'Sullivan EP, Avalos G, O'Reilly M, Dennedy MC, Gaffney G, Dunne F. Atlantic Diabetes in Pregnancy (DIP): the prevalence and outcomes of gestational diabetes mellitus using new diagnostic criteria. Diabetologia. 2011;54(7):1670–5.

22. Buckley BS, Harreiter J, Damm P, Corcoy R, Chico A, Simmons D, et al. Gestational diabetes mellitus in Europe: prevalence, current screening practice and barriers to screening. A review. Diabet Med. 2012;29(7):844–54.

23. Walsh JM, Mahony RM, Culliton M, Foley ME, McAuliffe FM. Impact of a low glycemic index diet in pregnancy on markers of maternal and fetal metabolism and inflammation. Reprod Sci. 2014;21:1378–81.

24. Group THSCR. Hyperglycemia and adverse pregnancy outcomes. N Engl J Med. 2008;358(19):1991–2002.

25. Walsh JM, Colby Milley J, Gilroy LC, Corcoran S. A stratified approach to the management of gestational diabetes – an effective alternative model of care? Am J Obstet Gynecol. 2016;214(1, Supplement):S185.

26. McDonnell R, Delany V, O'Mahony MT, Mullaney C, Lee B, Turner MJ. Neural tube defects in the Republic of Ireland in 2009–11. J Public Health. 2014;37(1):57–63.

27. Institute of Obstetricians and Gynaecologists, Royal College of Physicians of Ireland and Directorate of Clinical Strategy and Programmes, Health Service Executive. Nutrition for Pregnancy: Clinical practice guideline. Dublin: Health Service Executive; 2013. http://www.hse.ie/eng/about/Who/clinical/natclinprog/obsandgynaeprogramme/nutpreg.pdf.

28. Tarrant RC, Younger KM, Sheridan-Pereira M, Kearney JM. Maternal health behaviours during pregnancy in an Irish obstetric population and their associations with socio-demographic and infant characteristics. Eur J Clin Nutr. 2011;65(4):470–9.

29. McKeating A, Farren M, Cawley S, Daly N, McCartney D, Turner MJ. Maternal folic acid supplementation trends 2009–2013. Acta Obstet Gynecol Scand. 2015;94(7):727–33.

30. Cawley S, Mullaney L, McKeating A, Farren M, McCartney D, Turner MJ. An analysis of folic acid supplementation in women presenting for antenatal care. J Public Health. 2015;38:122–9.

31. Irish Universities Nutrition Alliance. National adult nutrition survey summary report on food and nutrient intakes, physical measurements, physical activity patterns and food choice motives. In: Dr Janette Walton editors. Irish Universities Nutrition Alliance: Cork; 2011. http://www.iuna.net/wp-content/uploads/2010/12/National-Adult-Nutrition-Survey-Summary-Report-March-2011.pdf.

32. McGowan CA, McAuliffe FM. Maternal dietary patterns and associated nutrient intakes during each trimester of pregnancy. Public Health Nutr. 2013;16(1):97–107.

33. Hopkins SM, Gibney MJ, Nugent AP, McNulty H, Molloy AM, Scott JM, et al. Impact of voluntary fortification and supplement use on dietary intakes and biomarker status of folate and vitamin B-12 in Irish adults. Am J Clin Nutr. 2015;101(6):1163–72.

34. Scientific Committee of the Food Safety Authority of Ireland. Update report on folic acid and the prevention of birth defects in Ireland. Dublin: Food Safety Authority of Ireland; 2016. http://www.fsai.ie/publications_folic_acid_update/.

35. Walsh JM, Kilbane M, McGowan CA, McKenna MJ, McAuliffe FM. Pregnancy in dark winters: implications for fetal bone growth? Fertil Steril. 2013;99(1):206–11.

36. Morgan K, McGee H, Watson D, Perry I, Barry M, Shelley E, Harrington J, Molcho M, Layte R, Tully N, van Lente E, Ward M, Lutomski J, Conroy R, Brugha R. SLÁN 2007: Survey of Lifestyle, Attitudes & Nutrition in Ireland. Main Report. Dublin; 2008. http://www.ucd.ie/t4cms/slan07_report.pdf.

37. Cashman KD, Muldowney S, McNulty B, Nugent A, FitzGerald AP, Kiely M, et al. Vitamin D status of Irish adults: findings from the national adult nutrition survey. Br J Nutr. 2013;109(7):1248–56.

38. Black LJ, Walton J, Flynn A, Cashman KD, Kiely M. Small increments in vitamin D intake by Irish adults over a decade show that strategic initiatives to fortify the food supply are needed. J Nutr. 2015;145(5):969–76.

39. McGowan CA, Byrne J, Walsh J, McAuliffe FM. Insufficient vitamin D intakes among pregnant women. Eur J Clin Nutr. 2011;65(9):1076–8.

40. O'Riordan MN, Kiely M, Higgins JR, Cashman KD. Prevalence of suboptimal vitamin D status during pregnancy. Ir Med J. 2008;101(8):240. 2–3

41. Zhang JY, Lucey AJ, Horgan R, Kenny LC, Kiely M. Impact of pregnancy on vitamin D status: a longitudinal study. Br J Nutr. 2014;112(7):1081–7.

42. Horan MK, McGowan CA, Gibney ER, Donnelly JM, McAuliffe FM. The association between maternal dietary micronutrient intake and neonatal anthropometry – secondary analysis from the ROLO study. Nutr J. 2015;14(1):1–11.

43. Dao MC, Sen S, Iyer C, Klebenov D, Meydani SN. Obesity during pregnancy and fetal iron status: is Hepcidin the link? J Perinatol. 2013;33(3):177–81.

44. Food Safety Authority of Ireland. Best practice for infant feeding in Ireland: from pre-conception through the first year of an infant's life. Dublin: Food Safety Authority of Ireland; 2012. https://www.fsai.ie/publications_infant_feeding/.

45. Best KP, Gold M, Kennedy D, Martin J, Makrides M. Omega-3 long-chain PUFA intake during pregnancy and allergic disease outcomes in the offspring: a systematic review and meta-analysis of observational studies and randomized controlled trials. Am J Clin Nutr. 2015;103(1):128–43.

46. Gould JF, Smithers LG, Makrides M. The effect of maternal omega-3 (n-3) LCPUFA supplementation during pregnancy on early childhood cognitive and visual development: a systematic review and meta-analysis of randomized controlled trials. Am J Clin Nutr. 2013;97(3):531–44.
47. Li K, McNulty BA, Tiernery AM, Devlin NF, Joyce T, Leite JC, et al. Dietary fat intakes in Irish adults in 2011: how much has changed in 10 years? Br J Nutr. 2016;115(10):1798–809.
48. EFSA NDA Panel (EFSA Panel on Dietetic Products NaA. Scientific opinion on dietary reference values for fats, including saturated fatty acids, polyunsaturated fatty acids, monounsaturated fatty acids, trans fatty acids, and cholesterol. EFSA J. 2010;8(3):107.
49. Working Group on Recommendations for Scientific Recommendations for a National Infant Feeding Policy – A Revision and Update. Scientific recommendations for a national infant feeding policy. 2nd ed. Dublin: Food Safety Authority of Ireland; 2011. https://www.fsai.ie/resources_publications/national_infant_feeding_policy/.
50. O'Keeffe LM, Kearney PM, McCarthy FP, Khashan AS, Greene RA, North RA, et al. Prevalence and predictors of alcohol use during pregnancy: findings from international multicentre cohort studies. BMJ Open. 2015;5(7):1–12.
51. Mullally A, Cleary BJ, Barry J, Fahey TP, Murphy DJ. Prevalence, predictors and perinatal outcomes of peri-conceptional alcohol exposure – retrospective cohort study in an urban obstetric population in Ireland. BMC Pregnancy Childbirth. 2011;11(1):1–7.
52. Daly SF, Kiely J, Clarke TA, Matthews TG. Alcohol and cigarette use in a pregnant Irish population. Ir Med J. 1992;85(4):156–7.
53. Mc Millan H, Smaarani S, Walsh T, Khawaja N, Collins C, Byrne P, et al. Smoking and alcohol in pregnancy. Survey in the immediate post-partum period. Ir Med J. 2006;99(9):283.
54. Department of Health. Steering group report on a national substance misuse strategy. Dublin: Department of Health; 2012. http://www.drugsandalcohol.ie/16908/2/Steering_Group_Report_on_a_National_Substance_Misuse_Strategy_-_7_Feb_11.pdf.
55. O'Leary CM, Bower C. Guidelines for pregnancy: what's an acceptable risk, and how is the evidence (finally) shaping up? Drug Alcohol Rev. 2012;31(2):170–83.

Chapter 30
Maternal Malnutrition, Fetal Programming, Outcomes, and Implications of Environmental Factors in Japan

Hideko Sone and Tin-Tin Win-Shwe

Key Points

- Prenatal nutrition influences the healthy development of multiple fetal organs. Delayed or abnormal mental, neural, and physical growth results from nutritional aberrations.
- Although fetal malformation was more common in the past, Japan has the highest longevity and lowest infant mortality rate worldwide. However, for over 20 years the proportion of low-birth weight infants has been greater in Japan than in other developed countries.
- The desire of young Japanese women to be thin has been identified as an underlying cause.
- This review provides an overview of the nutrients that may prevent or alleviate the development of neurologic disorders, diabetes, and allergies of childhood onset.
- This review also offers insight into the effects of prenatal nutritional interventions and environmental factors on fetal development.

Keywords Maternal malnutrition • Fetal programming • Low birth weight • Infant nutrient • Japanese women • Environmental factor

Introduction

Optimal maternal nutritional status should be maintained for normal fetal development. However, maternal nutrition is often compromised by inadequate nutrition and/or the consumption of hazardous substances from the environment—indoor or outdoor—such as through occupational exposure. It is extremely important to understand and reduce the physical and neurologic malformations that arise in the fetus as a result of an inappropriate prenatal diet. To explain how nutrition and the environment during development contribute to the risk of disease later in life, the Developmental Origins of Health and Disease (DOHaD) theory incorporates concepts such as developmental plasticity and programming mismatch. The consequences of nutritional and environmental factors are often seen as direct effects (e.g., low-birth weight [LBW] infants, premature parturition, or birth defects), whereas other adverse health outcomes associated

H. Sone, PhD (✉) • T.-T. Win-Shwe, MD, PhD
Center for Health and Environmental Risk Research, National Institute for Environmental Studies,
16-2 Onogawa, Tsukuba, Ibaraki 3058506, Japan
e-mail: hsone@nies.go.jp; tin.tin.win.shwe@nies.go.jp

© Springer International Publishing AG 2017   411
R. Rajendram et al. (eds.), *Diet, Nutrition, and Fetal Programming*,
Nutrition and Health, DOI 10.1007/978-3-319-60289-9_30

with early-life exposures do not manifest until years or decades later [1]. Birth cohort studies are popular in Europe and the United States because they are considered suitable epidemiologic studies to confirm the DOHaD theory. Currently, interdisciplinary studies are also in progress in Japan, but only at a few facilities. Healthy Parents and Children 21 is a health-promotion plan organized by the Ministry of Health, Labour and Welfare in Japan [2]. The Japan Environment and Children's Study organized by the Ministry of Environment is an ongoing nationwide birth cohort study launched in January 2011 [3]. In addition, individual birth cohort studies in Japan are underway at universities in Hamamatsu, Tohoku, and Hokkaido in accordance with the Birth Cohort Consortium of Asia [4].

The Lancet's World Report of 2007 [5] highlighted the growing epidemic of obesity in Japan, which may be relevant to future patterns of disease given the metabolic consequences of obesity identified by analyzing the association between LBW infants and adult diseases. The increasing prevalence of obesity is driven by changing patterns of nutrition and exercise, but other factors may also be worthy of consideration. Gluckman's report [6] suggested that a mismatch between intrauterine constraints, arising from small maternal stature and suboptimum fetal nutrition, and a nutritionally rich postnatal environment may explain the high levels of metabolic compromise seen in some adolescents. The proportion of LBW infants in Japan was 9.6% in 2013, whereas the mean proportion of LBW infants in Organization for Economic Co-operation and Development (OECD) member countries was only 6.6% [7]. Many researchers and physicians consider it a matter of concern that young women consume inadequate nutrition. In general, women with poor nutritional status during pregnancy have children with a LBW, poor health, physical abnormalities, behavioral disorders, and delayed cognitive and physical development [8]. Many population-based studies in other countries have shown that children suffering from a disease have a substantially reduced height, weight, head circumference, and body mass index (BMI) than healthy children.

Maintaining optimal nutrition during pregnancy is critical, which raises the questions of how much and what should be provided during pregnancy to deliver healthy babies and, consequently, healthy children and adults. Therefore, in this review, we surveyed the literature on nutritional studies performed in humans in Japan, and analyzed these publications based on the DOHaD theory.

Study Extraction and Overview

To analyze the association between alterations in fetal programming caused by nutritional status in pregnancy and outcomes in later life reported in Japan, we searched for relevant epidemiologic studies using the following key words: "pregnancy," "nutrition," "offspring," "infant," "child," "Japan," "Japanese," "cord blood," "fetal programming," "epigenetics," "histone acetylation," and "DNA methylation." We identified approximately 50 original articles on cross-sectional, cohort, and case studies conducted in Japan from the databases of PubMed (http://www.ncbi.nlm.nih.gov/pubmed), CiNii (http://ci.nii.ac.jp/), and Static Japan (http://www.stat.go.jp/) and the selected studies were summarized in Table 30.1. The focus of this review was on the following six topics:

- The current status of knowledge on vital statistics related to birth and young women in Japan;
- The current status of congenital anomalies (CAs) in Japan;
- Nutritional status in present-day Japan;
- The effects of nutritional factors on fetal and infant growth in Japan;
- Other factors related to fetal programming, such as the involvement of environmental substances; and
- Molecular aspects revealed by epigenetic studies in Japan.

We aimed to provide an overview of the nutrients (vitamins, lipids, folic acid [FA], and proteins) that may prevent or alleviate the development of neurologic disorders, diabetes mellitus (DM), and allergies of childhood onset because there is a lack of information on the role of nutrients and prenatal nutritional interventions in fetal programming in Japanese populations.

Table 30.1 Summary of studies for association between outcomes and nutritional status

	Nutrients and environmental factors	Exposed subject	Outcome (effects)	Study type and sample size	References
Eating and diet					
1	Caffeine intake from Japanese and Chinese tea	Pregnant woman	Preterm birth	Prospective cohort, Osaka Maternal and C hild Health Study (OMCHS), 858	Okubo et al. [57]
2	Dairy products and calcium	Pregnant woman and their children pairs	Dental caries in children	Prospective cohort OMCHS, 315 mother-child pairs, 687 base-line population	Tanaka et al. [58]
3	Diet history	Mother	Aged 3–6 years in Preschool Children	Cross-sectional, a brief type self-administered diet history questionnaire (BDHQ) 3 years, 61 children aged 3–4 years	Asakura et al. [59]
4	Dietary intake	Pregnant Japanese woman	Bodyweight and fetal growth	Cross-sectional, Hamamatsu University Hospital, 135 singleton pregnant Japanese women	Kubota et al. [14]
5	Dietary nutritional intake		Low birthweight infants	Cross-sectional, 15 extremely low biorth weight infant, mother milk	Itabashi et al. [20]
6	Eating habits	Primigravida	Weight gain	Cross-sectional, 237 pregnant women	Yokoyama et al. [60]
7	Eating habits skipping breakfast	Pregnant woman	Plasma total homocysteine levels	Cross-sectional, 254 singleton pregnant women	Shiraishi et al. [61]
8	Vegetable intake	Mothers and their children	10- to 12-year-old schoolchildren	Cross-sectional, 332 pairs of mothers and children	Tada et al. [62]
Fatty acids					
9	Fatty acid	Pregnant	Heterogeneity of the fatty acid composition of Japanese placentae	Methodological, 24 placenta	Yamazaki et al. [38]
10	Fatty acid, EPA, DHA	Pregnant	Energy-adjusted intakes of EPA, DHA, and EPA + DHA	Cross-sectional, 207 singleton pregnant women	Shiraishi et al. [39]
11	Fatty acid_ palmitoleic acid	Children	Plasma palmitoleic acid content and obesity	Cross-sectional, 59 obese children	Okada et al. [63]
Vitamines					
12	Folic acid	Mother and their newborns	Spina bifida	Case-control, 360 cases and 2333 controls	Kondo et al. [18]
13	Folic acid	Young Japanese women	Erythrocyte folate levels	Cross-sectional, 38 women	Shinozaki et al. [23]
14	Folic acid	Pregnant Japanese woman	Estimated average requirement intake	Cross-sectional, 192 pregnant and 38 delivered women	Shibata et al. [28]
15	Vitamin B6	Pregnancy	Vitamin B6 deficiency and anemia in pregnancy	Case-control, 56 pregnant women with anemia, 79 healthy pregnants	Hisano et al. [31]
16	Vitamin B6	Pregnant Japanese women	Plasma pyridoxal 5′-phosphate concentration of the VB6 biomarker	Cross-sectional, 192 pregnant and 38 delivered women	Shibata et al. [30]

(continued)

Table 30.1 (continued)

	Nutrients and environmental factors	Exposed subject	Outcome (effects)	Study type and sample size	References
17	Vitamin B-groups	Woman	Urinary excretion of the metabolites of the tryptophan-niacin	Case-control, 50 pregnant women with anemia, 10 nonpregnants	Fukuwatari et al. [63]
18	Vitamin D	Pregnant woman	Reduced risk of dental caries in young children	Cross sectional, Kyushu Okinawa Maternal and Child Health Study (KOMCHS). 267 mother with caries, 954 caries free	Tanaka et al. [33]
19	Vitamin D	Pregnant woman	Premature delivery	93 pregnant women	Shibata et al. [64]
20	Vitamin D	Neonates	Craniotabes in normal newborns: The earliest sign in Vitamin D deficiency	Prospective cohort, 1120 pregnant women and their neonates	Yorifuji et al. [32]
21	Vitamin D long-term hospitary	Pregnant woman	vitamin D deficiency in neonates	Case-control, 5 long-term hospitalized and 9 control pregnant women	Nishimura et al. [65]
22	Vitamin D	20-aged young males and females	Fok-I polymorphism in vitamin D receptor gene on serum 25-hydroxyvitamin D	Molecular aspect: epigenetics, 97 healthy Japanese males and 96 females	Tanabe et al. [66]
23	Vitamins	Pregnant and lactating women in Japan.	Urinary excretion levels of water-soluble vitamins	Cross-sectional, 192 pregnant and 38 delivered women	Shibata et al. [29]
24	Glucose	Japanese women diagnosed with gestational diabetes	Efficacy of nutrition therapy for glucose intolerance in Japanese women	Intervention, 41 pregnant women	Horie et al. [67]
25	Iodine status	Pregnant and postpartum Japanese women	Effect of iodine intake on maternal and neonatal thyroid function	Case-control, 683 pregnant women 532 postpartum women	Fuse et al. [40]
26	Phytoestrogens	mothers and newborns	The difference in phytoestrogen status between mother and fetus	Cross-sectional, 51 mothers and newborns	Todaka et al. [68]
27	Supplement	Pregnant women	Effects of inappropriate dietary due to supplement uses	Cross-sectional 1076 pregnant women	Sato et al. [26]
Not nutrition environmental factors					
28	Environemntal metals: mercury, lead, arsenic, cadmium and selenium	Neonates	Element exposures through breastfeeding does not pose any great concern in this population.	16 pregnant women and their newborns	Sakamoto et al. [69]
29	Environmental methyl mercury via fish consumption	Japanese population	MeHg intake for the Japanese population was estimated to be 6.76 μg/day or 0.14 μg/kg body weight per day (bw/day)	National Nutrition Survey in Japan, more than 15,000	Zhang et al. [42]

(continued)

Table 30.1 (continued)

	Nutrients and environmental factors	Exposed subject	Outcome (effects)	Study type and sample size	References
30	Environmental polychlorinated biphenyls, methylmercury, and polyunsaturated fatty acids	Neonates	Birth size	Cohort, Hokkaido study, 367 mother-newborn pairs	Miyashita et al. [44]
31	Environmental: hydroxylated PCBs and PCBs	Pregnant women and neonates	Blood thyroid hormone levels and body size of neonates	Cohort, 79 mother-child pairs	Hisada et al. [70]

Results of Literature Analysis

The Current Status of Knowledge on Vital Statistics Related to Birth and Young Women in Japan

Birth height and weight, premature birth, and congenital abnormalities are influenced by the nutritional status of mothers from around the 28th week of pregnancy until 1 week after birth. First, we intend to discuss the birth weight, premature birth, congenital abnormalities, and body weight of infants, and the BMI of young women, in the preceding 10 years in Japan. These data, shown in Tables 30.2, 30.3 and 30.4 and Figs. 30.1, 30.2, 30.3, and 30.4, derive from the national vital statistics data [9]. Yoshida et al. [10] reported that the proportion of LBW (1500–2499 g) babies in Japan is consistently increasing. LBW is a major public health problem worldwide and an indicator of social maturity and development.

Regarding the DOHaD theory that abnormal fetal programming influences the onset of obesity later in life, the Tanaka Women's Clinic Study [11] suggested that a low BMI at 20 years of age is predictive of gestational DM independent of BMI in early pregnancy in Japan. The study observed a statistically significant inverse association between BMI at 20 years of age and the incidence of gestational DM, and reported that second-trimester post-load glucose level is an important predictor of LBW infants and that first-trimester fasting plasma insulin levels contribute to the incidence of glucose intolerance in later pregnancy [12].

The Hamamatsu Birth Cohort Study [13] reported the identification of neurodevelopmental trajectories in infancy and risk factors that cause deviant development. This longitudinal study found that the markedly delayed class, characterized by an overall delay from early developmental stages, was predicted by male sex, being small for gestational age (SGA), low placenta:birth weight ratio, and low maternal education, suggesting that the presence of a small placenta relative to the birth weight may play an important role in the predisposition to delayed neurodevelopment. Nutritional conditioning during pregnancy may influence placental size [14].

In a multicenter retrospective cohort study using the database of the Neonatal Research Network Japan and including 9149 infants born between 2003 and 2010 at <28 weeks' gestation [15], the risks of mortality and some morbidity differed between birth weight standard deviation score (BWSDS) groups. Growth-restricted extremely preterm infants experienced additional risks of mortality and morbidity, such as chronic lung disease, retinopathy of prematurity, sepsis, and necrotizing enterocolitis, and these risks varied depending on BWSDS. The report provides evidence for an increasing natural stillbirth ratio, although the stillbirth rate in this period was decreasing, indicating that this tendency may be associated with the nutritional status of pregnant women.

Table 30.2 Japanese female (1–19 years) nutritional status in comparison between 2003 and 2013

		2003			2013		
	Unit	1–6 years	7–14 years	15–19 years	1–6 years	7–14 years	15–19 years
Energy	kcal	1261	1876	1880	1209	1818	1803
Protein	g	44.2	69.2	69.6	42.8	66.4	66.3
Animal	g	25.3	38.9	40.0	24.4	38.3	38.4
Lipids	g	40.2	61.4	64.0	38.4	60.8	62.7
Animal	g	21.4	32.3	33.4	20.6	33.0	33.3
Carbohydrate	g	177.8	256.4	249.2	169.7	245.2	236.2
Dietary fiber	g	8.40	13.30	12.20	8.35	12.63	11.86
Water soluble	g	2.10	3.30	2.90	2.05	3.10	2.84
Water insoluble	g	6.30	9.90	9.30	6.00	9.09	8.64
Vitamin A	μgRE[a]	636.0	945.0	858.0	355.2	533.9	450.7
Vitamin D	μg	3.50	6.20	7.20	3.94	5.45	6.03
Vitamin E	mg[b]	5.30	7.90	8.40	3.95	5.70	6.05
Vitamin K	μg	140.0	214.0	216.0	113.4	174.9	191.9
Vitamin B1	mg	0.59	0.94	1.11	0.55	0.85	0.83
Vitamin B2	mg	0.87	1.26	1.56	0.80	1.13	1.05
Niacin (vitamin B3)	mgNE[c]	7.30	11.80	12.70	7.18	11.46	12.23
Vitamin B6	mg	0.71	1.06	1.28	0.67	0.97	1.00
Vitamin B12	μg	3.90	6.10	6.40	2.88	4.75	4.16
Folate	μg	167.0	255.0	264.0	147.8	222.0	228.7
Pantothenic acid	mg	4.04	5.82	5.40	3.94	5.60	5.10
Vitamin C	mg	64.00	90.00	87.00	49.31	69.12	69.90
Sodium chloride equivalent	g/1000 kcal	5.80	9.30	10.00	4.19	4.72	4.88
Potassium	mg	1538	2261	2031	1442	2047	1850
Calcium	mg	465.0	649.0	518.0	413.1	606.9	430.7
Magnesium	mg	154.0	232.0	217.0	140.5	210.8	197.2
Phosphorus	mg	701.0	1045.0	982.0	659.5	1006.6	897.9
Iron	mg	4.60	6.90	7.30	4.13	6.31	6.77
Zinc	mg	5.30	8.30	8.40	5.17	8.01	8.08
Copper	mg	0.70	1.07	1.10	0.65	0.99	1.00
Fat energy ratio	%[d]	28.1	29.0	30.2	28.1	29.8	31.1
Carbohydrate energy ratio	%[d]	57.8	56.2	54.9	57.8	55.5	54.0
Animal protein ratio	%[d]	56.1	55.2	56.3	55.6	57.1	56.3

Data were extracted from the e-Stat portal site in the statics of Japan (http://www.e-stat.go.jp/SG1/estat/)
[a]RE: retinol equivalent
[b]Only a-tocopherol amounts
[c]NE: niacin equivalent
[d]These ratios were calculated mean values of the individual.

Current Status of Congenital Anomalies in Japan

We looked over data from international assessments of CAs in the 10 years from 2001 to 2010 in Japan by the Yokohama University monitoring data, but the frequencies of CA types showed few changes [16]. The top five CAs were: ventricular septal defects; cleft lip with cleft palate; low-set ears; hydrocephaly; and Down syndrome. Similarly, other phenotypes related to the top five CAs did not change dramatically. However, it should be noted that patent ductus arteriosus (PDA) was almost in the top five after 2007, whereas it was between 6th and 13th before 2006. This change in the

Table 30.3 Japanese male (1–19 years) nutritional status in comparison between 2003 and 2013

	Unit	2003			2013		
		1–6 years	7–14 years	15–19 years	1–6 years	7–14 years	15–19 years
Subject		347	472	272	197	314	175
Energy	kcal	1337	2148	2533	1275	2059	2510
Protein	g	47	77.9	91.2	44.5	74.8	85.6
Animal	g	27	43.6	53.9	25.0	43.4	48.7
Lipids	g	43.6	68.2	81.8	40.3	66.8	77.0
Animal	g	22.6	35.5	43.6	21.6	37.4	41.6
Carbohydrate	g	186.2	298.6	345.3	180.0	281.7	355.2
Dietary fiber	g	8.5	14.1	14.1	8.6	13.4	13.9
Water soluble	g	2.1	3.5	3.4	2.1	3.3	3.3
Water insoluble	g	6.4	10.5	10.7	6.2	9.7	10.2
Vitamin A	µgRE[a]	677	1004	980	412	542	563
Vitamin D	µg	4.4	6.1	8.2	3.8	6.2	6.9
Vitamin E	mg[b]	5.8	8.6	10.1	4.1	6.1	7.0
Vitamin K	µg	140	210	240	124	187	196
Vitamin B1	mg	0.6	1.12	1.22	0.58	0.93	1.08
Vitamin B2	mg	0.91	1.6	1.57	0.83	1.29	1.25
Niacin (Vitamin B3)	mgNE[c]	7.8	12.6	16.5	7.6	12.8	15.8
Vitamin B6	mg	0.73	1.59	1.36	0.68	1.08	1.21
Vitamin B12	µg	4.8	6.4	8.4	2.9	5.2	5.5
Folate	µg	175	273	303	151	232	261
Pantothenic acid	mg	4.25	6.64	7.16	3.93	6.42	6.43
Vitamin C	mg	62	89	88	53	68	72
Sodium chloride equivalent	g/1000 kcal	6.1	10	12.1	4.4	4.5	4.4
Potassium	mg	1590	2490	2559	1450	2259	2225
Calcium	mg	483	744	642	421	667	502
Magnesium	mg	158	255	269	146	230	240
Phosphorus	mg	735	1176	1274	681	1120	1140
Iron	mg	4.9	11.3	9.4	4.3	6.9	7.8
Zinc	mg	5.6	9.5	11.4	5.4	9.2	10.7
Copper	mg	0.73	1.2	1.4	0.68	1.12	1.35
Fat energy ratio	%[d]	28.9	28.4	28.9	27.5	29.1	27.6
Carbohydrate energy ratio	%[d]	57	57	56.7	58.5	56.3	58.6
Animal protein ratio	%[d]	56.2	55.3	57.1	54.1	56.8	55.4

Data were extracted from the e-Stat portal site in the statics of Japan (http://www.e-stat.go.jp/SG1/estat/)
[a]RE: retinol equivalent
[b]only a-tocopherol amounts
[c]NE: niacin equivalent
[d]These ratios were calculated mean values of the individual.

prevalence of PDA from 2007 to 2010 may indicate its association with an increasing proportion of LBW infants, because the known risk factors for PDA include preterm birth, congenital rubella syndrome, chromosomal abnormalities like Down syndrome, and genetic conditions, such as Loeys-Dietz syndrome (which would also present with other heart defects). A retrospective study conducted during 2004–2013 in Osaka showed that the prevalence of fetal congenital heart disease in 2009–2013 with 446 cases was significantly higher than that in 2004–2008 with 241 cases [17]. Thus, as for those data, it is thought that the identification of the background factor and trendy analysis will be necessary more in the future research.

Table 30.4 Japanese female (20–39 years) neutritional status in comparison between 2003 and 2013

		2003				2013			
		20–29 years		30–39 years		20–29 years		30–39 years	
		Average	SD	Average	SD	Average	SD	Average	SD
Subject	Unit	552		722		557		788	
Energy	kcal	1683	516	1708	484	1889	628	1898	582
Protein	g	63.8	21.4	62.7	21.2	67.3	24.3	68.6	23.3
Animal	g	35.5	17.1	32.9	16.9	37.4	19.4	36.5	18.5
Lipids	g	55.1	25.7	53.4	22.9	59.8	26.9	58.4	25.0
Animal	g	27.4	17.5	25.9	14.5	31.0	18.6	29.0	17.4
Carbohydrate	g	223.9	69.9	233.3	68.3	257.7	93.0	257.2	84.1
Cholesterol	mg	317	196	311	195	308	178	315	189
Dietary fiber	g	12	5.2	12.5	5.6	12.0	5.2	13.0	5.4
water soluble	g	2.9	1.4	3	1.5	2.9	1.4	3.1	1.4
Water insoluble	g	9.1	4.1	9.5	4.3	8.7	3.9	9.4	4.0
Vitamin A	μ gRE[a]	787	754	805	1052	417	376	523	871
Vitamin D	μ g	6.9	8.2	6.2	7.1	5.8	7.3	6.1	7.3
Vitamin E	mg[b]	9.1	19.1	9.9	22	6.0	3.1	6.1	3.1
Vitamin K	μg	221	186	242	209	180	137	211	158
Vitamin B1	mg	1.24	4.83	1.11	2.5	0.89	0.46	0.84	0.43
Vitamin B2	mg	3.23	42.66	1.43	2.65	1.03	0.49	1.05	0.53
Niacin (Vitamin B3)	mgNE[c]	12.9	6	13.1	6.3	13.7	7.0	14.1	6.4
Vitamin B6	mg	1.36	3.3	1.72	5.74	0.98	0.43	1.03	0.44
Vitamin B12	μ g	6.1	6.9	5.7	8	5.1	5.4	5.4	6.6
Folate	μ g	258	131	263	157	227	102	248	141
Pantothenic acid	mg	4.92	1.81	4.94	1.93	4.98	1.88	5.19	1.93
Vitamin C	mg	108	310	107	234	67	56	69	54
Sodium chloride equivalent	g	9.8	3.8	9.9	4	9.6	3.7	9.8	3.8
Potassium	mg	1973	762	2008	769	1881	770	1998	736
Calcium	mg	457	271	465	251	425	236	447	234
Magnesium	mg	211	77	219	83	206	76	226	83
Phosphorus	mg	887	313	895	316	900	323	936	319
Iron	mg	7	2.9	7.3	6	6.7	2.6	7.2	3.0
Zinc	mg	7.5	3.1	7.3	2.5	8.1	3.2	8.1	3.0
Copper	mg	1.01	0.36	1.03	0.37	1.04	0.37	1.09	0.39
Fat energy ratio	%[d]	28.9	7.7	27.6	7.3	28.3	7.6	27.4	7.1
Carbohydrate energy ratio	%[d]	55.7	8.5	57.6	8	57.2	8.7	58.0	8.1
Animal protein ratio	%[d]	53.9	13.9	50.4	14.5	53.6	14.1	51.1	14.2

Data were extracted from the e-Stat portal site in the statics of Japan (http://www.e-stat.go.jp/SG1/estat/)
[a]RE:retinol equivalent
[b]α-tocopheryl amount
[c]NE:niacin equivalent
[d]These ratios are the mean values that calculated value of the individual

Nutritional Status in Present-Day Japan

Maternal nutritional status during pregnancy is an important determinant of fetal growth. Although the effects of several nutrients and foods are well documented, little is known about the relationship between overall maternal diet in pregnancy and fetal growth. Vital statistics for nutrition, child growth, and Japanese health conditions derived from a nationwide survey are shown in Tables 30.2, 30.3, 30.4

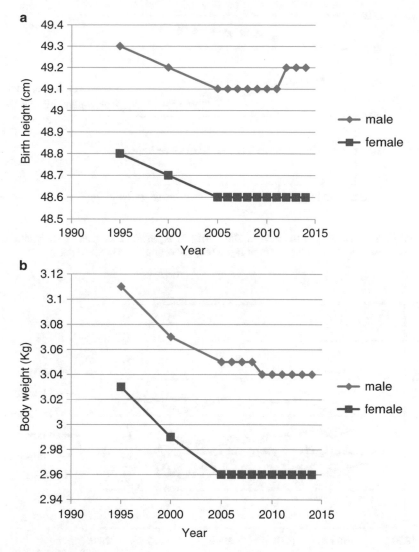

Fig. 30.1 Birth height (**a**) and body weight (**b**) in 1995–2015 in Japan from the data of vital statistics (Data were extracted from the e-Stat portal site in the statics of Japan (http://www.e-stat.go.jp/SG1/estat/))

and Fig. 30.4. In the 10 years during 2003–2013, alterations in the intake of most nutrients were evident at 1–6, 7–14, and 15–19 years of age in both males and females. More surprisingly, individuals aged 7–14 and 15–19 years in 2013 had a lower energy intake than their counterparts in 2003. However, at child-bearing age (20–39 years), individuals in 2013 had a higher energy intake but a lower vitamin intake than in 2003. These data substantiate the increasing concern about the components of the diets of teenagers—especially young women—and highlight the importance of education on nutrition and health in early life.

A prospective cohort study involving 135 Japanese women in Osaka investigated the associations between changes in dietary intake, maternal body weight, and fetal growth during pregnancy to identify the risk factors for spina bifida and evaluate how its prevalence has altered over the past three decades [18]. The results showed that the mean total calorie intake remained below 1600 kcal/day

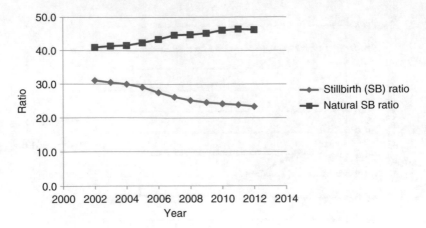

Fig. 30.2 Stillbirth ratio and Natural SB ratio in 2002–2012 in Japan from the data of vital statistics (Data were extracted from the e-Stat portal site in the statics of Japan (http://www.e-stat.go.jp/SG1/estat/))

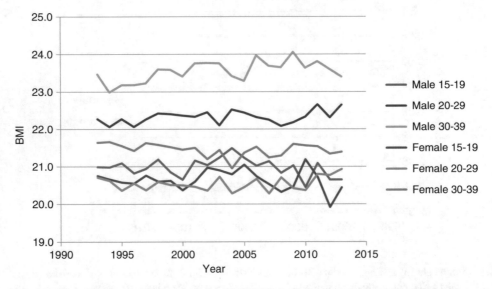

Fig. 30.3 Changes of BMI male and female during 1993–2013 in National vital data in Japan. Data values are means (Data were extracted from the e-Stat portal site in the statics of Japan (http://www.e-stat.go.jp/SG1/estat/))

during pregnancy, much lower than the value recommended in the 2010 edition of Dietary Reference Intakes for Japanese [19].

Itabashi et al. [20] retrospectively studied the relationship between the nutrient content of the milk of 15 mothers who delivered before term (preterm milk) until the 12th week of lactation and extremely LBW infants. The study suggested that the extremely LBW infants should be fed >100 mL milk/kg per day until the fourth week of life. The incidence of LBW infants has grown by nearly 10% in the last three decades in Japan: the highest rate among OECD member countries [7]. The incidences of pediatric obesity, hypertension, Type 2 DM, and autism have paralleled that of LBW. The theory of the fetal origins of adult disease is essential for understanding the pathophysiology of lifestyle-related adult diseases [21, 22]. There is concern that the next generation will face a higher future risk of adult

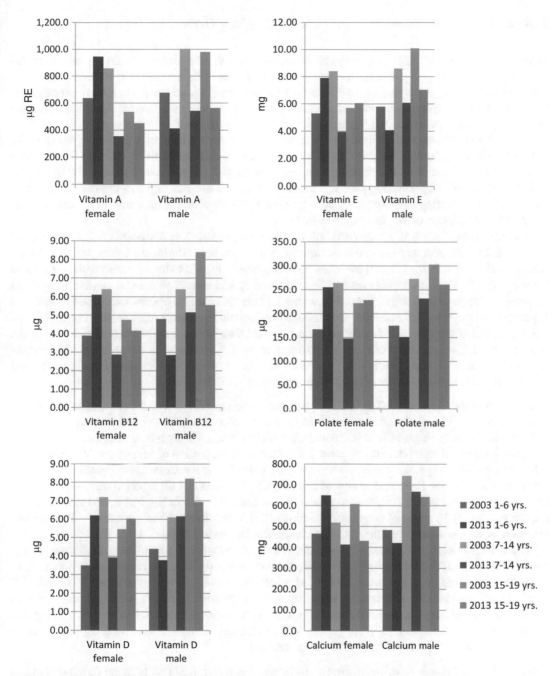

Fig. 30.4 Vitamins and calcium intake in comparison between 2003 and 2013 during 1–15 years of age from Japan national vital statics data (Data were extracted from the e-Stat portal site in the statics of Japan (http://www.e-stat.go.jp/SG1/estat/))

diseases, and maternal nutrition should be addressed to minimize this. Therefore, we must pay attention to childhood obesity.

Regarding inappropriate dietary supplement use among pregnant women in Japan, the nutrients that have the most influence and relevance to neuronal development are vitamins, lipids, fatty acids, FA, and zinc. These nutrients are discussed thoroughly in the following sections, and studies in humans related to them are summarized in Tables 30.2, 30.3, and 30.4.

Effects of Nutritional Factors on Fetal and Infant Growth in Japan

Folic acid In the 1990s, it was believed that most neural tube defects could be prevented by FA. Regarding dietary supplement use among young women [23] or pregnant women [24, 25] in Japan, however, only a few studies have estimated the amount of FA consumed in dietary supplements or meals. Of the 1076 pregnant Japanese women in mid-to-late pregnancy examined in the Hamamatsu study [26], most began to use supplements after recognizing that they were pregnant.

In 2000, the Japanese government recommended that women planning a pregnancy should take 400 µg of FA daily to decrease the risk of having an infant with spina bifida [17, 27]. The average amount of folate consumed by pregnant Japanese women was estimated to be about 250 µg/day by recent studies [24, 28]. This suggests that there is an urgent need to improve the diet of Japanese women of child-bearing age, especially during pregnancy. However, the incidence of spina bifida has not decreased in Japan during the past 20 years [25, 28].

In a case-control study that examined 360 women who gave birth to newborns afflicted with spina bifida and 2333 control women who gave birth to healthy newborns during a 12-year period in Japan, Kondo et al. (2013, 2015) [17, 27] evaluated the odds ratio (OR) of having an infant with spina bifida for women who took FA supplements periconceptionally and examined the association between an increase in supplement use and possible reasons for this increase. Newborns were divided into two 6-year periods: 2001–2006 and 2007–2012. Based on logistic regression analysis, the adjusted OR of having an infant with spina bifida for supplement users was 0.48 in the first period and 0.53 in the second period. The proportion of women who consumed supplements periconceptionally significantly increased from 10% in the first period to 30% in the second period. This increase in supplement use was due to increased awareness of the preventive role of FA [27].

Vitamins and related elements The folate-related one-carbon metabolism pathway regulates epigenetic modification via DNA methylation to modulate gene expression. Therefore, vitamins B_6 and B_{12} are key nutrients in the early stages of fetal development. Recent advances in analytic techniques have enabled the quantification of water-soluble vitamins [28, 29]. A high proportion of Japanese mothers have low folate and high homocysteine levels, possibly leading to babies with undesirable epigenetic changes, as described earlier in the Folic acid section of this chapter. Shibata et al. [30] reported that the water-soluble vitamins present in the urine, such as vitamin B_2, vitamin B_6, vitamin B_{12}, biotin, and vitamin C, did not change during the stages of pregnancy and did not differ from those of healthy individuals. However, pregnant women with anemia due to iron deficiency also had vitamin B_6 deficiency [31].

Vitamin D deficiency is a cause of craniotabes during development. Yorifuji et al. [32] reported that levels of a metabolite of vitamin D, 25-OHD, were significantly lower in breast-fed infants than in formula-/mixed-fed infants, whereas breast-fed infants had significantly higher serum PTH and ALP levels than formula-/mixed-fed infants. Higher maternal cheese intake during pregnancy was found to be significantly inversely associated with the risk of dental caries in children in a study involving 315 Japanese mother-child pairs [33], suggesting that inadequate vitamin D intake during pregnancy is strongly associated with dental caries in young children.

Fatty acids and lipids in relation to obesity In Japan, it is recognized that prenatal development is a critical period in the etiology of obesity and cardiometabolic disease [34]. Unhealthy thinness among female junior high-school girls in Japan reached 20% in 2014 [1, 35]. Several reports have examined changes in high-density lipoprotein and low-density lipoprotein (LDL) profiles during the neonatal period to evaluate the nutritional state related to lipids of preterm neonates with the aim of preventing the onset of obesity in adolescents and adult disease in later life [36, 37]. Gestational age and milk including breast and formula, rather than birth weight, determine postnatal changes in LDL profile. This suggests that cord blood may contain fatty acids derived from the maternal circulation via the placenta according to changes in de-novo lipogenesis.

Palmitoleic acid (16:1n − 7) is a product of endogenous lipogenesis. In human obesity, 16:1n − 7 reportedly correlates with indices of adiposity and insulin concentration. Excessive subcutaneous fat accumulation is often observed in LBW infants because of accelerating stearoyl-CoA desaturase activity. The fatty acid profiles of neonates can predict epigenetic conditions in the fetal period. Analysis of the placenta may be a useful way to determine the fatty acid status of pregnant women and neonates, because this large organ contains tissues from both the mother and fetus. A more recent report identified considerable variation in the fatty acid composition of the placenta, revealing low variation in central regions and high variation in peripheral regions [38]. 18:1n − 9 and 18:2n − 6 levels were higher on the fetal side, whereas 20:3n − 6, 20:4n − 6, and 22:6n − 3 levels were higher on the maternal side [39]. However, these data should be assessed by standardized methods.

Trace elements and other micronutrients   The effect of dietary iodine intake on maternal and infantile thyroid function in iodine-sufficient areas is poorly understood, and data are scarce on the appropriate gestational age-specific reference ranges for urinary iodine excretion during pregnancy and lactation in Japan despite the fact that iodine deficiency in pregnant and lactating women is known to induce serious damage in fetuses, newborns, and weaning infants [40]. However, iodine intake as assessed by the urine iodine concentration of pregnant Japanese women was considered sufficient and not excessive according to the World Health Organization criteria [40]. Selenium deficiency was also examined in children and adolescents with intestinal dysfunction and neurologic disabilities who were nourished through maternal. It was determined that the appearance of hair browning and nail whitening and presence of macrocythemia or cardiac dysfunction were important symptoms of selenium deficiency in such patients in Japan [41].

Other Factors Related to Fetal Programming: Alterations in Eating Habits and the Involvement of Environmental Substances

Two other factors impact the nutritional status of mothers and infants: lifestyle choices and exposure to environmental contaminants. We must consider the adverse effects on fetal growth of contaminants such as heavy metals, polychlorinated biphenyls (PCBs), and pesticides in the maternal environment, as well as inappropriate and insufficient nutrition.

Methyl mercury and polychlorinated biphenyls from fish consumption   Methyl mercury (MeHg) can get into in the breast milk of mothers, resulting in the lactational exposure of their infants. This is the cause of congenital Minamata disease in Japan. The levels of total mercury and MeHg in breast milk and maternal blood were determined using samples from the Tohoku Study of Child Development. An exposure assessment model described the relationship between fish consumption and body MeHg levels in the Japanese population, but not in infants [42]. Evidence on the effects on human health of low-level MeHg exposure by the daily consumption of foods such as fish, meat, vegetables, and milk has been reported in northern European countries [43]. However, there is a lack of information on the clear association between mercury and disease in children in Japan. Future large-scale studies on children and pregnant women are urgently needed. The effects of in-utero exposure to PCBs and MeHg on birth size in 367 mother-newborn pairs were assessed by Miyashita et al. [44] The study showed that the risk of having an SGA infant as assessed by weight was associated with mercury concentration, but that concentrations of PCBs had no association with birth size.

Polychlorinated biphenyls and environmental hormones   PCBs and their metabolites are known contaminants of seafood. Exposure to PCBs and consequent adverse health effects have been examined. The levels of PCBs or ratio of OH-PCBs:PCBs were determined not to be associated with neonatal free T4, or with the body size of neonates [45]. Mori et al. [46] measured PCB concentrations in blood samples from 507 Japanese individuals ranging from infants to those aged over 80 years. Interestingly, the PCB levels of multiparous women were lower than those of nulliparous women in their 30s, suggesting that the PCBs were transferred from the mothers to their children during pregnancy and lactation.

Phthalates have been used as plasticizers for various plastic compounds. Humans are constantly exposed to phthalates, and biomonitoring studies have demonstrated widespread exposure of the general population to these chemicals. Di(2-ethylhexyl) phthalate (DEHP) is one of the major phthalate compounds, and is mainly used in production in Japan. The Hokkaido Study Sapporo Cohort provided significant evidence of an association between maternal exposure to DEHP and the levels of reproductive hormones such as T/E2, P4, and inhibin B in fetal blood [47]. In 2012, a study by Suzuki et al. [48] also reported an association between fetal exposure to phthalate esters and anogenital distance in male newborns. These findings suggest that DEHP exposure in utero may have adverse effects on both Sertoli and Leydig cell development in males, because inhibin B and INSL3 are associated with Sertoli and Leydig cell function and their perturbation causes urogenital anomalies. Bisphenol has also been linked with reproductive disorders, and individual variations were evident in the genetic response to bisphenol A in human foreskin fibroblast cells derived from patients with cryptorchidism and hypospadias [49].

Air pollution and neurodevelopmental diseases The central nervous system is an important target for air pollution, which causes adverse health effects, such as neurodevelopmental disorders. Diesel exhaust is a major source of ambient particulate matter and a reported contaminant of food. In pregnant mice, exposure to air pollution may cause changes in maternal behavior and infant conditions [50]. The study showed that learning impairment was associated with modulation of the N-methyl-D-aspartate receptor and inflammatory markers in the hippocampus [51], suggesting that not only the nutritional status of the mother, but also the environmental factors during pregnancy and the lactational period, influence the neurobehavior of the offspring.

Molecular Aspects of Fetal Programming Revealed by Epigenetics Studies Conducted in Japan

Epigenetic modifications, such as DNA methylation and histone modification in offspring, are considered testament to the in-utero environment. However, few studies in humans have investigated the associations between maternal nutritional conditions during pregnancy and epigenetic alterations in the offspring in Japan. One report examined the genome-wide methylation profiles of 33 postpartum placentas from normal pregnancies and those with fetal growth restriction with varying degrees of maternal gestational weight gain [52]. The study showed that epigenetic alterations accumulated in the placenta under adverse in-utero conditions, and that hypermethylation frequently occurred at the promoter regions of transcriptional regulatory genes located in developmental regulator loci. This suggests that epigenetic alterations may elevate the risk of developing various diseases, including metabolic and mental disorders, later in life. Another interesting report about hazardous chemicals stated that elevated serum levels of many pesticide-related organochlorines and some PCBs were associated with global hypomethylation of leukocyte DNA in Japanese women [53].

Conclusion

Maternal obesity is a growing problem worldwide, but in Japan, there are two different problems: maternal obesity and unhealthy thinness. Being both overweight and underweight pre-pregnancy are risk factors for compromised maternal and child health outcomes. This review identified that maternal obesity alters fatty acid profiles, leading to fetal malformations, and that there is an association between being underweight during pregnancy and preterm birth and SGA babies. Surprisingly, energy intake has increased but the intake of various vitamins has decreased among teenagers and individuals in their 20s in Japan. This suggests that our present eating style does not equate to a balanced diet [54]. Because of the cultural trend among young Japanese women to be very slender, they try to remain underweight during pregnancy. Therefore, vitamin D deficiency is a serious problem in Japan. However, the outcomes of this deficiency in later life are unknown, and further study is needed in this area.

Other nutrition-specific interventions (e.g., iron, calcium, or balanced protein energy supplementation) have only been studied in pregnant women or, if studied during the preconception period, the outcomes were limited to changes in biochemical markers, and pregnancy and birth outcomes were not assessed. Strategies for the implementation of nutrition-specific interventions in the preconception period are necessary, especially in women in Japan. Furthermore, current epigenetic studies suggest an association between maternal nutrient intake during pregnancy and the epigenetic patterns of the offspring at birth. FA and other methyl donor nutrients appear to affect the DNA methylation pattern of the offspring. It is important that the characteristics of study cohorts, particularly current nutritional status and offspring sex, are considered when interpreting results used to explain fetal programming in pregnancy. Further research in this area may influence advice and guidelines regarding maternal nutrition during pregnancy and lactation.

Maternal nutritional status during the early gestational period is important for placental and fetal growth. Maternal under- or overnutrition during pregnancy can affect fetal growth. Therefore, new approaches that take into account the mechanisms that regulate fetal growth and development will be beneficial for designing new therapeutic strategies to prevent and treat intrauterine growth retardation [55, 56]. Understanding the many roles of nutrients in epigenetics will have a broad impact on the promotion of health and disease prevention. Finally, to prevent the "early origins of adult disease," pregnant mothers, health professionals, health educators, family members, maternal and child care teams, and the government should cooperate efficiently to achieve good health for the next generation. The potential contribution of environmental factors should be considered for both child and adult health in Japan, with recent dietary habits featuring much higher lipid concentrations and unknown environmental factors compared with those of a century ago.

Acknowledgements   The authors would like to thank Enago (www.enago.jp) for the English language review.

References

1. Tsukamoto H, Fukuoka H, Inoue K, et al. Restricting weight gain during pregnancy in Japan: a controversial factor in reducing perinatal complications. Eur J Obstet Gynecol Reprod Biol. 2007;133:53–9.
2. Ministry of Health, Labour and Welfare. http://sukoyaka21.jp/english.html, www.mhlw.go.jp/stf/shingi/0000030713.html (2016.4.12).
3. Kawamoto T, Nitta H, Murata K, et al. Working Group of the Epidemiological Research for Children's Environmental Health. Rationale and study design of the Japan environment and children's study (JECS). BMC Public Health. 2014;14:25.
4. The Birth Cohort Consortium of Asia. Workshop 2014 In Shanghai http://www.bicca.org/uploads/5/3/4/1/5341602/publication_lists_of_participating_cohorts.pdf.
5. McCurry J. Japan battles with obesity. Lancet. 2007;369:451–2.
6. Gluckman PD, Seng CY, Fukuoka H, Beedle AS, Hanson MA. Low birthweight and subsequent obesity in Japan. Lancet. 2007;369:1081–2.
7. OECD. Infant health: low birth weight. In: Health at a glance 2015: OECD indicators. Paris: OECD Publishing; 2015.
8. Ramakrishnan U, Imhoff-Kunsch B, Martorell R. Maternal nutrition interventions to improve maternal, newborn, and child health outcomes. Nestle Nutr Inst Workshop Ser. 2014;78:71–80.
9. Portal Site of Official Statistics of Japan is developed by Statistics Bureau, Ministry of Internal Affairs and Communications, in collaboration with ministries and agencies, and is managed by Incorporated Administrative Agency National Statistics Center. https://www.e-stat.go.jp/SG1/estat/GL02010101.do?method=init.

10. Yoshida H, Kato N, Yokoyama T. Current trends in low birth weight infants in Japan. J Natl Inst Public Health. 2014;63:2–16. (Japanese).

11. Yachi Y, Tanaka Y, Nishibata I, et al. Low BMI at age 20 years predicts gestational diabetes independent of BMI in early pregnancy in Japan: Tanaka Women's Clinic study. Diabet Med. 2013;30(1):70–3.

12. Yachi Y, Tanaka Y, Nishibata I, et al. Second trimester postload glucose level as an important predictor of low birth weight infants: Tanaka Women's Clinic Study. Diabetes Res Clin Pract. 2014;105:16–9.

13. Nishimura T, Takei N, Tsuchiya KJ, et al. Identification of neurodevelopmental trajectories in infancy and of risk factors affecting deviant development: a longitudinal birth cohort study. Int J Epidemiol. 2016;45(2):543–53.

14. Kubota K, Itoh H, Tasaka M, Hamamatsu Birth Cohort (HBC) Study Team, et al. Changes of maternal dietary intake, bodyweight and fetal growth throughout pregnancy in pregnant Japanese women. J Obstet Gynaecol Res. 2013;39:1383–90.

15. Yamakawa T, Itabashi K, Kusuda S, Neonatal Research Network of Japan. Mortality and morbidity risks vary with birth weight standard deviation score in growth restricted extremely preterm infants. Early Hum Dev. 2016;92:7–11.

16. International clearinghouse for birth defects monitoring systems in Japan at Yokohama City University. http://www.icbdsrj.jp/2001data.html – http://www.icbdsrj.jp/2010data.html.

17. Kawazu Y, Inamura N, Tanaka T, Department of Pediatric Cardiology, et al. Change in fetal echocardiography at our institution between 2004 and 2013. Ped Card Card Sur. 2016;32:31–7.

18. Kondo A, Morota N, Date H, et al. Awareness of folic acid use increases its consumption, and reduces the risk of spina bifida. Br J Nutrit. 2015;114:84–90.

19. Ministry of Health. Labour and Welfare of Japan (2010) dietary reference intake for Japanese. Tokyo: Daiichi Shuppan Publishing; 2009.

20. Itabashi K, Miura A, Okuyama K, et al. Estimated nutritional intake based on the reference growth curves for extremely low birthweight infants. Pediatr Int. 1999;41:70–7.

21. Yorifuji T, Naruse H, Kashima S, et al. Trends of preterm birth and low birth weight in Japan: a one hospital-based study. BMC Pregnancy Childbirth. 2012;12:162.

22. Sugiyama T, Saito M, Nishigori H, Japan Diabetes and Pregnancy Study Group, et al. Comparison of pregnancy outcomes between women with gestational diabetes and overt diabetes first diagnosed in pregnancy: a retrospective multi-institutional study in Japan. Diabetes Res Clin Pract. 2014;103:20–5.

23. Shinozaki K. Current status of folate intake and erythrocyte folate levels in young Japanese women. J Jpn Diet Assoc. 2010;53:13–7.

24. Okubo H, Miyake Y, Sasaki S, et al. Maternal dietary patterns in pregnancy and fetal growth in Japan: the Osaka maternal and child health study. Br J Nutrit. 2012;107:1526–33.

25. Watanabe H, Ishida S, Konno Y, et al. Impact of dietary folate intake on depressive symptoms in young women of reproductive age. J Midwifery Womens Health. 2012;57:43–8.

26. Sato Y, Nakanishi T, Chiba T, et al. Prevalence of inappropriate dietary supplement use among pregnant women in Japan. Asia Pac J Clin Nutr. 2013;22:83–9.

27. Kondo A, Morota N, Ihara S, et al. Risk factors for the occurrence of spina bifida (a case-control study) and the prevalence rate of spina bifida in Japan. Birth Defects Res A Clin Mol Teratol. 2013;97:610–5.

28. Shibata K, Tachiki A, Horiuchi H, et al. More than 50% of pregnant Japanese women with an intake of 150 μg dietary folate per 1,000 kcal can maintain values above the cut-off. J Nutr Sci Vitaminol (Tokyo). 2014;60:1–8.

29. Shibata K, Fukuwatari T, Sasaki S, et al. Urinary excretion levels of water-soluble vitamins in pregnant and lactating women in Japan. J Nutr Sci Vitaminol (Tokyo). 2013;59:178–86.

30. Shibata K, Tachiki A, Mukaeda K, et al. Changes in plasma pyridoxal 5′-phosphate concentration during pregnancy stages in Japanese women. J Nutr Sci Vitaminol (Tokyo). 2013;59:343–6.

31. Hisano M, Suzuki R, Sago H, et al. Vitamin B6 deficiency and anemia in pregnancy. Eur J Clin Nutr. 2010;64:221–3.

32. Yorifuji J, Yorifuji T, Tachibana K, et al. In normal newborns: the earliest sign of subclinical vitamin D deficiency. J Clin Endocrinol Metab. 2008;93:1784–8.

33. Tanaka K, Hitsumoto S, Miyake Y, et al. Higher vitamin D intake during pregnancy is associated with reduced risk of dental caries in young Japanese children. Ann Epidemiol. 2015;25:620.

34. Sata F. Developmental origins of health and disease (DOHaD) and epidemiology (mini review). Jpn J Hyg. 2016;71:41–6. (Japanese)

35. Tamura Y, Saito I, Asada Y, et al. A cross-sectional survey of factors influencing bone mass in junior high school students. Environ Health Prev Med. 2013;18:313–22.

36. Nagasaka H, Chiba H, Kikuta H, et al. Unique character and metabolism of high density lipoprotein (HDL) in fetus. Atherosclerosis. 2002;161:215–23.

37. Yonezawa R, Okada T, Kitamura T, et al. Very low-density lipoprotein in the cord blood of preterm neonates. Metabolism. 2009;58:704–7.

38. Yamazaki I, Kimura F, Nakagawa K, et al. Heterogeneity of the fatty acid composition of Japanese placentae for determining the perinatal fatty acid status: a methodological study. J Oleo Sci. 2015;64:905–14.

39. Shiraishi M, Haruna M, Matsuzaki M, et al. The biomarker-based validity of a brief-type diet history questionnaire for estimating eicosapentaenoic acid and docosahexaenoic acid intakes in pregnant Japanese women. Asia Pac J Clin Nutr. 2015;24:316–22.

40. Fuse Y, Ohashi T, Yamaguchi S, et al. Iodine status of pregnant and postpartum Japanese women: effect of iodine intake on maternal and neonatal thyroid function in an iodine-sufficient area. J Clin Endocrinol Metab. 2011;96:3846–54.

41. Yuri E, Nishimoto Y, Kawamoto K, et al. Selenium deficiency in children and adolescents nourished by parenteral nutrition and/or selenium-deficient enteral formula. J Trace Elem Med Biol. 2014;28:409–13.

42. Zhang Y, Nakai S, Masunaga S. An exposure assessment of methyl mercury via fish consumption for the Japanese population. Risk Anal. 2009;29:1281–91.

43. Karagas MR, Choi AL, Oken E, et al. Evidence on the human health effects of low-level methylmercury exposure. Environ Health Perspect. 2012;120:799–806.

44. Miyashita C, Sasaki S, Ikeno T, et al. Effects of in utero exposure to polychlorinated biphenyls, methylmercury, and polyunsaturated fatty acids on birth size. Sci Total Environ. 2015;533:256–65.

45. Reiko K, Seiko SASAKI. Status and perspective of birth cohort studies: lessons from the prospective Hokkaido study of the environment and Children's health: malformations, development, and allergies. J Natl Inst Public Health. 2010;59:366–71.

46. Mori C, Kakuta K, Matsuno Y, et al. Polychlorinated biphenyl levels in the blood of Japanese individuals ranging from infants to over 80 years of age. Environ Sci Pollut Res Int. 2014;21:6434–9.

47. Araki A, Mitsui T, Miyashita C, et al. Association between maternal exposure to di(2-ethylhexyl) phthalate and reproductive hormone levels in fetal blood: the Hokkaido study on environment and children's health. PLoS One. 2014;9:109039.

48. Suzuki Y, Yoshinaga J, Mizumoto Y, Serizawa S, Shiraishi H. Foetal exposure to phthalate esters and anogenital distance in male newborns. Int J Androl. 2012;35:236–44.

49. Qin XY, Sone H, Kojima Y, et al. Individual variation of the genetic response to bisphenol a in human foreskin fibroblast cells derived from cryptorchidism and hypospadias patients. PLoS One. 2012;7:52756.

50. Win-Shwe TT, Fujitani Y, Kyi-Tha-Thu C, Furuyama A, Michikawa T, Tsukahara S, Nitta H, Hirano S. Effects of diesel engine exhaust origin secondary organic aerosols on novel object recognition ability and maternal behavior in BALB/c mice. Int J Environ Res Public Health. 2014;11:11286–307.

51. Win-Shwe TT, Kyi-Tha-Thu C, Moe Y, Fujitani Y, Tsukahara S, Hirano S. Exposure of BALB/c mice to diesel engine exhaust origin secondary organic aerosol (DE-SOA) during the developmental stages impairs the social behavior in adult life of the males. Front Neurosci. 2016;9:524.

52. Kawai T, Yamada T, Abe K, Okamura K, Kamura H, Akaishi R, Minakami H, Nakabayashi K, Hata K. Increased epigenetic alterations at the promoters of transcriptional regulators following inadequate maternal gestational weight gain. Sci Rep. 2015;5:14224.

53. Itoh H, Iwasaki M, Kasuga Y, et al. Association between serum organochlorines and global methylation level of leukocyte DNA among Japanese women: a cross-sectional study. Sci Total Environ. 2014;490:603–9.

54. Kakutani Y, Kamiya S, Omi N. Association between the frequency of meals combining "Shushoku, Shusai, and Hukusai" (staple food, main dish, and side dish) and intake of nutrients and food groups among Japanese young adults aged 18–24 years: a cross-sectional study. J Nutr Sci Vitaminol (Tokyo). 2015;61:55–63.

55. Nagano R, Akanuma H, Qin XY, et al. Multi-parametric profiling network based on gene expression and phenotype data: a novel approach to developmental neurotoxicity testing. Int J Mol Sci. 2012;13:187–207.

56. Chango A, Pogribny IP. Considering maternal dietary modulators for epigenetic regulation and programming of the fetal epigenome. Forum Nutr. 2015;7:2748–70.

57. Okubo H, Miyake Y, Tanaka K, Sasaki S, Hirota Y. Maternal total caffeine intake, mainly from Japanese and Chinese tea, during pregnancy was associated with risk of preterm birth: the Osaka Maternal and Child Health Study. Nutr Res. 2015;35(4):309–16.

58. Tanaka K, Miyake Y, Sasaki S, Hirota Y. Dairy products and calcium intake during pregnancy and dental caries in children. Nutr J. 2012;11:33.

59. Asakura K, Haga M, Sasaki S. Relative validity and reproducibility of a brief-type self-administered diet history questionnaire for Japanese children aged 3-6 years: application of a questionnaire established for adults in pre-school children. J Epidemiol. 2015;25(5):341–50.

60. Associated with Weight Gain, Yokoyama Y, Nakamura M, Sugiura K. Current status of eating habits in primigravida and evaluation of factors. Bull Matsumoto Jr Coll. 2015;24(3):47–53. [Article in Japanese].

61. Shiraishi M, Haruna M, Matsuzaki M, Ota E, Murayama R, Sasaki S, Murashima S. Relationship between the plasma total homocysteine levels and skipping breakfast during pregnancy. J Jpn Acad Midwif. 2010;24(2):252–60.

62. Tada Y, Tomata Y, Sunami A, Yokoyama Y, Hida A, Furusho T, Kawano Y. Examining the relationship between vegetable intake of mothers and that of their children: a cross-sectional study of 10- to 12-year-old schoolchildren in Japan. Public Health Nutr. 2015;18(17):3166–71.

63. Fukuwatari T, Murakami M, Ohta M, Kimura N, Jin-No Y, Sasaki R, Shibata K. Changes in the urinary excretion of the metabolites of the tryptophan-niacin pathway during pregnancy in Japanese women and rats. J Nutr Sci Vitaminol (Tokyo). 2004;50(6):392–8.

64. Shibata M, Suzuki A, Sekiya T, Sekiguchi S, Asano S, Udagawa Y, Itoh M. High prevalence of hypovitaminosis D in pregnant Japanese women with threatened premature delivery. J Bone Miner Metab. 2011;29(5):615–20.

65. Nishimura K, Shima M, Tsugawa N, Matsumoto S, Hirai H, Santo Y, Nakajima S, Iwata M, Takagi T, Kanda Y, Kanzaki T, Okano T, Ozono K. Long-term hospitalization during pregnancy is a risk factor for vitamin D deficiency in neonates. J Bone Miner Metab. 2003;21(2):103–8.

66. Tanabe R, Kawamura Y, Tsugawa N, Haraikawa M, Sogabe N, Okano T, Hosoi T, Goseki-Sone M. Effects of Fok-I polymorphism in vitamin D receptor gene on serum 25-hydroxyvitamin D, bone-specific alkaline phosphatase and calcaneal quantitative ultrasound parameters in young adults. Asia Pac J Clin Nutr. 2015;24(2):329–35.

67. Horie I, Kawasaki E, Sakanaka A, Takashima M, Maeyama M, Ando T, Hanada H, Kawakami A. Efficacy of nutrition therapy for glucose intolerance in Japanese women diagnosed with gestational diabetes based on IADPSG criteria during early gestation. Diabetes Res Clin Pract. 2015;107(3):400–6.

68. Todaka E, Sakurai K, Fukata H, Miyagawa H, Uzuki M, Omori M, Osada H, Ikezuki Y, Tsutsumi O, Iguchi T, Mori C. Fetal exposure to phytoestrogens--the difference in phytoestrogen status between mother and fetus. Environ Res. 2005;99(2):195–203.

69. Sakamoto M, Chan HM, Domingo JL, Kubota M, Murata K. Changes in body burden of mercury, lead, arsenic, cadmium and selenium in infants during early lactation in comparison with placental transfer. Ecotoxicol Environ Saf. 2012;84:179–84.

70. Hisada A, Shimodaira K, Okai T, Watanabe K, Takemori H, Takasuga T, Koyama M, Watanabe N, Suzuki E, Shirakawa M, Noda Y, Komine Y, Ariki N, Kato N, Yoshinaga J. Associations between levels of hydroxylated PCBs and PCBs in serum of pregnant women and blood thyroid hormone levels and body size of neonates. Int J Hyg Environ Health. 2014;217(4-5):546–53.

Part VI
Effects of Fetal Programming in Childhood and Adulthood

Chapter 31
Growth Criteria and Predictors of Fetal Programming

Sandra da Silva Mattos and Felipe Alves Mourato

Key Points

- The purpose of growth restriction in humans is not well understood;
- Individuals who fall short or exceed their growth potential may be at risk for the development of chronic non-communicable diseases in adulthood;
- Standard growth criteria, although largely used, classify babies only through gestational age and gender;
- Customized growth criteria add variables such as maternal height, weight in the beginning of gestation, parity and ethnicity to the calculation of an individual's growth potential;
- Targeting subtle changes on neonatal pathophysiology better stratifies babies submitted to an adverse intrauterine environment;
- Applying standard and customized criteria to identify these subtle changes can better determine which criteria more accurately identifies babies at risk from foetal programming.

Keywords Fetal development • Gestational age • Small for gestational age • Growth charts • Prenatal programming

Abbreviations

AGA   Adequate for gestational age
IUGR Intrauterine growth restriction
LGA   Large for gestational age
SGA   Small for gestational age

S.S. Mattos, MD, PhD (✉) F.A. Mourato, MD, MSc
Royal Portuguese Hospital, Maternal Fetal Cardiac Unit, Recife, PE, Brazil
e-mail: ssmattos@cardiol.br; ssmattos@gmail.com

© Springer International Publishing AG 2017
R. Rajendram et al. (eds.), *Diet, Nutrition, and Fetal Programming*,
Nutrition and Health, DOI 10.1007/978-3-319-60289-9_31

Introduction

Low or excessive birth weights are considered the hallmark of an adverse intrauterine environment. This paradigm, however, has been disputed. Whether an adverse intrauterine environment does not always affect fetal weight gain, or standard criteria fail to evaluate the true growth potential of different individuals is unclear.

Customized growth criteria have been proposed to better differentiate between constitutional smallness from true growth restriction and constitutional largeness from macrosomia.

But much research on customized growth criteria focuses on neonatal morbidity and mortality.

And the complexity of intrauterine programming of adult diseases involves a myriad of pathways from the genetic message, through a complex system of transcriptions until the protein synthesis and the metabolic actions of proteins.

These subtle, pathophysiological changes may reflect fetal programming more accurately.

Weight may be too crude a measurement of intrauterine growth restriction, particularly if measured by population criteria.

Customized criteria identify individuals presenting with these subtle pathophysiological changes and, consequently, at risk from fetal programming.

Fetal Programming

The fetal programming hypothesis states that maternal malnourishment and other adverse conditions will set the fetus physiology, and depending on similarities or dissimilarities of the postnatal environments, its future propensity to health or disease [1].

While some controversy remains regarding the significance of low or excessive birth weight, the concept that an adverse intrauterine environment programs individuals to develop a range of chronic non-communicable diseases, throughout life, is universally accepted nowadays [2].

However, an accurate detection of these children remains a major challenge in maternal-fetal Medicine.

Besides, the outcome of these "intrauterine growth restricted" or "macrosomic" foetuses is usually measured as neonatal morbidity and mortality, rather than subtle pathophysiological changes that may point to an adverse intrauterine environment and to the development of chronic non-communicable diseases later in life.

Interpretation of Birth Weight

According to Wilcox, birth weight is one of the most poorly understood variables in epidemiology [3]. This variable has, for years, attracted the attention of researchers as a key component of human phenotype.

From an evolutionary perspective, birth weight represents the magnitude of maternal investment during foetal life, mediated by dynamics hormonal interactions between mother and foetus [4].

From the biomedical perspective birth weight is highly predictive of mortality in morbidity in infancy [5, 6] as well as the development of chronic non-communicable diseases throughout the life course of individuals [7–9], like hypertension and diabetes (Figs. 31.1 and 31.2).

However, the determination of what is an adequate or inadequate birth weight for a given individual is still a matter of debate. And consequently, to integrate all different perspectives to make use of birth weight as a predictor of health or disease remains a major challenge in current medical practice.

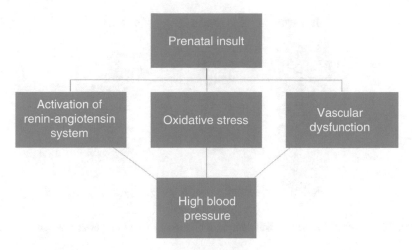

Fig. 31.1   Fetal origin for hypertension

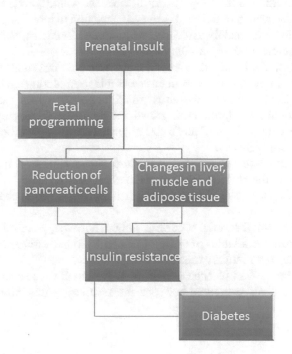

Fig. 31.2   Fetal origin for diabetes

Classification of Weight at Birth

In clinical practice, a baby is classified as small for gestational age (SGA) when it is born below the 10th weight percentile, adequate for gestational age (AGA) when it is born between the 10th and the 90th weight percentile, and large for gestational age when it born over de 90th weight percentile, for gender and gestational age [10].

Intra uterine growth restriction (IUGR) and macrosomia are terms used with to describe babies who fell short or exceeded their growth potential, and have a clinical connotation of abnormality.

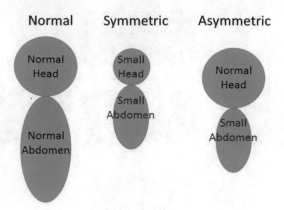

Fig. 31.3 Differences development between diferent types of neonates small for gestational age

Intra uterine growth restriction can be symmetrical, when the whole body is affected proportionately; or asymmetrical when the growth of the head is spared in relation to remaining of the body (Fig. 31.3). This last phenotype is more intimately associated with intrauterine damage during the second half of gestation, while the first insult usually occurs earlier [11].

As most babies who suffer intrauterine growth restriction are born small for gestational age, it is not unusual to associate an SGA baby with an unfavourable intra uterine environment [12].

But a clear distinction exists between the terms "small for gestational age" and "large for gestational age", and the clinical conditions "intrauterine growth restriction" and "macrosomia" [13].

The two former ones refer only to a baby's size at birth, being simple descriptions of its weight in relation to the duration of pregnancy.

Conversely, the two latter ones define babies who either did not reach or outran their growth potential and, consequently, refer to the physiopathology of the phenomenon.

In clinical practice, the distinction between them is it still a significant challenge for obstetricians and paediatricians [14].

Gestational age is the main determinant of birth weight, however, precise information over the last menstrual date is not often available. Because of this, ultrasound estimation of gestational age is considered more precise, and routinely used in clinical practice.

Ultrasound is also the method of choice to differentiate small for gestational age foetuses from those with intrauterine growth restriction; however, the accuracy of this information continues to be questioned [15–17].

Intrauterine Growth Curves

In 1963, Lubchenco et al. published the association of increased neonatal mortality with birth weight below the 10th percentile across all gestational ages [18].

This observation reinforced the concept of the implications from intrauterine growth restriction and impacted in obstetrical and neonatal management strategies for these babies.

Since then, Lubchenco curves have been largely used throughout the World. Many other curves of intrauterine grown have been published, some deriving data from larger databases, particularly for pregnant women [19, 20].

These curves were, for many years used as the guidelines to monitor intrauterine growth and classify foetal and neonatal weights.

Classical Growth Curves

The classical growth curves, based on population criteria, take into consideration only the baby's gestational age and gender. They define normal mean weights for all babies (within two standard deviation from the media) between the 10th and 90th percentile [21–24].

But birth weight results from complex interactions of numerous factors (Fig. 31.4), such as: gestational age and gender, mother's age, height, parity, ethnicity, initial weight and weight gain during gestation, nutritional status, social economic conditions and habits, such as smoking, among others [25–28].

It has been shown that, together, the baby's gender and mother's parity, height, weight and ethnicity are responsible for approximately 20–35% of the birth weight [29].

Other maternal conditions, such as hypertensive disease and congenital malformations, as well as paternal anthropometry, smoking and social economical conditions also affect the child's birth weight [30–35].

The mean birth weight varies among different ethnicities. Black babies weight less than Caucasians at birth; the Chinese are born smaller than Americans and Asians are smaller than Europeans at birth [36, 37].

Of note, birth weight has been strongly associated to maternal height, and this association is present throughout different ethnical groups [38].

The weight associated to an increased perinatal mortality varies from different populations, what suggests the existence of an "ideal birth weight", which could, however, be different to different individuals or groups of individuals.

The use of population curves to classify babies as small, adequate or large for gestational age ignores these factors and, inevitably, includes constitutionally small or large babies into the categories of SGA our LGA, respectively.

It can also miss babies who may not have reached or have extrapolated their growth potential, but in whom the birth weights fell within the limits of the general population curve.

If better, more reliable predictors of intrauterine growth restriction or macrosomia were defined and implemented in clinical practice, there would be a potential to reduce future perinatal morbidity and mortality, and long-term consequences among SGA ad LGA babies.

This is the main reason to continuously search for foetal growth curves and birth weight patterns that can be more meaningful to specific populations [39].

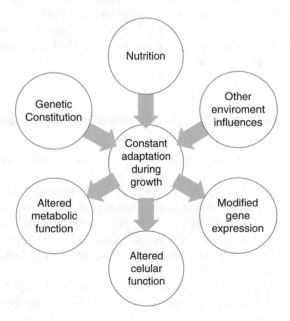

Fig. 31.4 Epigenetic factors influence in fetal growth

Customised Growth Criteria

Customised growth curves were proposed with the objective of better defining a foetus ability to reach its growth potential.

The initially proposed methods, used mathematical models to determined the estimated foetal weight from two ultrasonographic examinations performed before the 25th week [40].

The method was criticised because it assumed that foetal growth before this period would have been within normal range, because it required the performance of multiple ultrasound examinations and also because it did not seem to add many advantages to the current growth curves.

Subsequently, in the 1990s, new customised criteria were proposed, using maternal variables such as height, weight in the beginning of gestation, parity and ethnicity, besides the foetus' gender and gestational age [41, 42].

These researchers developed computer software that, by means of adjusted coefficients to each one of the previously mentioned variables, calculated the "ideal weight at birth". The coefficients were generated from multivariate analysis of large databases with well-documented birth weights.

A growth curve is then calculated using the logarithmic polynomial curve described by Hadlock et al. and derived from the transverse analysis of foetal weights estimated throughout different gestational ages [29, 43].

Studies from different ethnical groups have validated Gardosi's customised criteria and have been consistently superior to population growth curves for the detection of foetuses with intrauterine growth restriction [17, 27].

However prior to incorporating customised growth criteria into medical practice in different societies their validation, through large population studies, is necessary.

Some researchers have already adapted Gardosi's criteria to their populations.

One would expect that these criteria would perform better in societies with more ethnically homogeneous individuals, whereas in highly miscegenated cultures, the criteria may not be as specific.

Another aspect, which needs to be considered, is that most studies comparing the use of customized growth curves in relation to classical population curves focus on neonatal morbidity and mortality.

And customized growth curves may better identify neonates who may be well at birth but at higher risk to develop chronic non-communicable diseases throughout their life course.

Due to the potential impact from "undetected" intrauterine growth restriction on development of non-communicable diseases later in life, the correct identification of these individuals is key to promoting health and preventing disease.

Classical × Customized Growth Criteria and Neonatal Outcomes

Most studies address morbidity and mortality in SGA or LGA babies classified by classical or customized growth criteria.

However, few address the subtle effects from programming between these groups.

We have previously demonstrated that neonates classified as AGA by standard growth criteria, but who fall short of their true growth potential by customized criteria, show biochemical abnormalities compatible with an adverse intrauterine environment. In childhood, these biochemical abnormalities are predictive of adult health. We wonder what could be their long-term effects when they start at such an early and sensitive period of life [44].

Unpublished data from our laboratory also suggests that babies classified as SGA by customized growth criteria display an abnormal protein profile, which resembles that encountered in adults with chronic non-communicable diseases. This initial data unveils a window for exploring new mechanistic pathways for the developmental origins of health and disease.

Furthermore, our findings indicate that the effects from such adverse environment, follow a continuum from which some babies will show little clinical evidence and others will develop significant growth restriction or, possibly, excessive weight gain.

We suggest that the use of customized growth criteria, combined with maternal biochemistry, can be used as a screening approach for individuals at risk from adverse fetal programming.

And these findings have the potential to be used as biomarkers to detect individuals at risk from fetal programming.

Conclusions

The implications of programming reach all areas of physical and mental health in humans and break the paradigm of genetic immutality by showing us that, from the same code, diferente transcriptions can occur leading to diferente proteomes with consequently diverse metabolic activities.

Until now the pathways that transform the uterus from a protective organ into an adverse environment have not been clearly identified, nor have diagnostic tests been developed to screen patients at risk in the early stages.

Adequate somatic growth is the hallmark of fetal well being, however, the definition of what is adequate for a particular individual is still a matter of debate.

Customized growth criteria are more likely to reflect the true growth potential of individuals.

Their use may be particularly useful to identify babies who despite falling into "normal" weight ranges by standard criteria have suffered from an adverse intra-uterine environment. Targeting subtle physiopatological changes in these children is also more likely to stratify the high-risk group for programming.

In summary, while much still needs to be learned about programming, enough evidence has been accumulated to direct us to move past the stage of standardization and to understand that for the growth of an individual "one size may not fit all".

References

1. Barker DJ. The origins of the developmental origins theory. J Intern Med. 2007;261:412–7.
2. Chmurzynska A. Fetal programming: link between early nutrition, DNA methylation, and complex diseases. Nutr Rev. 2010;68:87–98.
3. Wilcox AJ. On the importance – and the unimportance – of birthweight. Int J Epidemiol. 2001;30(6):1233–41.
4. Haig D. Genetic conflicts in human pregnancy. Q Rev Biol. 1993;68(4):495–532.
5. Kramer MS. Determinants of low birth weight: methodological assessment and meta-analysis. Bull World Health Organ. 1987;65(5):663–737.
6. Horbar JD, Badger GJ, Carpenter JH, Fanaroff AA, Kilpatrick S, LaCorte M, Phibbs R, Soll RF. Trends in mortality and morbidity for very low birth weight infants, 1991–1999. Pediatrics. 2002;110(1):143–51.
7. Barker DJ, Osmond C. Low birth weight and hypertension. BMJ. 1988;297(6641):134–5.
8. Kanaka-Gantennein C. Fetal origins of adult diabetes. Ann NY Acad Sci. 2010;1205:99–105.
9. Varvarigou AA. Intrauterine growth restriction as a potential risk factor for disease onset in adulthood. J Pediatr Endocrinol Metab. 2010;23(3):215–24.
10. American Academy of Pediatrics. Committee on fetus and newborn. Nomenclature for duration of gestation, birth weight and intra-uterine growth. Pediatrics. 1967;39(6):935–9.
11. Rosenberg A. The IUGR newborn. Semin Perinatol. 2008;32(3):219–24.
12. Lee PA, et al. International small for gestational age advisory board consensus development conference statement: management of short children born small for gestational age, 2001 April 24-October 1, 2001. Pediatrics. 2003;111(6 Pt 1):1253–61.

13. Bernstein IG. Intrauterine growth restriction. In: Obstetrics: normal and problem pregnancies. v. 3rd ed. Philadelphia: Churchill Livingstone; 1996. p. 863–86.
14. Ananth CV, Vintzileos AM. Distinguishing pathological from constitutional small for gestational age births in population-based studies. Early Hum Dev. 2009;85(10):653–8.
15. McCowan LM, et al. Umbilical artery Doppler studies in small for gestational age babies reflect disease severity. BJOG. 2000;107(7):916–25.
16. Hershkovitz R, et al. Fetal cerebral blood flow redistribution in late gestation: identification of compromise in small fetuses with normal umbilical artery Doppler. Ultrasound Obstet Gynecol. 2000;15(3):209–12.
17. Figueras F, et al. Predictiveness of antenatal umbilical artery Doppler for adverse pregnancy outcome in small-for-gestational-age babies according to customised birthweight centiles: population-based study. BJOG. 2008;115(5):590–4.
18. Lubchenco LO, et al. Intrauterine growth as estimated from liveborn birth-weight data at 24 to 42 weeks of gestation. Pediatrics. 1963;32:793–800.
19. Alexander GR, et al. A United States national reference for fetal growth. Obstet Gynecol. 1996;87(2):163–8.
20. Bernstein IM, et al. Case for hybrid "fetal growth curves": a population-based estimation of normal fetal size across gestational age. J Matern Fetal Med. 1996;5(3):124–7.
21. Lubchenco LO. Assessment of gestational age and development of birth. Pediatr Clin N Am. 1970;17(1):125–45.
22. Brenner WE, et al. A standard of fetal growth for the United States of America. Am J Obstet Gynecol. 1976;126(5):555–64.
23. Williams RL, et al. Fetal growth and perinatal viability in California. Obstet Gynecol. 1982;59(5):624–32.
24. Marcondes E. The use of growth curves in child care. Rev Hosp Clin Fac Med Sao Paulo. 1987;42(5):218–21.
25. Wilcox AJ. Birth weight from pregnancies dated by ultrasonography m a multicultural British population. BMJ. 1993;308:588–91.
26. Ego A, et al. Customized versus population-based birth weight standards for identifying growth restricted infants: a French multicenter study. Am J Obstet Gynecol. 2006;194(4):1042–9.
27. Mongelli M, et al. A customized birthweight centile calculator developed for an Australian population. Aust N Z J Obstet Gynaecol. 2007;47(2):128–31.
28. Figueras F, et al. Customized birthweight standards for a Spanish population. Eur J Obstet Gynecol Reprod Biol. 2008;136(1):20–4.
29. Gardosi J, et al. An adjustable fetal weight standard. Ultrasound Obstet Gynecol. 1995;6(3):168–74.
30. Morrison J, et al. The influence of paternal height and weight on birth-weight. Aust N Z J Obstet Gynaecol. 1991;31(2):114–6.
31. Windham GC, et al. Prenatal active or passive tobacco smoke exposure and the risk of preterm delivery or low birth weight. Epidemiology. 2000;11(4):427–33.
32. Arntzen A, et al. Socioeconomic status and risk of infant death. A population-based study of trends in Norway, 1967-1998. Int J Epidemiol. 2004;33(2):279–88.
33. Arntzen A, Nybo Andersen AM. Social determinants for infant mortality in the Nordic countries, 1980–2001. Scand J Public Health. 2004;32(5):381–9.
34. Raatikainen K, et al. Marriage still protects pregnancy. BJOG. 2005;112(10):1411–6.
35. Nikkila A, et al. Fetal growth and congenital malformations. Ultrasound Obstet Gynecol. 2007;29(3):289–95.
36. James SA. Racial and ethnic differences in infant mortality and low birth weight. A psychosocial critique. Ann Epidemiol. 1993;3(2):130–6.
37. Fuller KE. Low birth-weight infants: the continuing ethnic disparity and the interaction of biology and environment. Ethn Dis. 2000;10(3):432–45.
38. Wells JC, Cole TJ. Birth weight and environmental heat load: a between population analysis. Am J Phys Anthropol. 2002;119(3):276–82.
39. Graafmans WC, et al. Birth weight and perinatal mortality: a comparison of "optimal" birth weight in seven western European countries. Epidemiology. 2002;13(5):569–74.
40. Deter RL, et al. Mathematic modeling of fetal growth: development of individual growth curve standards. Obstet Gynecol. 1986;68(2):156–61.
41. Gardosi J, et al. Customised antenatal growth charts. Lancet. 1992;339(8788):283–7.
42. Wilcox MA, et al. The individualised birthweight ratio: a more logical outcome measure than birthweight alone. Br J Obstet Gynaecol. 1993;100(4):342–7.
43. Hadlock FP, et al. In utero analysis of fetal growth: a sonographic weight standard. Radiology. 1991;181(1):129–33.
44. Mattos SS, et al. Which growth criteria better predict fetal programming? Arch Dis Child Fetal Neonatal Ed. 2013;98(1):F81–4.

Chapter 32
Effects of Fetal Programming on Metabolic Syndrome

Renata Pereira Alambert and Marcelo Lima de Gusmão Correia

Key Points

- Strong evidence indicates an association between small birth weight followed by "catch up" growth, the so-called "thrifty phenotype", and the development of metabolic diseases in adolescence and adulthood.
- Large birth weight after obese or diabetic mother's gestation is associated with metabolic diseases later in life. However, the association between large birth weight and the development of metabolic disease in the general population is inconsistent.
- The effect of specific nutrients deficiency (or abundance) during pregnancy on the offspring's development of metabolic syndrome in humans is poorly understood.
- Breast milk, as compared with formula feeding, appears to protect against the development of metabolic syndrome.
- Different rodent models of dietary manipulation during pregnancy and lactation induce metabolic changes in the offspring that resemble that of the metabolic syndrome in humans.
- Fetal programming through dietary manipulations in rodents has long-lasting effects that can be transmitted transgenerationally via epigenetic mechanisms.

Keywords Fetal programming • Metabolic syndrome • Nutrient • Human • Rodent

Abbreviations

HOMA-IR	Homeostatic model assessment-insulin resistance
HPA	Hypothalamic-pituitary-adrenocortical
ROS	Reactive oxygen species
SD	Sprague-Dawley
WIS	Wistar

R.P. Alambert • M.L. de Gusmão Correia (✉)
Department of Internal Medicine – Endocrinology and Metabolism, FOE Diabetes Research Center,
University of Iowa, Iowa City, IA, USA
e-mail: renata-pereira@uiowa.edu; marcelo-correia@uiowa.edu

Introduction

David Barker et al. introduced the concept of developmental origins of health and disease on their seminal manuscript published in *The Lancet* in 1989. They have shown that environmental factors that impair growth and development in early life could determine increased risk for ischemic heart disease. Since then, evidence from animal and epidemiological studies has expanded the scope of this concept to include a wide array of chronic diseases spanning from metabolic and cardiovascular illnesses to cognitive disorders, reproductive abnormalities and cancer. The theory of developmental origins of health and disease conveys the notion that the exposure to an unfavorable environment during pregnancy and lactation programs changes in fetal or neonatal metabolism, which in turn increases the risks of developing diseases in adult life. Developmental plasticity might explain the correlation between unfavorable events in early life exposures and adulthood diseases. This concept states that "one genotype can give rise to a range of different physiological or morphological states in response to different environmental conditions during development" [1]. Although the initial fetal programing hypothesis primarily dealt with undernutrition, recent epidemiological and animal studies have examined the effects of over-nutrition during fetal development and subsequent offspring's risk of developing chronic diseases. In this chapter we briefly review epidemiological and basic science literature covering the developmental origins of metabolic syndrome, with focus on nutritional factors.

Epidemiological Studies

The National Heart, Lung, and Blood Institute, American Heart Association and International Diabetes Foundation have proposed a harmonized definition of metabolic syndrome, which is diagnosed when a patient has at least three of the following five conditions:

- Fasting glucose ≥100 mg/dL (or receiving drug therapy for hyperglycemia)
- Blood pressure ≥130/85 mmHg (or receiving drug therapy for hypertension)
- Triglycerides ≥150 mg/dL (or receiving drug therapy for hypertriglyceridemia)
- HDL-C <40 mg/dL in men or <50 mg/dL in women (or receiving drug therapy for reduced HDL-C)
- Waist circumference ≥102 cm in men or ≥88 cm in women (if Asian American, ≥90 cm in men or ≥80 cm in women)

The definition of metabolic syndrome has been a matter of debate and varied according place and time. Therefore, the studies of developmental origins of metabolic syndrome often rely on variable definitions or discrete aspects of metabolic syndrome such as elevated blood pressure, hyperglycemia and excess adiposity. Other studies focus on potential pathophysiological factors, notably impaired insulin signaling and resistance. For instance, using a definition of the metabolic syndrome based on glucose intolerance, hypertension, and hypertriglyceridemia, the prevalence of the syndrome in Hertfordshire (UK) was sixfold higher in men aged 65 years who weighed ≤5.5 lbs. at birth than in those who weighed ≥9.5 lbs.

The risk of development of metabolic disease in adulthood is increased in small and perhaps in large to gestational age human newborns. An important finding is that both low and high birth weights are associated with insulin resistance. Indeed, the relation between birth weight and risk of type 2 diabetes appears to be U-shaped, with both small and large birth weight leading to an increased risk. Post-natal exposures also interact with birth weights and could determine risk of development of metabolic disease later in life.

Nutritional Deficiency During Pregnancy: Association with Small Birth Weight and Metabolic Disease

Birth weight is an indicator of fetal nutrient availability. Intrauterine undernutrition restricts fetal growth and leads to small for gestational age (<2.5 kg) offspring. It is estimated that approximately 9% of term newborns weight between 2 and 2.5 kg and about 1% weigh between 1.5 and 1.9 kg. It has been shown that the prevalence of metabolic syndrome was tenfold higher in the subjects with birth-weight <2.9 kg as compared to those weighting >4.3 kg. Several studies have provided evidence for a link between fetal undernutrition and increased risk of metabolic syndrome or its components (Table 32.1, adapted from Lakshmy [2] and Bacardi Gascon et al. [3]).

The first evidence that intrauterine undernutrition might be linked with metabolic disorders in adulthood came from the follow up of subjects exposed to intrauterine starvation during the Winter Dutch Famine, when the population survived on mere 400–800 kcal daily at the time of the German occupation of the Lower Countries between 1944 and 1945. Of note, normalization of food supply after the war led to catch-up growth of those infants born small for gestational age, giving rise to the concept of a "thrifty phenotype". It was observed that, after catch-up growth, the offspring of under-nourished mothers during the first and second trimesters was more likely to become obese and hypertensive as young adults. Furthermore, sexual dimorphism was observed given that women with low birth weight who experienced catch-up growth exhibited higher cardiovascular mortality. Glucose intolerance, microalbuminuria, atherogenic lipid profile and coronary heart disease were also documented in this population as it reached the middle age. More recently, a cohort of healthy children exposed to intra-uterine growth restriction experienced catch-up growth restricted to 1 year after birth without faster growth beyond infancy. Importantly, these children exhibited higher insulin levels and HOMA-IR, lower adiponectin levels, and a trend towards higher subcutaneous abdominal adipose tissue suggesting a condition of insulin resistance. This is another evidence of the "thrifty phenotype hypothesis" suggesting that fetuses make metabolic adaptations in response to nutritional deprivation in utero that benefit postnatal survival, but also predisposes them to insulin resistance and metabolic disease later in life [2, 4].

The Winter Dutch Famine was a situation of calorie, macro and micronutrient deprivation. The impact of specific nutrient deficiency during human pregnancy on the future metabolic health of the offspring is poorly understood. A complex relationship between the maternal protein/carbohydrate intake proportion during pregnancy and blood pressure in the offspring has been reported. Specifically, if maternal protein intake was <50 g, a higher carbohydrate intake was associated with blood pressure in adulthood. Maternal protein intake >50 g along with a low carbohydrate intake was also associated with blood pressure. More recently, maternal protein intake assessed by 24 h food diary during first trimester of pregnancy was negatively correlated with carotid-media intima thickness, a surrogate index of atherosclerosis. Surprisingly, current evidence of protein supplementation during pregnancy suggests a higher incidence of low birth weights and fetal demise through unclear mechanisms. Even though pre-existing or gestational diabetes are unequivocally associated with macrosomia, the Camden Study suggests that high sugar intake during pregnancy, at least in adolescents, is associated with twofold increase in the risk of low birth weight [2, 5].

The association of vitamins and other micronutrients deficiency during gestation and the future metabolic health of the offspring has been reported infrequently. Lower vitamin B_{12} and elevated folate during second trimester of pregnancy was associated with increased adiposity and insulin resistance in children whereas vitamin D deficiency during pregnancy can be associated with insulin resistance and gestational diabetes. Of note, vitamin A supplementation before, during and after pregnancy did not modulate blood pressure in pre-adolescents. In regard to minerals, observational studies have shown that calcium intake during pregnancy is inversely associated with systolic and diastolic blood pressures in neonates, which was confirmed in part in clinical trials [2].

Table 32.1 Retrospective studies correlating gestational malnutrition, birth weight and adult metabolic diseases

Author, country	Year	Age	n	Exposure	Main results
Wang et al., China	2012	46–53	12,065	Early gestational malnutrition	OR for HTN: 1.8 (95% CI 1.6–2.1)
					OR not increased for obesity
Van Abeelen et al., Holland	2012	49–70	7837	Gestational malnutrition	OR for T2DM: 1.4 (95% CI 1.1–1.7)
Van Abeelen et al., Holland	2012	49–70	8091	Gestational malnutrition:	
				Moderate	OR for overweight: 1.1 (95% CI 1.0–1.2)
				Severe	OR for overweight: 1.2 (95% CI 1.0–1.3)
Harville et al., US	2012	>18	2708	Birth weight	Small birth weight not associated with MS
					Large birth weight protects against MS
Li, et al., China	2011	49–53	7874	Gestational malnutrition	OR for MS: 3.1 (95% CI 1.2–7.9)
Hult et al., Biafra	2010	36–44	1339	Gestational malnutrition	OR for systolic HTN: 3.0 (95% CI 2.0–4.5)
					OR for severe HTN: 2.7 (95% CI 1.3–5.5)
					OR for IR: 1.8 (95% CI 1.1–2.8)
					OR for T2DM: 3.1 (95% CI 1.1–8.5)
Xiao et al., China	2010	59 ± 8	2019	Gestational malnutrition	Subjects who had a birthweight of <2.5 kg were 66%more likely to develop MS components in adulthood
Fall et al., India	2008	26–32	1526	Gestational malnutrition	Faster weight gain through infancy, childhood and adolescence associated with MS
Rooji et al., Holland	2007	58 ± 1	783	Gestational malnutrition	No association with MS
Mzayek et al., US	2007	18–44	2780	Small birth weight	Inverse correlation with blood pressure
Ramdhani et al., Holland	2006	26–31	744	Gestational malnutrition	Lowest tertile of birthweight associated with OR of 1.8 for MS
Painter et al., Holland	2005	48–53	741	Gestational malnutrition	Increased risk for IR, HLD, CAD
Fagerberg et al., Sweden	2004	58	396	Small birth weight	Inverse correlation with components of MS
Mzayek et al., US	2004	7–21	1155	Small birth weight	Inverse correlation with components of MS
Roseboom et al., Holland	2000	50	736	Early gestational malnutrition	OR for CAD: 3.0 (95% CI 1.1–8.1)
					OR for HTN: 3.2 (95% CI 1.2–8.6)
					OR for IR: 2.5 (95% CI 0.8–7.2)
					OR for HLD: 2.6 (95% CI 1.0–7.2)
Yarbrough et al., US	1998	50–84	303	Gestational malnutrition	Lowest tertile of birthweight was associated with a relative risk of 2.41 for MS
Barker et al., UK	1993	64	407	Small birth weight	>10-fold higher risk of developing MS, notably T2DM and HTN

Adapted from Lakshmy [2] and Bacardi Gascon et al. [3]

OR odds ratio, *CI* confidence interval, *HTN* hypertension, *T2DM* type 2 diabetes, *MS* metabolic syndrome, *IR* insulin resistance, *HLD* hyperlipidemia, *CAD* coronary artery disease

Over-Nutrition, Obesity and Diabetes During Pregnancy: Associations with Large Birth Weight and Metabolic Disease

Data from the Centers of Disease Control and Prevention indicate that 20% of women are obese at the start of pregnancy. Pre-pregnancy maternal obesity, defined as a body mass index ≥30 kg/m², confers an increased risk macrosomia (and also intrauterine growth restriction), gestational diabetes, pre-eclampsia and fetal death. Furthermore, over 40% of women exceed the Institute of Medicine Guidelines for optimal weight gain during pregnancy. In fact, obesity is now considered the most common clinical risk factor encountered in obstetric practice.

Likely due to maternal overweight and obesity, the weight at birth has been increasing over the past decades, and newborns presenting large birth weights are now more common than small to gestational age infants. Nevertheless, the link between fetal programming for metabolic syndrome in newborns with large birth weight (that is, >4 kg) appears to be weaker than that in low birth weight infants, at least in general population. However, ethnic differences are relevant. Furthermore, the offspring of diabetic mothers are clearly at increased risk of developing insulin resistance, diabetes and metabolic diseases. Illustrating these aspects, the effects of perinatal over-nutrition on metabolic programming have been thoroughly studied in Pima Indians which present the highest prevalence of diabetes in the world. Pima Indian newborns from obese mothers, independent of birthweight, exhibit tenfold greater risk of becoming obese during childhood and adolescence, and of developing impaired glucose tolerance as adolescents. By the age 20–24 years, 45% of Pima Indian offspring of diabetic mothers developed type 2 diabetes compared with 1.4% of the offspring of non-diabetic mothers.

In the general population, the combination of childhood obesity at 11 years old and large birth weight or maternal gestational diabetes was associated with insulin resistance, with odds ratios of 4.3 and 10.4, respectively. Furthermore, newborns with large birth weight and those whose mothers were obese (that is, body mass index >27 kg/m^2) before pregnancy had approximately twofold higher risk of developing metabolic syndrome at 11 years old. Notably, the offspring of obese women are 36% more likely to develop type 2 diabetes [6, 7]. It has also been shown that the adult offspring of Danish women with type 1 diabetes and gestational diabetes present an elevated risk of developing metabolic syndrome and overweight, respectively, which was associated with maternal blood sugars during pregnancy irrespective of gestational age or weight at birth [8].

The increased risk of large for gestational age infants to develop metabolic syndrome in adolescence and adulthood has been inconsistently reported, perhaps due to strong co-variates such as body mass index, body composition and fat distribution. In the Health Professionals Follow-Up Study, although large for gestational age newborns developed obesity more often, hypertension and type 2 diabetes were only correlated with low birth weight. One bi-racial cohort study (that is, Caucasians and African-americans) showed that large birth weight was indeed associated with a reduced risk of metabolic syndrome. These results contrast in part with reports showing that both low and high weight at birth are associated with increased risk of type 2 diabetes and higher blood pressure in adolescents. Metabolic diseases, notably associated with hypertension and high plasma triglycerides, were also more common in Chinese children with large birth weight [9, 10]. Contrasting with small birth weights, studies associating large birth weights with hard outcomes, such as major adverse coronary events and mortality, are lacking in the literature.

Post-natal Nutrition and the Risk of Development of Metabolic Disease

Epidemiological data exist supporting a role of the quantity and quality of neonatal nutrition in the development of overweight, type 2 diabetes, elevated blood pressure and dyslipidemia. The offspring of Pima Indians exclusively breastfed for the first 2 months of life were less likely to develop diabetes. By ages 20–24 years, 5% of breastfed offspring had developed diabetes versus 15% of formula-fed newborns, a benefit that was more pronounced in offspring of non-diabetic women during pregnancy. Meta-analyses have been conducted to explore the relationship between breastfeeding and risk of overweight. Data demonstrated that the duration of breastfeeding is dose-dependently associated with a decreased risk of overweight in later life. Up to 9 months of breastfeeding, each month of being breastfed is associated with a 4% decrease in overweight risk as compared to formula-feeding.

No studies have been published which investigated the possible effect of breastfeeding on composite elements of metabolic syndrome. However, some studies report the long-term effects of breastfeeding on single components of the syndrome such as blood pressure and lipid levels. In adulthood, breastfed subjects had lower total and LDL cholesterol levels than in formula-fed individuals. Likewise, systolic blood pressure was found to be lower in later life of breastfed participants than in formula-fed subjects. At least one clinical trial corroborates these observational results by showing that the blood pressure of adolescents born pre-term and breast fed was lower than that of those adolescents fed formula. In one meta-analysis, breast feeding has also been shown to reduce risk of developing type 2 diabetes by about 40% as compared to formula-feeding, with positive effects on fasting glucose and insulin levels on non-diabetic subjects. While formula-feeding might be detrimental due to its composition, it has also been shown that breastfed babies have lower daily caloric intake than formula-fed infants and, consequently, lower weight gain. Of note, increased early weight gain, as occurring in formula-fed infants, is a risk factor for later development of overweight and obesity [6, 11].

Children of mothers with diabetes during pregnancy have an increased risk of developing overweight and metabolic diseases, such as impaired glucose tolerance and increased blood pressure. Exposure to breast milk from diabetic mothers has been linked with the development of metabolic diseases in the offspring. Indeed, breast milk from diabetic women with diabetes contains higher levels of glucose, insulin and leptin, which can be absorbed by the gastrointestinal tract of newborns. Importantly, it has been demonstrated that a larger volume of breast milk ingested by newborns from diabetic mothers during the first week after delivery increases the risk of overweight during early childhood. Furthermore, newborn from glucose intolerant and diabetic mothers are protected from abnormal weight gain after ingesting banked breast milk from normal donors. Any imprinting mechanisms of protective influence by breast milk over formula are not currently known; but based on animal studies, macronutrient differences in carbohydrates and fats might play a role [11].

Animal Models

Despite the substantial epidemiological evidence for fetal origins of adult disease, there are intrinsic limitations in long-term retrospective studies, including potential confounding variables throughout an individual's lifetime. Therefore, several animal models have been developed to study the fetal programming of metabolic syndrome. Animal models allow evaluations of the effects of a specific controlled stress applied over a well-defined period of time. Although several animal species have been used experimentally for the study of fetal programming, the great majority of the studies in the literature utilized rodents as animal models [12]. For over 30 years, dietary manipulation has been an established model of fetal programming in humans and animal models. Different strategies have been used, including caloric restriction, low-protein diet, maternal high-fat feeding and maternal iron restriction at different points during pregnancy and lactation. These models are based on the observation that fetal nutrient supply is one of the most important environmental factors affecting pregnancy outcome [12]. Therefore, in this section, we will review the rodent models of dietary manipulation most commonly used to study fetal programming and will explore some of the mechanisms underlying the metabolic changes resulting from this phenomenon.

Caloric Restriction

A number of studies using different levels of global dietary restriction have been reported. The most common dietary intervention has been a 50% reduction in caloric intake. Total maternal food restriction to 50% of ad-lib in the last week of pregnancy [13] results in impairment of beta cell development.

Continued restriction of the mother during suckling results in a permanent reduction in beta-cell mass and number and impaired glucose tolerance [14] in the offspring. Caloric restriction programs hypertension, alteration in endothelial vasodilatation, decreased β-cell mass, islet number, decreased insulin response to an oral glucose tolerance test, and hepatic insulin resistance [15]. A more severe food restriction to 30% of ad libitum intake resulted in systolic hypertension and increased fasting insulin concentrations, hyperphagic behavior and obesity [16].

Low-Protein Diet

The low-protein model has emerged as one of the most extensively studied models of maternal dietary manipulation, which has been used to test the Thrifty Phenotype Hypothesis and to dissect molecular mechanisms. Initially described by Snoeck et al., in this model, pregnant rats are fed either a normal diet (20% protein) or an isocaloric low-protein diet (8% protein), from the first day of pregnancy to until the end of gestation. Neonates of protein-restricted dams were found to have lower birth weights, and there were effects on pancreas development, such that beta cell proliferation, islet size and islet vascularization were reduced [17]. In protein-deprived newborn rats, glucose intolerance is associated with diminished insulin secretion in response to the oral glucose loading test, which persists until adulthood, and with accelerated age-related islet cell insulin depletion [18]. Male offspring of Sprague-Dawley dams fed with 8% protein diet during gestation develop glucose intolerance, which was related with insulin resistance whereas, in female rats, glucose intolerance was associated with insulin deficiency, suggesting gender-specific mechanisms [19]. Maternal protein restriction also causes substantial changes in the liver, such as reduced hepatocyte number and steatosis, which are worsened after exposure of the offspring to a high-fat diet. These results highlight the importance of intra-uterine conditions and postnatal diet quality in the pathogenesis of chronic liver disease [20]. Additionally, maternal prenatal protein–calorie restriction in rats causes renal dysfunction and impaired glomerulogenesis in the adult offspring [21].

Maternal High-Fat Feeding

Metabolic programming leading to the development of obesity and related disorders is frequently associated with maternal undernutrition and low birth weight in animals and humans. However, it is well recognized that nutrition in most developed and developing countries is being undermined by western-style diets, which contain a high percentage of saturated fats. Studies have shown that high-levels of dietary fat intake during pregnancy are also related to an increase in the incidence of cardio-vascular risk factors in the offspring [22]. Animal studies have explored the development of such adverse effects. Studies using rodent models of maternal high-fat diet during pregnancy often result in the development of metabolic syndrome in the adult offspring. Particularly, the consumption of palatable processed foods with high-fat and/or high-sugar content causes hyperinsulinemia in pregnant rat dams and promotes the development of obesity and diabetes in the offspring [23–27]. Fetal programming of obesity and/or metabolic syndrome in this context results from complex interactions between maternal high-energy dietary intake and/or maternal fat mass. Several mechanisms could contribute to the development of overt metabolic syndrome or abnormalities in isolated components of the syndrome in the offspring. Those mechanisms include, abnormal feeding behavior, altered endocrine status and changes in pancreatic morphology and function [9]. Increased adiposity and cardiovascular dysfunction were also observed in the offspring of high-fat fed dams [28]. Insulin sensitivity and glucose tolerance in male offspring of dams fed a diet high in omega-6 polyunsaturated fat appeared to be unaffected at 3 months of age, although they were more hyperinsulinemic during an oral glucose challenge. Their liver triglyceride content was elevated and their pattern of insulin signaling protein expression was consistent with reduced hepatic insulin sensitivity, suggesting a predisposition to metabolic disease later in life [29]. Litter size reduction or cross-fostering growth-restricted offspring with normal dams is also considered postnatal overfeeding and have been associated with increased food intake in adult offspring [30, 31]. Overfeeding through litter size reduction also alters insulin and leptin signaling in the heart and induces hypertrophy in rats [32, 33].

Maternal Iron Restriction

About 20% of women in general and 50% of pregnant women are iron-deficient. Observational studies provide ample evidence for an association between maternal anemia and size at birth. Maternal anemia in early pregnancy seems to influence the pattern of placental vascularization, which may affect placental vascular impedance during early fetal life, thereby exerting effects on cardiovascular development [34]. Rodent models of maternal iron restriction also result in low birth weight offspring and programs hypertension throughout adult life, which is possibly due to a deficit in nephron number [35]. Maternal iron restriction has also been shown to program lipid metabolism in the liver [36]. Mechanistically, anemia by hypoxia or iron deficiency might exert their effects by inducing maternal and fetal stress. This is thought to stimulate corticotropin-releasing hormone synthesis, which is associated with major risk for preterm labor, pregnancy-induced hypertension and eclampsia, and premature rupture of the membranes, and also increase fetal cortisol production [37].

Transgenerational Studies

A key element of fetal programming is the existence of transgenerational effects, by which an early life exposure may affect health later in life not only of the F1 generation, but also of future generations (F2 and beyond). Different animal models have provided evidence for the transgenerational programming of adverse metabolic outcomes, including challenges such as nutrient restriction or overfeeding during pregnancy and lactation. Several studies have reported that glucose metabolism is altered in the offspring (F2) of F1 females undernourished in utero, even when the F1 females have been well-nourished after weaning [38, 39]. Moreover, glucose metabolism of the grand-offspring (F3) of female rats malnourished during development is also adversely affected, but these effects are reduced as compared to those observed for the F2 generation [40]. In mice, maternal undernutrition during pregnancy programs reduced birth weight, impaired glucose tolerance and obesity in both F1 and F2 offspring [41]. Regarding overfeeding, maternal high-fat diet consumed during the preconception period and throughout the gestation and lactation periods in mice promotes metabolism and pancreatic programming in F1 and F2 male offspring [42]. The impact of paternal obesity in transgenerational inheritance has also been reported. Paternal obesity was shown to initiate metabolic disturbances in two generations of mice albeit with incomplete penetrance to the F2 generation [43]. Dunn and Bale reported that maternal high-fat diet affects F3 female body size via the paternal lineage [44], which supports a stable germline-based transgenerational mode of inheritance, thus suggesting that imprinted genes may be involved in such epigenetic programming. Additional models of transgenerational fetal programming are provided in Table 2 (adapted from Aiken and Ozanne [45]).

Table 2 Rodent dietary studies of fetal programming where phenotype in offspring at least as far as the F2 generation was sought

Author	Year	Organism	Programming intervention	Phenotype examined	Generation with phenotype
Armitage et al.	2007	Rat (SD)	F0 high-fat diet/F1 and F2 no intervention	Aortic dysfunction, Na/K ATPase activity	Not F2
Benyshek et al.	2004	Rat (SD)	F0 low-protein or high-fat diet/F1 and F2 high-fat diet	Insulin resistance	Not F2
Benyshek et al.	2006	Rat (SD)	F0 low-protein diet/F1 and F2 energy restricted	Insulin/glucose metabolism	F2/F3
Benyshek et al.	2008	Rat (SD)	F0 low-protein diet/F1 and F2 energy restricted	Insulin/glucose metabolism	F2 not F3
Bertram et al.	2008	Guinea pig	F0 low-protein diet/F1 and F2 no intervention	HPA axis responses	F2
Blondeau et al.	2002	Rat (Wis)	F0 energy restriction/F1 and F2 no intervention	Beta cell mass	F2
Burdge et al.	2011	Rat (Wis)	F0 high-energy diet/F1 high-energy diet	Methylation status	F2/F3
Burdge et al.	2007	Rat (Wis)	F0 low-protein diet/F1 and F2 energy restricted	Methylation status	F2
Carone et al.	2010	Mouse	F0 low-protein diet/F1 and F2 no intervention	Hepatic cysteine metabolism	F2
Chernoff et al.	2009	Rat (SD)	F0 energy-restricted diet/no F1 and F2 intervention	Reproductive senescence	Not F2
Dunn and Bale	2011	Mouse	F0 high fat/F1 and F2 no intervention	Bodyweight and glucose tolerance	F2/F3
Frantz et al.	2011	Mouse	F0 low-protein diet/F1 and F2 no intervention	Insulin secretion and pancreatic beta cell mass	F2/F3
Fullston et al.	2012	Mouse	F0 high-fat paternal diet/F1 and F2 no intervention	Impaired gamete development	F2
Garg et al.	2012	Rat (SD)	F0 no intervention/F1 caloric restriction/F2 embryo-transfer	Body weight, glucose tolerance	F2
Gniuli et al.	2008	Mouse	F0 and F1 high fat/F2 no intervention	Glucose tolerance, pancreatic beta cell dysfunction	F2
Harrison and Langley-Evans	2009	Rat (Wis)	F0 low-protein diet/F1 and 2 no intervention	Systolic blood pressure, nephron number, body composition	F2 not F3
Jimenez-Chillaron et al.	2009	Mouse	F0 50% caloric restriction/F1 and 2 no intervention	Birthweight, glucose tolerance and obesity	F2
Martin et al.	2000	Rat (SD)	F0 low-protein diet/F1 and 2 high fat or control diet	Plasma glucose and insulin	F2
Peixoto-Silva et al.	2011	Mouse	F0 low-protein diet/F1 and F2 no intervention	Birthweight, glucose tolerance and adipocyte size	F2
Pentinat et al.	2011	Mouse	F0 early over-nutrition/F1 and F2 no intervention	Peripheral glucose tolerance	F2
Pinheiro et al.	2008	Rat (Wis)	F0 low-protein diet/F1 and F2 no intervention	Birthweight, glucose, leptin	F2
Radford et al.	2012	Mouse	F0 50% caloric restriction/F1 and F2 no intervention	DNA methylation	F2
Slamberova et al.	2005	Rat (SD)	F0 morphine exposure/F1 and F2 no intervention	Righting reflex	F2
Stone and Bales	2010	Prairie vole	F0 handling/F1 and F2 no intervention	Social behavioral indices	F2
Thamotharan et al.	2007	Rat (SD)	F0 50% caloric restriction/F1 and F2 no intervention	Glucose:insulin ratio, GLUT4	F2
Torrens et al.	2008	Rat (Wis)	F0 low-protein diet/F1 and F2 no intervention	Vascular endothelial changes	F2
Zambrano et al.	2005	Rat (Wis)	F0 low-protein diet/F1 and F2 no intervention	Glucose and insulin metabolism	F2

Adapted from Aiken and Ozanne [45]

SD Sprague Dawley, *Wis* Wistar, *HPA*, hypothalamic-pituitary-adrenocortical

Common Mechanisms for Fetal Programming of Metabolic Syndrome

Two main mechanistic theories have been proposed by which disparate intrauterine insults go on to exert effects on various different physiological systems in the offspring. One common postnatal outcome for various experimental conditions utilized to induce fetal programming is alterations in corticosterone/cortisol and/or adrenocorticotropic hormone levels in response to stress, glucocorticoid receptor expression within the hypothalamic-pituitary-adrenocortical (HPA) axis and in peripheral tissues, and hypothalamic corticotropin-releasing hormone mRNA levels [46], all of which are thought to adapt development of the fetus and slow down its growth to meet with reduced nutrient availability. The experimental evidence therefore seems to supports a hypothesis that adult metabolic disease arises in utero as a result of programming of the HPA axis, at least for a large range of maternal insults. One other mechanism proposed is the "oxidative stress" hypothesis [47]. Excessive reactive oxygen species (ROS) can cause modulation of gene expression and/or direct damage to cell membranes and other molecules at critical developmental windows. Many believe that oxidative stress is the primary link between adverse fetal growth and later elevated risks of the metabolic syndrome, type 2 diabetes, and other disorders. The experimental evidence for a role for oxidative stress in adverse programming is sparse however. Two separate groups have demonstrated its role in the in-utero programming of hypertension [48, 49]. Furthermore, dietary supplements, which support nitric oxide formation and scavenge ROS, administered to spontaneously hypertensive rats during pregnancy and lactation, resulted in a persistent lowering of blood pressure in the offspring [49]. Regarding the transgenerational effects of fetal programming, many authors have argued in favor of epigenetic mechanisms [45], which refers to all modifications to genes other than changes in the DNA sequence itself and includes alterations in DNA methylation, histone modification or small RNA molecules. Most studies have focused on changes in DNA methylation patterns invoked by nutritional or other environmental stimuli. Such changes are sought in diverse transgenerational developmental programming models. Fetal programming via histone modification is less well described. Histones can be modified by methylation, phosphorylation and acetylation, all of which can change the interaction between histones and DNA to alter gene expression. Additionally, transgenerational epigenetic effects may be mediated via alteration of microRNA (miRNA) expression, which is known to be modulated in response to environmental factors such as cigarette smoke and dietary factors. However, there is little evidence yet, that such changes can be transmitted through generations [5].

Conclusions

Epidemiological and animal studies have been conducted to investigate the maternal milieu, which directs fetal programming and the molecular mechanisms adversely altered in the metabolic syndrome (Fig. 32.1). The idea that phenotypic changes brought about by fetal programming are inherited is supported by transgenerational studies, which show that the effects of an adverse fetal environment influence both the exposed offspring and subsequent non-exposed generations. In the past few years, many studies aimed to understand the significance of epigenetic patterns and their role on early life-programmed disease. More studies are required to identify effective strategies to prevent deleterious effects of fetal programming and reduce the adverse effects of poor maternal nutrition on the offspring's health.

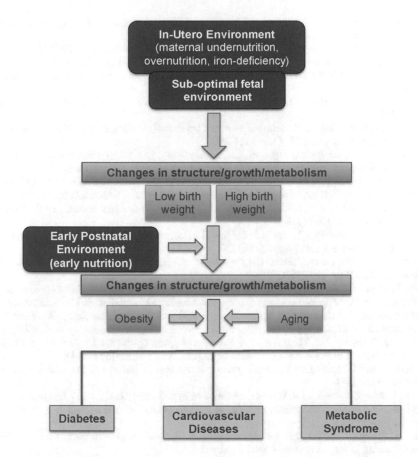

Fig. 32.1 Adverse intrauterine and early post-natal environments program metabolic disorders. Understanding the mechanisms underlying these metabolic alterations would enable identification of molecular markers of disease risk and identification of individuals at risk (Adapted from Martin-Gronert and Ozanne [50])

References

1. Barker DJ. The developmental origins of insulin resistance. Horm Res. 2005;64(Suppl 3):2–7.
2. Lakshmy R. Metabolic syndrome: role of maternal undernutrition and fetal programming. Rev Endocr Metab Disord. 2013;14(3):229–40.
3. Bacardi Gascon M, Jimenez Moran E, Santillana Marin E, Jimenez Cruz A. Effect of pre and post natal undernutrition on components of metabolic syndrome later in life; systematic review. Nutr Hosp. 2014;29(5):997–1003.
4. Crume TL, Scherzinger A, Stamm E, et al. The long-term impact of intrauterine growth restriction in a diverse U.S. cohort of children: the EPOCH study. Obesity (Silver Spring). 2014;22(2):608–15.
5. Brenseke B, Prater MR, Bahamonde J, Gutierrez JC. Current thoughts on maternal nutrition and fetal programming of the metabolic syndrome. J Pregnancy. 2013;2013:368461.
6. Dyer JS, Rosenfeld CR. Metabolic imprinting by prenatal, perinatal, and postnatal overnutrition: a review. Semin Reprod Med. 2011;29(3):266–76.
7. Boney CM, Verma A, Tucker R, Vohr BR. Metabolic syndrome in childhood: association with birth weight, maternal obesity, and gestational diabetes mellitus. Pediatrics. 2005;115(3):e290–6.
8. Clausen TD, Mathiesen ER, Hansen T, et al. Overweight and the metabolic syndrome in adult offspring of women with diet-treated gestational diabetes mellitus or type 1 diabetes. J Clin Endocrinol Metab. 2009;94(7):2464–70.
9. de Gusmao Correia ML, Volpato AM, Aguila MB, Mandarim-de-Lacerda CA. Developmental origins of health and disease: experimental and human evidence of fetal programming for metabolic syndrome. J Hum Hypertens. 2012;26(7):405–19.

10. Harville EW, Srinivasan S, Chen W, Berenson GS. Is the metabolic syndrome a "small baby" syndrome?: the bogalusa heart study. Metab Syndr Relat Disord. 2012;10(6):413–21.

11. Plagemann A, Harder T, Schellong K, Schulz S, Stupin JH. Early postnatal life as a critical time window for determination of long-term metabolic health. Best Pract Res Clin Endocrinol Metab. 2012;26(5):641–53.

12. Vuguin PM. Animal models for small for gestational age and fetal programming of adult disease. Horm Res. 2007;68(3):113–23.

13. Garofano A, Czernichow P, Breant B. In utero undernutrition impairs rat beta-cell development. Diabetologia. 1997;40(10):1231–4.

14. Garofano A, Czernichow P, Breant B. Beta-cell mass and proliferation following late fetal and early postnatal malnutrition in the rat. Diabetologia. 1998;41(9):1114–20.

15. Ergaz Z, Avgil M, Ornoy A. Intrauterine growth restriction-etiology and consequences: what do we know about the human situation and experimental animal models? Reprod Toxicol. 2005;20(3):301–22.

16. Vickers MH, Breier BH, Cutfield WS, Hofman PL, Gluckman PD. Fetal origins of hyperphagia, obesity, and hypertension and postnatal amplification by hypercaloric nutrition. Am J Physiol Endocrinol Metab. 2000;279(1):E83–7.

17. Snoeck A, Remacle C, Reusens B, Hoet JJ. Effect of a low protein diet during pregnancy on the fetal rat endocrine pancreas. Biol Neonate. 1990;57(2):107–18.

18. Dahri S, Snoeck A, Reusens-Billen B, Remacle C, Hoet JJ. Islet function in offspring of mothers on low-protein diet during gestation. Diabetes. 1991;40(Suppl 2):115–20.

19. Shepherd PR, Crowther NJ, Desai M, Hales CN, Ozanne SE. Altered adipocyte properties in the offspring of protein malnourished rats. Br J Nutr. 1997;78(1):121–9.

20. Souza-Mello V, Mandarim-de-Lacerda CA, Aguila MB. Hepatic structural alteration in adult programmed offspring (severe maternal protein restriction) is aggravated by post-weaning high-fat diet. Br J Nutr. 2007;98(6):1159–69.

21. Almeida JR, Mandarim-de-Lacerda CA. Maternal gestational protein-calorie restriction decreases the number of glomeruli and causes glomerular hypertrophy in adult hypertensive rats. Am J Obstet Gynecol. 2005;192(3):945–51.

22. Newman WP 3rd, Freedman DS, Voors AW, et al. Relation of serum lipoprotein levels and systolic blood pressure to early atherosclerosis. The Bogalusa Heart Study. N Engl J Med. 1986;314(3):138–44.

23. Patel MS, Srinivasan M. Metabolic programming due to alterations in nutrition in the immediate postnatal period. J Nutr. 2010;140(3):658–61.

24. Plagemann A, Harder T, Rake A, et al. Perinatal elevation of hypothalamic insulin, acquired malformation of hypothalamic galaninergic neurons, and syndrome x-like alterations in adulthood of neonatally overfed rats. Brain Res. 1999;836(1–2):146–55.

25. Holemans K, Caluwaerts S, Poston L, Van Assche FA. Diet-induced obesity in the rat: a model for gestational diabetes mellitus. Am J Obstet Gynecol. 2004;190(3):858–65.

26. Napoli C, de Nigris F, Welch JS, et al. Maternal hypercholesterolemia during pregnancy promotes early atherogenesis in LDL receptor-deficient mice and alters aortic gene expression determined by microarray. Circulation. 2002;105(11):1360–7.

27. Zhang J, Wang C, Terroni PL, Cagampang FR, Hanson M, Byrne CD. High-unsaturated-fat, high-protein, and low-carbohydrate diet during pregnancy and lactation modulates hepatic lipid metabolism in female adult offspring. Am J Physiol Regul Integr Comp Physiol. 2005;288(1):R112–8.

28. Khan IY, Dekou V, Douglas G, et al. A high-fat diet during rat pregnancy or suckling induces cardiovascular dysfunction in adult offspring. Am J Physiol Regul Integr Comp Physiol. 2005;288(1):R127–33.

29. Buckley AJ, Keseru B, Briody J, Thompson M, Ozanne SE, Thompson CH. Altered body composition and metabolism in the male offspring of high fat-fed rats. Metabolism. 2005;54(4):500–7.

30. Plagemann A. Perinatal programming and functional teratogenesis: impact on body weight regulation and obesity. Physiol Behav. 2005;86(5):661–8.

31. Desai M, Gayle D, Han G, Ross MG. Programmed hyperphagia due to reduced anorexigenic mechanisms in intrauterine growth-restricted offspring. Reprod Sci. 2007;14(4):329–37.

32. Pereira RO, Moreira AS, de Carvalho L, Moura AS. Overfeeding during lactation modulates insulin and leptin signaling cascade in rats' hearts. Regul Pept. 2006;136(1–3):117–21.

33. Moreira AS, Teixeira Teixeira M, da Silveira Osso F, et al. Left ventricular hypertrophy induced by overnutrition early in life. Nutr Metab Cardiovasc Dis. 2009;19(11):805–10.

34. Kadyrov M, Kosanke G, Kingdom J, Kaufmann P. Increased fetoplacental angiogenesis during first trimester in anaemic women. Lancet. 1998;352(9142):1747–9.

35. Lisle SJ, Lewis RM, Petry CJ, Ozanne SE, Hales CN, Forhead AJ. Effect of maternal iron restriction during pregnancy on renal morphology in the adult rat offspring. Br J Nutr. 2003;90(1):33–9.

36. Zhang J, Lewis RM, Wang C, Hales N, Byrne CD. Maternal dietary iron restriction modulates hepatic lipid metabolism in the fetuses. Am J Physiol Regul Integr Comp Physiol. 2005;288(1):R104–11.

37. Allen LH. Biological mechanisms that might underlie iron's effects on fetal growth and preterm birth. J Nutr. 2001;131(2S-2):581S–9S.

38. Benyshek DC, Johnston CS, Martin JF. Post-natal diet determines insulin resistance in fetally malnourished, low birth-weight rats (F1) but diet does not modify the insulin resistance of their offspring (F2). Life Sci. 2004;74(24):3033–41.
39. Martin JF, Johnston CS, Han CT, Benyshek DC. Nutritional origins of insulin resistance: a rat model for diabetes-prone human populations. J Nutr. 2000;130(4):741–4.
40. Benyshek DC, Johnston CS, Martin JF. Glucose metabolism is altered in the adequately-nourished grand-offspring (F3 generation) of rats malnourished during gestation and perinatal life. Diabetologia. 2006;49(5):1117–9.
41. Jimenez-Chillaron JC, Isganaitis E, Charalambous M, et al. Intergenerational transmission of glucose intolerance and obesity by in utero undernutrition in mice. Diabetes. 2009;58(2):460–8.
42. Graus-Nunes F, Dalla Corte Frantz E, Lannes WR, da Silva Menezes MC, Mandarim-de-Lacerda CA, Souza-Mello V. Pregestational maternal obesity impairs endocrine pancreas in male F1 and F2 progeny. Nutrition. 2015;31(2):380–7.
43. Fullston T, Ohlsson Teague EM, Palmer NO, et al. Paternal obesity initiates metabolic disturbances in two genera-tions of mice with incomplete penetrance to the F2 generation and alters the transcriptional profile of testis and sperm microRNA content. FASEB J. 2013;27(10):4226–43.
44. Dunn GA, Bale TL. Maternal high-fat diet effects on third-generation female body size via the paternal lineage. Endocrinology. 2011;152(6):2228–36.
45. Aiken CE, Ozanne SE. Transgenerational developmental programming. Hum Reprod Update. 2014;20(1):63–75.
46. Fowden AL, Giussani DA, Forhead AJ. Endocrine and metabolic programming during intrauterine development. Early Hum Dev. 2005;81(9):723–34.
47. Luo ZC, Fraser WD, Julien P, et al. Tracing the origins of "fetal origins" of adult diseases: programming by oxida-tive stress? Med Hypotheses. 2006;66(1):38–44.
48. Franco Mdo C, Dantas AP, Akamine EH, et al. Enhanced oxidative stress as a potential mechanism underlying the programming of hypertension in utero. J Cardiovasc Pharmacol. 2002;40(4):501–9.
49. Racasan S, Braam B, van der Giezen DM, et al. Perinatal L-arginine and antioxidant supplements reduce adult blood pressure in spontaneously hypertensive rats. Hypertension. 2004;44(1):83–8.
50. Martin-Gronert MS, Ozanne SE. Mechanisms underlying the developmental origins of disease. Rev Endocr Metab Disord. 2012;13(2):85–92.

Chapter 33
Fetal Programming of Food Preferences and Feeding Behavior

Adrianne Rahde Bischoff, Roberta DalleMolle, and Patrícia Pelufo Silveira

Key Points

- Poor fetal growth is associated with increased risk for glucose intolerance and metabolic disease later in life. Although increased appetite has been largely described as a part of the "thrifty phenotype", only more recently researchers have dedicated their studies to describe the specific food preferences and feeding behavior of this population.
- Clinical studies demonstrate that individuals born with low birth weight demonstrate increased preferences for highly palatable foods (those rich in carbohydrates and fat) at different ages.
- It is also shown that these subjects have particular eating behaviors and demonstrate more feeding difficulties in infancy.
- Several animal models of poor fetal growth also have shown food preferences towards palatable foods in IUGR vs. controls. More heterogeneity is found regarding conditioning properties of sugar in the different models.
- Brain systems involved in these alterations are those from mesocorticolimbic dopaminergic pathways and opioid systems. Differential modulation by peripheral hormones such as insulin and leptin also seem to play a role in these behaviors.
- Environmental variation (e.g. quality of maternal care, n-3 PUFAs consumption) seem to moderate the association between being born small and having increased preference for palatable foods, and may offer insights into the development of preventive measures to avoid metabolic disease in this population.

Keywords Food preferences • Low birth weight • Feeding behavior • IUGR • Appetitive traits • SGA

A.R. Bischoff, MD (✉)
Division of Neonatology in the Department of Pediatrics, University of Toronto and the Hospital for Sick Children, Toronto, ON, Canada
e-mail: adrianne.bischoff@sickkids.com

R. DalleMolle, MSc, PhD
McGill Center for the Convergence of Health and Economics and Montreal Neurological Institute McGill University, Montreal, QC, Canada

P.P. Silveira, MD, PhD
Departamento de Pediatria – FAMED – Universidade Federal do Rio Grande do Sul, Porto Alegre, RS, Brazil

Ludmer Centre for Neuroinformatics and Mental Health, Douglas Mental Health University Institute, McGill University, Montreal, QC, Canada

© Springer International Publishing AG 2017
R. Rajendram et al. (eds.), *Diet, Nutrition, and Fetal Programming*, Nutrition and Health, DOI 10.1007/978-3-319-60289-9_33

Abbreviations

AGA	Adequate for gestational age
AgRP	Agouti-related peptide
ARC	Arcuate nucleus
ASST	Attentional Set-Shifting Task
BMI	Body mass index
BWR	Birth weight ratio (birth weight/mean populational birth weight, sex and gestational age specific)
D2	Dopamine type 2 receptor
DA	Dopamine
DAT	Dopamine reuptake transporter
DHA	Docosahexaenoic acid
fMRI	Functional magnetic resonance imaging
HOMA-IR	Homeostatic model assessment for insulin resistance
HPA	Hypothalamus – pituitary – adrenal
IUGR	Intrauterine growth restriction
LMPT	Late and moderately preterm children
LPEarly, LPMid, LPLate	Low-protein diet in different gestational periods: day 0–7 (LPEarly), day 8–14 (LPMid) or day 15–22 (LPLate)
MOR	Mu-opioid receptor
n-3 PUFAs	n-3 polyunsaturated fatty acids
NAcc	Nucleus accumbens
NPY	Neuropeptide Y
ObRb	Leptin receptor
OFC	Orbitofrontal cortex
PENK	Preproenkephalin
PFC	Prefrontal cortex
PI3K	Phosphoinositide 3-kinase
POMC	Pro-opiomelanocortin
pTH	Phospho-tyrosine hydroxylase
SGA	Small for gestational age
TH	Tyrosine-hydroxylase
VLBW	Very low birth weight
VTA	Ventral tegmental area

Introduction

Feeding behavior is essential to maintain homeostasis, and therefore it is tightly regulated by a complex net of mechanisms. The neurobiology involved in the control of feeding behavior and food choices, in a very simplistic way, can be divided into homeostatic, hedonic and executive influences. Basically, the hypothalamus is the central brain region involved in regulating appetite and guaranteeing the energy intake needed for survival. However, beyond the homeostatic needs, the pleasurable sensations associated with the intake of highly palatable foods – usually rich in sugar and fat – are controlled mostly by the mesocorticolimbic dopaminergic pathway, although many inputs from other brain systems such as the opioids also play a role in this behavior. Finally, impulse control and decision- making processes, largely based on the prefrontal cortex, are important determinants of

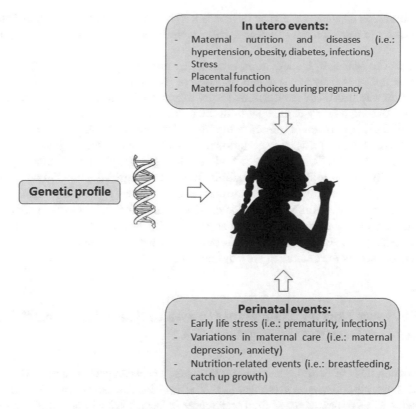

Fig. 33.1 Early life determinants of food choices and feeding behaviors. *Legend*: Genetic heritage, adverse events happening in utero and early postnatal exposures contribute to the development of food preferences

food choices. All these brain areas are enriched with receptors for peripheral hormones involved in energy intake and expenditure, such as insulin, leptin and ghrelin, and therefore signals from the gastrointestinal tract and adipose tissue depots are able to modulate the central responses, in a finely regulated fashion.

Our group has been focusing in comprehending the early life determinants of feeding behavior and food choices [1, 2], Fig. 33.1. Some studies show that the genetic profile has a main effect on food choices in children [3], and they interact with the environment [4]. Early postnatal experience also influences the different brain mechanisms involved in the modulation of feeding behaviors and preferences [5, 6]. Furthermore, the amazing brain development occurring during fetal life is a wide-open opportunity for the establishment of programming effects, therefore the exposure to adverse events in utero also has a major impact on these behaviors – and this is the focus of this Chapter. Several studies have shown that food preferences are related to physical health and will affect the risk for conditions such as cardiovascular diseases, type II diabetes and even some types of cancer [7–9]. Therefore, understanding the early life determinants of feeding behaviors and food choices may offer insights on targets for the development of interventions and prevention of these very prevalent diseases.

Aberrant fetal growth – either poor or exaggerated – has also been linked to the development of metabolic syndrome in later life. Many authors describe a U-shaped curve linking both low and high birth weights with these conditions [10, 11]. Moreover, adversities happening in utero, even those that do not affect birth weight, program the functioning of several organs and systems – and those controlling appetite, feeding behavior and food preferences are no exception. Unfortunately, little is known about the effects of being born large for gestational age on appetite and food choices later in life. Therefore, in this Chapter, we review the evidence (both clinical and experimental) linking poor fetal growth and the development of specific food preferences and feeding behaviors over the life course.

It is important to note that, by definition, intrauterine growth restriction (IUGR) is a condition in which the fetus does not grow at a rate that will lead to its full potential size at birth. This concept, involving growth rate, has clear implications for its diagnosis. In most cases, birth weight (a single point in time) is used as a proxy of the quality of the intrauterine environment. Children are classified by comparison to the population of reference into those born small (SGA, below the 10th percentile) or adequate (AGA, above) for a specific gestational age and sex. It is assumed that SGA children were the ones who suffered IUGR. However, not all fetuses that are SGA are pathologically growth restricted. Similarly, not all fetuses that have failed to meet their growth potential are in less than the 10th percentile for estimated fetal weight, or can be classified as low birth weight (i.e., less than 2500 g) [12]. In most cases, birth cohorts have only the information on birth weight, not growth during gestation. As a result, expressions such as SGA, IUGR and low birth weight have been vastly used interchangeably as synonymous in this literature. In this chapter, we decided to keep the terminology primarily used by the authors in the original papers.

Clinical Evidence Linking Poor Fetal Growth to Altered Feeding Behavior and Preferences Over the Life Course

There is a growing body of evidence showing an association between poor fetal growth and differential eating behaviors over the life course in humans [13]. The available clinical data has focused on two major aspects related to either programming of food preferences or feeding behavior in different age groups.

Food Preferences

The effects of fetal programming on food preferences are apparent at very early ages as demonstrated by Ayres et al. [14] and Rotstein et al. [15]. Using the birth weight ratio (BWR) as a continuous variable to define intrauterine growth restriction (IUGR), Ayres et al. recorded facial responses of preterm newborns that received either water or a sucrose solution during their very first day of life. They found a positive correlation between the BWR and the hedonic response to a sweet solution (sucrose) meaning that the more restricted the newborn, the less hedonic responses to sucrose they'd demonstrate, although no differences were seen in response to water. The authors suggested that IUGR may lead to a decreased sensibility to the pleasurable sensation related to the sweet taste, which would prone them to an increased consumption of palatable foods in order to achieve the same degree of pleasure [14].

Using a similar method, Rotstein et al. evaluated term newborn's facial recognition patterns for taste and smell, using repeated exposures to water or sucrose that were born small for gestational age (SGA) or not. The authors suggested that there were no differences in the facial reaction to sweet stimuli between small and appropriate for gestational age newborns [15]. However, as the responses to water were different between the two groups and since water is tasteless and odorless, the pattern of response to water should be considered as baseline. Had Rotstein et al. used a ratio sucrose:water, the mean reactivity values would almost double for the control group, as opposed to the SGA group where responses to water and sucrose were similar. This is in agreement to Ayres findings [14], confirming that SGAs had diminished sensitivity to the sucrose taste [16].

Besides the above-mentioned evidence regarding sweet taste, studies in different age groups have shown that low birth weight individuals show different behaviors for other types of palatable foods.

For instance, Silveira et al. demonstrated that 3-year old IUGR girls are more impulsive towards a sweet reward using the Snack Delay Task [17]. In addition, the ability to wait for the sweet reward at 3 years of age was inversely related to the amount of fat consumed and the body mass index at 4 years of age [17]. Similarly, Crume et al. demonstrated that IUGR children at 10 years of age have significantly higher percent energy intake derived from fat when compared to controls [18]. Besides, IUGR children had higher waist circumference and altered metabolic state, demonstrated by higher insulin and HOMA-IR and lower adiponectin levels [18].

At 23–25 years, women born with severe IUGR have a higher intake of carbohydrates, and increased carbohydrate to protein ratio in their diets [19]. Women born with IUGR have also a higher waist to hip ratio, even though the prevalence of metabolic syndrome was not different between severe IUGR, moderate IUGR and non-IUGRs [19]. In young adults born with very low birth weight (VLBW), a markedly reduced consumption of vegetables, fruits, berries, milk products and low-fat dairy products was observed, when compared with controls [20]. Although there were 35.8% SGA in the VLBW group, there were no differences in macro and micronutrient intake between VLBW-AGA and VLBW-SGA in this study, suggesting that in this sample prematurity was a major key player in the development of specific food preferences.

In older adults exposed to famine during fetal life, Steiner et al. reported a higher total energy intake and higher dietary fat density at 58 years [21] while Lussana et al. found that those exposed to famine in early gestation were twice more likely to consume a high-fat diet in older ages [22]. The same correlation of increased consumption of fats in those with small size at birth was demonstrated by Perälä et al. in their study [23]. There was also a lower consumption of fruits, berries, rye and rye products, carbohydrates, sucrose, fructose and fiber in adults of 56–70 years old that were born small [23].

Another interesting aspect refers to maternal smoking during pregnancy, which is highly associated with poor fetal growth; therefore, it may be difficult to tear the effects of smoking per se and of IUGR on the programming of feeding behavior. Smoking alters caloric consumption, energy expenditure, preference for different flavors and body weight, but little is known about the potential programming effect of smoking during pregnancy on the feeding behavior of the offspring. Experimental data suggests that nicotine influences the ontogeny of hypothalamic pathways in the fetus; however, there is only scattered data in humans. For instance, individuals exposed to smoking during fetal life have a higher preference for carbohydrates over protein in adult life, even after adjusting for variables that influence feeding behavior such as socio-economic status, current smoking, physical activity, current body mass index (BMI) and especially birth weight [24]. Smoking may program food preferences independently of the effects of IUGR; however, more studies are needed to clarify this association.

Despite the apparent discrepancies of food preferences in terms of the type of food that is preferred by SGA individuals or for the effect being apparent in males or females, all studies converge to the development of altered food preferences towards highly palatable foods in those born with low birth weight. Prenatal programming modifies eating patterns for both sexes, but the timing and nature of the preferences may vary as a function of the age and the tools used to measure consumption. The causality of events is also uncertain, but studies performed at very young ages, before the development of altered metabolic states, suggest that obesogenic alterations in feeding behavior and spontaneous food choices may precede and contribute to the development of metabolic diseases in populations at risk [14, 17–19].

Feeding Behavior

Low birth weight, although far from being a perfect marker of fetal adversity, is usually widely available in large birth cohorts. Indeed, several studies in different age groups have shown that poor fetal growth is associated with altered eating behaviors. For instance, Hvelplund et al. reported that in children younger than 3 years, being born SGA is a risk factor for feeding and eating disorders [25].

These findings contribute to a growing body of evidence showing an association between poor fetal growth and differential eating behaviors over the life course [13].

Migraine et al. evaluated two French cohorts regarding their eating behavior at 2 years of age. The initial finding revealed that preterm children had a lower drive-to-eat and a tendency for lower-food-repertoire. Further analysis, adjusted for maternal age, BMI, education level, breastfeeding, sex and birth weight z score, revealed that the association of gestational age with an impaired eating behavior was no longer significant. However, the study identified that a birth weight z score less than -1 was associated with eating difficulties, regardless of gestational age, showing that those born small appear to be at a greatest risk for eating difficulties, even in term infants [26]. Birth weight and gestational age may each have a separate influence on infant development of the neuronal circuitry that controls eating behaviors. This circuitry could be exquisitely sensitive to minute alterations in the intrauterine growth rate [26], as we further discuss below.

A study by Oliveira et al. involved three European cohorts to evaluate the impact of birth weight in eating behaviors of young children. Problematic eating behaviors were assessed at 4–6, 12–15, 24 and 48–54 months. The main finding was that those born SGA were more likely to have feeding difficulties and poor eating, particularly at 4–6 months of age [27]. More recently, Johnson et al. reported that late and moderately preterm children (LMPT) (born 32–36 weeks gestational age) had an increased risk of eating difficulties, particularly related to refusal/picky eating problems. Although this study did not adjust the analysis according to birth weight z score, it is noticeable that the proportion of SGA was higher among those LMPT when compared to those born at term (17.7% versus 12.3%), which may partially explain these findings [28]. Since the study was designed to evaluate children born preterm, other factors that are more prevalent in this population should also be accounted for the development of eating difficulties, for instance prolonged nasogastric feeding, neurodevelopmental and behavioral sequelae.

One recent study performed using a large cohort found no association between birth weight and energy intake or satiety responses at 5 years of age [29]. Interestingly, the study describes that conditional weight gain both in early and late childhood was associated with lower satiety responsiveness and a higher energy intake. The authors propose that an earlier adiposity rebound could be involved in these findings, considering that early adiposity rebound is linked to poorer outcomes such as obesity risk [29]. This suggests a role for catch up growth on the development of altered feeding behaviors in children.

As described above, we have previously investigated impulsive behavior through a snack-delay task at 3 years of age [17]. We showed that boys in general are more impulsive than girls in this task, having a poorer ability to delay responses to an eating impulse. However, SGA girls behave similarly to boys, being significantly more impulsive than the normal birth weight girls. That is, IUGR girls have a more impulsive behavior towards a sweet reward [17]. Furthermore, poor fetal growth interacts with poor inhibitory control, enhancing food fussiness at 72 months of age [30]. Interestingly, the reported consumption of n-3 polyunsaturated fatty acids (n-3 PUFAs) seems to be a protective factor, decreasing food fussiness especially in SGA children [30]. More recently, we showed that the serum level of docosahexaenoic acid (DHA, a marker of n-3 PUFAs consumption) is inversely correlated with External Eating scores in IUGR subjects, but not in normal birth weight subjects [31]. In other words, a higher intake of n-3 PUFAs diminishes food intake in response to external cues (logos, advertising) in IUGR adolescents. Therefore, n-3 PUFAs seem to be able to protect vulnerable individuals from developing inappropriate feeding behaviors, such as external eating in adolescents and food fussiness in young children.

The assumption that the exposure to a poor fetal environment correlates with differential eating behaviors is supported by epidemiological evidence such as Hveplund et al. article [25] as well as several clinical studies despite the heterogeneity of the studied populations in terms of age, sex, economic development and type of adversity. More recent brain fMRI studies have started to explore the mechanisms involved in the altered feeding behaviors in IUGR individuals. For instance, Reis et al. showed that birth weight adjusted for gestational age and sex predicted right superior frontal gyrus

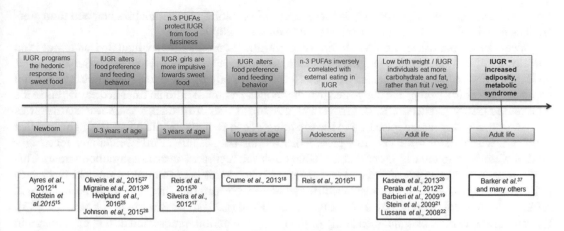

Fig. 33.2 Summary of the evidence showing the association between poor fetal growth and altered food preferences and feeding behavior at different ages. *Legend: Numbers* represent the references cited in the reference list

activation in response to the visualization of palatable foods, a brain area involved in inhibitory control [31], supporting previous evidence that impulsivity is an important feature in this association.

Apart from adequate prenatal care in order to diminish risk factors for a poor fetal environment, an adequate and careful pediatric follow-up of infants with identifiable vulnerabilities may represent a window for intervention prior to the development of metabolic consequences of chronic altered feeding behaviors. An increased awareness for the association between perinatal history and differential eating behaviors and feeding preferences is imperative to focus counseling on the positive impacts of breastfeeding, healthy foods and adequate growth, particularly in this at-risk population. Furthermore, impulsivity appears to be an important characteristic in these children and n-3 PUFAs intake may be a promising protection factor for this population.

Future research is needed to identify possible mechanisms involved and potential targets of interventions. Since IUGR is a dynamical process, larger birth cohorts, with appropriate IUGR definition and prospective long-term follow-up may further clarify the relation and causality of these findings. In addition, controlled intervention studies would further explore the clinical applications of n-3 PUFAs to modulate feeding behaviors in this population. Considering that children born with IUGR have increased risk for chronic adult diseases such as type 2 diabetes, hypertension and metabolic syndrome, acknowledging eating difficulties and altered feeding behavior is crucial for the development of health strategies targeted to this particularly vulnerable group.

Figure 33.2 depicts the different studies showing an association between small size at birth and altered feeding behavior and preferences over the life course.

Experimental Evidence

Feeding Behavior and Food Preferences

The literature shows that fetal growth-restricted animals have increased food intake and greater weight and fat mass gain throughout life, often accompanied by altered glucose dynamics, insulin and leptin resistance, hypertriglyceridemia and hyperactivity of the hypothalamus-pituitery-adrenal (HPA) axis [32–36]. These studies support the thrifty phenotype hypothesis – behavioral and metabolic adaptations to an environment that was supposed to be scarce in nutrients – which contributes to the development of chronic diseases [37, 38]. The interest in exploring the eating behavior and food preferences in animal models in more detail started in the early 2000.

Vickers et al. published the first studies exploring the consequences of maternal undernutrition (30% of ad libitum diet during pregnancy) on the offspring's eating behavior. They observed greater food intake and reduced physical activity, as well as higher body fat in the fetal undernourished group compared to control group, and suggested that the "couch potato" syndrome can have its origins in the fetal period [39, 40]. Afterwards, Bellinger et al. developed a series of studies to investigate the effect of a low-protein diet during gestation in the offspring's food preferences. The first study showed that adult rats, whose dams received a low-protein diet throughout gestation, had a preference for a high-fat diet when having three types of diet available (high-fat, high-protein and high carbohydrate). This food preference was observed in young adult rats (12-week-old) but not in older rats (30-week-old) [41]. In subsequent studies, they tested a different protocol by offering the dams a low-protein diet in different gestational periods: day 0–7 (LPEarly), day 8–14 (LPMid) or day 15–22 (LPLate) [42, 43]. Prenatal protein restriction, independently of the restriction period, programmed food preferences in female offspring at 12 weeks of age, but not in males. Females from all the low-protein groups consumed less fat than the control group when in a self-selection regimen [42]. In older rats (18 months of age), they observed a greater food intake in LPMid males and hypophagia in females [43].

More recently, Whitaker et al. observed that IUGR females, born from dams fed with a low protein diet (8% protein) through pregnancy and lactation, have greater food intake after weaning than control females regardless of the diet offered (standard or high-fat diet). However, IUGR males have increased food intake only when fed with the high-fat diet [44]. Nielsen et al. investigated the consequences of gestational undernutrition in a sheep model and found that fetal undernourished young lambs prefer to eat a high-fat diet (dairy cream) until 3 weeks of age, whereas the fetal well-nourished young lambs prefer to eat the less palatable and less energy dense diet (starch-rich popped maize). This food preference pattern was not observed in older lambs. The results point out that the timing of the nutrient insult during gestation, sex and age are important factors in the fetal programming of food preferences and feeding behavior [45].

Interestingly, Vuceticet also observed an increased addiction risk as a result of reduced protein availability during fetal development. IUGR rats derived from an animal model based on protein restriction during gestation exhibited hyperactivity after consuming a high fat diet, reduced preference for sucrose and exacerbated response to cocaine. The results show that intrauterine growth-restricted rats present characteristics that can put them at higher risk for addiction [46].

In our research group, we have been investigating the fetal programming of food preferences and feeding behavior using an animal model of IUGR based on caloric restriction of 50% starting on gestational day 10 [32]. In our model, pups from both groups (food restricted and controls dams) are fostered to control dams within 24 h of life, which ensures growth restriction only during the fetal period [47–49]. Our experiments revealed a higher preference for palatable food in IUGR animals when having standard and palatable chow (diet with higher contents of sugar and fat) available [49]. In addition, we see increased sweet food consumption in IUGR males compared to control males in an experiment in which the rats were acutely exposed to Froot Loops® [47]. Despite the lack of differences in females, IUGR female rats needed fewer trials to reach criterion in the Attentional Set-Shifting Task (ASST), using the same sweet food as reward. Thus, IUGR females have a greater ability to deal with the difficulty of finding a sweet food [47], even though it is known that IUGR animals can have difficulties in learning [50]. Unexpectedly, we also observed that IUGR rats have a reduced conditioned place preference to sweet food when compared to controls (see explanation in the next section – *Fetal programming mechanisms*) [49]. Interestingly, other studies, which evaluated IUGR animals' food motivation and food consumption in adulthood, observed that perinatal protein restriction (IUGR) is associated with increased motivation for food rewards [50–52]. In addition, it was also shown that these animals have greater intake of a high fat diet with added simple carbohydrates in females, despite the lack of alterations in the taste reactivity to sucrose [52]. Together these results suggest that IUGR animals are more driven towards food reward and have enhanced skills to find rewarding food, which seems to be an adaptation to deal with scarcity.

Using the same animal model based on 50% food restriction during gestation we also explored the hedonic responses to sucrose and water in newborns and adult rats. IUGR newborns demonstrate more persistent hedonic responses to sucrose when compared to control newborns. In adulthood, the differences were subtle: control rats decrease the hedonic responses to sucrose 40 s after receiving the solution while IUGR responses did not change overtime [53]. These results emphasize the hypothesis of the fetal programming of food preferences since an altered response to sucrose was observed already in the first day of life.

Table 33.1 describes the different experimental studies exploring the association between IUGR and feeding preferences over the life course.

Proposed Mechanisms for the Fetal Programming of Food Preferences

Food intake is a complex process, which involves hedonic, homeostatic and executive components. In addition, the body sends many signals to various brain regions capable of modulating specific neurotransmitters systems [2]. Therefore, understanding the mechanisms involved in the fetal programming of eating behavior and food preferences is challenging.

There are many studies focused on understanding the modulation of the homeostatic control system as one of the mechanisms involved in the fetal programming of eating behavior. Scarcity of nutrients in early life (prenatal or perinatal) is related to diminished expression of anorexigenic neuropeptides (Pro-opiomelanocortin – POMC), and increased expression of orexigenic neuropeptides (Neuropeptide Y – NPY, Agouti-related peptide – AgRP) and of the leptin receptor (ObRb) in the hypothalamus [54–59]. In addition, reduced satiety responses to leptin, with leptin resistance in the arcuate nucleus (ARC) [33, 58, 60–62], and increased responses to ghrelin [63] were observed. Cell counts in three hypothalamic regions involved in food intake regulation (paraventricular, arcuate, and ventromedial nuclei) are increased in fetal growth-restricted rats [56], and alterations in leptin and insulin levels during gestation may contribute to this cell cycle dysregulation in the hypothalamus [64]. Another study investigated the effect of protein restriction during gestation and lactation in the hypothalamic intracellular signaling and observed an upregulation of the insulin and leptin intracellular transduction cascade (phosphoinositide 3-kinase – PI3K pathway) in adult rats of the low-protein group [65]. Thus, caloric restriction or low protein diet during gestation can impact the offspring's neuroendocrine levels and signaling, neuropeptide levels and/or neurogenesis, as well as differential sensitivity to nutrients' sensory properties, which affect food intake (for review see [66]).

Vucetic et al. observed that the behavioral results derived from the experiments based on maternal protein restriction were related to alterations in the brain systems involved in hedonic responses. They showed increased levels of tyrosine-hydroxylase (TH) as well as dopamine in the ventral tegmental area (VTA) and prefrontal cortex (PFC), respectively, and enhanced expression of genes responsible for TH and dopamine reuptake transporter (DAT) production in areas of the mesocorticolimbic system [46]. Together with the hyperdopaminergic tone (TH overactivity and compensatory increases in DAT) they found changes in the opioid system. IUGR rats have decreased expression of opioid-related genes [preproenkephalin (PENK) in the PFC and mu-opioid receptor (MOR) in the NAcc] [67], which corroborate the reduced sucrose preference observed in the behavioral tasks.

Our research group has also focused in the dopaminergic and opioid systems as target systems involved in the fetal programming of food preferences by maternal malnutrition. Our animal model of IUGR showed alterations in both systems. Firstly, we investigated changes in the dopaminergic sys-

Table 33.1 Feeding behavior and food preferences results from experimental studies

Author/year	Intervention	Sex	Age	Outcome
Vickers et al. (2000) [39, 40]	30% of an *ad libitum* diet throughout gestation	Male	Pre-pubertal/ Post-pubertal/ Mature adult	Fetal growth restricted offspring showed hyperphagia at each age period. After puberty, statistical interactions between programming and diet offered to the offspring were observed
Bellinger et al. (2004) [41]	Low protein diet throughout gestation	Male and female	12 weeks and 30 weeks	Male and female rats (12-week-old) from the low protein group consumed significantly more high-fat and significantly less high-carbohydrate food when having three types of diet available (high-fat, high-protein and high carbohydrate)
Bellinger and Langley-Evans (2005) [42]	Low-protein diet in different gestational periods: day 0–7 (LPEarly), day 8–14 (LPMid) or day 15–22 (LPLate)	Male and female	12 weeks	Females from all low-protein groups consumed less fat than the control group. Male offspring showed no changes
Bellinger et al. (2006) [43]	Low-protein diet in different gestational periods: day 0–7 (LPEarly), day 8–14 (LPMid) or day 15–22 (LPLate) and also throughout gestation (LPAll) (days 0–22)	Male and female	18 months	Greater food intake in LPMid males and hypophagia in LPAll and LPLate females
Vucetic et al. (2010) [46]	8.5% low protein diet during breeding, pregnancy and lactation	Male and female	18–20 weeks	All mice preferred sucrose over water, but IUGR mice had decreased preference for sucrose
Whitaker et al. (2012) [44]	Low protein diet (8% protein) through pregnancy and lactation	Male and female	11 through 20 weeks	IUGR females have greater food intake after weaning regardless of the diet offered (standard or high-fat diet) and IUGR males have increased food intake only when fed with the high-fat diet
Da Silva et al. (2013) [50]	Low protein diet (8% protein) during pregnancy and lactation	Male and female	60 days	Increased motivation for food reward (chocolate-flavored cookies) in IUGR offspring
Nielsen et al. (2013) [45]	50% of a normal diet during the last trimester of gestation	Male and female	From day 3 postpartum to 6 months	Undernourished young lambs prefer to eat a high-fat diet (dairy cream) until 3 weeks of age, whereas the fetal well-nourished young lambs prefer to eat the diet less palatable and less energy dense (starch-rich popped maize)
Dalle Molle et al. (2015) [49]	50% of a regular chow starting on day 10 of gestation	Male and female	80 days	Higher preference for palatable food in IUGR offspring when having standard chow and palatable chow available
				IUGR offspring have a reduced conditioned place preference to palatable food when compared to controls

(continued)

Table 33.1 (continued)

Author/year	Intervention	Sex	Age	Outcome
Alves et al. (2015) [47]	50% of a regular chow starting on day 10 of gestation	Male and female	70 days	Increased sweet food consumption in IUGR males when acutely exposed to it, no differences in females. IUGR females needed fewer trials to reach criterion in the Attentional Set-Shifting Task (ASST), using sweet food as reward
De Melo Martimiano et al. (2015) [51]	Low protein diet (8% protein) during pregnancy and lactation	Male	70 days	IUGR offspring consumed more palatable food and demonstrated increased motivation for food reward (chocolate-flavored cookies)
Da Silva et al. (2016) [52]	Low protein diet (8% protein) during pregnancy and lactation	Female	145 days	Greater intake of a high fat diet with added simple carbohydrates in IUGR females, even without alterations in the taste reactivity to sucrose
Laureano et al. (2016) [53]	50% of a regular chow starting on day 10 of gestation	Male and female	1 day and 90 days	More persistent hedonic responses to sucrose solution in IUGR newborns Adult control rats decrease the hedonic responses to sucrose 40 s after receiving the solution, while IUGR rats do not show changes in the responses overtime

tem and observed altered TH and phospho-tyrosine hydroxylase (pTH) levels in the nucleus accumbens (NAcc) of IUGR rats in different metabolic status: at baseline and after 1 h of sweet food intake. The alterations in TH and pTH were shown to be sex-specific [49]. Interestingly, the IUGR females that needed fewer trials to reach criterion in the ASST had enhanced TH content in the orbitofrontal cortex (OFC) in response to sweet food intake [47]. In addition to changes in the enzyme involved in dopamine production, whose phosphorylated levels are positively related to the speed of dopamine synthesis [68], we also observed alterations in dopaminergic receptors. IUGR rats have reduced levels of dopamine-2 (D2) receptors in the NAcc when compared to controls [49], which explains IUGR deficiency in conditioning to a place paired with palatable food [69]. Secondly, we explored changes in the opioid system by exposing the animals to water or sucrose, and differences between IUGR and controls were found according to the age. IUGR pups have diminished phosphorylation of the μ-opioid-receptor in the NAcc independently of the received solution (water or sucrose). However, μ-opioid-receptor differences between IUGR and controls were not observed in older rats (3-months-age). Because of the importance of the opioid system in the ontogeny of early feeding pathways [70], we believe that the changes observed in the opioid system of IUGR newborns may set the stage for the differential dopaminergic functioning found later in life in IUGR animals, and finally contribute to their altered food preferences. Changes in DA and opioid systems described in IUGR offspring are summarized in Table 33.2.

According to Da Silva et al. perinatal undernutrition alters neural responses to a high fat diet [52]. The experiments showed increased neuronal activation in perinatal undernourished females compared with control females in amygdala, caudate putamen and paraventricular nucleus of the hypothalamus. Therefore, high fat diet seems to have a higher impact in IUGR by activating hedonic areas followed by compensatory responses via the hypothalamus. One could propose that an imbalance between the homeostatic and hedonic control systems seems to be involved in the increased food consumption, especially palatable/rewarding foods, in IUGR animals.

Furthermore, studies show that the functioning of the HPA axis might be also involved in the disruptive eating behavior of IUGR animals, as they have higher corticosterone levels [35, 36, 71], as

Table 33.2 Changes in dopamine and opioid brain systems in IUGR offspring compared to control

Brain marker/brain area	Age/Sex	Baseline	Aftersweetfood
TH/VTA [46]	Adult/Male	↑	−
TH/PFC [46]	Adult/Male	↑	−
DAT gene expression/VTA and NAcc [46]	Adult/Male	↑	−
mu-opioid receptor (MOR) gene expression/NAcc [46]	Adult/Male	↓	−
D2 receptors/NAcc [49]	Adult/Male and female	↓	−
TH/NAcc [49] [47]	Adult/Male	↑	=
pTH/NAcc [49]	Adult/Male	↑	=
TH/NAcc [49] [47]	Adult/Female	=	↑
pTH/NAcc [49]	Adult/Female	=	↑
TH/OFC [47]	Adult/Female	=	↑
Phospho mu-opioid/NAcc [53]	Newborn/Male and female	↓	↓
Phospho mu-opioid: mu-opioid/NAcc [53]	Newborn/Male and female	↓	↓

TH tyrosine-hydroxylase, *VTA* ventral tegmental area, *DAT* dopamine reuptake transporter, *NAcc* nucleus accumbens, *pTH* phospho tyrosine-hydroxylase, *OFC* orbitofrontal cortex

well as altered mineralocorticoid and glucocorticoid receptors expression in the hippocampus [72] and hypothalamus [73, 74]. These features can lead to chronic hyperactivity of the HPA axis with altered responses to acute stress, with consequent impact on food choices and higher intake of palatable foods [6].

The literature is advancing in exploring the mechanisms involved in the fetal programming of eating behavior and food preferences, nevertheless studies aimed at a deeper investigation of the interaction between the sensitivity to metabolic signals (insulin, leptin and ghrelin) and their modulation of neurotransmitters' release and neurons' activity in areas related to reward, pleasure and decision making are still needed. In addition, assessment of in vivo functional changes during food intake is another important step for this research area.

Moderators of the Association Between Poor Fetal Growth and Food Choices: Possible Targets for Developing Interventions

Besides the study of mechanisms, it is important to explore the factors that modify the association between poor fetal growth and later food preferences. For example, Vega et al. demonstrated that resveratrol administration to dams fed with a low protein diet during gestation can partially prevent adverse metabolic outcomes in the adult offspring [75], with decreased leptin and insulin levels, as well as HOMA index in the undernourished offspring whose dams received resveratrol compared to their control counterparts. In addition, leptin replenishment from postnatal day 2–8 decreases the expression of orexigenic neuropeptides (NPY, AgRP) via enhanced leptin receptor (ObRb) signaling, which led to increase oxygen consumption, carbon dioxide production, and physical activity, with consequent increase in milk intake but with no change in body weight on postnatal day 14 in IUGR rats [76].

There are few human studies also searching for such moderators. For example, the quality of maternal care, as well as its improvement, seems to modify the relationship between IUGR and emotional eating, as well as sucrose intake, especially in girls. Moreover, as commented above, the studies from Reis et al. [30, 31] observed that the consumption of n-3 polyunsaturated fatty acids (n-3 PUFAs) decreases non-adaptive feeding behaviors in IUGR children and adolescents. n-3PUFAs modulate mood and inhibitory control [77], possibly by diminishing the activation of the mesolimbic DA path-

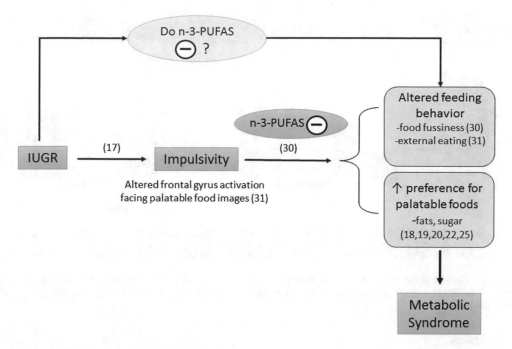

Fig. 33.3 n-3 PUFAs as a possible intervention to decrease non-adaptive feeding behaviors in IUGR individuals. *Legend*: The studies done so far used simply observed an association between the regular n-3 PUFAs intake and better feeding behaviors. Controlled clinical trials using n-3 supplementation (*yellow*) could clarify the potential role of these molecules in modulating food preferences in vulnerable children. *Numbers* represent the references cited in the text

way while increasing the activation of the mesocortical DA pathway [78]. Therefore, the consumption of n-3 PUFAs potentially decreases reward sensitivity, impulsivity and palatable food intake [79, 80], being a possible interesting molecular candidate for influencing feeding behavior in IUGR individuals towards a more healthy style (see Fig. 33.3).

Conclusions

Aside from the early determinants of food preferences, there are many other aspects that will affect an individuals' propensity to consume palatable foods. In addition, early and late determinants interact over the life course (see Fig. 33.4). For instance, we recently showed that the same individuals who carry a risk allele for having obesogenic behaviors when facing environmental adversity, are also most likely to benefit from enriched environmental conditions. Therefore, a genetic differential susceptibility to the environment that affects the development of unhealthy behaviors in children exists [4]. However, other personal features, such as being born IUGR, may turn individuals more or less vulnerable to developing obesogenic behaviors depending on how good or bad is the environment in which they will grow up, which may be called a "phenotypic differential susceptibility" [81]. It remains to be clarified if IUGR individuals have a differential susceptibility to external influences (such as advertisement or stress) or to better environments (such as exposure to exercise), and this may serve as a basis for developing preventive measures that will have a protective role against the development of metabolic syndrome in this vulnerable population.

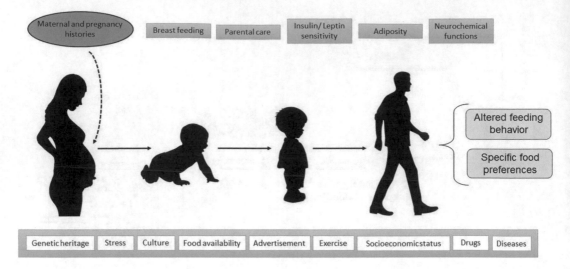

Fig. 33.4 Internal and external influences on food preferences over the life course. *Legend*: As an individual age, different constitutional features and environmental factors, as well as the interaction between these variables, will affect his feeding behavior

References

1. Portella AK, Kajantie E, Hovi P, Desai M, Ross MG, Goldani MZ, et al. Effects of in utero conditions on adult feeding preferences. J Dev Orig Hlth Dis. 2012;3(3):140–52. PubMed PMID: WOS:000307183200002. English.
2. Portella AK, Silveira PP. Neurobehavioral determinants of nutritional security in fetal growth-restricted individuals. Ann N Y Acad Sci. 2014;1331:15. PubMed PMID: 24650246.
3. Silveira PP, Portella AK, Kennedy JL, Gaudreau H, Davis C, Steiner M, et al. Association between the seven-repeat allele of the dopamine-4 receptor gene (DRD4) and spontaneous food intake in pre-school children. Appetite. 2014;73:15–22. PubMed PMID: 24153108. Pubmed Central PMCID: 3872500.
4. Silveira PP, Gaudreau H, Atkinson L, Fleming AS, Sokolowski MB, Steiner M, et al. Genetic differential susceptibility to socioeconomic status and childhood obesogenic behavior. JAMA Pediatr. 2016;170:359.
5. Colman JB, Laureano DP, Reis TM, Krolow R, Dalmaz C, Benetti Cda S, et al. Variations in the neonatal environment modulate adult behavioral and brain responses to palatable food withdrawal in adult female rats. Intern J Dev Neurosc Off J Intern Soc Dev Neurosci. 2015;40:70–5. PubMed PMID: 25450525.
6. Machado TD, Dalle Molle R, Laureano DP, Portella AK, Werlang IC, Benetti Cda S, et al. Early life stress is associated with anxiety, increased stress responsivity and preference for "comfort foods" in adult female rats. Stress. 2013;16(5):549–56. PubMed PMID: 23781957. Epub 2013/06/21. eng.
7. Brunner EJ, Mosdol A, Witte DR, Martikainen P, Stafford M, Shipley MJ, et al. Dietary patterns and 15-y risks of major coronary events, diabetes, and mortality. Am J Clin Nutr. 2008;87(5):1414–21. PubMed PMID: 18469266.
8. Mekary RA, Giovannucci E, Willett WC, van Dam RM, Hu FB. Eating patterns and type 2 diabetes risk in men: breakfast omission, eating frequency, and snacking. Am J Clin Nutr. 2012;95(5):1182–9. PubMed PMID: 22456660. Pubmed Central PMCID: 3325839.
9. Flood A, Rastogi T, Wirfalt E, Mitrou PN, Reedy J, Subar AF, et al. Dietary patterns as identified by factor analysis and colorectal cancer among middle-aged Americans. Am J Clin Nutr. 2008;88(1):176–84. PubMed PMID: 18614739. Pubmed Central PMCID: 2495056.
10. Grattan DR. Fetal programming from maternal obesity: eating too much for two? Endocrinology. 2008;149(11):5345–7. PubMed PMID: 18936494.
11. McCance DR, Pettitt DJ, Hanson RL, Jacobsson LT, Knowler WC, Bennett PH. Birth weight and non-insulin dependent diabetes: thrifty genotype, thrifty phenotype, or surviving small baby genotype? BMJ. 1994;308(6934):942–5. PubMed PMID: 8173400. Pubmed Central PMCID: PMC2539758. eng.
12. Chatelain P. Children born with intra-uterine growth retardation (IUGR) or small for gestational age (SGA): long term growth and metabolic consequences. Endocr Regul. 2000;34(1):33–6. PubMed PMID: 10808251.
13. Dalle Molle R, Bischoff AR, Portella AK, Silveira PP. The fetal programming of food preferences: current clinical and experimental evidence. J Dev Orig Health Dis. 2016;7(3):222–30. PubMed PMID: 26412563. Eng.

14. Ayres C, Agranonik M, Portella AK, Filion F, Johnston CC, Silveira PP. Intrauterine growth restriction and the fetal programming of the hedonic response to sweet taste in newborn infants. Int J Pediatr. 2012;2012:657379. PubMed PMID: 22851979. Pubmed Central PMCID: PMC3407636.
15. Rotstein M, Stolar O, Uliel S, Mandel D, Mani A, Dollberg S, et al. Facial expression in response to smell and taste stimuli in small and appropriate for gestational age newborns. J Child Neurol. 2015;30(11):1466–71. PubMed PMID: 25694467.
16. Laureano DP, Molle RD, Portella AK, Silveira PP. Facial expressions in small for gestational age newborns. J Child Neurol. 2015;31:398. PubMed PMID: 26129978.
17. Silveira PP, Agranonik M, Faras H, Portella AK, Meaney MJ, Levitan RD, et al. Preliminary evidence for an impulsivity-based thrifty eating phenotype. Pediatr Res. 2012;71(3):293–8. PubMed PMID: 22278183.
18. Crume TL, Scherzinger A, Stamm E, McDuffie R, Bischoff KJ, Hamman RF, et al. The long-term impact of intrauterine growth restriction in a diverse U.S. cohort of children: the EPOCH study. Obesity. 2014;22(2):608–15.
19. Barbieri MA, Portella AK, Silveira PP, Bettiol H, Agranonik M, Silva AA, et al. Severe intrauterine growth restriction is associated with higher spontaneous carbohydrate intake in young women. Pediatr Res. 2009;65(2):215–20. PubMed PMID: 19047956.
20. Kaseva N, Wehkalampi K, Hemiö K, Hovi P, Järvenpää AL, Andersson S, et al. Diet and nutrient intake in young adults born preterm at very low birth weight. J Pediatr. 2013;163(1):43–8. PubMed PMID: 23391045. eng.
21. Stein AD, Rundle A, Wada N, Goldbohm RA, Lumey LH. Associations of gestational exposure to famine with energy balance and macronutrient density of the diet at age 58 years differ according to the reference population used. J Nutr. 2009;139(8):1555–61. PubMed PMID: 19549753. Pubmed Central PMCID: PMC2709303. eng.
22. Lussana F, Painter RC, Ocke MC, Buller HR, Bossuyt PM, Roseboom TJ. Prenatal exposure to the Dutch famine is associated with a preference for fatty foods and a more atherogenic lipid profile. Am J Clin Nutr. 2008;88(6):1648–52. PubMed PMID: 19064527. eng.
23. Perälä MM, Männistö S, Kaartinen NE, Kajantie E, Osmond C, Barker DJ, et al. Body size at birth is associated with food and nutrient intake in adulthood. PLoS One. 2012;7(9):e46139. PubMed PMID: 23049962. Pubmed Central PMCID: PMC3458835. eng.
24. Ayres C, Silveira PP, Barbieri MA, Portella AK, Bettiol H, Agranonik M, et al. Exposure to maternal smoking during fetal life affects food preferences in adulthood independent of the effects of intrauterine growth restriction. J Dev Orig Hlth Dis. 2011;2(3):162–7. PubMed PMID: WOS:000291564200004. English.
25. Hvelplund C, Hansen BM, Koch SV, Andersson M, Skovgaard AM. Perinatal risk factors for feeding and eating disorders in children aged 0 to 3 years. Pediatrics. 2016;137:e20152575. PubMed PMID: 26764360.
26. Migraine A, Nicklaus S, Parnet P, Lange C, Monnery-Patris S, Robert CD, et al. Effect of preterm birth and birth weight on eating behavior at 2 y of age. Am J Clin Nutr. 2013;97:1270–7.
27. Oliveira A, de Lauzon-Guillain B, Jones L, Emmett P, Moreira P, Ramos E, et al. Birth weight and eating behaviors of young children. J Pediatr. 2015;166(1):59–65. PubMed PMID: 25444001.
28. Johnson S, Matthews R, Draper ES, Field DJ, Manktelow BN, Marlow N, et al. Eating difficulties in children born late and moderately preterm at 2 y of age: a prospective population-based cohort study. Am J Clin Nutr. 2015;103:406–14. PubMed PMID: 26718420.
29. van Deutekom AW, Chinapaw MJ, Vrijkotte TG, Gemke RJ. The association of birth weight and postnatal growth with energy intake and eating behavior at 5 years of age – a birth cohort study. Int J Behav Nutr Phys Act. 2016;13(1):15. PubMed PMID: 26847088. Pubmed Central PMCID: PMC4743237.
30. Reis RS, Bernardi JR, Steiner M, Meaney MJ, Levitan RD, Silveira PP, et al. Poor infant inhibitory control predicts food fussiness in childhood – a possible protective role of n-3 PUFAs for vulnerable children. Prostaglandins Leukot Essent Fat Acids. 2015;97:21–5. PubMed PMID: 25892188.
31. Reis RS, Dalle Molle R, Machado TD, Mucellini AB, Rodrigues DM, Bortoluzzi A, Bigonha SM, Toazza R, Salum GA, Minuzzi L, Buchweitz A, Franco AR, Pelúzio MCG, Manfro GG, Silveira PP. Impulsivity-based thrifty eating phenotype and the protective role of n-3 PUFAs intake in adolescents. Transl Psyhchiatry. 2016;6:e755.
32. Desai M, Gayle D, Babu J, Ross MG. Programmed obesity in intrauterine growth-restricted newborns: modulation by. Am J Phys Regul Integr Comp Phys. 2005;288(1):R91–6. PubMed PMID: 15297266. Epub 2004/08/07. eng.
33. Desai M, Gayle D, Han G, Ross MG. Programmed hyperphagia due to reduced anorexigenic mechanisms in intrauterine growth-restricted offspring. Reprod Sci. 2007;14(4):329–37. PubMed PMID: WOS:000248324500008. English.
34. George LA, Zhang L, Tuersunjiang N, Ma Y, Long NM, Uthlaut AB, et al. Early maternal undernutrition programs increased feed intake, altered glucose metabolism and insulin secretion, and liver function in aged female offspring. Am J Phys Regul Integr Comp Phys. 2012;302(7):R795–804. PubMed PMID: 22277936. eng.
35. Dellschaft NS, Alexandre-Gouabau MC, Gardner DS, Antignac JP, Keisler DH, Budge H, et al. Effect of pre- and postnatal growth and post-weaning activity on glucose metabolism in the offspring. J Endocrinol. 2015;224(2):171–82. PubMed PMID: 25416820. eng.

36. Ovilo C, Gonzalez-Bulnes A, Benitez R, Ayuso M, Barbero A, Perez-Solana ML, et al. Prenatal programming in an obese swine model: sex-related effects of maternal energy restriction on morphology, metabolism and hypothalamic gene expression. Br J Nutr. 2014;111(4):735–46. PubMed PMID: 24528940. eng.

37. Hales CN, Barker DJ. Type 2 (non-insulin-dependent) diabetes mellitus: the thrifty phenotype hypothesis. Diabetologia. 1992;35(7):595–601. PubMed PMID: 1644236.

38. Hales CN, Barker DJ. Type 2 (non-insulin-dependent) diabetes mellitus: the thrifty phenotype hypothesis. 1992. Int J Epidemiol. 2013;42(5):1215–22. PubMed PMID: 24159065. eng.

39. Vickers MH, Breier BH, Cutfield WS, Hofman PL, Gluckman PD. Fetal origins of hyperphagia, obesity, and hypertension and postnatal amplification by hypercaloric nutrition. Am J Physiol Endocrinol Metab. 2000;279(1):E83–7. PubMed PMID: 10893326.

40. Vickers MH, Breier BH, McCarthy D, Gluckman PD. Sedentary behavior during postnatal life is determined by the prenatal environment and exacerbated by postnatal hypercaloric nutrition. Am J Phys Regul Integr Comp Phys. 2003;285(1):R271–3. PubMed PMID: 12794001. eng.

41. Bellinger L, Lilley C, Langley-Evans SC. Prenatal exposure to a maternal low-protein diet programmes a preference for high-fat foods in the young adult rat. Br J Nutr. 2004;92(3):513–20. PubMed PMID: 15469656.

42. Bellinger L, Langley-Evans SC. Fetal programming of appetite by exposure to a maternal low-protein diet in the rat. Clin Sci. 2005;109(4):413–20. PubMed PMID: 15992360.

43. Bellinger L, Sculley DV, Langley-Evans SC. Exposure to undernutrition in fetal life determines fat distribution, locomotor activity and food intake in ageing rats. Int J Obes. 2006;30(5):729–38. PubMed PMID: 16404403. Pubmed Central PMCID: 1865484.

44. Whitaker KW, Totoki K, Reyes TM. Metabolic adaptations to early life protein restriction differ by offspring sex and post-weaning diet in the mouse. Nutr Metab Cardiovasc Dis. 2012;22(12):1067–74. PubMed PMID: 21704502. Pubmed Central PMCID: PMC3183163. Epub 2011/06/28. eng.

45. Nielsen MO, Kongsted AH, Thygesen MP, Strathe AB, Caddy S, Quistorff B, et al. Late gestation undernutrition can predispose for visceral adiposity by altering fat distribution patterns and increasing the preference for a high-fat diet in early postnatal life. Br J Nutr. 2013;109(11):2098–110. PubMed PMID: 23069212. Epub 2012/10/17. eng.

46. Vucetic Z, Totoki K, Schoch H, Whitaker KW, Hill-Smith T, Lucki I, et al. Early life protein restriction alters dopamine circuitry. Neuroscience. 2010;168(2):359–70. PubMed PMID: WOS:000278262100004. English.

47. Alves MB, Dalle Molle R, Desai M, Ross MG, Silveira PP. Increased palatable food intake and response to food cues in intrauterine growth-restricted rats are related to tyrosine hydroxylase content in the orbitofrontal cortex and nucleus accumbens. Behav Brain Res. 2015;287:73–81. PubMed PMID: 25796489.

48. Cunha Fda S, Dalle Molle R, Portella AK, Benetti Cda S, Noschang C, Goldani MZ, et al. Both food restriction and high-fat diet during gestation induce low birth weight and altered physical activity in adult rat offspring: the "Similarities in the Inequalities" model. PLoS One. 2015;10(3):e0118586. PubMed PMID: 25738800. eng.

49. Dalle Molle R, Laureano DP, Alves MB, Reis TM, Desai M, Ross MG, et al. Intrauterine growth restriction increases the preference for palatable foods and affects sensitivity to food rewards in male and female adult rats. Brain Res. 2015;1618:41–9. PubMed PMID: 26006109.

50. da Silva AA, Borba TK, de Almeida LL, Cavalcante TC, de Freitas MF, Leandro CG, et al. Perinatal undernutrition stimulates seeking food reward. Int J Dev Neurosci. 2013;31(5):334–41. PubMed PMID: 23669181. Epub 2013/05/15. eng.

51. de Melo Martimiano PH, da Silva GR, Coimbra VF, Matos RJ, de Souza BF, da Silva AA, et al. Perinatal malnutrition stimulates motivation through reward and enhances drd receptor expression in the ventral striatum of adult mice. Pharmacol Biochem Behav. 2015;134:106. PubMed PMID: 25933794. Epub 2015/05/03. Eng.

52. da Silva AA, Oliveira MM, Cavalcante TC, Do Amaral Almeida LC, de Souza JA, da Silva MC, et al. Low protein diet during gestation and lactation increases food reward seeking but does not modify sucrose taste reactivity in adult female rats. Int J Dev Neurosci. 2016;49:50–9. PubMed PMID: 26805766. Epub 2016/01/26. eng.

53. Laureano DP, Dalle Molle R, Alves MB, Luft C, Desai M, Ross MG, et al. Intrauterine growth restriction modifies the hedonic response to sweet taste in newborn pups – role of the accumbal mu-opioid receptors. Neuroscience. 2016;322:500–8. PubMed PMID: 26926962. Epub 2016/03/02. eng.

54. Remmers F, Verhagen LA, Adan RA, Delemarre-van de Waal HA. Hypothalamic neuropeptide expression of juvenile and middle-aged rats after early postnatal food restriction. Endocrinology. 2008;149(7):3617–25. PubMed PMID: 18372335.

55. Garcia AP, Palou M, Priego T, Sanchez J, Palou A, Pico C. Moderate caloric restriction during gestation results in lower arcuate nucleus NPY- and alphaMSH-neurons and impairs hypothalamic response to fed/fasting conditions in weaned rats. Diabetes Obes Metab. 2010;12(5):403–13. PubMed PMID: 20415688.

56. Plagemann A, Harder T, Rake A, Melchior K, Rohde W, Dorner G. Hypothalamic nuclei are malformed in weanling offspring of low protein malnourished rat dams. J Nutr. 2000;130(10):2582–9. PubMed PMID: 11015493.

57. Fukami T, Sun X, Li T, Desai M, Ross MG. Mechanism of programmed obesity in intrauterine fetal growth restricted offspring: paradoxically enhanced appetite stimulation in fed and fasting states. Reprod Sci. 2012;19(4):423–30. PubMed PMID: 22344733. eng.

58. Fraser M, Dhaliwal CK, Vickers MH, Krechowec SO, Breier BH. Diet-induced obesity and prenatal undernutrition lead to differential neuroendocrine gene expression in the hypothalamic arcuate nuclei. Endocrine. 2016;53:839–47. PubMed PMID: 26979526. Epub 2016/03/17. Eng.

59. Manuel-Apolinar L, Rocha L, Damasio L, Tesoro-Cruz E, Zarate A. Role of prenatal undernutrition in the expression of serotonin, dopamine and leptin receptors in adult mice: implications of food intake. Mol Med Rep. 2014;9(2):407–12. PubMed PMID: 24337628. Pubmed Central PMCID: 3896523.

60. Shin BC, Dai Y, Thamotharan M, Gibson LC, Devaskar SU. Pre- and postnatal calorie restriction perturbs early hypothalamic neuropeptide and energy balance. J Neurosci Res. 2012;90(6):1169–82. PubMed PMID: 22388752. Pubmed Central PMCID: PMC4208917. Epub 2012/03/06. eng.

61. Puglianiello A, Germani D, Cianfarani S. Exposure to uteroplacental insufficiency reduces the expression of signal transducer and activator of transcription 3 and proopiomelanocortin in the hypothalamus of newborn rats. Pediatr Res. 2009;66(2):208–11. PubMed PMID: 19390493. Epub 2009/04/25. eng.

62. Delahaye F, Breton C, Risold PY, Enache M, Dutriez-Casteloot I, Laborie C, et al. Maternal perinatal undernutrition drastically reduces postnatal leptin surge and affects the development of arcuate nucleus proopiomelanocortin neurons in neonatal male rat pups. Endocrinology. 2008;149(2):470–5. PubMed PMID: WOS:000252506800006. English.

63. Yousheng J, Nguyen T, Desai M, Ross MG. Programmed alterations in hypothalamic neuronal orexigenic responses to ghrelin following gestational nutrient restriction. Reprod Sci. 2008;15(7):702–9. PubMed PMID: 18562700.

64. Desai M, Li T, Ross MG. Fetal hypothalamic neuroprogenitor cell culture: preferential differentiation paths induced by leptin and insulin. Endocrinology. 2011;152(8):3192–201. PubMed PMID: 21652728. eng.

65. Orozco-Solis R, Matos RJ, Guzman-Quevedo O, Lopes de Souza S, Bihouee A, Houlgatte R, et al. Nutritional programming in the rat is linked to long-lasting changes in nutrient sensing and energy homeostasis in the hypothalamus. PLoS One. 2010;5(10):e13537. PubMed PMID: 20975839. Pubmed Central PMCID: PMC2958833. Epub 2010/10/27. eng.

66. Ross MG, Desai M. Developmental programming of appetite/satiety. Ann Nutr Metab. 2014;64(Suppl 1):36–44. PubMed PMID: 25059804. eng.

67. Grissom NM, Reyes TM. Gestational overgrowth and undergrowth affect neurodevelopment: similarities and differences from behavior to epigenetics. Intern J Dev Neurosci Off J Intern Soc Dev Neurosci. 2013;31(6):406–14. PubMed PMID: 23201144.

68. Dunkley PR, Bobrovskaya L, Graham ME, von Nagy-Felsobuki EI, Dickson PW. Tyrosine hydroxylase phosphorylation: regulation and consequences. J Neurochem. 2004;91(5):1025–43. PubMed PMID: 15569247. Epub 2004/12/01. eng.

69. Smith JW, Fetsko LA, Xu R, Wang Y. Dopamine D2L receptor knockout mice display deficits in positive and negative reinforcing properties of morphine and in avoidance learning. Neuroscience. 2002;113(4):755–65. PubMed PMID: 12182883.

70. Gugusheff JR, Ong ZY, Muhlhausler BS. Naloxone treatment alters gene expression in the mesolimbic reward system in 'junk food' exposed offspring in a sex-specific manner but does not affect food preferences in adulthood. Physiol Behav. 2014;133:14–21. PubMed PMID: 24727340.

71. Vieau D, Sebaai N, Leonhardt M, Dutriez-Casteloot I, Molendi-Coste O, Laborie C, et al. HPA axis programming by maternal undernutrition in the male rat offspring. Psychoneuroendocrinology. 2007;32(Suppl 1):S16–20. PubMed PMID: 17644270. eng.

72. Lesage J, Blondeau B, Grino M, Breant B, Dupouy JP. Maternal undernutrition during late gestation induces fetal overexposure to glucocorticoids and intrauterine growth retardation, and disturbs the hypothalamo-pituitary adrenal axis in the newborn rat. Endocrinology. 2001;142(5):1692–702. PubMed PMID: 11316731. Epub 2001/04/24. eng.

73. Li C, McDonald TJ, Wu G, Nijland MJ, Nathanielsz PW. Intrauterine growth restriction alters term fetal baboon hypothalamic appetitive peptide balance. J Endocrinol. 2013;217(3):275–82. PubMed PMID: 23482706. Pubmed Central PMCID: PMC4018765. Epub 2013/03/14. eng.

74. Begum G, Stevens A, Smith EB, Connor K, Challis JR, Bloomfield F, et al. Epigenetic changes in fetal hypothalamic energy regulating pathways are associated with maternal undernutrition and twinning. FASEB J. 2012;26(4):1694–703. PubMed PMID: 22223754. Pubmed Central PMCID: PMC3316895. Epub 2012/01/10. eng.

75. Vega CC, Reyes-Castro LA, Rodriguez-Gonzalez GL, Bautista CJ, Vazquez-Martinez M, Larrea F, et al. Resveratrol partially prevents oxidative stress and metabolic dysfunction in pregnant rats fed a low protein diet and their offspring. J Physiol. 2016;594(5):1483–99. PubMed PMID: 26662841. Pubmed Central PMCID: PMC4771783. Epub 2015/12/15. eng.

76. Gibson LC, Shin BC, Dai Y, Freije W, Kositamongkol S, Cho J, et al. Early leptin intervention reverses perturbed energy balance regulating hypothalamic neuropeptides in the pre- and postnatal calorie-restricted female rat offspring. J Neurosci Res. 2015;93(6):902–12. PubMed PMID: 25639584. Pubmed Central PMCID: PMC4533910. Epub 2015/02/03. eng.

77. Balanza-Martinez V, Fries GR, Colpo GD, Silveira PP, Portella AK, Tabares-Seisdedos R, et al. Therapeutic use of omega-3 fatty acids in bipolar disorder. Expert Rev Neurother. 2011;11(7):1029–47. PubMed PMID: 21721919.
78. Zimmer L, Vancassel S, Cantagrel S, Breton P, Delamanche S, Guilloteau D, et al. The dopamine mesocorticolimbic pathway is affected by deficiency in n-3 polyunsaturated fatty acids. Am J Clin Nutr. 2002;75(4):662–7. PubMed PMID: 11916751.
79. Mathieu G, Denis S, Lavialle M, Vancassel S. Synergistic effects of stress and omega-3 fatty acid deprivation on emotional response and brain lipid composition in adult rats. Prostaglandins Leukot Essent Fat Acids. 2008;78(6):391–401. PubMed PMID: 18579362.
80. Ferreira CF, Bernardi JR, Krolow R, Arcego DM, Fries GR, de Aguiar BW, et al. Vulnerability to dietary n-3 polyunsaturated fatty acid deficiency after exposure to early stress in rats. Pharmacol Biochem Behav. 2013;107:11–9. PubMed PMID: 23537731.
81. Agranonik M PA, Hamilton J, Fleming AS, Steiner M, Meaney MJ, Levitan RD, Silveira PP. Breastfeeding in the 21st century, good for all, even better for the small. Lancet. 2016;387(10033):(p2088-2089).

Chapter 34
Effects of Fetal Programming on Osteoporosis

George M. Weisz and William Randall Albury

Key Points

- Starvation during gestation has a programming effect leading to premature lipid, glucose, endocrine and bone mineral metabolism disorders in adolescents and adults.
- Intrauterine starvation predisposes the individual not only to osteoporosis, but also to obesity and sarcopenia which contribute to the risk of osteoporotic fracture.
- Rapid compensatory growth in the neonatal or infant periods may exacerbate the negative effects of intrauterine starvation by producing obesity without significantly improving bone quality, thus increasing the risk of osteoporotic fractures.
- Survivors of famine conditions such as those experienced in Europe during WWII and in underdeveloped countries thereafter, provide clinical proof of the immediate and late effects of intrauterine nutritional deprivation on bone quality.
- Immigrants coming to developed countries from famine-affected backgrounds are at risk of osteoporosis and related disorders caused both by their previous deprivation and by subsequent compensatory growth, presenting a serious public health issue for their adopting countries.

Keywords Osteoporosis • Osteopenia • Metabolic bone syndrome • Early life starvation • Rapid compensatory over-feeding

Abbreviations

ACTH   Adreno-corticotropic hormone
BMD   Bone mineral density
BMI   Body mass index
DES   Diethylstilboestrol

G.M. Weisz, MD, BA, MA, FRACS (Ortho) (✉)
School of Humanities and Languages, University of New South Wales, Sydney, NSW, Australia

School of Humanities, University of New England, Armidale, NSW, Australia
e-mail: gmweisz1@aol.com

W.R. Albury, BA, PhD
School of Humanities, University of New England, Armidale, NSW, Australia
e-mail: walbury2@une.edu.au

© Springer International Publishing AG 2017   471
R. Rajendram et al. (eds.), *Diet, Nutrition, and Fetal Programming*,
Nutrition and Health, DOI 10.1007/978-3-319-60289-9_34

DEXA   Dual energy x-ray absorptiometry
DNA   Deoxyribonucleic acid
HRT   Hormone replacement therapy
WWII   World War Two

Introduction: The Nature of Osteoporosis, Its Prophylaxis and Treatment

Osteoporosis (porous bone) is a loss of bone mineral density (BMD), mainly through calcium deprivation, and a loss of the normal architecture of the bone. The honeycomb structure of the calcified bone is degraded, depleted of minerals and brittle, thus significantly increasing the risk of fracture. This condition can occur in women as an acute transitional osteoporosis during pregnancy, when pelvic bones are demineralised, or as a permanent change to bones throughout the body in the post-menopausal stage. It can also occur in both sexes as the result of prolonged cortisone or anticonvulsant therapy, prolonged immobilisation or, as the present chapter documents, intrauterine starvation which programmes the developing fetus for premature bone density loss in later life.

The *diagnosis* of osteoporosis is made by DEXA scan, which results in a numerical figure known as a T-score. This score compares the BMD of the subject with the expected BMD of a healthy 30-year-old of the same sex, and expresses the difference in terms of standard deviations. A T-score between −1and +1, which is less than one standard deviation below or above the norm, indicates normal BMD. Below this range, a T-score from −1 to −2.5 indicates osteopenia (reduced bone), a loss of density which increases the risk of fracture and is often the precursor to osteoporosis. A T-score of −2.5 or lower indicates osteoporosis and the high risk of fracture associated with this condition [1].

In the *prophylaxis* of osteoporosis, emphasis should be placed on daily physical activity with light to moderate weight exercises, and exposure to the sun for 15 min to promote vitamin D formation. Oral supplements are appropriate for those with vitamin and mineral deficiencies. Persons with a known risk of osteoporosis, and those experiencing repeated falls and fractures, should be investigated with a DEXA scan. In Australia, where the prevalence of osteoporosis doubled (after adjusting for age) between 1995 and 2008 [2] due to lack of sufficient attention to the problem in the past, the public health effort also includes clinical and radiographic screening to discover "silent" cases and to ensure adequate calcium and vitamin D intake for persons who are potentially at risk.

Subjects diagnosed with osteoporosis, as a result of a T-score of −2.5 or lower, ought to receive *treatment* with hormone replacement therapy (HRT) or with bone metabolites administered through tablets or intravenous infusion [3]. Patients with osteopenia should be counselled and individually treated, with or without medications according to their situation.

In the case of *osteoporotic fractures*, surgical intervention would be similar to that appropriate for other fractures, but with internal fixation using extended plates and longer stems in hip prosthesis. Bone grafting will often be required and a delay in healing can be expected.

Historical Background to the Theory That Early Life Nutrition Programmes Adult Diseases

The intrauterine pathogenesis of adult disorders is a fairly recent discovery, mostly dating from the late twentieth century. The brief outline given in sections "Historical Background to the Theory That Early Life Nutrition Programmes Adult Diseases" and "Extension of the Theory to Include Musculo-Skeletal Pathology" of this chapter illustrates some key points in the development of the theory and is not intended as a comprehensive historical study.

Initial Studies on Survivors of Mass Famines During WWII

The effect of early life malnutrition on the development of adult diseases was discovered in studies conducted on European populations which had been exposed to hunger during their embryonic, fetal, neonatal or early childhood periods some 40–50 years earlier as a result of wartime conditions.

During WWII there were food shortages throughout Europe, but these were especially acute in occupied countries where the conquering Axis powers confiscated food and sometimes removed fertilising earth. In some occupied countries such as Greece or the British Channel Islands plundering by the occupying Axis forces was aggravated by Allied blockades. Starvation was also used by the German authorities as a weapon to force submission or administer punishment, as in the siege of Leningrad, the Dutch embargo, and the harsh conditions imposed on the inmates of ghettos and concentration camps.

These circumstances produced large cohorts of survivors who had experienced starvation perinatally and as children. In later years studies of the Channel Islands, Leningrad and the Dutch cohorts showed an association between early life starvation and the development of adult metabolic disorders leading to increased mortality [4–6].

Development of the Theory of Fetal Programming

Subsequently, the theory of the effect of early life nutrition on the development of adult diseases was confirmed. Important studies, led by researchers under Lucas starting in the 1980s, were comprehensive and scientific, and were done initially from a paediatric point of view focussed on the nutrition of the developing human [7].

The adult aspect of the theory was elaborated in a series of multi-professional studies. Work on the metabolic syndromes resulting from starvation was done at Southampton Hospital under Barker and Hales, leading to the *"thrifty phenotype hypothesis"* in 1992 [8]. The "Barker theory" was at times revised or criticised, but all in all, as the theory of a "programming" mechanism, it was globally accepted and published as the *"developmental origins of well-being"* [9]. The same phenomenon of pathogenesis was studied by epidemiologists from the 1990s [10–12]. Later, in 2014 Vaiserman established the connection between early life nutrition and longevity [13].

The theory of fetal programming was supported experimentally in various animal species, in different geographical areas and by different researchers. But it nevertheless attracted some criticism, mainly invoking the lack of explanation for the time lag between gestation and adult diagnosis, and advocating additional environmental influences during adulthood. More recently, the epigenetic mechanism leading to an adult susceptibility to disease has been presented as a DNA modification causing insulin resistance, atherogenesis and osteoporosis [14]. According to this explanation, these conditions would be a result of *"the phenomenon of developmental plasticity whereby a simple genotype may give rise to a different phenotype depending on the prevailing environment"* [15].

Extension of the Theory to Include Musculo-Skeletal Pathology

In early studies of the long-term effects of early life malnutrition – for example, those focusing on the survivors of the Channel Islands occupation, the Leningrad siege, and the Dutch embargo – issues relating to musculo-skeletal pathology were not considered. The relation between gestational development and the initially suspected intrauterine origin of adult musculo-skeletal pathology (adipose tissue, sarcopenia, osteopenia) was therefore elucidated somewhat later compared to the general metabolic studies, but was eventually well defined.

Early Life Starvation and Bone Metabolism

In the 1990s Cooper and associates gradually developed the theory that changes in early stages of bone development due to starvation and reduced provision of nutrition, minerals and growth factors, will lead to bone metabolic changes in adults [16]. This theory was further elaborated in the following decade, when the pathogenesis of osteoporosis was described and a role was attributed to intrauterine programming, confirming the earlier analysis of growth in infancy and bone mass in adult life [17–19]. Important connections were shown to exist between maternal life style, maternal body mass and vitamin D dependence, which could predict bone mass in offspring and the risk of future fracture [20–22].

A detailed review in 2012 re-emphasized the epigenetic programming of metabolic disorders, including osteoporosis [15]. And in 2015 further descriptions were published giving clear confirmations of the bone metabolic aberrations resulting from intrauterine macro- and micro-nutritional deprivation [23].

Recent Studies on Survivors of WWII Ghettos and Concentration Camps

Recently, small scale studies of survivors of WWII ghettos and concentration camps have demonstrated an increased incidence of adult osteoporosis not only in those subjects who experienced perinatal starvation but also in those who were severely malnourished as children and young adults [24, 25].

The immediate effects of starvation on bone metabolism and fractures were established in 1941–1942 in a clandestine study carried out over 17 months in the Warsaw Ghetto by the equally clandestine Ghetto Medical School [26]. Their studies on bone histology showed both architectural bone changes and depleted matrix, namely osteoporosis and osteomalacia. Fractures in children were found not to heal, making surgical treatment inexpedient.

To illustrate the long-term effects of such starvation in survivors of WWII concentration camps and ghettos, the metabolic details of 14 cases are presented in Table 34.1, a small sample out of the cohort of survivors in Australia, the country with the third largest such population in the post war period.

In the above mentioned table (Table 34.1) and those which follow (Tables 34.2 and 34.3) the risk of fractures within 5 and 10 years were calculated from the results obtained with DEXA scanners, and all were compared with age and gender general values. The Garvan nomogram, also used here, is an individual risk assessment based on clinical parameters, number of fractures/falls, combined with BMD and/or T-score values [27]. The predicted risk and the prognostic values suggest, as expected, that the more intense the osteoporosis, the higher the fracture incidence will be.

To further illustrate the long-term effects of early life starvation, the metabolic details of three siblings (cases 7–9 in Table 34.1 above) from the same family of survivors of the Budapest Ghetto are used (Table 34.2). A fourth sibling (not included in Table 34.1), born post-liberation, serves as a control. The fracture risk in this small group of survivors is indicative of moderate risk predicted in 5 and 10 years.

Studies on this small group of WWII survivors cannot be statistically significant, so a rigorous epidemiological study on a larger population of child survivors will be required to confirm these findings.

Table 34.1 Late adult metabolic changes in survivors of early life starvation

Subject and age when tested	Age at time of starvation	Duration of starvation	Lipids	Blood pressure	Diabetes	Osteoporosis (≥++) or osteopenia (+)	% risk any fracture in 5/10 years
1. M1, age 61	21, hiding in mountains, Slovakia	10 months, only corn intake	?	?	+	+++	13/26%
2. D1, age 73	14, Ghetto Lwow; then "aryan" side of Warsaw	3 years under-nutrition, with 4 months starvation	−	+	−	+++	16/29%
3. B1, age 70	6, in Ghetto Budapest	6 months	+	+	+	++	10/20%
4. R1, age 68	Born in Terezin camp Czechia	Last trimester of pregnancy	+	+	+	?	?
5. S1, age 69	2, born Ghetto Szabadka, Hungary	6 months	+	+	−	++	4.9/9.0%
6. I1, age 67	Born Viehofen camp, Austria	In utero last trimester	+	+	−	?	?
7. M2, age 64	4	12 months	−	+	−	+	6.0/11%
8. H1, age 62	1.5	12 months	−	+	−	+	5.0/10%
9. M3, age 60	In utero	Last trimester	−	−	−	++	13/26%
10. D2, age 62	Born Vienna; aged 2 in Terezin camp orphanage	4 months	+	+	−	+	3.9/8.1%
11. E1, age 69	1	6 months	−	+	−	++	8.4/15.5%
12. V1, age 58	Born 1946	Preterm, 4 months in Prague hospital	+	+	−	++	23/44%
13. R2, age 58	Born 1944	3 months	+	+	−	+	5.0/10%
14. M4, age 60	Born 1943 Ghetto Debrecen, Hungary; in January 1945 Rothschild Hospital, Vienna	In ghetto last trimester, 8 months severe starvation in 1944	+	+	−	++	13/26%

Material from the original version of this table, now expanded with additional data, is reprinted here with permission of *Aust J Prim Health*, http://www.publish.csiro.au/nid/261/paper/PY12004.htm

Table showing the presence (+) or absence (−) of abnormalities in lipids, blood pressure, glucose metabolism and bone mineral density in 14 adults who were child survivors of WWII concentration camps and ghettos

Table 34.2 Fracture risk in one family

Subject and age when tested	Age at time of starvation	Duration of starvation	Osteoporosis (≥ ++) or osteopenia (+)	% risk any fracture in 5/10 years	% risk hip fracture in 5/10 years
M2, age 64	4	12 months	+	6.4/11.8%	1.1/2.1%
H1, age 62	1.5	12 months	+	5.0/10.3%	0.6/1.2%
M3, age 60	From last trimester in utero to 6 months postnatal	9 months	++	13/26%	5.0/9.0%
S2, age 60	Born 1947	Nil	–	2.0/4.2%	0.1/0.2%

From Weisz and Albury [25]; © 2014 Weisz and Albury, under the terms of the Creative Commons Attribution License (http://creativecommons.org/licenses/by/3.0), with some numerical errors in the original table corrected
Table showing the presence (+) or absence (–) of late adult bone mineral abnormality and fracture risk in three siblings who were malnourished as children during WWII and one control sibling born after the war

Table 34.3 Metabolic changes in a female survivor of early life starvation and her son

Subject and age when tested	Perinatal history	Duration of starvation	Lipids	Blood pressure	Glucose intolerance	Osteoporosis (≥++) or osteopenia (+)	% risk any fracture in 5/10 years
M4, age 60	Born 1943 in Ghetto Debrecen, Hungary; in January 1945 Rothschild Hospital, Vienna	In ghetto last trimester, 8 months severe starvation in 1944	+	+	–	++	13/26%
Son of M4, age 39–41	Born 1972 in Sydney	Nil	+	+	+	+	0.5/1.0%

Source: private practice of the author, GMW
Table showing the presence (+) or absence (–) of abnormalities in lipids, blood pressure, glucose metabolism and bone mineral density in a mother who was exposed to perinatal starvation and her son who experienced normal perinatal nutrition

Possible Transgenerational Effect of Intrauterine Starvation

Of additional interest in the study of this cohort is evidence which supports the view that the effects of intrauterine starvation might be found in later generations. This phenomenon would be consistent with epidemiological studies which have established that the *"adverse consequences of altered intrauterine environments can be passed from first generation to second generation offspring"* [28].

A female subject in one of the studies cited above [25] has a son whose history would suggest a transgenerational effect (Table 34.3). At age 39 he had hyperlipidaemia, high blood pressure, coronary infarct, and glucose intolerance, all typical adult outcomes of fetal starvation although it was the mother who was undernourished perinatally, not her son. At age 41 the son was found to have osteopenia with a DEXA bone density T-score of −1.5. This outcome could be the result of a genetic predisposition in one family, or it could be an early sign of the transgenerational transfer of inherited metabolic disease. Once again, further research is needed to clarify this point.

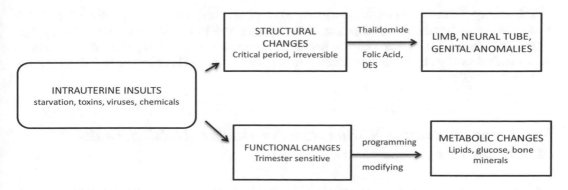

Fig. 34.1 Pathological influences on osteogenesis. *Legend*: Illustration of the effects of toxins on bone formation (Designed by author, GMW)

Intrauterine Nutrition as a Programmer of Bone Development

General Principles

The concept of trimester based intrauterine development has become essential for an understanding of fetal programming, including the programming of bone development. The effects of many environmental and intrauterine conditions upon the fetus are trimester sensitive, although the relationship is not absolute as some overlapping developments between trimesters have also been found (Fig. 34.1).

Intrauterine conditions during the first 12 weeks from conception, the embryonic trimester, were found to affect neuron [29] and *mesenchymal-cartilaginous tissue* development, between weeks 4 and 9 in particular. Cell formation could be affected by external ionising radiation, hypo- or hyper-glycaemia, zinc or folic acid deficiency (predisposing to neural arch malformation such as spina bifida, with or without externally protruding myelocoele) and by viral infection in the mother, such as rubella affecting the myocardium and most recently Zika virus affecting brain development (microcephaly).

It is in the first trimester that thalidomide disturbs limb development, that opioid drugs, alcohol and nicotine affect neurological development (including the effects of alcohol on Corpus Callosum Disorder), and that DES contributes to genital malformations and malignancy.

The following 6 months of pregnancy, namely the two fetal trimesters, were found to be critical to the multiplication and growth of existing cells. It was determined that various organs grow at a different pace, the periods being both sensitive and critical.

The second trimester is most sensitive to metabolic intake, affecting *adipose, muscle and bone tissue formation*; whilst glucose and cortisol are most critical in the third trimester with effects on the developing child's kidney formation, *birth weight, limb length and head circumference at birth*, as well as on post-partum maternal weight changes.

During nutritional deprivation, the body adapts to the food shortage in various ways. The number of developing cells is selectively controlled, while oxygen and nutrition are redirected toward the vital organs (brain, heart, arteries). These changes in growth and function are economically or "thriftily" developed to make the best use of vital resources. The resulting neonate will be small sized and low in weight (BMI, head, chest and abdominal circumferences), which establishes the basis for future neonatal, childhood, or adult diseases.

Conversely, it was found that an excessive food supply in the neonatal period, intended to provide a morphological "catch-up" development, in fact predisposes to obesity and early metabolic syndromes of diabetes, hypertension and cardiac disease, with an impact on longevity and potentially on bone metabolism also. Even with the "catch-up phenomenon," not all bones return to their normal line of growth [30–33].

Specifics on Intrauterine Nutrition as a Programmer of Adult Musculo-Skeletal Diseases

Adipose tissue development occurs mainly in the third trimester (around 30 weeks). Starvation or various degrees of sub-nutrition will predispose to low birth weight, compensated by a "catch-up" metabolism. Both experimental and epidemiological studies suggest that fetal nutritional deprivation programmes *obesity* in adulthood. The issue of obesity is important to any consideration of osteoporosis and fracture risk, since excessive body mass places an abnormal strain on weight-bearing bones.

Myogenesis Maternal and fetal under-nutrition were found to be programmers of muscle development, and are also trimester sensitive. The development of the muscular system arises from the somites region of the embryo's paravertebral region. The myocytes first produce *myofibril I* (second trimester) then *myofibril II* (third trimester), each developing with an attached peripheral nerve. Restriction of glucose and cortisol will redirect nutrients from muscle formation to more essential organs.

It has been documented, both experimentally and epidemiologically, that fetal nutritional deprivation programmes adult *sarcopenia* (reduced flesh) a condition in which both muscle mass and muscle strength are diminished [34]. Like obesity, sarcopenia increases the fracture risk associated with osteoporosis, since a subject with weak muscles would be more likely to experience falls than would a person with normal strength.

Osteogenesis As noted above, the recognition of intrauterine starvation and its effect on *bone metabolism* was subsequent to studies on general metabolism. Numerous researchers made contributions to the theory of intrauterine *starvation resulting in premature adult osteoporosis*. The theory was reproduced experimentally, re-affirmed epidemiologically and is now generally accepted.

Specifics on Fetal Programming and the Mechanism of Osteoporosis Development

According to the 1962 classification of Casuccio [35], still applicable today, *osteoporosis* develops in several ways: by

(a) Primary Osteoblastic deficiency, which is congenital (osteogenesis imperfecta); by
(b) Reduced Osteoblastic activity in the absence of trophic stimuli (inactivity, ovarian agenesis, testicular agenesis, menopause); by
(c) Reduced Osteoblastic activity from inhibitory stimuli (Cushing cortico-steroidism, excess ACTH, thyrotoxicosis); or,
(d) In the case of Normal Osteoblastic activity, by an insufficiency in construction material.

It is necessary to recall the process of *normal osteogenesis* and its requirements in order to appreciate how starvation programmes the adult onset of osteoporosis and sarcopenia [36] (Fig. 34.2).

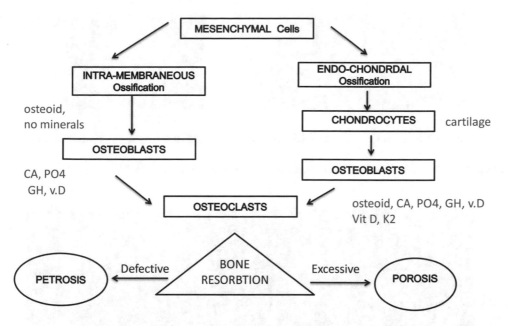

Fig. 34.2 Osteogenesis. *Legend*: The extent of normal and pathological bone formation (Designed by author, GMW)

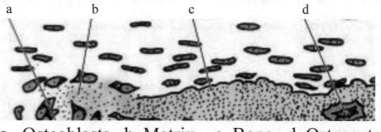

a. Osteoblasts b. Matrix   c. Bone   d. Osteocyte

Fig. 34.3 Bone formation 1. *Legend*: Schematic illustration of bone cell development (Designed by author, GMW)

The concept of "*sensitive period*" or critical trimester dependence was also applied in bone mineral studies. While there are overlapping trimester effects, the particularly vulnerable trimester is the one in which a particular "*development occurs with greatest ease*" [29]. It was found that intrauterine osteogenesis is under hormonal control, as well as dependent upon the availability of minerals and vitamins D and K [37] (Fig. 34.2). Vitamin K in particular has wide-ranging effects on bone formation, a matter which is discussed further in section "Vitamin K-Anticoagulant Antagonism During Gestation and the "Paradoxical Calcification" Phenomenon: Osteoporosis Versus Arterial Wall Calcifications in Adults" below.

Bone ontogenesis is already evident in the fourth week of the embryonic period with some bone formation, but a soft structure. *Mesenchymal* cells are transformed into *osteoblasts,* which soon lead to *osteoclasts* within the *intra-membranous axial ossification* (skull, mandible, clavicle, ribs, sternum genesis) (Fig. 34.3).

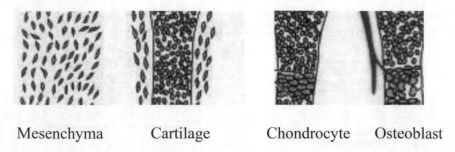

Mesenchyma   Cartilage   Chondrocyte   Osteoblast

Fig. 34.4 Bone formation 2. *Legend*: Normal osteogenesis (Designed by author, GMW)

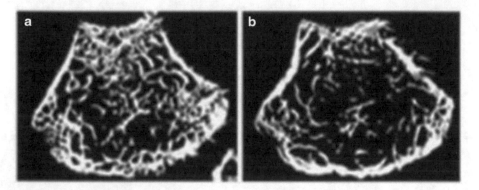

Fig. 34.5 Bone architecture seen in transverse cross-section. *Legend*: (**a**) normal bone architecture. (**b**) Osteoporosis (Computer design by author, GMW)

More frequent is *endochondral appendicular ossification* of long bones, pelvis and vertebrae (Fig. 34.4). During the second and the third trimesters, limb development (muscle and bone) continues with intra-membranous ossification: osteoblasts secrete the non-mineralised bone matrix, and then they transform into osteocytes.

The enchondral path appears first as chondrocytes (cartilage) at the end of the first trimester, then they partially apoptose (self-destroy), but some transform into osteoblasts, from where the path leads to osteoclasts. These osteoclasts contribute to bone marrow formation by destruction of the central bone matrix, leaving a cavity for the hematopoietic marrow. Although the matrix continues to absorb calcium, the central bone space is emptied, whilst the bone grows externally toward the cortex/periosteum.

A balance is maintained between osteoblast and osteoclast activities under the influences of minerals (sulphur, calcium, phosphates, magnesium, selenium, strontium, zinc) and vitamins D and K; of hormones (pituitary growth and parathyroid secretion); of glucose, cortisol and the important osteoproteins. Vascularisation of the bone leads to the blast/clast equilibrium, producing normal bone architecture (Fig. 34.5a).

Any derangement of the chondrocytes leads to chondroplastic pathology. A disturbance in the blast/clast equilibrium in the direction of excessive osteoclastic activity will lead to osteopenia or osteoporosis (Figs. 34.5b and 34.6a), whilst reduced osteoclastic activity will lead to osteopetrosis (excessive mineralisation of the bone) (Fig. 34.6b).

The development will continue during the neonatal stage, as bone growth is not complete at birth. It was found to continue, albeit in diminished blast/clast (production/destruction), balance, even in adults.

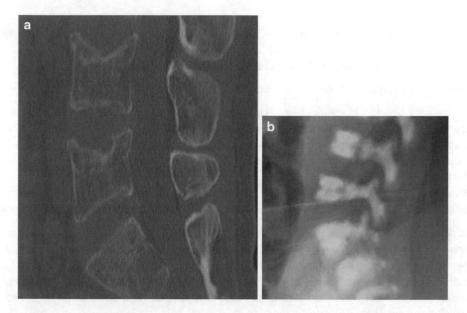

Fig. 34.6 Osteoporosis and osteopetrosis. *Legend*: Radiographic images of osteoporosis and osteopetrosis (From private practice of author, GMW, 1970s)

The need for a strong osteogenic line was confirmed in bone healing experiments: an unstable fracture fixation will allow chondrocytes to develop along the chondrogenic lineage resulting in fibrous union, whilst a stable bone fixation leads to early mesenchymal cell invasion and development along the osteogenic lineage.

Vitamin K-Anticoagulant Antagonism During Gestation and the "Paradoxical Calcification" Phenomenon: Osteoporosis Versus Arterial Wall Calcifications in Adults

The vitamin K complex is essential for a normal osteogenesis. Any deficiency through malnutrition, lack of congenital enzymatic production, lack of intestinal absorption or antagonism by anti-coagulants, leads to various bone metabolic abnormalities [37, 38].

Normal osteogenesis requires carboxylation of bone proteins, a process which is vitamin K dependant. Vitamin K complex was proven to be promoted by enzymatic carboxyl reductase and is essential in the production of three basic bone proteins [39–42]. The substances making up this complex [43, 44] are:

(a) *Matrix Gla protein* or K1, a potent protector against arterial wall and cartilage calcification.
(b) *Osteocalcin* or K2, the most potent, promotes osteoblast stimulation and osteoclast inhibition. An insufficiency of K2 leads to osteopathy.
(c) *Protein S* promotes coagulation, and its deficiency leads to childhood osteoporosis with vertebral compressions.

The pathological features resulting from vitamin K deficiency, apart from haemorrhagic events are [37, 40, 45, 46]:

- *Cerebral*: microcephalus, hydrocephalus, mental retardation;
- *Ocular*: microphthalmia, cataracts, blindness;

- *Acoustic*: deafness;
- *Skeletal*: stappling of epiphysis, shortened limbs, shortened fingers, nail bed deformities, scoliosis, facial bone anomalies (depressed nasal bridge and nasal hypoplasia);
- *Cardiac*, with various congenital anomalies.

Several clinical syndromes result from vitamin K deficiency.

1. From lack of vitamin K production: *Bone reductase deficiency syndrome* (known as pseudo-warfarin embryopathy) is an imbalance due to a congenital defect of vitamin K metabolism. It leads to insufficient carboxylase and to the "calcification paradox," namely to calcifications of epiphyseal areas and arterial walls at the same time as the bones become demineralized leading to osteoporosis [47–50].

2. From lack of absorption: *Malabsorption vitamin K deficiency embryopathy* is an imbalance due to intestinal malabsorption or to malnutrition, with similar cartilage and neurological complications.

(a) *Malabsorption* is due either to a small intestine inflammatory or autoimmune disease (Crohn disease, Coeliac disease, Lupus, etc.) or to short bowel syndrome. The latter is a result of bariatric by-pass surgery performed for morbid obesity. Vitamin K1 deficiency is specific to the upper small bowel (ileal) level, with by-pass exclusion or resection for malignancy. Alternatively, vitamin K2 deficiency results from distal small bowel level (end-ileal) or large bowel (colon) exclusion or resection [43].

(b) The K2 *malnutrition* syndrome is a nutritional deficiency in the pre-gestational and gestational periods leading to the same clinical syndrome as the previous embryopathy.

Both syndromes present with abnormalities detectable by means of ultrasound or x-ray investigations during gestation, imaging the growth plate (punctate chondrodystrophy of hips, ankles, etc.) and stunted sizes in new-born parameters. Both are curable with vitamin K2 supplementation.

3. From antagonism by anti-coagulants: *warfarin embryopathy*. Treatment with warfarin can be required during pregnancy for mothers with thrombotic vein pathology (leg or embolic) or heart disease (valve replacement or arrhythmia). Warfarin is toxic to the osteocalcin devoid embryo or to the partially protected fetus. A vitamin K/warfarin imbalance leads to severe embryonic/fetal haemorrhages and neurological complications.

The effect of warfarin is trimester sensitive: in the first trimester there is no antagonism to the administered warfarin. Indeed the malformations following warfarin treatment appear in weeks 6–9 of gestation, when most of the intracranial bleeding occurs. During the second and third trimester, the balance between vitamin K and anticoagulants is also vulnerable.

The role of vitamin K deficiency in the pathogenesis of osteoporosis and vascular calcification has been raised in the literature but it remains disputed, an unresolved topic [37]. Experimental reproduction of early closure of epiphyseal growth plates was documented [51] and supported by several, but not unanimous clinical studies [46].

Experimentally, the osteocalcin (K2) deficiency in mice led to an increased bone formation, with calcification of growth plate, whilst the matrix Gla protein deficiency (K1) led to the "calcification paradox" [37, 40–43]. The prophylactic values of vitamin K2 supplement showed improved bone strength, preventing fracture re-occurrence [52, 53].

The temporal gap between the intrauterine period and the late effect in adulthood needs a scientific explanation. One theory accepts the direct relationship between the effect of warfarin on the mother and the development of bone and arterial pathology in the embryo/fetus. This is similar to the effect of nutritional deficiency in the fetus as a programmer of later adult glucose, lipid and mineral metabolism. This hypothesis was reinforced recently in a study of children treated for congenital heart disease with warfarin, which found osteocalcin in the arterial wall calcifications and also found decreased bone density [54].

A daily vitamin K supplement of 1 µg/kg would prevent or treat the warfarin osteopathy [42]. A replacement anticoagulant therapy using heparin is effective, with its large sized molecule unable to be filtered through the placenta, but it carries other specific risks for the mother.

The effect of the more recent and as yet only experimental oral anticoagulants on intrauterine life has not been sufficiently tested. Experimental studies on rats and rabbits indicate a similar haemorrhagic syndrome, since Xarelto (rivaroxaban) and others are of small molecular weight and are filtered through the placenta [55]. Clinical studies are awaiting the results of the antidote studies, prior to their approval. The authors could find no detailed studies regarding the effect of these new anticoagulants on osteogenesis, but it is expected that small molecular weight drugs would filter through the placenta and lead to the same complications as warfarin does.

Postnatal Compensatory Growth and Adult Bone Quality

The situation with regard to individuals who experience intrauterine starvation and then undergo "catch up overfeeding", or "*compensatory growth*," after birth is still unclear. McCance in the early 1960s, using an animal model, indicated that recovery is limited, with prolonged over-nutrition leading only to partial bone quality improvement [56]. On the other hand, more recent animal experiments on post-starvation overfeeding showed that "*reduction in bone quality is a transient and reversible phenomenon*" [32].

In studies focussed on human longitudinal bone growth after malnutrition, rather than on bone quality, Prader et al. concluded in 1963 that even with catch up growth "*recovery is nearly always retarded*" [30]; whereas in the following year Golden found evidence that with an adequate diet "*almost complete reversal of stunting is possible [and] children can reach their own height potentials*" [31]. What are needed are direct, long-term studies of human bone quality in the circumstances of intrauterine starvation followed by compensatory growth. In the absence of these, the evidence cited in section "Extension of the Theory to Include Musculo-Skeletal Pathology" above makes it prudent to assume that compensatory growth cannot fully reverse the effects of the fetal programming of osteoporosis. There is also a possibility that compensatory growth could potentially exacerbate these effects.

Fetal Programming of Osteoporosis as a Public Health Issue

In countries where food shortages are common, the public health challenge is to provide for large numbers of people with programmed osteopathy. Wealthier countries, on the other hand, must prepare to care adequately for immigrant populations from these backgrounds who can also be expected to undergo compensatory growth.

The risk to these migrant populations, many with infants, neonates and pregnant women, apart from their previous exposure to starvation (partial, selective or full), is also an eventual exposure to overfeeding in their new countries. A Swedish report published in 2010 on survivors of the civil war in Biafra (1967–1970), who were born nutritionally deprived 40 years earlier and who subsequently had a sufficient nutritional supply, documented their high levels of obesity [57].

Although this study and others like it do not explicitly address the issue of bone metabolism, the balance of evidence from the research cited above gives reason to expect that these populations experiencing compensatory growth would suffer from bone mineral deficiencies as well as other metabolic disorders. Obesity in particular, as noted in section "Specifics on Intrauterine Nutrition as a Programmer of Adult Musculo-Skeletal Diseases" above, adds significantly to the risk of osteoporotic fractures.

Societies receiving large numbers of nutritionally deprived immigrants will face a medical and organisational demand for the provision of extensive public health services within a few decades. Public health initiatives will need to be directed toward the prevention of osteoporosis as well as early diagnosis and treatment in order to reduce the incidence of fractures and other disabilities resulting from this condition.

Conclusions

Nutritional deprivation during pregnancy or in the post-natal period can have a programming effect on the development of an adult, leading to complex disturbances in glucose, lipid and bone mineral metabolism. The theory that intrauterine nutritional status can programme an adult onset of osteoporosis has been proven clinically, epidemiologically and experimentally.

Decreased bone mineral content and bone mineral density of the femoral neck, with increased risk of fractures, was recently found in a small group of survivors of intrauterine starvation (in particular, case 2, Table 34.1), an indicative finding although statistically not significant. Outcomes of this kind, if confirmed by broader studies, would provide support for Cooper's theory of a link between intrauterine development and early adult osteoporosis.

The *fetal programming of adult osteoporosis* has a multi-factorial pathogenesis that despite several proposed plausible theories, is not yet definitely established. A good explanation may be found in the description given by Kueper of pregnant women whose exposure to hunger was connected with early onset of osteoporosis in their offspring [23].

A patient's history of intrauterine malnutrition should raise the suspicion of a tendency toward osteoporosis and should be used in the early detection of adult osteoporosis, apart from obesity and sarcopenia.

References

1. Monash University. http://www.med.monash.edu.au/sphpm/womenshealth/health-information/definition-diagnosis-of-osteoporosis.html. Accessed 11 May 2016.
2. Australian Bureau of Statistics. http://www.abs.gov.au/ausstats/abs@.nsf/Lookup/4843.0.55.001main+features 32007-08. Accessed 11 May 2016.
3. Osteoporosis Australia. www.osteoporosis.org.au/therapeutic-management. Accessed 11 May 2016.
4. Head R, Gilthorpe M, Byrom A, et al. Cardiovascular disease in a cohort exposed to the 1940–45 Channel Islands occupation. BMC Public Health. 2008;8:303–7.
5. Sparen P, Vagero D, et al. Long term mortality after severe starvation during the siege of Leningrad. BMJ. 2004;384(1):11–4.
6. Susser M, Stein Z. Timing in prenatal nutrition: a reprise of the Dutch famine study. Nutr Rev. 1994;52(3):84–93.
7. Lucas A. Programming by early nutrition in man. In: Bock GR, Whelan J, editors. The childhood environment and adult disease, Ciba Foundation Symp. 156. Chichester: Wiley; 1991. p. 38–55.
8. Hales CN, Barker DJ. Type 2 (non-insulin-dependent) diabetes mellitus: the thrifty phenotype hypothesis. Diabetologia. 1992;35(7):595–601.
9. Barker DJP. The developmental origins of well-being. Philos Trans R Soc Lond B. 2004;359(1449):1359–66.
10. Kuh D, Ben Shlomo Y. A life course approach to chronic disease epidemiology. 2nd ed. Oxford: OUP; 1997. 2004.
11. Gluckman PD, Hanson MA. Environmental influences during development and their later consequences for health and disease. Proc R Soc Lond B. 2005;272:671–7.
12. Gluckman PD, Hanson MA, Cooper C, Thornburg KL. Effect of in utero and early-life conditions on adult health and diseases. N Engl J Med. 2008;359(3):61–73.
13. Vaiserman AM. Early life nutritional programming of longevity. J Dev Orig Health Dis. 2014;5(5):325–8.
14. Laker RC, Wlodek ME, Connelly JJ, Yan Z. Epigenetic origins of metabolic disease: the impact of the maternal condition to the offspring epigenome and later health consequences. Food Sci Human Wellness. 2013;2:1–11.

15. Holroyd C, Harvey N, Dennison E, Cooper C. Epigenetic influences in the developmental origins of osteoporosis. Osteoporos Int. 2012;23(2):401–10.
16. Cooper C, Fall C, Egger P, Hobbs R, Eastell R, Barker D. Growth in infancy and bone mass in later life. Ann Rheum Dis. 1997;56:17–21.
17. Cooper C, Walker-Bone K, Arden N. Novel insights into the pathogenesis of osteoporosis: the role of intrauterine programming. Rheumatology. 2000;39:1312–5.
18. Cooper C, Erikson JG, Forsen T, Osmon C, Tuomilehto J, Barker DJP. Maternal height, childhood growth and risk of hip fracture in later life, a longitudinal study. Osteoporos Int. 2001;12(8):623–9.
19. Javaid K, Taylor P, et al. The fetal origins of osteoporotic fractures. Calcif Tissue Int. 2002;70:391–4.
20. Dennison EM, Arden NK, et al. Birth weight, vitamin D receptor genotype and the programming of osteoporosis. Pediatr Perinat Epidemiol. 2001;15:211–9.
21. Harvey N, Cooper C. The developmental origins of osteoporotic fracture. Menopause Int. 2004;10:14–29.
22. Cooper C, Javaid K, et al. Developmental origins of osteoporotic fracture: the role of maternal vitamin D insufficiency. J Nutr. 2005;135(11):2728S–34S.
23. Kueper J, Beyth S, Lebergall M, Kaplan L, Schroeder JE. Evidence for the adverse effect of starvation on bone quality: a review. Int J Endocrinol. 2015;2015:628740. http://dx.doi.org/10.1155/2015/628740.
24. Weisz GM, Albury WR. Osteoporosis in survivors of early life starvation. Aust J Prim Health. 2013;19(1):3–6. http://dx.doi.org/10.1071/PY12004.
25. Weisz GM, Albury WR. Hunger whilst "in utero" programming adult osteoporosis. Rambam Maimonides Med J. 2014;5(1):1–4.
26. Winnick MD. Hunger disease: studies by Jewish physicians in the Warsaw ghetto. New York: Wiley-Interscience; 1979.
27. Garvan Institute. www.garvan.org.au/bone-fracture-risk. Accessed 11 May 2016.
28. Zambrano E. The transgenerational mechanisms in developmental programming of metabolic diseases. Rev Investig Clin. 2009;61(1):41–52.
29. Smart JL. Critical periods in brain development. In: Bock GR, Whelan J, editors. The childhood environment and adult disease, Ciba Foundation Symp 156. Chichester: Wiley; 1991. p. 109–28.
30. Prader A, Tanner JM, Harnack GA. Catch up growth following illness or starvation. J Pediatr. 1963;62(5):646–59.
31. Golden MH. Is complete catch-up possible for stunted, malnourished children? Eur J Clin Nutr. 1994; 48(Suppl.1):S58–71.
32. Pando R, Masarwi M, Shtaif B, Idelevich A, Ornan EM, Shahar R, Phillip M, Gat-Yablonski G. Bone quality is affected by food restrictions and by nutrition-induced catch up growth. J Endocrinol. 2014;223:227–39.
33. Gat-Yablonski G, Philip M. Nutritional-induced catch up growth. Forum Nutr. 2015;7(1):517–51.
34. Cooper C, Sayer AA, et al. Developing origins of musculoskeletal disease. In: Newnham JP, Ross MG, editors. Early life origins of human health and disease. Basel: Karger; 2009. p. 100–12.
35. Casuccio C. Concerning osteoporosis. J Bone Joint Surg. 1962;44B(3):453–63.
36. Moore KL, Persaud TVN, Torchia MG. The developing human: clinically oriented embryology. 10th ed. Philadelphia: Elsevier; 2016.
37. Shearer MJ. Role of vitamin K and Gla proteins in the pathophysiology of osteoporosis and vascular calcification. Curr Opin Clin Nutr Metab Care. 2000;3(6):433–8.
38. Hall JG, Paull RM, Wilson KM. Maternal and fetal sequelae of anticoagulation during pregnancy. Am J Med. 1989;68:122–40.
39. Vermeer C, Jie KSG, Knapen MHJ. Role of vitamin K in bone metabolism. Annu Rev Nutr. 1995;15:1–22.
40. Koshihara Y, Hoshi K, et al. Vitamin K2 promotes 1α,25(OH)2 vitamin D3-induced mineralisation in human periosteal osteoblasts. Calcif Tissue Int. 1996;59(6):466–73.
41. Booth SL. Skeletal functions of vitamin K-dependent proteins: not just for clotting anymore. Nutr Rev. 1997; 55(7):282–4.
42. Shearer MJ, Vitamin K. Lancet. 1995;345:229–34.
43. Silaghi CN, et al. Matrix Gla protein: the inhibitor of vascular and osteoarticular calcifications. HVM Bioflux. 2011;3(3):178–90.
44. Hou JW. Fetal warfarin syndrome. Chang Gung Med J. 2004;27(9):691–4.
45. Raghav S, Reutens D. Neurological sequelae of intrauterine warfarin exposure. J Clin Neurosci. 2007;27:99–103.
46. Rosen HN, Maitland LA, et al. Vitamin K and maintenance of skeletal integrity in adults. Am J Med. 2003;94: 62–8.
47. Cockayne S, Adamson J, et al. Vitamin K and the prevention of fractures: systematic review and meta-analysis of randomised controlled trials. Arch Intern Med. 2006;166(12):1256–61.
48. Wessels MJ, Hollander NJD, et al. Fetus with an unusual form of nonrhizomelic chondrodysplasia punctata. Am J Med Genet. 2003;120A:97–104.
49. Menger H, Lin AE, et al. Vitamin K deficiency embryopathy. Am J Med Genet. 1997;72:129–34.
50. Pauli RM, Madden JD, et al. Warfarin therapy initiated during pregnancy and phenotypic chondrodysplasia punctata. J Pediatr. 1976;88(3):506–8.

51. Price PA, Williamson MK, et al. Excessive mineralization with growth plate closure in rats on chronic warfarin treatment. Proc Natl Acad Sci U S A. 1982;79(24):7734–8.
52. Shiraki M, Shiraki Y, et al. Vitamin K2 effectively prevents fractures and sustains lumbar bone mineral density in osteoporosis. J Bone Miner Res. 2000;15(3):515–21.
53. Iwamoto J, Takeda T. Effect of combined administration of vitamin D3 and K2 on bone mineral density. J Orthop Sci. 2000;5(6):546–51.
54. Barnes C, Newall F, et al. Reduced bone density in children on long term warfarin. Pediatr Res. 2005;17(4):578–81.
55. Königsbrügge O, Langer M, Hayde M, Ay C, Pabinger I. Oral anticoagulation with rivaroxaban during pregnancy: a case report. Thromb Haemost. 2014;112(6):1323–4.
56. McCance RA, Widdowson EM. Nutrition and growth. Proc R Soc Lond B. 1962;156(964):326–37.
57. Hult M, Tomhammar P, et al. Hypertension, diabetes and overweight: looming legacies of the Biafran famine. PLoS One. 2010;5(10):e13582.

Chapter 35
Childhood Sleep After Fetal Growth Restriction

Stephanie R. Yiallourou

Key Points

- Fetal growth restriction is associated with increased risk of preterm birth, perinatal mortality and neurodevelopmental delay.
- The growth restricted fetus employs a number of adaptations to preserve energy and ensure oxygen and nutrient delivery to vital organs, including alteration of sleep state architecture.
- The development of sleep begins in utero, when identifiable sleep states emerge. Sleep undergoes marked maturational changes after birth within the first 6 months of life.
- Infants and children born both preterm and growth restricted have altered maturation of sleep.
- Poor sleep in childhood is associated with neurocognitive and behavioural deficits.
- The long-term consequences of altered sleep in preterm and FGR children are unknown and require future follow-up.

Keywords Fetal growth restriction • Sleep • Preterm birth • Sleep architecture • Circadian rhythms

Abbreviations

AGA	Appropriate birth weight for gestational age
AS	Active sleep
EEG	Electroencephalogram
EMG	Electromyogram
EOG	Electrooculogram
FGR	Fetal growth restriction
IS	Indeterminate sleep
N1	Non-rapid eye movement stage 1 sleep
N2	Non-rapid eye movement stage 2 sleep
N3	Non-rapid eye movement stage 3 sleep

S.R. Yiallourou, BSc (Hons), PhD (✉)
Centre for Primary Care and Prevention, Mary MacKillop Institute for Health Research,
Australian Catholic University, Melbourne, VIC, Australia
e-mail: Stephanie.yiallourou@acu.edu.au; MacKillopInstitute@acu.edu.au

© Springer International Publishing AG 2017
R. Rajendram et al. (eds.), *Diet, Nutrition, and Fetal Programming*,
Nutrition and Health, DOI 10.1007/978-3-319-60289-9_35

NREM   Non-rapid eye movement sleep
PNA   Postnatal age
QS   Quiet sleep
REM   Rapid eye movement sleep
SCN   Suprachiasmatic nucleus

Introduction

Fetal growth restriction (FGR) complicates 5–10% of pregnancies and is associated with increased risks of preterm birth (<37 weeks gestation), perinatal mortality, and short and long term morbidity [1]. FGR is associated with a high risk of neurodevelopmental impairment, including motor and sensory deficits, cognitive and learning difficulties, and cerebral palsy [2]. Underpinning these deficits, FGR is associated with altered brain structure with reduced total brain and cortical gray matter volume [3]. In particular, both the hippocampus and the cerebellum are known to be effected [4]. Much later in life, during adulthood, it is also well established that FGR is associated with high risk of metabolic disorders such as hypertension and diabetes leading to heart disease [5].

In addition to the well-known neurodevelopmental and cardiovascular consequences of FGR, there is a growing body of evidence showing that FGR alters the development of sleep in utero [6, 7]. Also, being born preterm, whether the infant is growth restricted or not, can alter the maturation of sleep after birth. Thus, FGR may program the fetus for life-long sleep related sequelae. This is of particular concern as it is well described that poor sleep in childhood is related to neurocognitive impairment [8] and in adulthood metabolic disorders and cardiovascular disease [5].

Fetal Growth Restriction (FGR)

FGR describes the fetus that does not reach its genetic growth potential and primarily results from placental insufficiency, which compromises the delivery of oxygen and essential nutrients to the fetus. FGR is defined as an estimated fetal weight and/or birth weight at or below the fifth percentile for gestation and sex. FGR can manifest from poor maternal nutrition or a number of fetal and maternal disorders, such as maternal vascular disease, fetal infections, multiple gestations and exposure to maternal smoking during pregnancy. Severe FGR results in fetal asymmetry, where head growth is spared relative to body growth; known as the 'head sparing' effect. These fetal adaptations are critical to optimise oxygen and nutrient delivery to the brain and heart of a compromised fetus and involves complex cardiovascular and metabolic changes. In regards to sleep, we know that the compromised fetus alters its organization of sleep states, favouring a state that requires reduced energy needs, in an effort to further preserve energy in a reduced oxygen environment [6, 7]. While these adaptations are beneficial in the short-term they may program the fetus for long-term morbidities [9]. In the long-term, it is well known that FGR is associated with heightened risk of adult onset of cardiovascular disease, including coronary heart disease and hypertension [5, 9, 10]. We also know, though human data is scarce, that FGR alters the maturation of sleep circadian rhythms in neonatal life and sleep efficiency later in life [11]. Understanding the long-term effect of FGR on sleep is of particular importance, as sleep is the main behavioural state during the neonatal period and is known to be important for neurological development [12]. Currently, there is no therapy to treat these long-term dysfunctions.

Sleep and Its Development

Function of Sleep

Approximately one-third of an adult's day is spent asleep, and this proportion is even larger in infants and children, who spend approximately two-thirds of each 24-h day asleep [13]. Whilst no consensus has been reached, the function of sleep is thought to be involved in the homeostatic maintenance of key body systems. Sleep is thought to be fundamental for memory consolidation [13], peak immunological performance [14], restoration of somatic function [15], and neurological growth and repair [16]. The hypothesis that sleep is essential for brain connectivity/plasticity has recently been suggested to be the leading contender for the primordial function of sleep [17]. In support of this concept, studies show that neuronal connectivity changes with sleep, sleep loss, and with changing afferent input [18]. Thus it is not surprising that obtaining adequate sleep is imperative to sustaining optimal day time functioning and health [13].

Sleep States

Children and Adults

In order to understand the development of sleep, a brief understanding of sleep states is crucial. In children and adults, sleep is divided into two distinct states known as rapid eye movement (REM) and non-rapid eye movement (NREM) sleep. NREM is further divided into sleep stages N1, N2 and N3. These stages are distinguished by a succession of changes in electroencephalographic (EEG) activity. EEG terminology defines waves by their frequency in cycles per second, or Hertz (Hz). Defined frequency ranges include: delta (1–4 Hz), theta (4–7 Hz), alpha (8–13 Hz), and beta (>13 Hz). Polysomnographic recordings are used to asses sleep stages determined by differences in EEG activity, the presence or absence of eye movements (electrooculographic activity, EOG) and changes in muscle tone (electromyographic activity, EMG).

Humans enter sleep via N1 which is characterised by rolling eye movements along with low voltage mixed frequency theta activity (Fig. 35.1). In stage 2, theta activity continues and fast sleep spindles (an oscillatory burst of EEG activity of 12–15 Hz and at least 0.5 s) and k-complexes (a well-defined EEG pattern consisting of a sharp negative wave followed by a slow positive component lasting at least 0.5 s) appear (Fig. 35.2). Following stage 2 we enter our deepest sleep known as stage 3 (also called slow wave sleep, SWS). Stage 3 is characterized by high amplitude, low-frequency delta waves and spindle activity (Fig. 35.3). From NREM sleep, we transition to REM sleep, a "lighter sleep state" where dreaming usually occurs. REM sleep is characterised by a sudden loss in muscle tone and the presence of rapid eye movements. The EEG is similar to wake patterns characterized by low-voltage, high frequency EEG activity as well as theta rhythms (Fig. 35.4). NREM sleep and REM sleep continue to alternate throughout the night in a cyclic fashion. The majority of NREM sleep occurs within the first half of the night and REM sleep episodes generally become longer throughout the night.

As evidenced by its physiological characteristics, sleep in children and adults is a highly complex and regulated process, with distinct states. This mature form of sleep is not present at birth, however, and sleep undergoes marked maturational changes in both fetal life and within the first year of life as it forms adult-like states and patterns. The following section outlines the maturation of sleep during fetal life and infancy.

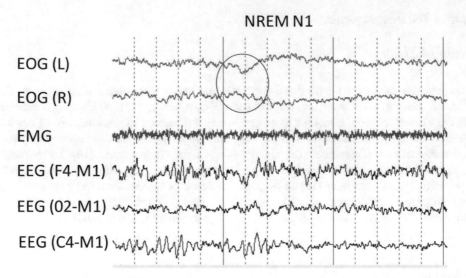

Fig. 35.1 Polysomnographic recording of N1 sleep. A typical example of a polysomnographic recording of a child in non-rapid eye movement stage 1 sleep (*N1*). Electroencephalographic (*EEG*) activity is recorded at frontal (*F4*), occipital (*O2*) and central (*C4*) regions and referenced to mastoid regions (*M1*). Note the EEG recording is dominated by theta activity. There is the presence of rolling eye movements (*circled in red*) in the electrooculograph (left (*L*) and right (*R*) *EOG*) and muscle tone recorded by the electromyography (*EMG*) is also relatively high

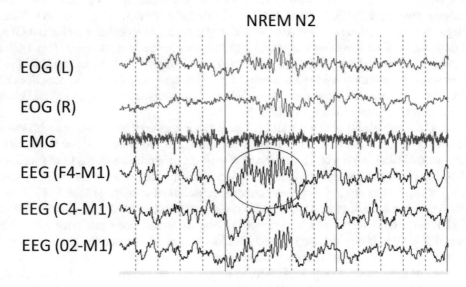

Fig. 35.2 Polysomnographic recording of N2 sleep. A typical example of a polysomnographic recording of a child in non-rapid eye movement stage 2 sleep (*N2*). Electroencephalographic (*EEG*) activity is recorded on frontal (*F4*), occipital (*O2*) and central (*C4*) regions and referenced to mastoid regions (*M1*). Note the presence of sleep spindles (*circled in red*) in the EEG. There is the absence of eye movements recorded by the electrooculograph (left (*L*) and right (*R*) *EOG*) and high muscle tone recorded by the electromyograph (*EMG*)

Fetal Life

The development of sleep begins in fetal life. Sleep can be identified in the human fetus as early as 28 weeks gestation [19] and at 32 weeks of gestation fetal sleep can be clearly differentiated into three defined states; Active sleep (AS), Quiet sleep (QS) and Indeterminate sleep (IS). AS is thought to be the precursor for REM sleep and is defined by continuous mixed EEG activity consisting mostly of theta

NREM N3

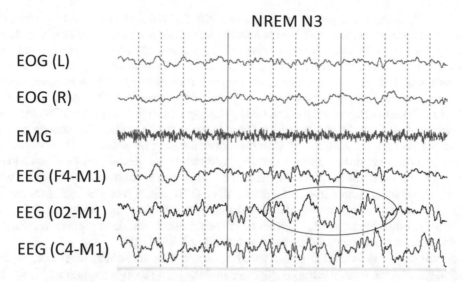

Fig. 35.3 Polysomnographic recording of N3 sleep. A typical example of a polysomnographic recording of a child in non-rapid eye movement stage 3 sleep (*N3*). Electroencephalographic (*EEG*) activity is recorded on frontal (*F4*), occipital (*O2*) and central (*C4*) regions and referenced to mastoid regions (*M1*). Note the EEG recording is dominated by slow wave delta activity. There is an absence of eye movements recorded by electrooculograph (left (*L*) and right (*R*) *EOG*) and high muscle tone recorded by the electromyograph (*EMG*)

REM

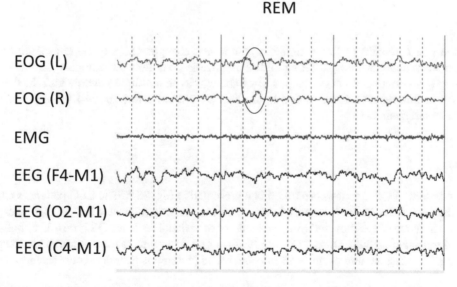

Fig. 35.4 Polysomnographic recording of REM sleep. A typical example of a polysomnographic recording of a child in rapid eye movement sleep (*REM*). Electroencephalographic (*EEG*) is recorded on frontal (*F4*), occipital (*O2*) and central (*C4*) regions and referenced to mastoid regions (*M1*). Note the EEG recording is characterised by low-amplitude high frequency activity. There is the presence of rapid eye movements (*circled in red*) recorded by the electrooculograph (left (*L*) and right (*R*) *EOG*) and low muscle tone recorded by the electromyograph (*EMG*)

brain waves and irregular breathing. QS is thought to be the precursor for NREM sleep which emerges at 32 weeks of gestation [15]. QS is defined by bursts of slow wave EEG activity (delta waves) amongst otherwise discontinuous EEG activity, and regular breathing. Indeterminate sleep (IS) refers to sleep that cannot be classified as either AS or QS. The proportion of time a fetus spends within each sleep state is a function of gestational age. Generally, the human fetus will spend approximately 80% of the sleep-wake cycle in the sleep period, with this consisting of twice the amount of AS compared to QS. Early in the pregnancy, the fetus spends a large amount of time in IS [20]. This decreases as the pregnancy progresses, with a significant increase in QS seen from 32 to 40 weeks of gestation, with AS time unchanged [21]. Once at term age, time spent in AS and QS equalises.

The entrainment of circadian rhythms also begins before birth [21–23]. Circadian rhythms are physiological changes that occur based on an intrinsic 24-h cycle, usually influenced by light and darkness [15]. Circadian rhythms are controlled by the suprachiasmatic nucleus (SCN) in the anterior hypothalamus. In the fetus, SCN cells are known to have intrinsic circadian rhythmicity, and respond to periodic fluctuations in the release of maternal hormones such as melatonin [24]. Melatonin is an endogenous neuroendocrine compound primarily produced by the pineal gland and has a major role in regulating circadian rhythms. In adults, melatonin production is controlled by the SCN, with high levels of synthesis at night, and low levels during the day. The SCN receives light information from the retina and sends information to the pineal gland to modulate the production of melatonin. Melatonin plays a role in sleep state regulation, where specific blockade of melatonin receptors (M1 or M2) can alter the percentage of time spent in NREM and REM [25].

The developing fetus is reliant on maternal fluctuations in melatonin to entrain rhythmicity. Maternal melatonin can readily cross the placenta and the fetal blood-brain-barrier. While the SCN develops throughout gestation, it is still functionally immature after birth. Thus, before birth, it is thought that the mother entrains the developing fetus circadian rhythm to the light-dark cycle. This entrainment is evidenced in the fetus, with a night-day rhythm of fetal heart rate being synchronised with maternal rest-activity and melatonin rhythms [23].

Infancy

Within the first 6 months of life, dramatic maturational changes occur to sleep as adult-like sleep states and sleep patterns emerge. This rapid reorganization parallels the complex maturation of the central nervous system and hence sleep is often thought to be a unique window into the developing brain. Within this period of maturation both sleep state architecture and 24 h sleep-wake cycles undergo marked changes.

Quiet Sleep

A typical pattern of QS in a newborn infant is represented in Fig. 35.5. The EEG pattern is characterised by frequent notched, high amplitude slow waves occurring against a low voltage background. There is an absence of eye movements and except for occasional twitches QS is devoid of body movements and muscular activity. During QS, the EMG is high and remains tonic throughout. Respiratory rate during QS is regular and mean heart rate and blood pressure is decreased compared to AS.

Active Sleep

Figure 35.6 presents a typical pattern of AS in a newborn infant. During AS the EEG is characterised by a low amplitude, mixed frequency signal. As illustrated in Fig. 35.6, the presence of discontinuous ocular deflections in the EOG (rapid eye movements) is prominent. In contrast to QS, AS is characterised by frequent body movements and regular muscle contractions. Grimaces, whimpers, smiles and twitches of the face and extremities are common during the AS state. Gross shifts of position of the limbs in addition to frequent 10–15 s episodes of tonic, athetoid writhing of the torso, limbs and digits also occur. Tonic muscle tone is significantly reduced compared to QS. The respiratory rate is very irregular and can be associated with, but not limited to, brief periods of apnoea, hypopnoea and tachypnoea. Heart rate and blood pressure are generally higher in AS compared to QS and is also more variable.

Quiet Sleep

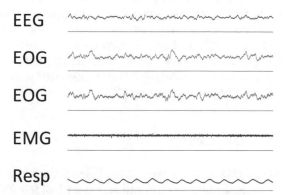

Fig. 35.5 Polysomnographic recording of QS sleep. A typical example of a polysomnographic recording of a newborn infant in quiet sleep (*QS*). Note the electroencephalographic (*EEG*) recording is dominated by theta activity. There is absence of rapid eye movements recorded by the electrooculograph (*EOG*); muscle tone recorded by the electromyograph (*EMG*) is also relatively high and respiration (*Resp*) is regular

Active Sleep

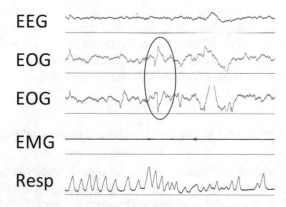

Fig. 35.6 Polysomnographic recording of AS sleep. A typical example of a polysomnographic recording of a newborn infant in active sleep (*AS*). Note the electroencephalographic (*EEG*) recording is characterised by low amplitude mixed frequency activity. There is the presence of rapid eye movements (*circled in red*) recorded by the electrooculograph (*EOG*), muscle tone recorded by the electromyograph (*EMG*) is low and respiration (*Resp*) is irregular

Maturation of Infant Sleep State Architecture

The duration and cycling of sleep states throughout sleep is termed as sleep state architecture. Typically newborn infants enter sleep via AS and cycle between AS and QS, with sleep cycles lasting 45–60 min [26]. Within each sleep cycle, infants spend approximately half their time in each sleep state. Between 10 and 12 week postnatal age (PNA), a critical period of reorganization occurs when infant sleep patterns shift to a more mature form [27]. After 12 weeks PNA, the onset of sleep via AS switches to QS and the proportion of AS gradually decreases while the proportion of QS and wakefulness increases. By 6 months PNA the amount of AS comprises one-third of total sleep time, approaching adult REM proportions [28].

Maturation of EEG Patterns

In infancy as the brain matures, marked changes are also seen in the development of EEG activity in the first 6 months after birth. Within the first 3 months the disappearance of discontinuity or "tracè alternant" pattern in the EEG occurs and is replaced by a continuous slow-wave pattern. Between 2 and 3 months PNA sleep spindles begin to emerge which are a distinctive feature of adult N2 sleep. By 5–6 months PNA, K-complexes and delta waves are present in the EEG and NREM stages 1, 2 and 3 can be identified. In AS, a reduction in the amplitude and increase in the mixture of EEG frequencies occur as the more mature REM-like pattern emerges [27].

Maturation of Infant Sleep-Wake Cycling

Changes in sleep-wake cycling also occur across infancy. Diurnal sleep wake patterns develop within the first 12 weeks of life. Around the time of birth and during the first few months after birth the cells within the human SCN increase in number and size [29] and melatonin levels become rhythmic by 9–12 weeks after birth [30]. Due to maturation of circadian rhythms, the distribution of sleep across the 24-h cycle changes with PNA. Within the first 6 weeks, newborns average five episodes of sleep in 3–4 h blocks. After this time, longer periods of sleep are sustained, particularly at night and by 9–16 weeks, diurnal patterns are established, with sleep at nights lasting 8–9 h [31]. The amount of total sleep time within a 24-h cycle also decreases with PNA. Newborns spend approximately 16 h of each 24 h period and this gradually decreases to 13–14 h by 6–8 months PNA [31].

In summary, during fetal life and infancy, rapid maturational changes in sleep state architecture and the organization of sleep-wake patterns occur. In the fetus, the development of circadian rhythms relies on maternal melatonin cues. Thus, sleep undergoes significant maturational changes in utero and continues into the neonatal period. Therefore, as the development of sleep begins in utero, it is not surprising that sleep would be particularly vulnerable to conditions of prenatal and postnatal stress, where intrauterine environment is poor such as FGR and preterm birth.

Effects of Preterm Birth and FGR on the Development of Sleep

FGR is associated with increased risk of preterm birth as preterm delivery is the only treatment option to prevent fetal death and hypoxia. Preterm birth, with an appropriate weight for gestational age (AGA), is known alter the development of sleep and the compounding effect of FGR is known to augment these features. Of note, the long-term separate effects of preterm birth and FGR on sleep are difficult to differentiate. Many long-term investigations have studied cohorts of infants born with "low birth weight". The term "low birth weight" is a broad description of infants born <2500 g regardless of gestational age and therefore includes infants born preterm AGA and infants that are FGR. Nonetheless, the effects of (1) preterm birth alone and (2) FGR in preterm and term infants on sleep are discussed separately in the following sections.

Effect of Preterm Birth

Preterm newborns spend much more of their time asleep compered to term born infants, with 90% of their 24-h day spent sleeping. In preterm infants born <30 weeks gestation, development of sleep state architecture parallels that of the fetus [21]. Between 32 and 42 weeks postconceptional age, the amount of QS more than triples, the amount of IS more than halves, and the amount of wake time increases by a factor of four while the time spent in AS remains constant [21]. After term equivalent age, the development of sleep state architecture does not appear to be altered by prematurity [32]. Percentages of time spent in QS, AS and IS are similar between preterm-born infants compared to term-born infants aged between 38 and 55 weeks postconceptional age [32].

In contrast to sleep state architecture, prematurity is known to effect the development of circadian rhythms in infancy. While exposed to bright (and sometimes continuous) light in the neonatal nursery, the premature infant must complete crucial stages of SCN maturation ex utero [33]. This environment is in stark contrast to the in utero environment, where the fetus receives maternal melatonin cues for the development of rhythmicity. Consequently, preterm birth alters the developmental trajectory of circadian rhythms, with studies identifying that prematurity delays the development of melatonin rhythmicity in preterm infants aged between 23 and 34 weeks gestation age [33].

Effect of Fetal Growth Restriction

Fetus

In severe FGR, Doppler and behavioural studies have shown altered organization of behavioral states in the fetus. These alterations are thought to arise from either adaptive responses to placental insufficiency or cellular brain damage as a result of chronic hypoxia and/or malnutrition in human fetuses [34]. Compared to appropriately grown fetuses, FGR fetuses have reduced amounts of AS and increased amounts of QS and IS [34]. This re-organisation of sleep state architecture is thought to be an adaptive response to a hypoxic environment, as the brain shifts its time spent in a state with higher oxygen needs (AS) to one with lower oxidative needs (QS) [6, 7]. Differences in in utero development of sleep in FGR fetuses compared to appropriately grown fetuses have been confirmed in animal studies. Compared to appropriately-grown fetuses, chronically hypoxic sheep fetuses, had significantly lower amounts of low voltage/high frequency electrocortical activity (reflecting AS sleep) and the incidence and duration of sleep state transitions was altered. [35].

Preterm FGR Infants

The compounding effects of both preterm birth and FGR are known to effect both sleep state architecture and circadian rhythmicity in neonatal and post-neonatal periods. Within the immediate neonatal period, studies using power spectral analysis techniques have identified that FGR may affect EEG activity in preterm infants [36]. Single channel EEG studies revealed a higher amount of delta activity in FGR neonates compared to matched preterms born with appropriates birth weights [36]. In addition, FGR neonates had lower amounts of beta, alpha and theta power, however no differences in sleep state architecture were found between the two groups [36]. Beyond the neonatal period, Hoppenbrouwers et al. [32] showed that a delay in sleep state architecture is evident in preterm infants born growth restricted. In this study growth restricted infants (defined as <10th percentile for weight) had higher amounts of AS compared with age matched preterm infants with appropriate birth weights [32]. Interestingly the average duration of wakefulness, as well as the longest episode of wakefulness, was prolonged in infants born to smoking mothers. This interaction between smoking and sleep state percentages, however, disappeared in babies who were ventilated [32].

In regards to 24 h day/night patterning, Kenneway et al. studied the development of melatonin rhythmicity in preterm infants born growth restricted. Emergence of melatonin rhythmicity was studied between 46 and 55 weeks postconception by monitoring the excretion of the urinary melatonin metabolite 6-sulfatoxymelatonin. Levels of 6-sulfatoxymelatonin were 67% lower at night in preterm infants born growth restricted, showing the delay in circadian rhythmicity that occurs in preterm infants is exacerbated by FGR [33].

Long-Term Effects of Preterm Birth and FGR on Sleep

Effect of Preterm Birth

Based on subjective measures of sleep, results from face-face interview reveal that preterm children born <37 weeks gestation at age 10 ($N = 130$) had no differences in sleep duration, bed sharing, night awakenings, bed resistance and sleep onset difficulties compared to term born children [37]. In contrast, objective measures of sleep, including actigraphy and gold-standard polysomnography reveal different results. In a study in very preterm (<32 weeks gestation) children aged between 7 and 12 years, polysomnographic studies revealed that preterm children had earlier sleep onset times compared to term-born children, suggesting that very preterm children have an earlier sleep phase [38]. Sleep architecture in childhood was also altered with preterm children spending more time in N2 sleep, less time in N3 and more nocturnal awakenings [39].

In contrast, other studies have shown that sleep architecture is not altered by preterm birth in childhood, however rates of sleep disordered breathing are high along with periodic limb movements [40, 41]. In addition, studies based on questionnaire data, show adolescents born preterm have a higher propensity to morningness, again indicating advanced sleep phase compared to term-born individuals [42].

Effect of Fetal Growth Restriction

Few studies have investigated the long-term effect of FGR on sleep. Of the studies available, actigraphy and not gold standard polysomnography has been used to assess sleep patterns and quality. Consequently, a paucity of data on the long-term effect of FGR on sleep architecture exists. Actigraphy studies in children aged between 4 and 7 years, compared 26 term-born FGR to 47 term-born AGA children have been performed [43]. Compared to their appropriately grown peers, FGR children had reduced amounts of sleep and a higher percentage of children categorised as poor sleepers, defined by a lower sleep efficiency and more awakenings during the sleep period [43].

Adult studies investigating sleep/wake patterns indicate that very low birth weight (<1500 g) alters circadian rhythms. In adulthood, being born very low birth weight was associated with earlier rise times, with a wake up time 45 min earlier compared to term born controls, suggesting that preterm birth may permanently alter sleep by advancing sleep phase [44]. However, in the former study the global definition of "low birth weight" grouped FGR and preterm adults together and the full effects of FGR could not be discerned. Nonetheless, Kenneway et al. showed that low overnight melatonin excretion was associated with low birth weight and this effect amplified in adults that had a low ponderal index (where a low ponderal index reflects asymmetric FGR) and who were obese in adulthood [11].

Animal models in rats, using fetal protein restriction as a model of FGR, show that fetal undernutrition can result in long-term alterations of sleep in adulthood. Though the proportion of sleep states were not altered, increases in delta activity was observed in the FGR mice over a 24-h period [45]. Similarly, prenatally malnourished adult rats spent 20% more time in slow-wave sleep and 61% less in REM sleep compared to control adult rats when studied at 90–120 days of age [46].

In summary, both preterm birth and FGR alters the maturation of sleep. In the long-term, being born preterm leads to significant alterations in sleep architecture and circadian rhythms phase. In FGR fetuses, sleep state organization is significantly altered, perhaps as an adaptive response to preserve energy. Though studies in children and adults are lacking, in utero changes that occur due to FGR may program the fetus for lifelong alterations in sleep, particular impacting sleep quality in children and circadian phases in adulthood.

Future Research

Both preterm birth and FGR   alter the development of sleep. The exact mechanisms of how these permanent alterations are unknown. The combination of both chronic hypoxia and undernutrition in fetal life along with ex-utero development in an intensive care setting may play a role. In response to a hypoxic environment, reduced time spent in AS during fetal life could potentially effect brain maturation. AS is thought to play a significant role in the stimulation of central nervous system development in the fetus and the neonate [47]. In particular, animal studies indicate that muscle twitches during REM sleep are highly organised behaviours and induce specific cortical activity during sleep [48]. It is though that AS, in particular, provides endogenous stimulation to sensory processing areas in the central nervous system via fetal movements, breathing movements, sucking, swallowing, yawns, stretches and eye movements [49].

We also know that FGR has long-term effects on brain structure, in particular the hippocampus and the cerebellum [4]. EEG theta activity can be recorded from both the hippocampus and cortical regions and is prominent during REM sleep. Though the function of theta activity is unclear and difficult to study in humans, it has been proposed that theta activity during REM sleep plays a role in learning and memory consolidation [50]. However, whether or not theta activity is permanently altered by FGR in REM sleep remains unknown.

In children, sleep disruption and poor sleep quality are known to impair cognitive functioning, concentration, daytime alertness and overall behaviour [8]. NREM and REM sleep are known to be important for memory consolidation and neurological growth and repair [16]. It has been well established that infants born preterm and FGR go on to have neurodevelopmental and behavioural impairments. Few studies have investigated the inter-relationship between prematurity, sleep and neurodevelopmental impairment during childhood. One study showed, in toddlers born preterm with appropriate birth weights, those with sleep/wake patterns that closely aligned with the 24-h circadian cycle had higher abbreviated intelligence quotient scores at 3 years of age [51]. Additionally, at 6 years these children had a lower risk for illness-related medical visits [51]. To date, the relationship between poor sleep and neurodevelopment in children born preterm and FGR, has not been explored. Indeed, there is the potential that poor sleep could exacerbate neurodevelopmental deficits in this population.

Conclusions

Sleep undergoes marked maturational changes in fetal life and infancy. Stress to the fetus, as occurs with FGR, may disrupt this development. Consequently, altered sleep has been reported in children and adults born FGR. Future studies are required to determine the long-term impact of FGR on sleep, both in childhood and adulthood. In particular, a detailed investigation of circadian rhythms and sleep state architecture in combination with neurodevelopmental assessment in childhood may provide unique insight into the life-long outcomes of being born FGR.

References

1. Figueras F, Eixarch E, Gratacos E, Gardosi J. Predictiveness of antenatal umbilical artery Doppler for adverse pregnancy outcome in small-for-gestational-age babies according to customised birthweight centiles: population-based study. BJOG. 2008;115(5):590–4.
2. Bernstein IM, Horbar JD, Badger GJ, Ohlsson A, Golan A. Morbidity and mortality among very-low-birth-weight neonates with intrauterine growth restriction. The Vermont Oxford network. Am J Obstet Gynecol. 2000;182(1 Pt 1):198–206.
3. Tolsa CB, Zimine S, Warfield SK, Freschi M, Sancho Rossignol A, Lazeyras F, et al. Early alteration of structural and functional brain development in premature infants born with intrauterine growth restriction. Pediatr Res. 2004;56(1):132–8.
4. Padilla N, Falcon C, Sanz-Cortes M, Figueras F, Bargallo N, Crispi F, et al. Differential effects of intrauterine growth restriction on brain structure and development in preterm infants: a magnetic resonance imaging study. Brain Res. 2011;1382:98–108.
5. Barker DJ. In utero programming of chronic disease. Clin Sci. 1998;95(2):115–28.
6. Richardson BS, Carmichael L, Homan J, Gagnon R. Cerebral oxidative metabolism in lambs during perinatal period: relationship to electrocortical state. Am J Phys. 1989;257(5 Pt 2):R1251–7.
7. Richardson GS, Moore-Ede MC, Czeisler CA, Dement WC. Circadian rhythms of sleep and wakefulness in mice: analysis using long-term automated recording of sleep. Am J Phys. 1985;248(3 Pt 2):R320–30.
8. Sadeh A. Consequences of sleep loss or sleep disruption in children. Sleep Med Clin. 2007;2(3):513–20.
9. Barker DJ, Osmond C, Golding J, Kuh D, Wadsworth ME. Growth in utero, blood pressure in childhood and adult life, and mortality from cardiovascular disease. BMJ. 1989;298(6673):564–7.
10. Ojeda NB, Grigore D, Alexander BT. Intrauterine growth restriction: fetal programming of hypertension and kidney disease. Adv Chronic Kidney Dis. 2008;15(2):101–6.
11. Kennaway DJ, Flanagan DE, Moore VM, Cockington RA, Robinson JS, Phillips DI. The impact of fetal size and length of gestation on 6-sulphatoxymelatonin excretion in adult life. J Pineal Res. 2001;30(3):188–92.
12. Weisman O, Magori-Cohen R, Louzoun Y, Eidelman AI, Feldman R. Sleep-wake transitions in premature neonates predict early development. Pediatrics. 2011;128(4):706–14.
13. Mindell JA, Owens JA. A clinical guide to sleep: diagnosis and management of sleep problems. 2nd ed. Philadelphia: Lippincott Williams & Wilkins; 2010. 27 p.
14. Everson CA. Sustained sleep deprivation impairs host defense. Am J Phys. 1993;265(5 Pt 2):R1148–54.
15. Sheldon SH, Ferber R, Kryger MH, Gozal D. Principles and practice of pediatric sleep medicine. 2nd ed. Chicago: Elsevier; 2014.
16. Davis KF, Parker KP, Montgomery GL. Sleep in infants and young children: part one: normal sleep. J Pediatr Health Care. 2004;18(2):65–71.
17. Krueger JM, Frank MG, Wisor JP, Roy S. Sleep function: toward elucidating an enigma. Sleep Med Rev. 2016;28:46–54.
18. Yang G, Lai CS, Cichon J, Ma L, Li W, Gan WB. Sleep promotes branch-specific formation of dendritic spines after learning. Science. 2014;344(6188):1173–8.
19. Dreyfus-Brisac C. Sleep ontogenesis in early human prematurity from 24 to 27 weeks of conceptional age. Dev Psychobiol. 1968;1(3):162–9.
20. Groome LJ, Singh KP, Bentz LS, Holland SB, Atterbury JL, Swiber MJ, et al. Temporal stability in the distribution of behavioral states for individual human fetuses. Early Hum Dev. 1997;48(1–2):187–97.
21. Mirmiran M, Maas YG, Ariagno RL. Development of fetal and neonatal sleep and circadian rhythms. Sleep Med Rev. 2003;7(4):321–34.
22. Kennaway DJ. Programming of the fetal suprachiasmatic nucleus and subsequent adult rhythmicity. Trends Endocrinol Metab. 2002;13(9):398–402.
23. Mirmiran M, Lunshof S. Perinatal development of human circadian rhythms. Prog Brain Res. 1996;111:217–26.
24. Zemdegs IZ, McMillen IC, Walker DW, Thorburn GD, Nowak R. Diurnal rhythms in plasma melatonin concentrations in the fetal sheep and pregnant ewe during late gestation. Endocrinology. 1988;123(1):284–9.
25. Comai S, Ochoa-Sanchez R, Gobbi G. Sleep-wake characterization of double MT(1)/MT(2) receptor knockout mice and comparison with MT(1) and MT(2) receptor knockout mice. Behav Brain Res. 2013;243:231–8.
26. Anders T, Sadeh A, Appareddy V. In: Kryger M, Roth T, Dement W, editors. Principles and practice of sleep medicine. Philadelphia: Elsevier Saunders; 1995. 169–84 p.
27. Sheldon S, Spire J, Levy H. Normal sleep in children and young adults. Paediatric sleep medicine. Philadelphia: WB Saunders Company; 1992. p. 14–27.
28. Curzi-Dascalova L, Challamel M. Neurophysiological basis of sleep development. In: Loughlin G, Carroll J, Marcus C, editors. Sleep and breathing in children. New York: Marcal Dekker; 2000. p. 3–37.

29. Swaab DF, Hofman MA, Honnebier MB. Development of vasopressin neurons in the human suprachiasmatic nucleus in relation to birth. Brain Res Dev Brain Res. 1990;52(1–2):289–93.
30. Kennaway DJ, Stamp GE, Goble FC. Development of melatonin production in infants and the impact of prematurity. J Clin Endocrinol Metab. 1992;75(2):367–9.
31. Parmelee A, Stern E. Development of states in infants. In: Clemente C, Purpura D, Mayer F, editors. Sleep and the maturing nervous system. New York: Academic; 1972. p. 199–228.
32. Hoppenbrouwers T, Hodgman JE, Rybine D, Fabrikant G, Corwin M, Crowell D, et al. Sleep architecture in term and preterm infants beyond the neonatal period: the influence of gestational age, steroids, and ventilatory support. Sleep. 2005;28(11):1428–36.
33. Kennaway DJ, Goble FC, Stamp GE. Factors influencing the development of melatonin rhythmicity in humans. J Clin Endocrinol Metab. 1996;81(4):1525–32.
34. Gazzolo D, Visser GH, Santi F, Magliano CP, Scopesi F, Russo A, et al. Behavioural development and Doppler velocimetry in relation to perinatal outcome in small for dates fetuses. Early Hum Dev. 1995;43(2):185–95.
35. Keen AE, Frasch MG, Sheehan MA, Matushewski B, Richardson BS. Maturational changes and effects of chronic hypoxemia on electrocortical activity in the ovine fetus. Brain Res. 2011;1402:38–45.
36. Yerushalmy-Feler A, Marom R, Peylan T, Korn A, Haham A, Mandel D, et al. Electroencephalographic characteristics in preterm infants born with intrauterine growth restriction. J Pediatr. 2014;164(4):756–61. e1
37. Iglowstein I, Latal Hajnal B, Molinari L, Largo RH, Jenni OG. Sleep behaviour in preterm children from birth to age 10 years: a longitudinal study. Acta Paediatr. 2006;95(12):1691–3.
38. Maurer N, Perkinson-Gloor N, Stalder T, Hagmann-von Arx P, Brand S, Holsboer-Trachsler E, et al. Salivary and hair glucocorticoids and sleep in very preterm children during school age. Psychoneuroendocrinology. 2016;72:166–74.
39. Perkinson-Gloor N, Hagmann-von Arx P, Brand S, Holsboer-Trachsler E, Grob A, Weber P, et al. The role of sleep and the hypothalamic-pituitary-adrenal axis for behavioral and emotional problems in very preterm children during middle childhood. J Psychiatr Res. 2015;60:141–7.
40. Marcus CL, Meltzer LJ, Roberts RS, Traylor J, Dix J, D'Ilario J, et al. Long-term effects of caffeine therapy for apnea of prematurity on sleep at school age. Am J Respir Crit Care Med. 2014;190(7):791–9.
41. Raynes-Greenow CH, Hadfield RM, Cistulli PA, Bowen J, Allen H, Roberts CL. Sleep apnea in early childhood associated with preterm birth but not small for gestational age: a population-based record linkage study. Sleep. 2012;35(11):1475–80.
42. Natale V, Sansavini A, Trombini E, Esposito MJ, Alessandroni R, Faldella G. Relationship between preterm birth and circadian typology in adolescence. Neurosci Lett. 2005;382(1–2):139–42.
43. Leitner Y, Bloch AM, Sadeh A, Neuderfer O, Tikotzky L, Fattal-Valevski A, et al. Sleep-wake patterns in children with intrauterine growth retardation. J Child Neurol. 2002;17(12):872–6.
44. Bjorkqvist J, Paavonen J, Andersson S, Pesonen AK, Lahti J, Heinonen K, et al. Advanced sleep-wake rhythm in adults born prematurely: confirmation by actigraphy-based assessment in the Helsinki study of very low birth weight adults. Sleep Med. 2014;15(9):1101–6.
45. Shimizu N, Chikahisa S, Nishi Y, Harada S, Iwaki Y, Fujihara H, et al. Maternal dietary restriction alters offspring's sleep homeostasis. PLoS One. 2013;8(5):e64263.
46. Datta S, Patterson EH, Vincitore M, Tonkiss J, Morgane PJ, Galler JR. Prenatal protein malnourished rats show changes in sleep/wake behavior as adults. J Sleep Res. 2000;9(1):71–9.
47. Roffwarg HP, Muzio JN, Dement WC. Ontogenetic development of the human sleep-dream cycle. Science. 1966;152(3722):604–19.
48. Kurth S, Olini N, Huber R, LeBourgeois M. Sleep and early cortical development. Curr Sleep Med Rep. 2015;1(1):64–73.
49. Peirano P, Algarin C, Uauy R. Sleep-wake states and their regulatory mechanisms throughout early human development. J Pediatr. 2003;143(4 Suppl):S70–9.
50. Montgomery SM, Sirota A, Buzsaki G. Theta and gamma coordination of hippocampal networks during waking and rapid eye movement sleep. J Neurosci. 2008;28(26):6731–41.
51. Schwichtenberg AJ, Christ S, Abel E, Poehlmann-Tynan JA. Circadian sleep patterns in toddlers born preterm: longitudinal associations with developmental and health concerns. J Dev Behav Pediatr. 2016;37(5):358–69.

Part VII
Mechanisms of Programming

Chapter 36
Biomarkers of Abnormal Birth Weight in Pregnancy

Beata Anna Raczkowska, Monika Zbucka-Kretowska, Adam Kretowski,
and Michal Ciborowski

Key Points

- Abnormal birth weight is a risk factor for several diseases in adulthood including cancer, cardiovascular disease, diabetes, overweight or mental disorders.
- "Omics" techniques are powerful tools in the quest for biomarkers.
- The following genes have been linked with abnormal birth weight: IGF-I, IGF-II, ADCY5, CDKAL1, ADRB1, HMGA2, LCORL, CMPXM2, CLDN1, TXNDC5, LRP2, PHLDB2, LEP, and GCH1.
- The following proteins have been proposed as abnormal birth weight biomarkers: IL-8, TNF-alpha, IFN-gamma, IL-10, alpha fetoprotein, free beta hCG, PAPP-A, MMP-9, VEGF, endothelin peptides, and A-FABP.
- Phospholipids, monoglycerides and vitamin D3 metabolites have been found as potential metabolic biomarkers of abnormal birth weight.

Keywords Low birth weight • High birth weight • Biomarkers • Omics • Genomics • Transcriptomics • Proteomics • Metabolomics

Abbreviations

11B-HSD-2	Hydroxysteroid (11-beta) dehydrogenase 2
2D-DIGE	Two-dimensional difference gel electrophoresis
A-FABP	Adipocyte fatty acid-binding protein
ADCY5	Adenylate cyclase 5

B.A. Raczkowska, MSc
Department of Endocrinology, Diabetology and Internal Medicine, Medical University of Bialystok, Bialystok, Poland
e-mail: beata-anna.raczkowska@umb.edu.pl

M. Zbucka-Kretowska, MD, PhD
Department of Reproduction and Gynecological Endocrinology, Medical University of Bialystok, Bialystok, Poland

A. Kretowski, MD, PhD • M. Ciborowski, PhD (✉)
Clinical Research Centre, Medical University of Bialystok, Bialystok, Poland
e-mail: michal.ciborowski@umb.edu.pl

© Springer International Publishing AG 2017
R. Rajendram et al. (eds.), *Diet, Nutrition, and Fetal Programming*,
Nutrition and Health, DOI 10.1007/978-3-319-60289-9_36

ADRB1   Adrenoceptor beta 1
BCL6   B-cell CLL/lymphoma 6
beta-hCG   Beta-human chorionic gonadotropin
CDK19   Cyclin-dependent kinase 19
CDKAL1   Cyclin-dependent kinase 5 regulatory subunit associated protein 1-like 1
CE   Capillary electrophoresis
CLDN1   Claudin-1
CNVs   Copy number variations
CPXM2   Carboxypeptidase X 2 (M14 family)
CRP   C-reactive protein
DNA   Deoxyribonucleic acid
ENG   Endoglin
ESI-LC-MS/MS   Electrospray ionization-liquid chromatography-tandem mass spectrometry
FLNB   Filamin B
FLT1   fms-related tyrosine kinase 1
FSTL3   Follistatin-like 3
GC   Gas chromatography
GCH1   Guanosine-5′-triphosphate cyclohydrolase 1
GDM   Gestational diabetes mellitus
HBW   High birth weight
HMGA2   High mobility group AT-hook 2
hPGH   Human placental growth hormones
ICAM-1   Intercellular adhesion molecule 1
IFN-gamma   Interferon gamma
IGF-I   Insulin-like growth factor I
IGF-II   Insulin-like growth factor II
IGFBP-1   Insulin-like growth factor-binding protein 1
IGFBP-3   Insulin-like growth factor-binding protein 3
IHD   Ischaemic heart disease
IL-8   Interleukin 8
IL-10   Interleukin 10
INHA   Inhibin alpha subunit
INHBA   Inhibin beta A subunit
IUGR   Intrauterine growth restriction
KCNQ1   Potassium voltage-gated channel subfamily Q member 1
LBW   Low birth weight
LC   Liquid chromatography
LC-MS   Liquid chromatography-mass spectrometry
LCORL   Ligand-dependent nuclear receptor corepressor-like
LEP   Leptin
LGA   Large for gestational age
LRP2   Low-density lipoprotein receptor-related protein 2
LYN   Proto-oncogene, Src family tyrosine kinase
MALDI-TOF   Matrix-assisted laser desorption/ionization-time-of-flight
MMP-1   Matrix metalloproteinase-1
MMP-9   Matrix metalloproteinase-9
MMPs   Matrix metalloproteinases
MS   Mass spectrometry
NDRG1   N-myc downstream regulated 1
NFIA   Nuclear factor I/A
NGS   Next-generation sequencing

NMR	Nuclear magnetic resonance
PAPP-A	Pregnancy-associated plasma protein A
PE	Preeclampsia
PHLDA2	Pleckstrin homology-like domain family A member 2
PHLDB2	Pleckstrin homology-like domain family B member 2
PlGF	Placental growth factor
PROCR	Protein C receptor
PTMs	Post-translational modifications
QSOX	Putative quiescin sulfhydryl oxidase
RNA	Ribonucleic acid
SDS-PAGE	Sodium dodecyl sulphate-polyacrylamide gel electrophoresis
SELDI-TOF	Surface-enhanced laser desorption/ionization-time-of-flight
SGA	Small for gestational age
SMG8	Nonsense-mediated mRNA decay factor
SNA	*Sambucus nigra* agglutinin
SNPs	Single nucleotide polymorphisms
TNF-alpha	Tumour necrosis factor alpha-like
TPBG	Trophoblast glycoprotein
TXNDC5	Thioredoxin domain-containing protein 5
VCAM-1	Vascular cell adhesion molecule 1
VEGF-A	Vascular endothelial growth factor A
VLBW	Very low birth weight
WHO	World Health Organization
XBP1	X-box binding protein 1
ZNF127	Zinc finger protein 127

Introduction

According to the World Health Organization (WHO), biomarkers are defined as "almost any measurement reflecting an interaction between a biological system and a potential hazard, which may be chemical, physical, or biological. The measured response may be functional and physiological, biochemical at the cellular level, or a molecular interaction" [1]. Finding parameters that could (at early stage of gestation) indicate which pregnant women are at risk to deliver an infant with birth weight higher or lower than assumed acceptable range would allow modification of the pregnancy management to optimise foetal growth and achieve desired birth weight [2]. Moreover, knowledge about the biochemical components and processes related to abnormal birth weight may indicate nutrition, lifestyle or pharmacology-related solutions that can be introduced to prevent delivery of abnormal birth weight neonate.

Regarding birth weight, the normal range is between 2500 and 4000 g [3]. A normal birth weight is one of the factors indicating a proper foetus development. Different genetic and environmental factors may alter the foetus growth affecting birth weight, what may have the long-term effects on human health. Such lasting changes in the biological functions and structures during the foetal and early infancy development, induced by distinct factors and affecting individual health later in life, are called the foetal programming [4]. This concept was introduced almost 30 years ago by Barker et al. who reported an association between low birth weight and increased risk of ischaemic heart disease (IHD) in adulthood and increased incidence of death from IHD [5]. Nowadays the evidence of foetal programming concept is clear as researchers have developed numerous studies reporting the impact of early life to disease development in adulthood [6–12]. One of the most important assumptions regarding foetal programming is the thrifty phenotype hypothesis. The idea is based on the association between aetiology of type 2 diabetes and poor nutrition during the prenatal and postnatal development [4]. It suggests that malnutrition during the foetal and early infancy causes lasting changes in glucose and insulin metabolism reflected by poor foetal and infant growth and subsequent development of type 2 diabetes in adulthood [13]. Inappropriate organ development in LBW infants may be responsible for future diabetes, as dysfunction of multiple organs (i.e. liver, pancreas, gut, muscle, adipose tissue, kidney and brain) is involved in the process of glucose intolerance, prediabetes and finally type 2 diabetes development [8]. The association between the low birth weight and risk of type 2 diabetes, impaired insulin secretion and insulin resistance in adulthood are considered as predominantly non-genetic. Nevertheless, poor nutrition causes modifications in foetal development which may comprise postnatal survival, particularly in challenging environmental conditions.

Increasing evidence suggest that low birth weight is associated with an increased risk of adult disease. LBW may lead to hypercholesterolemia, development of endothelial dysfunction and atherosclerotic process at a young age or higher blood pressure in adulthood [6]. Furthermore, a meta-regression analysis performed on data from 27 studies indicates association between LBW and adult depression [7]. A potential contribution of very low birth weight (VLBW), below 1500 g, to childhood cancer was examined by unconditional logistic regression performed based on combined case-control datasets of the cancer and birth registries of California, Minnesota, New York, Texas and Washington states. The dataset comprised of 17,672 children up to 14 years old who were diagnosed with cancer and 57,966 randomly selected controls. The data indicate that VLBW is a strong risk factor for hepatoblastoma development in childhood and moderate risk factor for other gliomas and retinoblastoma [9]. Based on the prospective analysis of 193,306 children (born from 1936 to 1972) registered in the Copenhagen School Health Record, it was established that LBW is associated with a decreased risk for colon cancer, while HBW is associated with an increased risk for colon cancer and decreased risk for rectal cancer [14]. In another report the effect of prenatal development on hearing, vision and cognition in adulthood was investigated. The study was performed based on UK biobank data, and depending on the studied factor, different numbers of participants completed each measure. The results indicate that participants with the smallest and the largest birth weights had significantly poorer function than others [15]. High birth weight (HBW) carries also an increased risk for several diseases in adulthood. Gillman et al. analysed combined results from two cohort studies (one included nurses and other their children) to evaluate the association between birth weight and adolescent BMI. Based on the analysis of data from 14,881 participants, it was concluded that HBW increases a risk of overweight in adolescence [10]. Another population-based study was conducted in a group of 15,600 children aged from 3 to 6 years. The purpose of this study was to determine whether association between high birth weight and hypertension exists. Obtained results indicated that HBW or postnatal weight gain is associated with childhood hypertension [11]. Several studies have shown a positive association between HBW and cancer. HBW has been reported as a risk factor for childhood leukaemia and astrocytoma, as well as breast, prostate, endometrial and colon cancer in adulthood [12]. Moreover, HBW is associated with difficult labour and delivery. Birthweight of a child greater than 4000 g is the indication for operative birth or caesarean section. Caesarean delivery places also the mother at a higher risk for blood transfusion, infections, hysterectomy or even death [16]. Also that large baby can suffer during a vaginal delivery. A child is at risk of fractures, trauma, shoulder dystocia and brachial plexus injury [17]. Interestingly, the birth weight may also influence the mother's future life. Based on the data from Framingham Offspring Birth History Study, it was shown that "giving birth to an infant with high birth weight was associated with increased breast cancer risk in later life, independently of mother's own birth weight and breast cancer risk factors" [18]. In case of a VLBW child, maternal anxiety may compromise lactation [19]. Lactation may also be perturbed by caesarean delivery, due to reported differences in oxytocin and prolactin when comparing maternal levels between those delivering via caesarean section and vaginally. Consequently, caesarean delivery may affect early breastfeeding [20]. Health consequences of abnormal birth weight for mother and offspring are presented in Table 36.1.

Table 36.1   Health **consequences** of abnormal birth weight for mother and **offspring**

	Consequences	Ref.
Very low birth weight	**Maternal**	
	Maternal anxiety may compromise lactation	[19]
	Offspring	
	Strong risk of hepatoblastoma and moderate risk of retinoblastoma and other gliomas in childhood	[9]
Low birth weight	**Offspring**	
	Cardiovascular disease, hypercholesterolemia, development of endothelial dysfunction and atherosclerotic process in adolescence or higher blood pressure in adulthood	[5, 6]
	Increased risk of type 2 diabetes in adulthood	[13]
	Increased risk of depression in adulthood	[7]
	Deterioration of hearing, vision and cognition in adulthood	[15]
	Decreased risk of colon cancer	[14]
High birth weight	**Maternal**	
	Difficult labour and delivery/caesarean delivery – higher risk for blood transfusion, infections, hysterectomy, death for mother and lactation disorders	[16]
	Increased risk of breast cancer	[18]
	Offspring	
	Deterioration of hearing, vision and cognition in adulthood	[15]
	Increased risk of fractures, trauma, shoulder dystocia and brachial plexus injury for the child during delivery	[17]
	Increased risk of leukaemia and astrocytoma in childhood	[12]
	Increased risk of breast, prostate, endometrial and colon cancer in adulthood	[12]
	Increased risk of hypertension in childhood	[11]
	Increased risk of overweight in adolescence	[10]
	Increased risk of colon cancer and decreased risk of rectal cancer	[14]

The table presents the reported consequences for mother and offspring's health in childhood, adolescence and adulthood resulting from high or low birth weight in pregnancy

Birthweight and foetal development may be affected by maternal health. One of the main factors leading to macrosomia – defined as an excessive birth weight – is maternal obesity or immoderate weight gain during the pregnancy [21]. In a Danish study, the effect of maternal weight gain on birth weight was investigated. It was found that the risk of birth weight <3000 g is increased when maternal weight gain is below recommended level and the risk of birthweight >4000 is almost twice higher when the women gained more than what was recommended [22]. Macrosomia is also characteristic to mothers who are diabetic before pregnancy or develop gestational diabetes mellitus (GDM). Infants born to GDM mother have significantly higher percentage of body fat than infants born to lean women [21]. On the other hand, maternal underweight and mentioned low weight gain during pregnancy are risk factors for LBW [22]. Another maternal factors contributing to LBW are placental pathology [23], hypertension and preeclampsia (PE) [24] or exposure to social stress during pregnancy [25]. LBW or small for gestational age (SGA) may also appear as a consequence of heterogeneous syndrome associated with multiple factors like hypertensive disorders, smoking, infection, undernutrition or unexplained factors, generally named as intrauterine growth restriction (IUGR) [26]. Risk factors for abnormal birth weight are presented in Table 36.2.

Table 36.2 Causes of LBW and HBW

	Causes	Ref.
Low birth weight	Hypertension	[24]
	Placenta and vascular abnormalities	[23]
	Foetal infections (toxoplasmosis, rubella, HIV, parvovirus 19)	[26]
	Genetic abnormalities	[42]
	Underweight/low weight gain during pregnancy	[22]
	Social stress	[25]
High birth weight	Maternal obesity/immoderate weight gain during pregnancy	[21]
	GDM	

The table presents maternal diseases and other conditions which predispose pregnant women to deliver high or low birth weight child

Technologies for the Discovery of Biomarkers

The above-mentioned data indicate the importance of searching for biomarkers of abnormal birth weight. A huge development of biomarker discovery field was possible thanks to the development of high-throughput analytical methods which allow for rapid and accurate measurement of multiple parameters [27]. Over the last three decades, we can observe an immense development of large-scale technologies among which the four major ones are genomics, transcriptomics, proteomics and metabolomics (Fig. 36.1). "Omics" suffix refers to a large-scale approach applied to study the complete set of deoxyribonucleic acid (DNA) molecules, ribonucleic acid (RNA) transcripts, proteins and metabolites, respectively. The term "genomics" was first proposed by geneticist Thomas H. Roderick in 1986 as the name of a new scientific journal devoted to the research on sequencing, gene mapping and new technologies in genetics [28]. Since that time, genomics has begun the new epoch of considering the particular biological systems at different levels (e.g. genome) as a whole. Then, in 1995, Wilkins et al. and Wasinger et al. published the first papers using the term proteomics and described both methods of global protein detection as well as the data analysis [29–31]. Finally in 1999, Jeremy K. Nicholson defined metabonomics as "the quantitative measurement of the dynamic multiparametric metabolic response of living systems to pathophysiological stimuli or genetic modification" [32]. Two years later Oliver Fiehn devoted his paper to describe metabolomics and different approaches used in this field [33]. Even though initially terms metabonomics and metabolomics referred to slightly different approaches in metabolite analyses, nowadays these two terms are used interchangeably. In order to analyse the biological samples in the most comprehensive manner, omics technologies require the usage of sophisticated tools that are characterized by high resolution, sensitivity and reproducibility. Furthermore it is crucial to design experiments carefully, starting with proper biobanking of the biological materials, followed by accurate sample treatment, choosing a proper analytical platform and finally by performing appropriate data filtering together with statistical and bioinformatics analyses. The revolutionary technology used nowadays in genomics and transcriptomics is called next-generation sequencing (NGS). This high-throughput technology allows for rapid and deep analyses of huge amount of data which has to be then analysed using different bioinformatics tools. NGS has many applications in genomics (e.g. copy number variations (CNVs), single nucleotide polymorphisms (SNPs)) and transcriptomics (e.g. gene expression, microRNA profiling, splicing variants). It permits searching for specific DNA methylation and histone modifications responsible for the epigenetic regulation [34]. Proteins are the effector molecules of cell functions and therefore play a key role in determining the phenotype. Two main proteomics approaches exist, termed "top-down" and "bottom-up" proteomics. The main advantage of top-down proteomics is a possibility to obtain protein sequences and detection of post-translational modifications (PTMs); however it has got also many limitations such as sensitivity or limited availability of bioinformatics tools [35]. On the contrary, the

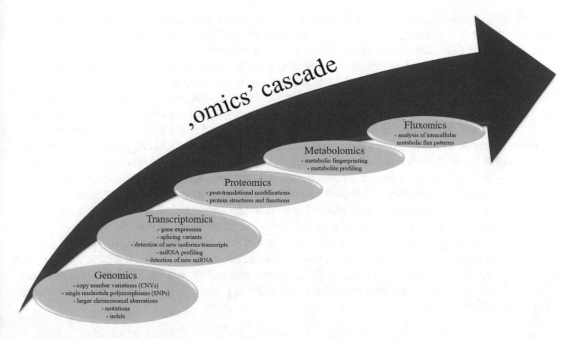

Fig. 36.1 The "omics" cascade. Particular "omics" technique has different approaches to sample analysis. In the field of biomarkers research, a global analysis is used mostly in discovery phase, whereas a target analysis is utilized for validation of potential biomarkers. Fluxomics is a powerful tool to study biochemical pathways

bottom-up proteomics is more mature and more often used. Its main application is the protein identification and quantification. In proteomics the most commonly used technique for biomarker discovery is mass spectrometry (MS). Before analysis in MS, the proteins have to be first digested. In this regard, there are two main strategies which are in-solution digestion using trypsin as a proteolytic enzyme or SDS-PAGE (sodium dodecyl sulphate – polyacrylamide gel electrophoresis) followed by in-gel digestion. Finally the resulting peptide mixture is separated using the liquid chromatography (LC), and the obtained spectra are identified using the available databases. Protein quantification might be performed using stable isotope labelling or label-free approach [36, 37]. Among all of the omics technologies, metabolomics represents the actual biological outcome most strongly as it is the last in the cascade of omics and most sensitive in terms of the phenotype response to genetic or external factors [38]. The two major techniques used in metabolomics are nuclear magnetic resonance (NMR) and mass spectrometry. The samples that are analysed with NMR do not require any previous treatment, whereas sample treatment for MS analysis depends on the separation technique which is coupled to MS, i.e. liquid chromatography, gas chromatography (GC) and capillary electrophoresis (CE). Taking into account that each separation technique allows for detection of different classes of compounds to increase the metabolites coverage, it is crucial to use all of the available analytical platforms, if feasible. After completing the run in equipment, the raw data have to be first reprocessed and aligned, followed by the data treatment including normalization, filtering and statistical analyses [39]. Identification of the obtained significant features can be done at different confidence levels using the existing spectral databases and eventually chemical reference standards (in order to confirm the metabolite assignment) [40]. Once metabolites are identified and assigned to the biochemical pathways, they can serve as the potential diagnostic biomarkers of a particular disease or condition. Application of metabolomics in biomarker discovery can give the information about the pathomechanisms underlying diseases and can improve their diagnosis or even predict the short- and long-term consequences. Each particular omics approach can bring the novel information about the biological processes at different levels independently. However integration of high-throughput experimental and computational technologies from the field of genomics, transcriptomics, proteomics and metabolomics allows for comprehensive analysis of the system biology. This is a holistic approach which seeks to obtain a complex information about the human or animal biology. Recent advances in the omics field provide insight into the molecular mechanisms of different diseases and conditions, with precise and complex information about the interactions between genetic and environmental factors. System biology holds a great potential in elucidating the risk of disease devolvement, individual susceptibility, predicting the response to drugs, etc. In this regard, large-scale technologies lead to the development of personalized medicine and thus enable to progress with the targeted drug therapies for patients. Nevertheless integrating the omics data in the context of system biology is an emerging field. Hence novel techniques for acquiring and analysis of the data obtained through the research of genome, transcriptome, proteome and metabolome are still evolving. Among all components of systems biology, epigenetics plays an important role in the foetal programming. It regulates the gene expression via DNA methylation and histone modifications without changing the underlying DNA sequence. Despite the fact that epigenetics modifications regulate the physiological development, they can also be induced in response to several environmental factors (e.g. diet, drugs) [41]. Epigenetics together with genomics, transcriptomics, proteomics and metabolomics studies is a powerful tool able to provide the knowledge about the molecular networks that are responsible for metabolic programming at different stages of prenatal and postnatal life, having also a potential to discover biomarkers of abnormal birth weight.

Biomarkers of Abnormal Birth Weight

Until now, "omics" techniques were used in several studies to search for biomarkers of abnormal birth weight. Genetic background cannot be omitted while considering factors influencing a birth weight. Based on the epidemiological studies, it was estimated that genetic factor may be responsible for birth weight in up to 80%. In humans, several genes were found to be related to birth weight. A defect in the insulin-like growth factor (IGF-I) gene was found in small-for-gestational-age subjects. Moreover another insulin-related genes (e.g. insulin receptor, insulin receptor substrates 1 and 2 or IGF-II) were found critical for normal foetal growth [42, 43]. Furthermore, based on the study of almost 70,000 individuals, additional loci responsible for birth weight were discovered. Some of them were previously known as related to type 2 diabetes (ADCY5 and CDKAL1), adult blood pressure (ADRB1) and adult height (HMGA2 and LCORL) [44]. Measurement of placental gene expression in pregnancies with growth dysfunction revealed upregulation of CPXM2 and CLDN1 and downregulation of TXNDC5 and LRP2 genes in case of foetal growth restriction. In case of macrosomia, PHLDB2 and CLDN1 genes were upregulated while LEP and GCH1 downregulated [45]. A recent study has found that placental 11B-hydroxysteroid dehydrogenase type 2 (11B-HSD-2) mRNA is a potential placental biomarker of foetal smallness [46]. Regarding proteomics markers, a shotgun plasma proteomics approach was used to evaluate maternal biochemical pathways regulating infant birth weight. The results show that in the third trimester, plasma of mothers who will later deliver low birth weight infants was richer in several pro-inflammatory cytokines (IL-8, TNF-alpha and IFN-gamma), while the anti-inflammatory cytokine IL-10 was decreased. Moreover, matrix metalloproteinases (MMPs) were upregulated in mothers with low birth weight infants [47]. In a different study, serum alpha fetoprotein (msAFP), free β-hCG and pregnancy-associated plasma protein A (PAPP-A) were retrospectively evaluated as potential biomarkers for adverse pregnancy outcomes. Combination of all three proteins was found predictive for pre-term delivery and LBW [48]. Recently published paper demonstrates the use of the multiplex protein array assay targeting vascular endothelial growth factor (VEGF-A), acute phase proteins C-reactive protein (CRP), soluble intracellular adhesion molecule (ICAM-1), soluble vascular cell adhesion molecule (VCAM-1) and matrix metalloproteinases

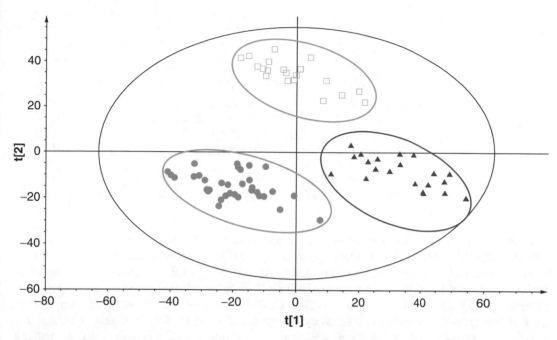

Fig. 36.2 Classification of pregnant women according to neonate's birth weight based on serum metabolic fingerprints. Partial least square discriminant analysis (PLS-DA) score plot generated based on the data obtained by serum LC-QTOF-MS fingerprinting analysis in positive ion mode [3]. Colours indicate neonate's birth weight: normal (*green*), high (*red*) and low (*blue*)

(MMPs) to evaluate biomarkers of adverse birth outcome including abnormal birth weight. In this study MMP-9 and VEGF proteins, endothelin peptides and 8-isoprostane were proposed as markers associated with birth weight [49]. An adipocyte fatty acid-binding protein (A-FABP) is one of the proteins in maternal serum that was found to be related to neonate's birth weight. The hypothesis linking this protein with birth weight has originated from a metabolomics research. Based on serum metabolic fingerprinting, several metabolites (phospholipids, monoglycerides and vitamin D3 metabolites) were found correlated with birth weight. Detected lipids were diminished in the serum of mothers who delivered large neonates, while A-FABP was found negatively correlated with the level of serum lipids and directly related to the birth weight of the future neonate [3]. Multivariate model showing classification of pregnant women according to neonate's birth weight based on the serum metabolic fingerprint is presented in Fig. 36.2. Currently reported molecular biomarkers which enable to predict abnormal birth weight are presented in Table 36.3.

Biomarkers for Maternal Diseases Influencing Birth Weight

As already mentioned there are several maternal conditions which influence birth weight. Some of them (e.g. GDM, preeclampsia or IUGR) may develop in the course of pregnancy; therefore finding biomarkers that can predict their development may help to assure a normal birth weight. Genetic background of GDM is partly similar to those predisposing to type 2 diabetes. Polymorphisms in genes such as TCF7L2, CDKAL1 and KCNQ1 may increase the risk of GDM [50]. Maternal plasma microRNA has also a potential to predict gestational diabetes. Five miRNAs (hsa-miR-16-5p, hsa-miR-17-5p, hsa-miR-19a-3p, hsa-miR-19b-3p, hsa-miR-20a-5p) differentially expressed in GDM are potential non-invasive biomarkers [51]. Proteomics biomarkers of GDM have been reviewed by Singh

Table 36.3 Different types of abnormal birth weight molecular biomarkers

Type of biomarker	Biomarker	Ref.
Genes	IGF-I, IGF-II	[42, 43]
	ADCY5, CDKAL1, ADRB1, HMGA2, LCORL	[44]
	CMPXM2, CLDN1, TXNDC5, LRP2, PHLDB2, LEP, GCH1	[45]
Transcripts	11B-HSD-2	[46]
Proteins	IL-8, TNF-alpha, IFN-gamma, IL-10, MMPs	[47]
	Alpha fetoprotein, free beta hCG, PAPP-A	[48]
	MMP-9, VEGF, endothelin peptides	[49]
	A-FABP	[3]
Metabolites	Phospholipids, monoglycerides, vitamin D3 metabolites	[3]

The table shows potential prognostic biomarkers of abnormal birth weight at different molecular levels, i.e. genes, transcripts, proteins and metabolites

et al. Several proteomics techniques were used in the quest for GDM protein biomarker including two-dimensional difference gel electrophoresis (2D-DIGE), matrix-assisted laser desorption/ionization-time-of-flight-mass spectrometry (MALDI-TOF-MS), surface-enhanced laser desorption/ionization-time-of-flight-mass spectrometry (SELDI-TOF-MS) and the electrospray ionization-liquid chromatography-tandem mass spectrometry (ESI-LC-MS/MS) techniques. By use of these approaches, the following protein biomarkers for GDM were proposed: fibronectin-SNA, clusterin, apolipoprotein CII, fibrinogen alpha chain precursor, haptoglobin, protein SMG8, apoptosis-inducing factor and others [52]. Metabolomics has also been used to search for GDM biomarkers. In one of the studies, serum fingerprints of GDM patients were compared with controls showing differences in lysophospholipids, taurine-bile acids and long-chain polyunsaturated fatty acid derivatives [53]. However in this study, women with already developed GDM were compared to controls. Consequently, significant metabolites can be considered as GDM biomarkers, but their ability for GDM prediction requires further investigations. Attempts to find prognostic biomarkers of gestational diabetes have been made in another metabolomics study. By use of NMR-based plasma metabolomics, Pinto et al. have found that glucose, amino acids, betaine, urea, creatine, cholesterol as well as plasma lipoproteins, fatty acids, triglycerides and metabolites related to gut microflora are potential prognostic biomarkers of GDM [54]. Preeclampsia may also have a genetic background. Currently multiple genes (FLT1, LEP, INHA, ENG, PROCR, MMP1, XBP1, FSTL3 as well as FLNB, INHBA, BCL6, TPBG, NDRG1, LYN and QSOX) were found predisposing to preeclampsia [55]. Preeclampsia is closely related to hypertension; however, in recently published article, it has been shown that genetic risk scores for hypertension and blood pressure are not associated with preeclampsia [56]. Several studies have been performed in order to find proteomics biomarkers of PE. The results indicate that the most frequently reported proteomics biomarkers of preeclampsia were alpha-2-HS-glycoprotein, endoglin, fibrinogen alpha chain, fibronectin, fibulin-1, haemoglobin subunit alpha, haemoglobin subunit zeta, plasminogen, pregnancy-specific beta-1-glycoprotein 3, pregnancy-specific beta-1-glycoprotein 4, thyroid hormone-binding protein and vitronectin [57]. In order to search for small molecule biomarkers of preeclampsia, several studies using NMR [58] and LC-MS [59] were performed. Based on the NMR metabolic profiles of urine and serum, potential biomarkers present in both body fluids were proposed. Hippurate was found the most important metabolite for the prediction of preeclampsia based on the analysis of urine, while lipid (including an atherogenic lipid profile) based on the analysis of plasma samples. LC-MS serum acylcarnitines were measured in the first trimester of pregnancy in maternal serum of PE group and controls. Performed study enabled to identify stearoylcarnitine as a novel biomarker of PE [59]. Likewise, in case of IUGR, researchers were searching for potential biomarkers at different omics levels. Genetic determinants of IUGR have been reviewed by Zhang [60]. Significantly lower expression of growth factor genes (hPGH, IGF-I, IGFBP-1 and IGFBP-3) was found in placentas from human IUGR in comparison to the ones with normal foetal growth. It has been also demonstrated that IUGR is associated with maternal and foetal angiotensinogen Thr235 genotype, what might be

Table 36.4 Prognostic biomarkers for maternal diseases influencing birth weight

Type of biomarker	Disease	Ref.
GDM		
Genes	TCF7L2, CDKAL1, KNCQ1	[50]
Transcripts	hsa-miR-16-5p, hsa-miR-17-5p, hsa-miR-19a-3p, hsa-miR-19b-3p, hsa-miR-20a-5p	[51]
Proteins	Fibronectin-SNA, clusterin, apolipoprotein CII, fibrinogen alpha chain precursor, haptoglobin, protein SMG8, apoptosis-inducing factor	[52]
Metabolites	Glucose, amino acids, betaine, urea, creatine, cholesterol as well as plasma lipoproteins, fatty acids, triglycerides	[54]
Preeclampsia		
Genes	FLT1, LEP, INHA, ENG, PROCR, MMP1, XBP1, FSTL3, FLNB, INHBA, BCL6, TPBG, NDRG1, LYN and QSOX	[55]
Proteins	Alpha-2-HS-glycoprotein, endoglin, fibrinogen alpha chain, fibronectin, fibulin-1, haemoglobin subunit alpha, haemoglobin subunit zeta, plasminogen, pregnancy-specific beta-1-glycoprotein 3, pregnancy-specific beta-1-glycoprotein 4, thyroid hormone-binding protein, vitronectin	[57]
	msAFP, PAPP-A	[48]
Metabolites	Hippuric acid, lipids	[58]
	Stearoylcarnitine	[59]
IUGR		
Genes	hPGH, IGF-I, IGFBP-1 and IGFBP-3, CDK19, NFIA	[60]
	Changes in methylation of ZNF127 and PHLDA2 genes	
Proteins	Placental growth factor, soluble fms-like tyrosine kinase-1, soluble endoglin, vascular endothelial growth factor, angiopoietin-2, endothelial cell adhesion molecules, fibronectin, lactate dehydrogenase, pentraxin 3, cytokines, C-reactive protein	[26]
Metabolites	Homocysteine, 8-oxo-7,8 dihydro-2-deoxyguanosine, isoprostanes, asymmetric dimethylarginine	

The table shows potential biomarkers of such maternal conditions that may influence on neonate's birth weight. Biomarkers are divided into genes, transcripts, proteins and metabolites, according to their molecular type

responsible for insufficient placental circulation. Among other genes related to IUGR, inversion of chromosome 6 of the CDK19 gene or deletion of chromosome 1p32-p31 of the NFIA gene was reported. Epigenetic studies have shown differential methylation changes in growth-restricted placenta genes, ZNF127 gene expression was upregulated and PHLDA2 downregulated [60]. Proteomics and metabolomics biomarkers of IUGR have been reviewed by Conde-Agudelo et al. and divided them based on their functions on angiogenesis, endothelial/oxidative stress and placental related biomarkers. In the group of proteins, placental growth factor (PlGF), soluble fms-like tyrosine kinase-1, soluble endoglin, vascular endothelial growth factor, angiopoietin-2, endothelial cell adhesion molecules, fibronectin, lactate dehydrogenase, pentraxin 3, cytokines and C-reactive protein were reported as potential biomarkers of IUGR, whereas, regarding metabolites homocysteine, 8-oxo-7,8 dihydro-2-deoxyguanosine, isoprostanes and asymmetric dimethylarginine were proposed [26]. Biomarkers for maternal diseases influencing birth weight are summarized in Table 36.4.

Conclusions

Development of high-throughput analytical platforms and chemometric tools allowed for "omics" field inception. Genomics, transcriptomics, proteomics and metabolomics have been extensively used to search for disease biomarkers. Considering the importance of foetal programming and neonate's proper birth weight, these techniques were also applied to search for predictive biomarkers of possible birth weight abnormalities. Until now several potential biomarkers of abnormal birth weight were reported. However, before introducing them into routine clinical diagnostics, proposed biomarkers require validation on large cohorts and in distinct medical centres, independently. Nevertheless, studies on the mechanisms underlying foetal growth disorders are meaningful, as they may indicate how to assure a normal foetal growth.

Acknowledgements Authors acknowledge funding from the Centre for Innovative Research—the Leading National Research Centre in Poland (112/KNOW/15).

References

1. WHO, International Programme on Chemical Safety. Biomarkers and risk assessment: concepts and principles. Geneva: World Health Organization; 1993. Available from: http://www.inchem.org/documents/ehc/ehc/ehc155.htm
2. Shaheen R, de Francisco A, El Arifeen S, Ekström E-C, Persson LÅ. Effect of prenatal food supplementation on birth weight: an observational study from Bangladesh. Am J Clin Nutr. 2006;83(6):1355–61.
3. Ciborowski M, Zbucka-Kretowska M, Bomba-Opon D, Wielgos M, Brawura-Biskupski-Samaha R, Pierzynski P, et al. Potential first trimester metabolomic biomarkers of abnormal birth weight in healthy pregnancies. Prenat Diagn. 2014;34(9):870–7.
4. Hales CN, Barker DJ. Type 2 (non-insulin-dependent) diabetes mellitus: the thrifty phenotype hypothesis. Diabetologia. 1992;35(7):595–601.
5. Barker DJ, Winter PD, Osmond C, Margetts B, Simmonds SJ. Weight in infancy and death from ischaemic heart disease. Lancet. 1989;2(8663):577–80.
6. Mercuro G, Bassareo PP, Flore G, Fanos V, Dentamaro I, Scicchitano P, et al. Prematurity and low weight at birth as new conditions predisposing to an increased cardiovascular risk. Eur J Prev Cardiol. 2013;20(2):357–67.
7. Loret de Mola C, Araújo de França GV, Quevedo LDA, Horta BL. Low birth weight, preterm birth and small for gestational age association with adult depression: systematic review and meta-analysis. Br J Psychiatr. 2014;205(5):340–7.
8. Vaag AA, Grunnet LG, Arora GP, Brøns C. The thrifty phenotype hypothesis revisited. Diabetologia. 2012;55(8):2085–8.
9. Spector LG, Puumala SE, Carozza SE, Chow EJ, Fox EE, Horel S, et al. Cancer risk among children with very low birth weight. Pediatrics. 2009;124(1):96–104.
10. Gillman MW, Rifas-Shiman S, Berkey CS, Field AE, Colditz GA. Maternal gestational diabetes, birth weight, and adolescent obesity. Pediatrics. 2003;111(3):e221–e6.
11. Bowers K, Liu G, Wang P, Ye T, Tian Z, Liu E, et al. Birth weight, postnatal weight change, and risk for high blood pressure among Chinese children. Pediatrics. 2011;127(5):e1272–9.
12. Ross JA. High birthweight and cancer: evidence and implications. Cancer Epidemiol Biomark Prev. 2006;15(1):1–2.
13. Hales CN, Barker DJ. The thrifty phenotype hypothesis. Br Med Bull. 2001;60:5–20.
14. Smith NR, Jensen BW, Zimmermann E, Gamborg M, Sørensen TIA, Baker JL. Associations between birth weight and colon and rectal cancer risk in adulthood. Cancer Epidemiol. 2016;42:181–5.
15. Dawes P, Cruickshanks KJ, Moore DR, Fortnum H, Edmondson-Jones M, McCormack A, et al. The effect of prenatal and childhood development on hearing, vision and cognition in adulthood. PLoS One. 2015;10(8):e0136590.
16. Rifai RA. Rising cesarean deliveries among apparently low-risk mothers at university teaching hospitals in Jordan: analysis of population survey data, 2002–2012. Glob Health Sci Pract. 2014;2(2):195–209.
17. Boulvain M, Irion O, Dowswell T, Thornton JG. Induction of labour at or near term for suspected fetal macrosomia. Cochrane Database Syst Rev. 2016;5:CD000938.
18. Bukowski R, Chlebowski RT, Thune I, Furberg A-S, Hankins GDV, Malone FD, et al. Birth weight, breast cancer and the potential mediating hormonal environment. PLoS One. 2012;7(7):e40199.
19. Sisk PM, Lovelady CA, Dillard RG, Gruber KJ. Lactation counseling for mothers of very low birth weight infants: effect on maternal anxiety and infant intake of human milk. Pediatrics. 2006;117(1):e67–75.
20. Prior E, Santhakumaran S, Gale C, Philipps LH, Modi N, Hyde MJ. Breastfeeding after cesarean delivery: a systematic review and meta-analysis of world literature. Am J Clin Nutr. 2012;95(5):1113–35.
21. Santangeli L, Sattar N, Huda SS. Impact of maternal obesity on perinatal and childhood outcomes. Best Pract Res Cl Ob. 2015;29(3):438–48.

22. Rode L, Hegaard HK, Kjærgaard H, Møller LF, Tabor A, Ottesen B. Association between maternal weight gain and birth weight. Obstet Gynecol. 2007;109(6):1309–15.
23. Odibo AO, Patel KR, Spitalnik A, Odibo L, Huettner P. Placental pathology, first-trimester biomarkers and adverse pregnancy outcomes. J Perinatol. 2014;34(3):186–91.
24. Odell DC, Kotelchuck M, Chetty VK, Fowler J, Stubblefield GP, Orejuela M, et al. Maternal hypertension as a risk factor for low birth weight infants: comparison of Haitian and African-American women. Matern Child Health J. 2006;10(1):39–46.
25. Brunton PJ. Effects of maternal exposure to social stress during pregnancy: consequences for mother and offspring. Reproduction. 2013;146(5):R175–R89.
26. Conde-Agudelo A, Papageorghiou AT, Kennedy SH, Villar J. Novel biomarkers for predicting intrauterine growth restriction: a systematic review and meta-analysis. BJOG Int J Obstet Gynecol. 2013;120(6):681–94.
27. Blankenburg M, Haberland L, Elvers HD, Tannert C, Jandrig B. High-throughput omics technologies: potential tools for the investigation of influences of EMF on biological systems. Curr Genomics. 2009;10(2):86–92.
28. Kuska B. Beer, Bethesda, and biology: how "Genomics" came into being. J Natl Cancer Inst. 1998;90(2):93.
29. Wilkins MR, Sanchez JC, Gooley AA, Appel RD, Humphery-Smith I, Hochstrasser DF, et al. Progress with proteome projects: why all proteins expressed by a genome should be identified and how to do it. Biotechnol Genet Eng. 1996;13:19–50.
30. Wilkins MR, Pasquali C, Appel RD, Ou K, Golaz O, Sanchez JC, et al. From proteins to proteomes: large scale protein identification by two-dimensional electrophoresis and amino acid analysis. Biotechnology (N Y). 1996;14(1):61–5.
31. Wasinger VC, Cordwell SJ, Cerpa-Poljak A, Yan JX, Gooley AA, Wilkins MR, et al. Progress with gene-product mapping of the Mollicutes: mycoplasma genitalium. Electrophoresis. 1995;16(7):1090–4.
32. Nicholson JK, Lindon JC, Holmes E. 'Metabonomics': understanding the metabolic responses of living systems to pathophysiological stimuli via multivariate statistical analysis of biological NMR spectroscopic data. Xenobiotica. 1999;29(11):1181–9.
33. Fiehn O. Combining genomics, metabolome analysis, and biochemical modelling to understand metabolic networks. Comp Funct Genom. 2001;2(3):155–68.
34. Park PJ. ChIP-seq: advantages and challenges of a maturing technology. Nat Rev Genet. 2009;10(10):669–80.
35. Armirotti A, Damonte G. Achievements and perspectives of top-down proteomics. Proteomics. 2010;10(20):3566–76.
36. Altelaar AF, Munoz J, Heck AJ. Next-generation proteomics: towards an integrative view of proteome dynamics. Nat Rev Genet. 2013;14(1):35–48.
37. Aebersold R, Mann M. Mass spectrometry-based proteomics. Nature. 2003;422(6928):198–207.
38. Nicholson JK, Lindon JC. Systems biology: metabonomics. Nature. 2008;455(7216):1054–6.
39. Dunn WB, Broadhurst D, Begley P, Zelena E, Francis-McIntyre S, Anderson N, et al. Procedures for large-scale metabolic profiling of serum and plasma using gas chromatography and liquid chromatography coupled to mass spectrometry. Nat Protoc. 2011;6(7):1060–83.
40. Sumner LW, Amberg A, Barrett D, Beale MH, Beger R, Daykin CA, et al. Proposed minimum reporting standards for chemical analysis Chemical Analysis Working Group (CAWG) Metabolomics Standards Initiative (MSI). Metabolomics. 2007;3(3):211–21.
41. Vo T, Hardy DB. Molecular mechanisms underlying the fetal programming of adult disease. J Cell Commun Sig. 2012;6(3):139–53.
42. Johnston LB, Clark AJL, Savage MO. Genetic factors contributing to birth weight. Arch Dis Child Fetal. 2002;86(1):F2–3.
43. Andraweera PH, Gatford KL, Dekker GA, Leemaqz S, Russell D, Thompson SD, et al. Insulin family polymorphisms in pregnancies complicated by small for gestational age infants. Mol Hum Reprod. 2015;21(9):745–52.
44. Horikoshi M, Yaghootkar H, Mook-Kanamori DO, Sovio U, Taal HR, Hennig BJ, et al. New loci associated with birth weight identify genetic links between intrauterine growth and adult height and metabolism. Nat Genet. 2013;45(1):76–82.
45. Sabri A, Lai D, D'Silva A, Seeho S, Kaur J, Ng C, et al. Differential placental gene expression in term pregnancies affected by fetal growth restriction and macrosomia. Fetal Diagn Ther. 2014;36(2):173–80.
46. Gómez-Roig MD, Mazarico E, Cárdenas D, Fernandez MT, Díaz M, Ruiz de Gauna B, et al. Placental 11B-Hydroxysteroid dehydrogenase type 2 mRNA levels in intrauterine growth restriction versus small-for-gestational-age fetuses. Fetal Diagn Ther. 2016;39(2):147–51.
47. Kumarathasan P, Vincent R, Das D, Mohottalage S, Blais E, Blank K, et al. Applicability of a high-throughput shotgun plasma protein screening approach in understanding maternal biological pathways relevant to infant birth weight outcome. J Proteome. 2014;100:136–46.
48. Cohen JL, Smilen KE, Bianco AT, Moshier EL, Ferrara LA, L. Stone J. Predictive value of combined serum biomarkers for adverse pregnancy outcomes. Eur J Obstet Gynecol R B. 2014;181:89–94.

49. Kumarathasan P, Vincent R, Bielecki A, Blais E, Blank K, Das D, et al. Infant birth weight and third trimester maternal plasma markers of vascular integrity: the MIREC study. Biomarkers. 2016;21(3):257–66.
50. Wung SF, Lin PC. Shared genomics of type 2 and gestational diabetes mellitus. Annu Rev Nurs Res. 2011;29:227–60.
51. Zhu Y, Tian F, Li H, Zhou Y, Lu J, Ge Q. Profiling maternal plasma microRNA expression in early pregnancy to predict gestational diabetes mellitus. Int J Gynecol Obstet. 2015;130(1):49–53.
52. Singh A, Subramani E, Datta Ray C, Rapole S, Chaudhury K. Proteomic-driven biomarker discovery in gestational diabetes mellitus: a review. J Proteome. 2015;127(Pt A):44–9.
53. Dudzik D, Zorawski M, Skotnicki M, Zarzycki W, Kozlowska G, Bibik-Malinowska K, et al. Metabolic fingerprint of gestational diabetes mellitus. J Proteome. 2014;103:57–71.
54. Pinto J, Almeida LM, Martins AS, Duarte D, Barros AS, Galhano E, et al. Prediction of gestational diabetes through NMR metabolomics of maternal blood. J Proteome Res. 2015;14(6):2696–706.
55. Tejera E, Bernardes J, Rebelo I. Co-expression network analysis and genetic algorithms for gene prioritization in preeclampsia. BMC Med Genet. 2013;6(1):1–10.
56. Smith CJ, Saftlas AF, Spracklen CN, Triche EW, Bjonnes A, Keating B, et al. Genetic risk score for essential hypertension and risk of preeclampsia. Am J Hypertens. 2016;29(1):17–24.
57. Law KP, Han T-L, Tong C, Baker PN. Mass spectrometry-based proteomics for pre-eclampsia and preterm birth. Int J Mol Sci. 2015;16(5):10952–85.
58. Austdal M, Tangerås LH, Skråstad RB, Salvesen KÅ, Austgulen R, Iversen A-C, et al. First trimester urine and serum metabolomics for prediction of preeclampsia and gestational hypertension: a prospective screening study. Int J Mol Sci. 2015;16(9):21520–38.
59. Koster MP, Vreeken RJ, Harms AC, Dane AD, Kuc S, Schielen PC, et al. First-trimester serum acylcarnitine levels to predict preeclampsia: a metabolomics approach. Dis Markers. 2015;2015:857108.
60. Zhang XQ. Intrauterine growth restriction and genetic determinants – existing findings, problems, and further direction. World J Obstet Gynecol. 2012;1(3):20–8.

Chapter 37
Mechanisms of Programming: Pancreatic Islets and Fetal Programming

Luiz F. Barella, Paulo C.F. Mathias, and Júlio C. de Oliveira

Key Points

- Type 2 diabetes is a worldwide global health concern and its development is closely associated with perinatal insults, such as undernutrition or overnutrition.
- Pancreatic islets are among the main targets of early life nutritional insults, which can eventually result in significant islet impairments.
- Skeletal muscle and white adipocytes are the major peripheral insulin-dependent tissues injured by metabolic malprogramming effects, leading to type 2 diabetes later in life.
- Malprogramming effects, which lead to phenotypes like obese individual with insulin resistance or lean with insulin hypersensitivity later in life, are highly dependent on the time and severity of the nutritional insults.
- Imbalanced autonomous nervous system, especially through changes in muscarinic acetylcholine receptor signaling in pancreatic islets, contributes to the type 2 diabetes development later in life.
- Recent studies show relevant epigenetic modifications in pancreatic islets to explain the early life impairments due to nutritional insults.

Keywords Pancreatic islets • Nutritional insults • Sensitive periods of life • Fetal programming • Developmental Origins of Health and Disease (DOHaD) • Metabolic programming • Epigenetic

L.F. Barella, PhD (✉)
Laboratory of Secretion Cell Biology, Department of Biotechnology, Genetics and Cell Biology, State University of Maringa, Maringa, PR, Brazil

Molecular Signaling Section, Laboratory of Bioorganic Chemistry, National Institute of Diabetes and Digestive and Kidney Diseases, National Institutes of Health (NIDDK/NIH), Bethesda, MD, USA
e-mail: lfbarella@gmail.com; luiz.barella@nih.gov

P.C.F. Mathias, PhD
Laboratory of Secretion Cell Biology, Department of Biotechnology, Genetics and Cell Biology, State University of Maringa, Maringa, PR, Brazil

J.C. de Oliveira, PhD
Institute of Health Sciences, Federal University of Mato Grosso, Sinop, MT, Brazil

© Springer International Publishing AG 2017
R. Rajendram et al. (eds.), *Diet, Nutrition, and Fetal Programming*,
Nutrition and Health, DOI 10.1007/978-3-319-60289-9_37

Abbreviations

ANS   Autonomous nervous system
CNS   Central nervous system
DOHaD   Developmental Origins of Health and Disease
mAChR   Muscarinic acetylcholine receptor
T2D   Type 2 diabetes

Introduction

Numerous experimental [1, 2] and epidemiological [3, 4] studies have highlighted the metabolic diseases as a major threat to global health. Metabolic dysfunctions commonly related to prenatal and postnatal nutritional insults, such as undernutrition or ingestion of high caloric diets, are one of the triggers of the development of obesity, hypertension, and type 2 diabetes (T2D), among other disorders.

Studies have confirmed the importance of the thrifty phenotype hypothesis, which states that low birth weight is one of the major risk factors for the development of metabolic syndrome later in life. Based on this hypothesis, the idea of the Developmental Origins of Health and Disease (DOHaD) was proposed, and this concept has been extensively discussed and accepted by numerous researchers around the world [5]. The DOHaD concept pursues to explain how insults (e.g., malnourishment) during critical windows of body development, such as perinatal phase, can lead to metabolic dysfunctions later in life. Normally, the early life effects of malnourishment on metabolism will be observed in the adult offspring if their diet improves or if overnutrition occurs [6, 7]. In sum, the DOHaD concept can be defined as a malprogramming of the metabolism, which induces diseases when children become adults. The DOHaD notion is not only limited to nutritional insults but also focuses on insults caused by several drugs, such as nicotine, which is an important trigger of metabolic dysfunctions in adulthood [8].

The central nervous system (CNS) is affected by undernutrition leading to its malformation and this is particularly due to its sensitive developmental phase [9, 10]. However, the CNS is not the only affected system and several other tissues, such as the liver and the endocrine pancreas [11–13], are also impaired by nutritional restriction during the perinatal phase. The pancreatic islets are believed to be a key target of metabolic programming [12, 14–16]. Such impairments might lead the endocrine cells of the pancreas, especially beta cells, to exhaustion, which will eventually result in T2D that is when the beta cells are not able to produce enough insulin to overcome the insulin resistance developed as consequence of the disease impairments. During the last decade, numerous studies have linked overnutrition and undernutrition effects on beta-cell dysfunction with epigenetic mechanisms, which appear to induce the onset of T2D [17, 18]. Given the importance of pancreatic islets in metabolic programming, this chapter aims to focus on the current advances to understanding the role of pancreatic islets and perinatal programming, particularly due to nutritional insults.

The Intrauterine and Suckling Phases as Very Sensitive Windows for Metabolic Programming

The endocrine pancreas development is an important biological process that will constitute the pancreatic islets of Langerhans. This critical stage (Fig. 37.1) makes this organ very sensitive to changes in hormone, macro- and micronutrients, metabolites and growth factors in their surrounding environment [19]. The T2D is one of the major dysfunctions of the pancreatic islets, it has been closely

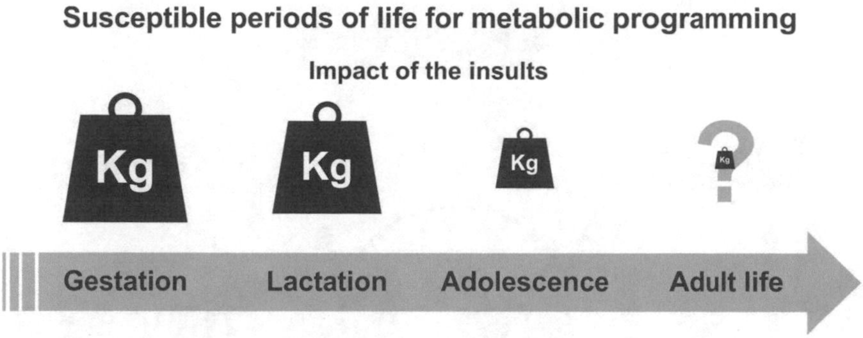

Susceptible periods of life for metabolic programming

Impact of the insults

Fig. 37.1 Impact of insults during the sensitive periods of life. The impact of insults is greater during gestation and lactation and leads to more severe metabolic dysfunctions later in life. Moreover, recent studies indicate that adolescence is also a susceptible period for programming and may imbalance metabolic homeostasis later in life

associated with maternal exposition to nutritional insults, both overnutrition and undernutrition, in critical stages of offspring development [20, 21]. In this section, we will focus on the effects of maternal undernutrition both during pregnancy and lactation as well as the outcome presented by the offspring later in life, once these changes are greatly contributing to the T2D.

In early life, especially when pregnant and lactating dams undergo a low-protein or low-calorie dietary regimen, the lack of amino acids to guarantee metabolic demand affects maternal endocrine systems in mothers, via placenta or change in milk composition, malprogramming the pancreas physiology of their offspring [22, 23]. In addition, changes in metabolism as well as in pancreatic islet function are also found in the offspring, as a long-term consequence, when perinatal overnutrition occurs [20, 24].

Thus, for a healthy and functioning endocrine pancreas, an equilibrated-homeostatic environment is necessary during its formation/maturation. It is important because the pancreatic endocrine cells, especially glucagon-containing α-granules are observed since the 9th embryonic day (E9; *in the mouse*); on the other hand, insulin-containing β-granules are not typically seen at this period. Even though the endocrine pancreatic cells could be seen at this time, they are not completely isolated as an endocrine cell line; all of them are associated together with the epithelial and/or exocrine cells and the *pancreatic and duodenal homeobox factor 1 (Pdx1)*, a key factor for the early pancreatic progenitor cells differentiation, does not seem to be expressed yet. In fact, the pancreas originates from the dorsal and ventral regions of the foregut endoderm at the embryonic day E9.5 *in the mouse*, E11 *in the rat*, and 25–26 days of gestational age *in the human* [19].

Following the progression of pregnancy (around of E14 and E18; *in the mouse pancreas*), a surge of new endocrine cells, separated from the exocrine cells, begins to accumulate along the ducts and blood vessels. Interestingly, the morphogenesis and differentiation process continue after birth, when these new pancreatic endocrine cells adhere and form an aggregation that represents the first islets of Langerhans (consisting of insulin-producing β-cells, glucagon-producing α-cells, somatostatin-producing δ-cells, ghrelin-producing ε-cells and pancreatic polypeptide-producing PP-cells) [25]. Considering the physiological importance of this process, an inadequate maternal nutrition either in pregnancy or in suckling phase is a determinant for the unhealthy shaping of pancreatic beta cell in early life.

Regarding metabolic malprogramming effects upon the endocrine pancreas, there are many studies reporting that the intrauterine and suckling phases are critical windows for malprogramming, leading to metabolic dysfunction associated to pancreas due to environmental injuries through the maternal dietary. Among the changes in organ and/or neuroendocrine systems, the maternal undernutrition in experimental animal models, either in pregnancy or in lactation, show many subtle malfunctioning effects on metabolism. Altogether, they appear as risk factors for the metabolic syndrome (Fig. 37.2).

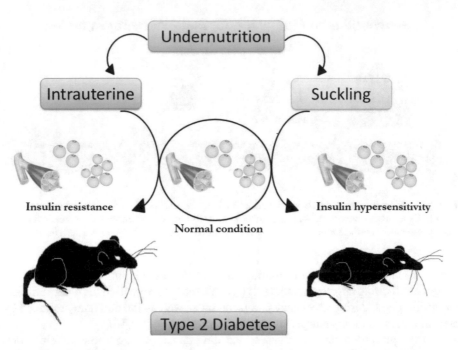

Fig. 37.2 Metabolic malprogramming by maternal undernutrition in critical phase of life upon the peripheral insulin action in the adult offspring. Offspring whose dams experienced protein/calorie deprivation during pregnancy (especially later) and lactation (especially earlier) malprograms insulin-dependent tissues to different changes that converges with a high risk of type 2 diabetes onset. If malnutrition occurs during pregnancy, it can disrupt mechanisms that lead to insulin resistance in both skeletal muscle and white adipose tissues. On the other hand, if malnutrition occurs during suckling phase, a similar mechanism is also disrupted, but in this case, leading to insulin hypersensitivity in both skeletal muscle and white adipose tissues. Altogether, maternal malnourishment in critical stages of life malprograms the offspring to a high risk of developing type 2 diabetes

In fact, there are many variations regarding the studies of malfunctioning effects on metabolic parameters, but it can be explained by the duration of insult, severity of food restriction, time where the insult occurs, sex, species and/or the moment in which data are evaluated. However, in general the phenotypic outcome depends on when mothers experience food deprivation (protein-, calorie-, and/or protein-calorie restriction), e.g., only in pregnancy, pregnancy plus lactation, or only in lactation.

In line with that, we can visualize the following effects:

1. When food deprivation occurs at pregnancy, high peripheral insulin resistance, which is associated with an obese phenotype at adulthood in offspring, is usually present. At this point, the physiological changes as long-term consequence of the effects of metabolic malprogramming in the important regulatory proteins that is involved in different signaling pathways controlling key functions in the cell have been found. Given that, impaired activation of the *phosphatidylinositol-3 kinase* (*PI3-K*) and *protein kinase B* (*PKB*, also known as *Akt*) pathway [26] and low protein expression and/or translocation activity of *glucose transporter 4* (*GLUT4*) in white adipose tissue have been reported [27]. In addition, in this experimental model of food deprivation during pregnancy, it was observed a downregulation of the isoform *zeta* of *protein kinase C* (*PKC ζ*) that is directly involved in insulin-mediated metabolic processes by positively influencing glucose uptake through the stimulation of the GLUT4 translocation in the cell [28]. Together with the *p85α*, a non-catalytic subunit associated with catalytic subunit *p110β* of the PI3K, in both white adipocytes and skeletal muscle, it was found decreased in adult rat offspring from mothers that underwent protein restriction during pregnancy

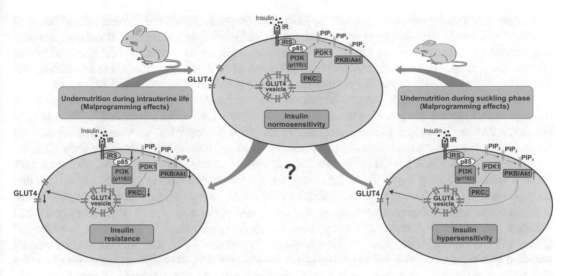

Fig. 37.3 Metabolic malprogramming by maternal undernutrition in critical phases of life upon the insulin pathway in skeletal muscle and white adipose tissue in the adult offspring. Offspring whose dam experienced protein/calorie deprivation exhibit a disrupted insulin pathway, which leads to a metabolic syndrome pattern (not yet elucidated) with insulin resistance if malnourishment was during pregnancy and insulin hypersensitivity if malnourishment was during lactation. Insulin is a pivotal hormone that controls critical energy functions such as glucose metabolism, among other signaling pathways. When the insulin molecule binds and activates its insulin receptor tyrosine kinase (IR), a phosphorylation activity occurs by recruiting different substrate proteins such as the IRS family of proteins. Subsequently, the phosphorylated IRS bind to various other different signaling proteins (including PI3K, which plays an important role in insulin function, primarily through the activation of the Akt/PKB and the PKCζ signaling cascades. In summary, the insulin-stimulated glucose uptake in muscle and/or adipocytes, via the GLUT4 vesicles translocation to the plasma membrane, involving the PI3K/Akt pathway, is altered (downregulation in malprogramming induced during intrauterine phase) and (upregulation in malprogramming induced during suckling phase), and this has been demonstrated to be associated with the activation/expression of these insulin-dependent signaling proteins

[27, 29–31]. These changes are strong contributors to metabolic dysfunction, like insulin resistance, leading to high risk of T2D (Fig. 37.3).

2. On the other hand, when dams are undernourished only during lactation (especially at the early lactation period) their offspring display high peripheral insulin sensitivity associated with a lean phenotype. In this case, the malprogramming effects, as long-term consequences, are influenced by the physiological changes in insulin signaling pathway like the one shown above. In line, autonomous nervous system imbalance [32], especially low parasympathetic tonus, can attenuate the effects upon glucose-induced insulin secretion in pancreatic beta cell [14]. In an experimental model, an increased translocation of GLUT4 associated with high activation of *mammalian target of rapamycin (mTOR)/Akt* pathway in white adipose tissue [33] and a high protein expression of *insulin receptor substrate-1 (IRS-1)*, PI3K, and GLUT4 in skeletal muscle was also found [34]. Altogether, these cell-signaling changes are strong contributors to metabolic dysfunctions, primarily leading to an insulin hypersensitivity pattern in peripheral tissues. Even though the insulin hypersensitivity is present as a primary effect, a second disturbance may develop, leading to a high risk of an impairment of the insulin secretion response on the beta cells and, eventually, the development of T2D. The development of T2D in this case might be triggered by an increased availability of food in individuals that underwent poor-energy diets in early periods of life [7] (Fig. 37.3).

It is evident that beyond the disturbances in the insulin production/secretion (pancreatic beta-cell impairment), the insulin action in peripheral tissues (adipose tissue and skeletal muscle) are also imbalanced by malprogramming effects due to maternal nutrients scarcity in critical stages of life. In consequence, it appears as subtle changes in metabolism later in life, and all of these alterations converge in metabolic dysfunctions that corroborates for the metabolic syndrome and T2D onset.

In a similar way as to gestation and lactation, many studies have supported that insults occurring during the adolescence can program the metabolism to exhibit dysfunctions later in life. Thus, beyond the pregnancy and suckling phases, adolescence is also a pivotal window where individuals that undergo nutritional insults may develop metabolic dysfunctions later in life. It has been shown that the adolescence is a sensitive period for the final maturation of neuroendocrine circuits, which includes those involved in energy expenditure [35]. Rats fed a high-fat diet during a period of 60 days that encompasses their peripubertal period exhibit more drastic effects (e.g., increased adipose tissue accumulation, impaired glucose tolerance. and decreased peripheral insulin sensitivity) compared with rats fed a high-fat diet during 60 days after the adolescence period, i.e., only during adulthood [36]. In the same line, when rats are fed a low-protein diet during adolescence, impaired beta-cell function and imbalanced metabolism homeostasis are observed [6]. This latter study points out to the alteration in the activity of *muscarinic acetylcholine receptor* (*mAChR*) subtypes as a possible mechanism to explain, at least in part, where metabolic programming is acting through. Although the evidence for adolescence as an additional window for metabolic programming is in place, it is still lacking mechanistic studies showing how this occurs.

Early Nutritional Insults Malprogram Pancreatic Islet Function

At adulthood, endocrine pancreas is composed by around one million islets of Langerhans with variable sizes (from 40 up to 900 μm). In fact, the location of smaller and larger islets of Langerhans is dependent on the metabolic availability during their development, whereas the smaller islets of Langerhans are deeply embedded in the pancreas' parenchyma, the larger islets are found to be closely to the major arterioles, which points out that failure in nutrient delivery can affect drastically the endocrine pancreas development [19, 37]. In general, most of islets are constituted by around 3000–4000 cells of the five major types, as described above. Human pancreatic islets consist of around 50% β-cells, ~40% α-cells, ~10% δ-cells, and few PP-cells, while rodent pancreatic islets comprise around of 60–80% β-cells, ~15–20% α-cells, less than 10% δ-cells, and less than 1% PP-cells [38].

Maternal scarcity of nutrients, during pregnancy and/or suckling phase, creates a larger energy demand in dams' metabolism. Consequently it can lead to undernourishment in the offspring in these critical stages of life development, which is translated as lack of glucose, amino acids, hormone signaling and/or the action of growth factors that are critical for the development of the endocrine pancreas in the offspring [19, 22, 39]. Moreover, insulin itself might modulate the endocrine pancreatic cell development. As elegantly reported in a previous study, the appropriate modulation of insulin signaling as feedback loop into the pancreas is pivotal for the optimal generation of pancreatic beta cells, where insulin signaling by itself can regulate the differentiation of pancreatic progenitor cells during the islet development and regeneration [40]. The physiological ability of pancreatic beta cells to synthesize and secrete insulin is regulated primarily by blood glucose levels, additionally neural and paracrine signals are important factors that influence pancreatic islet function. In fact, pancreatic islets from prediabetic obese mice, with an early malprogramming for metabolic disturbances, present failure in the autocrine effects of insulin, especially on the insulin receptor and insulin receptor substrate-1 level [41]. Interestingly, this functional failure can be attenuated by exercise training, which modulates pathways, improving the metabolic parameters of exercised mice, particularly if the intervention is performed in early developmental stages of life.

Regarding the metabolic malprogramming effects, directly influencing pancreatic beta cells, it has been well demonstrated that the weak ability of pancreatic beta cells to secrete insulin is associated with lower activity of the *autonomous nervous system (ANS)* in potentiating glucose-induced insulin secretion. It has been reported that ANS is disrupted in adult rat offspring whose mothers were malnourished during the first half of lactation [14, 32]. In addition, as shown previously, this functional disability of pancreatic beta cells to secrete insulin is, in part, intrinsically associated with an early malprogramming effect that leads to downregulation of the *insulinotropic mAChR subtype M₃* and upregulation of the *insulinostatic mAChR subtype M₂* [16]. These two subtypes of mAChRs belong to the superfamily of the *G protein-coupled receptors*. While the M_3 subtype is a $G_{q/11}$-coupled receptor [42], the M_2 subtype couples to $G_{i/o}$ [43]. These two mAChRs are the major receptor subtypes modulating signaling pathways in pancreatic beta cells. Moreover, the insulinotropic effect of mAChR subtype M_3 as well as the insulinostatic effect of mAChR subtype M_2 from adult rat offspring whose mothers were protein deprived just in the last third of pregnancy is shown to be functionally decreased; thus, acetylcholine-responsiveness of pancreatic islets to physiological stimuli is found to be drastically reduced [44].

In another rodent model of early malprogramming, besides the unbalanced function of the ANS by acting on the pancreatic beta cells potentiating insulin secretion [45, 46], the insulinotropic mAChR subtype M_3 was found to be upregulated, while the insulinostatic mAChR subtype M_2 was downregulated in adult rat offspring [47], which is an important predictor for the onset of T2D.

It is important to highlight that in the critical stage in which pancreatic beta cells are developing, disturbances in the environment are a powerful factor addressing changes in several mechanisms involving transcription factors. These transcription factors underlie the architecture of the pancreas formation, as well as their maturation and function. As previously shown the capacity of beta cells to proliferate is critical for their ability to adapt either to physiological [48] or nonphysiological changes [22] in metabolic demands, which has been closely linked to epigenetic changes, as well described in the next section.

Epigenetics and the Fetal Programming of the Pancreatic Beta Cells

Epigenetic has emerged as a key factor contributing to metabolic programming and may explain a substantial part of the mechanisms involved in the early life nutritional insults that manifest later in life as metabolic dysfunctions (Fig. 37.4). Interestingly, in humans, a study showed that children of mothers who were pregnant during the Dutch famine of 1944 (occurred in Netherlands at the end of the World War II) presented less DNA methylation of the *Igf2* gene, a major factor in human growth and development, in blood cells during adulthood [49]. Recently, several studies, both in humans and animal models, have clearly shown that the maternal nutritional status has a key importance causing differential epigenetic changes in the offspring methylome, and these changes may lead to phenotypic consequences [50, 51].

T2D manifests when the secreted amount of insulin is not able to overcome the peripheral insulin resistance that diabetic individuals exhibit. For this reason, deciphering the epigenetic patterns in pancreatic islets is essential for understanding how the impairment of insulin release occurs and at which extent epigenetics contribute to this impairment, opening possibilities to more effectively tackle this disease (Fig. 37.5). A comprehensive study was recently developed to describe the human methylome in pancreatic islets [52]. In this study, the authors analyzed almost 500,000 CpG islands in pancreatic islets from T2D and nondiabetic individuals, providing a global map of the DNA methylation pattern in human islets, as well as potential novel candidates susceptible to methylation changes that may lead to T2D. In previous studies, the authors found increased DNA methylation of INS and PDX-1 in islets from T2D patients compared with controls [53, 54].

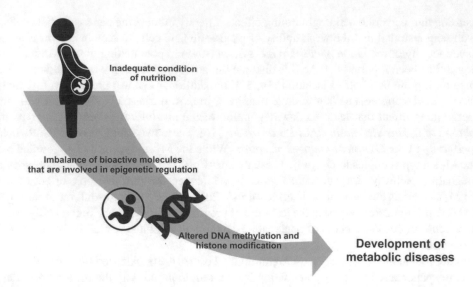

Fig. 37.4 Maternal environment and nutrition. Maternal environment is affected by nutrition, which results in altered availability of bioactive molecules (e.g., folate) involved in epigenetic regulation. Altered epigenome occurs in the fetus making him/her susceptible to the development of metabolic diseases later in life

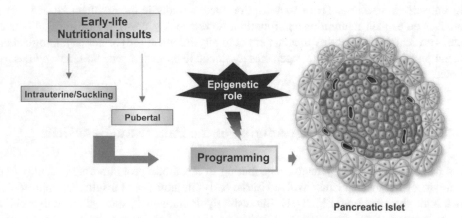

Fig. 37.5 Pancreatic islets as targets of metabolic programming. Stressors disturb the normal development of the endocrine cells of the pancreas leading to dysfunctions and consequent impaired glucose homeostasis. Numerous studies have pointed out epigenetics as a main role in these programming events (as described in the text)

The search for gene targets involved in islet health and disease that can be epigenetically altered by environmental inputs, such as nutrition, has been constant. The hepatocyte nuclear factor 4-α (HNF-4α) is a transcription factor required for proper beta-cell differentiation and glucose homeostasis [55]. It has been shown that maternal protein restriction leads to decreased HNF-4α mRNA levels in islets of the adult offspring, and this was due to a slight increase of DNA methylation at the promoter region and a considerable change in the histone marks specifically at the enhancer region [56]. In addition, T2D patients show decreased HNF-4α expression [57], which makes this gene a potential target for epigenetic therapy.

In an interesting study, Ding et al. [58] show that the F1 and F2 offsprings from dams that exhibited intrauterine hyperglycemia, i.e., gestational diabetes, presented impaired glucose tolerance, and impaired insulin secretion. In addition, they show downregulation of Igf2 and H19 from isolated islets from both F1 and F2 lineages of gestational diabetes. Igf2 and H19 are involved in islet development and pathogenesis of diabetes; moreover, they are well-described targets of reciprocal imprinting leading to their gene expression or repression, depending on their epigenetic imprinting inheritance from parents [59–61]. Interestingly, the authors show altered methylation pattern of the differentially methylated regions (DMRs) in both Igf2 and H19, which can be one of the mechanisms involved in their abnormal gene expression [58].

The key features for the establishment of T2D is impaired beta-cell function combined with the decrease in beta-cell mass and the development of peripheral insulin resistance [62]. *Pdx1* is a pancreatic transcription factor responsible for the early development and maintenance of the endocrine pancreas and the decrease in its expression, either in human or animals, has been associated with the development of T2D [63, 64]. Substantial epigenetic modifications were shown to affect pancreatic islet development by silencing the Pdx1 locus of adult animals that underwent an uteroplacental insufficiency (IUGR). Their Pdx1 expression is diminished by 50% early in life and by 80% when adults [65]. In this elegant study, Park et al. [65] showed a cascade of epigenetic modifications including increased methylation of the Pdx1 gene promoter and significant reduction of acetylated H3 and H4 that encompasses CpG islands at Pdx1 in IUGR animals. DNA methylation leads to transcriptional silencing whereas histone deacetylation is associated with the repression of chromatin structure [66], which explains the striking decrease in Pdx1 expression in IUGR animals.

Interestingly, the metabolic programming is not limited to the impact of nutrition on the mothers, but also obese fathers have their own contribution. In this study, Ng et al. [67] showed that fathers exposed to high-fat diet program beta-cell dysfunction of their rat female offspring. Among the several altered expression of pancreatic islet genes, they analyzed whether these alterations could be associated with epigenetic changes. They found that *Il13ra2,* the gene that exhibited the greatest fold difference in expression and is involved in some key metabolic networks, was hypomethylated, and thus indicates that these changes can be explained, at least in part, by modification of the offspring epigenome.

Therefore, it is clear that understanding and unraveling the epigenome pathways, which lead to disease due to under- or overnutrition during sensitive periods of life, will help understand islet function and possibly lead to novel therapies to prevent diabetes progression.

Conclusion

The mechanisms of programming have been associated to a great extent to epigenetic modifications. In line, it might be associated with an early epigenetic mechanism imprinting where adaptations due to environmental adversity, which tries to ensure survival for the individual and promotes persistent alterations in the physiology and metabolism of developing tissues, including structural and functional alterations in the endocrine pancreas, as well as changes in the insulin-sensitive target tissues. Consequently, it may persist throughout life, predisposing individuals to the onset of T2D. Although the understanding of epigenetic patterns regulating pancreatic islet development and function has advanced quickly, the precise mechanisms that regulate tissue function or disease risk remain largely unknown and a large amount of work needs to be done in order to expand our knowledge and find helpful and potential therapeutic targets.

References

1. Vickers MH, Reddy S, Ikenasio BA, et al. Dysregulation of the adipoinsular axis – a mechanism for the pathogenesis of hyperleptinemia and adipogenic diabetes induced by fetal programming. J Endocrinol. 2001;170(2):323–32.
2. Moura AS, Carpinelli AR, Barbosa FB, et al. Undernutrition during early lactation as an alternative model to study the onset of diabetes mellitus type II. Res Commun Mol Pathol Pharmacol. 1996;92(1):73–84.
3. Barker DJ. Intrauterine programming of adult disease. Mol Med Today. 1995;1(9):418–23.

4. van Abeelen AF, Elias SG, Bossuyt PM, et al. Famine exposure in the young and the risk of type 2 diabetes in adulthood. Diabetes. 2012;61(9):2255–60.
5. Hales CN, Barker DJ. The thrifty phenotype hypothesis. Br Med Bull. 2001;60:5–20.
6. de Oliveira JC, Lisboa PC, de Moura EG, et al. Poor pubertal protein nutrition disturbs glucose-induced insulin secretion process in pancreatic islets and programs rats in adulthood to increase fat accumulation. J Endocrinol. 2013;216(2):195–206.
7. Gosby AK, Maloney CA, Caterson ID. Elevated insulin sensitivity in low-protein offspring rats is prevented by a high-fat diet and is associated with visceral fat. Obesity (Silver Spring). 2010;18(8):1593–600.
8. Lisboa PC, de Oliveira E, de Moura EG. Obesity and endocrine dysfunction programmed by maternal smoking in pregnancy and lactation. Front Physiol. 2012;3:437.
9. Morgane PJ, Mokler DJ, Galler JR. Effects of prenatal protein malnutrition on the hippocampal formation. Neurosci Biobehav Rev. 2002;26(4):471–83.
10. Resnick O, Miller M, Forbes W, et al. Developmental protein malnutrition: influences on the central nervous system of the rat. Neurosci Biobehav Rev. 1979;3(4):233–46.
11. Plagemann A, Harder T, Rake A, et al. Hypothalamic nuclei are malformed in weanling offspring of low protein malnourished rat dams. J Nutr. 2000;130(10):2582–9.
12. Rodriguez-Trejo A, Ortiz-Lopez MG, Zambrano E, et al. Developmental programming of neonatal pancreatic beta-cells by a maternal low-protein diet in rats involves a switch from proliferation to differentiation. Am J Physiol Endocrinol Metab. 2012;302(11):E1431–9.
13. Altmann S, Murani E, Metges CC, et al. Effect of gestational protein deficiency and excess on hepatic expression of genes related to cell cycle and proliferation in offspring from late gestation to finishing phase in pig. Mol Biol Rep. 2012;39(6):7095–104.
14. de Oliveira JC, Scomparin DX, Andreazzi AE, et al. Metabolic imprinting by maternal protein malnourishment impairs vagal activity in adult rats. J Neuroendocrinol. 2011;23(2):148–57.
15. Arantes VC, Teixeira VP, Reis MA, et al. Expression of PDX-1 is reduced in pancreatic islets from pups of rat dams fed a low protein diet during gestation and lactation. J Nutr. 2002;132(10):3030–5.
16. Oliveira JC, Miranda RA, Barella LF, et al. Impaired beta-cell function in the adult offspring of rats fed a protein-restricted diet during lactation is associated with changes in muscarinic acetylcholine receptor subtypes. Br J Nutr. 2014;111(2):227–35.
17. Berends LM, Ozanne SE. Early determinants of type-2 diabetes. Best Pract Res Clin Endocrinol Metab. 2012;26(5):569–80.
18. Pinney SE, Simmons RA. Epigenetic mechanisms in the development of type 2 diabetes. Trends Endocrinol Metab. 2010;21(4):223–9.
19. Green AS, Rozance PJ, Limesand SW. Consequences of a compromised intrauterine environment on islet function. J Endocrinol. 2010;205(3):211–24.
20. de Souza Rodrigues Cunha AC, Pereira RO, Dos Santos Pereira MJ, et al. Long-term effects of overfeeding during lactation on insulin secretion – the role of GLUT-2. J Nutr Biochem. 2008;20:435–42.
21. Lopes Da Costa C, Sampaio De Freitas M, Sanchez Moura A. Insulin secretion and GLUT-2 expression in under-nourished neonate rats. J Nutr Biochem. 2004;15(4):236–41.
22. Holness MJ, Langdown ML, Sugden MC. Early-life programming of susceptibility to dysregulation of glucose metabolism and the development of type 2 diabetes mellitus. Biochem J. 2000;349(Pt 3):657–65.
23. Reusens B, Remacle C. Programming of the endocrine pancreas by the early nutritional environment. Int J Biochem Cell Biol. 2006;38(5–6):913–22.
24. Plagemann A, Heidrich I, Gotz F, et al. Obesity and enhanced diabetes and cardiovascular risk in adult rats due to early postnatal overfeeding. Exp Clin Endocrinol. 1992;99(3):154–8.
25. Gittes GK. Developmental biology of the pancreas: a comprehensive review. Dev Biol. 2009;326(1):4–35.
26. Ozanne SE, Dorling MW, Wang CL, et al. Impaired PI 3-kinase activation in adipocytes from early growth-restricted male rats. Am J Physiol Endocrinol Metab. 2001;280(3):E534–9.
27. Gardner DS, Tingey K, Van Bon BW, et al. Programming of glucose-insulin metabolism in adult sheep after maternal undernutrition. Am J Physiol Regul Integr Comp Physiol. 2005;289(4):R947–54.
28. Considine RV, Caro JF. Protein kinase C: mediator or inhibitor of insulin action? J Cell Biochem. 1993;52(1):8–13.
29. Ozanne SE, Olsen GS, Hansen LL, et al. Early growth restriction leads to down regulation of protein kinase C zeta and insulin resistance in skeletal muscle. J Endocrinol. 2003;177(2):235–41.
30. Ozanne SE, Nave BT, Wang CL, et al. Poor fetal nutrition causes long-term changes in expression of insulin signaling components in adipocytes. Am J Phys. 1997;273(1 Pt 1):E46–51.
31. Fernandez-Twinn DS, Wayman A, Ekizoglou S, et al. Maternal protein restriction leads to hyperinsulinemia and reduced insulin-signaling protein expression in 21-mo-old female rat offspring. Am J Physiol Regul Integr Comp Physiol. 2005;288(2):R368–73.
32. Gravena C, Andreazzi AE, Mecabo FT, et al. Protein restriction during lactation alters the autonomic nervous system control on glucose-induced insulin secretion in adult rats. Nutr Neurosci. 2007;10(1–2):79–87.

33. Garcia-Souza EP, Da Silva SV, Felix GB, et al. Maternal protein restriction during early lactation induces GLUT4 translocation and mtor/akt activation in adipocytes of adult rats. Am J Physiol Endocrinol Metab. 2008;295:E626–36.
34. Sampaio de Freitas M, Garcia De Souza EP, Vargas da Silva S, et al. Up-regulation of phosphatidylinositol 3-kinase and glucose transporter 4 in muscle of rats subjected to maternal undernutrition. Biochim Biophys Acta. 2003;1639(1):8–16.
35. Sisk CL, Zehr JL. Pubertal hormones organize the adolescent brain and behavior. Front Neuroendocrinol. 2005;26(3–4):163–74.
36. Barella LF, de Oliveira JC, Branco RC, et al. Early exposure to a high-fat diet has more drastic consequences on metabolism compared with exposure during adulthood in rats. Horm Metab Res. 2012;44(6):458–64.
37. Gatford KL, Simmons RA, De Blasio MJ, et al. Review: placental programming of postnatal diabetes and impaired insulin action after IUGR. Placenta. 2010;31(Suppl):S60–5.
38. Steiner DJ, Kim A, Miller K, et al. Pancreatic islet plasticity: interspecies comparison of islet architecture and composition. Islets. 2010;2(3):135–45.
39. Heywood WE, Mian N, Milla PJ, et al. Programming of defective rat pancreatic beta-cell function in offspring from mothers fed a low-protein diet during gestation and the suckling periods. Clin Sci (Lond). 2004;107(1):37–45.
40. Ye L, Robertson MA, Mastracci TL, et al. An insulin signaling feedback loop regulates pancreas progenitor cell differentiation during islet development and regeneration. Dev Biol. 2016;409(2):354–69.
41. Miranda RA, Branco RC, Gravena C, et al. Swim training of monosodium L-glutamate-obese mice improves the impaired insulin receptor tyrosine phosphorylation in pancreatic islets. Endocrine. 2013;43(3):571–8.
42. Ruiz de Azua I, Gautam D, Guettier JM, et al. Novel insights into the function of beta-cell M3 muscarinic acetylcholine receptors: therapeutic implications. Trends Endocrinol Metab. 2011;22(2):74–80.
43. Haga K, Kruse AC, Asada H, et al. Structure of the human M2 muscarinic acetylcholine receptor bound to an antagonist. Nature. 2012;482(7386):547–51.
44. de Oliveira JC, Gomes RM, Miranda RA, et al. Protein restriction during the last third of pregnancy malprograms the neuroendocrine axes to induce metabolic syndrome in adult male rat offspring. Endocrinology. 2016;157(5):1799–812.
45. Grassiolli S, Gravena C, de Freitas Mathias PC. Muscarinic M2 receptor is active on pancreatic islets from hypothalamic obese rat. Eur J Pharmacol. 2007;556(1–3):223–8.
46. Scomparin DX, Gomes RM, Grassiolli S, et al. Autonomic activity and glycemic homeostasis are maintained by precocious and low intensity training exercises in MSG-programmed obese mice. Endocrine. 2009;36:510–7.
47. Miranda RA, Agostinho AR, Trevenzoli IH, et al. Insulin oversecretion in MSG-obese rats is related to alterations in cholinergic muscarinic receptor subtypes in pancreatic islets. Cell Physiol Biochem. 2014;33(4):1075–86.
48. Xie R, Carrano AC, Sander M. A systems view of epigenetic networks regulating pancreas development and beta-cell function. Wiley Interdiscip Rev Syst Biol Med. 2015;7(1):1–11.
49. Heijmans BT, Tobi EW, Stein AD, et al. Persistent epigenetic differences associated with prenatal exposure to famine in humans. Proc Natl Acad Sci U S A. 2008;105(44):17046–9.
50. Dominguez-Salas P, Moore SE, Baker MS, et al. Maternal nutrition at conception modulates DNA methylation of human metastable epialleles. Nat Commun. 2014;5:3746.
51. Radford EJ, Ito M, Shi H, et al. In utero effects. In utero undernourishment perturbs the adult sperm methylome and intergenerational metabolism. Science. 2014;345(6198):1255903.
52. Dayeh T, Volkov P, Salo S, et al. Genome-wide DNA methylation analysis of human pancreatic islets from type 2 diabetic and non-diabetic donors identifies candidate genes that influence insulin secretion. PLoS Genet. 2014;10(3):e1004160.
53. Yang BT, Dayeh TA, Volkov PA, et al. Increased DNA methylation and decreased expression of PDX-1 in pancreatic islets from patients with type 2 diabetes. Mol Endocrinol. 2012;26(7):1203–12.
54. Yang BT, Dayeh TA, Kirkpatrick CL, et al. Insulin promoter DNA methylation correlates negatively with insulin gene expression and positively with HbA(1c) levels in human pancreatic islets. Diabetologia. 2011;54(2):360–7.
55. Odom DT, Zizlsperger N, Gordon DB, et al. Control of pancreas and liver gene expression by HNF transcription factors. Science. 2004;303(5662):1378–81.
56. Sandovici I, Smith NH, Nitert MD, et al. Maternal diet and aging alter the epigenetic control of a promoter-enhancer interaction at the Hnf4a gene in rat pancreatic islets. Proc Natl Acad Sci U S A. 2011;108(13):5449–54.
57. Gunton JE, Kulkarni RN, Yim S, et al. Loss of ARNT/HIF1beta mediates altered gene expression and pancreatic-islet dysfunction in human type 2 diabetes. Cell. 2005;122(3):337–49.
58. Ding GL, Wang FF, Shu J, et al. Transgenerational glucose intolerance with Igf2/H19 epigenetic alterations in mouse islet induced by intrauterine hyperglycemia. Diabetes. 2012;61(5):1133–42.
59. Calderari S, Gangnerau MN, Thibault M, et al. Defective IGF2 and IGF1R protein production in embryonic pancreas precedes beta cell mass anomaly in the Goto-Kakizaki rat model of type 2 diabetes. Diabetologia. 2007;50(7):1463–71.
60. Hark AT, Schoenherr CJ, Katz DJ, et al. CTCF mediates methylation-sensitive enhancer-blocking activity at the H19/Igf2 locus. Nature. 2000;405(6785):486–9.

61. Kaffer CR, Grinberg A, Pfeifer K. Regulatory mechanisms at the mouse Igf2/H19 locus. Mol Cell Biol. 2001;21(23):8189–96.
62. Prentki M, Nolan CJ. Islet beta cell failure in type 2 diabetes. J Clin Invest. 2006;116(7):1802–12.
63. Brissova M, Blaha M, Spear C, et al. Reduced PDX-1 expression impairs islet response to insulin resistance and worsens glucose homeostasis. Am J Physiol Endocrinol Metab. 2005;288(4):E707–14.
64. Holland AM, Gonez LJ, Naselli G, et al. Conditional expression demonstrates the role of the homeodomain transcription factor Pdx1 in maintenance and regeneration of beta-cells in the adult pancreas. Diabetes. 2005;54(9):2586–95.
65. Park JH, Stoffers DA, Nicholls RD, et al. Development of type 2 diabetes following intrauterine growth retardation in rats is associated with progressive epigenetic silencing of Pdx1. J Clin Invest. 2008;118(6):2316–24.
66. Jaskelioff M, Peterson CL. Chromatin and transcription: histones continue to make their marks. Nat Cell Biol. 2003;5(5):395–9.
67. Ng SF, Lin RC, Laybutt DR, et al. Chronic high-fat diet in fathers programs beta-cell dysfunction in female rat offspring. Nature. 2010;467(7318):963–6.

Chapter 38
Pancreatic GABA and Serotonin Actions in the Pancreas and Fetal Programming of Metabolism

David J. Hill

Key Points

- Both GABA and serotonin are synthesized within the pancreatic islets of Langerhans as well as the central nervous system and exert local actions on insulin synthesis and release.
- GABA is synthesized within the β-cells of the islets and can have both a direct inhibitory action on insulin secretion and a stimulatory action on glucagon from adjacent α-cells.
- GABA can also promote proliferation and survival of β-cells.
- Intrauterine growth retardation causes long-term changes in GABA receptor subtype expression in the pancreas of the offspring that can have lifelong implications for metabolic control and the risk of metabolic disease.
- Serotonin is synthesized in β-cells by the tryptophan hydroxylase genes, and serotonin receptors are found on β-cells throughout life.
- The 5-HTr2b serotonin receptor promotes β-cell proliferation, while 5-HTr3a potentiates glucose-stimulated insulin release.
- During pregnancy placental lactogen and prolactin increase the expression of tryptophan hydroxylases within β-cells, resulting in β-cell proliferation as part of a maternal adaptation to the insulin resistance of pregnancy.
- Serotonin receptor gene expression is altered during suboptimal intrauterine growth by epigenetic modification, resulting in long-term changes of pancreatic serotonin action in the offspring that could provide a risk for metabolic disease.

Keywords Pancreas • β-cell • Islets of Langerhans • Serotonin • Gamma-aminobutyric acid • GABA receptor • Serotonin receptor

Abbreviations

5-HT	5-hydroxytryptophan
ACTH	Adrenocorticotrophic hormone
DNMT1	DNA methyltransferase 1

D.J. Hill, BSc, DPhil, FCAHS (✉)
Lawson Health Research Institute, St. Joseph's Health Care London, London Health Sciences Centre, and Western University, London, ON, Canada
e-mail: david.hill@lhrionhealth.ca

© Springer International Publishing AG 2017
R. Rajendram et al. (eds.), *Diet, Nutrition, and Fetal Programming*,
Nutrition and Health, DOI 10.1007/978-3-319-60289-9_38

GABA   Gamma-aminobutyric acid
GAD   Glutamic decarboxylase
GLP-1   Glucagon-like polypeptide 1
Glut2   Glucose transporter 2
IL-6   Interleukin-6
MCP1   Monocyte chemotactic protein 1
Pdx1   Pancreatic and duodenal homeobox 1
SERT   Serotonin transporter
SSRIs   Selective serotonin reuptake inhibitors
TNFα   Tumor necrosis factor-α
Tph   Tryptophan hydroxylase
VEGF   Vascular endothelial growth factor
VMAT2   Vesicular monoamine transporter 2

Epidemiological studies have clearly demonstrated associated risks for either impaired growth in utero or relative overgrowth of the fetus at term and chronic diseases in adulthood such as type 2 diabetes and cardiovascular disease [1]. The contributing phenotype includes both a relative insulin resistance within insulin-target tissues in the offspring and anatomical and functional deficiencies in the endocrine pancreas [2]. We, and others, have utilized rodent models to show that a relative dietary protein restriction administered to the mother during pregnancy and lactation [3–5] has long-term effects on the development of the endocrine pancreas and contributes to impaired glucose homeostasis in adulthood [6]. Maternal LP diet resulted in changes to the pancreatic islet morphology and a reduction of β-cell mass in the neonates [5, 7] through a decrease in β-cell proliferation, increased apoptosis, and diminished intra-islet vascularity [5, 8, 9]. The mechanisms responsible for long-lasting changes in pancreatic function include altered developmental expression of transcription factors and the presence of paracrine growth factors [10]. However, the endocrine pancreas also expresses neurotransmitters that are more commonly associated with synaptic function and development in the central and nervous system, but which have important paracrine actions within the islets of Langerhans. This review explores potential changes to the presence and actions of two such molecules, gamma-aminobutyric acid (GABA) and serotonin, that might contribute to fetal programming of adult metabolic disease.

GABA acts as an important inhibitory neurotransmitter that is found throughout the neurons of the cerebral cortex where it plays a role in vision, motor control, and higher cortical functions. A variety of GABA receptor agonists, such as the benzodiazepines, potentiate the GABA-induced reduction in neural activity and are useful in the treatment of anxiety, while drugs that induce GABA production are used for the control of epilepsy and Huntington's disease. Paradoxically, GABA has an excitatory role during brain development and drives the proliferation of neural progenitor cells and maturation of neurons in areas such as the hippocampus [11].

Conversely, serotonin (5-hydroxytryptophan) generally acts as a stimulator of neuronal activity and is involved with mood, appetite, pain recognition, cognition, and sleep cycle, among many other functions. Selective serotonin reuptake inhibitors (SSRIs) are widely used to raise synaptic levels of serotonin and elevate mood for the treatment of depression. Serotonin and other neurotransmitters are also involved in the hypothalamic control of the release of several pituitary hormones including ACTH, growth hormone, and prolactin. Both GABA and serotonin are also produced in non-neural tissues. The greatest generation of serotonin, approximately 80%, occurs in the gastrointestinal tract where it is produced by the enterochromaffin cells and contributes to gut motility [12]. Similar to GABA, serotonin contributes to peripheral tissue growth and development. Damage to the human liver is associated with an upregulation of the serotonin receptors 5-HT2a and 5-HT2b, which mediate a direct proliferative action of circulating serotonin on hepatocytes to enable a regeneration of liver mass [13].

Similarly, 5-HT2b receptors on osteocytes mediate an anabolic action of serotonin on bone accretion [14], while 5-HT1b receptors on endothelial cells mediate angiogenic effects of serotonin [15].

Both GABA and serotonin are expressed in the endocrine pancreas. GABA was shown to be enriched in the pancreas by Gerber and Hare in 1979 in rat [16] and was reduced following depletion of β-cells with streptozotocin. However, it was not until 1984 that GABA was linked physiologically to insulin secretion [17]. Although serotonin was shown to be present in pancreatic β-cells five decades ago [18], only recently has the potential importance to glucose homeostasis been recognized through a variety of mechanisms. Inappropriate presence or actions of both GABA and serotonin during intra-uterine and neonatal development can potentially cause long-term perturbations to the metabolic axis.

The GABA Signaling Pathway in the Endocrine Pancreas

As in the central nervous system, GABA expressed in the endocrine pancreas [19] is synthesized by glutamate decarboxylase (GAD) through the decarboxylation of L-glutamate [20]. The deactivating enzyme GABA transaminase [21] and GABA transporter proteins [22, 23] are similarly found associated with islets of Langerhans. GABAergic neurons present within the pancreas are closely associated and can penetrate the islet mantle [24, 25], but GABA is synthesized independently within the islet β-cells.

GABA is both utilized in an autocrine fashion and is released into the extracellular fluid and micro-circulation of the islets of Langerhans where it has paracrine actions to cross regulate islet hormone synthesis and release [26–29]. The majority of GABA is expressed and co-released from pancreatic β-cells together with insulin in response to hyperglycemia [23] and secretogogues such as glucagon-like polypeptide 1 (GLP-1) [30]. GABA is co-located within the large dense core vesicles of β-cells, from where it is exocytosed. In rodents considerably less GABA is synthesized within the islet endocrine cell types other than β-cells. However, in human islets the levels of GABA approach those found in the brain [31] due to synthesis in β-, α-, and δ-cells [32].

There are three GABA receptor forms present in the endocrine pancreas, the GABA-A, GABA-B, and GABA-C receptors. The GABA-A/GABA-C receptors belong to the superfamily of ligand-gated ion channels. The GABA-A receptor is an oligomeric chloride ion channel composed of up to five subunits. In rodent islets the subunits consist of α1, α4, β1, β2, β3, and γ3, and they are localized mainly in α-cells [33–36]. In human islets GABA-A receptors are found on all islet endocrine cell types [32]. Insulin can enhance GABA-A receptor presence on cells by causing translocation to the plasma membrane [37] through the Akt kinase second messenger system. Binding of GABA to the GABA-A receptor results in membrane hyperpolarization of the α-cell and a suppression of glucagon secretion [36] (Fig. 38.1). GABA-B receptors assemble as heteromers from GABA-B1 and GABA-B2 subunits [38–42], and two isoforms of GABA-B1 exist, GABA-B1a and GABA-B1b. These are generated by differential promoter usage of the GABA-B1 gene [39]. The GABA-B receptors are G-protein-coupled receptors that activate Gi/o second messenger proteins and mediate slower metabolic responses than GABA-A/GABA-C receptors. They are predominantly localized to β-cells in rat islets [43] (Fig. 38.2).

GABA regulates both insulin and glucagon release within the islets [26]. It has been proposed to have an inhibitory effect on insulin secretion through an autocrine negative feedback at high glucose concentrations [28]. In support of this role, activation of GABA-B receptors has been demonstrated to inhibit insulin secretion and suppress exocytosis of both insulin and GABA [43] (Fig. 38.1). Similarly, the administration of the GABA-B receptor agonist, baclofen, caused an inhibition of glucose-stimulated insulin secretion in rat islets [43] and the mouse MIN6 β-cell line [28]. Studies with GABA-B1 gene knockout mice showed that functional GABA-B receptors are essential for maintaining insulin content and secretion as well as glucose homeostasis [44] (Fig. 38.3). Such animals demonstrated a

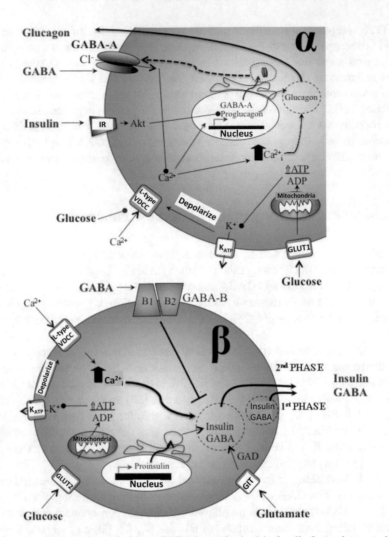

Fig. 38.1 GABA actions in the pancreatic islets. GABA is synthesized in β-cells from glutamate by glutamic acid decarboxylase (*GAD*) and co-secreted within granules with insulin upon stimulation by glucose. Glucose uptake by the GLUT2 transporter increases ATP causing ATP-dependent potassium (K_{ATP}) channels to close, preventing potassium (K^+) efflux, and results in membrane depolarization. The depolarization opens voltage-gated calcium (Ca^{2+}) channels and increases Ca^{2+} conductance. Increased intracellular Ca^{2+} allows for Ca^{2+}-dependent exocytosis of insulin-/GABA-containing granules within first and second phases. GABA can act on GABA-B receptors on the β-cells to inhibit insulin secretion. Insulin can inhibit proglucagon synthesis within the α-cells at a direct transcriptional level, acting through the insulin receptor and the activation of Akt. Also, insulin can inhibit glucagon secretion by promoting GABA-A receptor translocation to the plasma membrane resulting in an inhibition of hormone secretion by GABA. GABA-A receptor activation results in increased chloride ion (*Cl-*) conductance, hyperpolarization of α-cells, and prevention of glucagon secretion. Conversely, islet α-cells respond to an elevation of extracellular glucose levels by increasing the intracellular ATP/ADP ratio following glucose entry into the cell via GLUT1. The increase in ATP blocks the K_{ATP} channels and depolarizes the membrane potential, which activates voltage-gated Na^+ and Ca^{2+} channels, stimulating Ca^{2+} influx and eventually glucagon secretion

greater β-cell insulin content and secretion and also insulin resistance [44]. However, the actions of GABA on glucose-stimulated insulin release may be biphasic, since insulin secretion from isolated islets was inhibited by GABA over a 1-h incubation (Fig. 38.3), but a prior exposure to GABA for 45 min before incubation with a high glucose concentration enhanced insulin release [45]. This divergence may be due, in part, to an independent ability of GABA to increase somatostatin release from

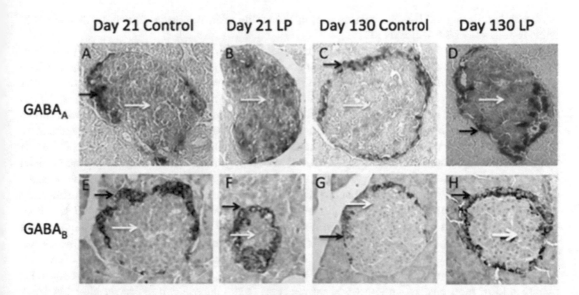

Fig. 38.2 Immunohistochemical localization of GABA-A and GABA-B receptors in pancreatic islets from rats born to mothers exposed to a low-protein diet during pregnancy. Representative micrographs of pancreatic islets at age 21 and 130 days from animals previously exposed to control or low-protein (*LP*) diet and stained for GABA-Aβ2/GABA-Aβ3 (**a–d** [*blue*]) and GABA-B2 (**e–h** [*gray*] and counterstained for glucagon [*brown*]). GABA-Aβ2/GABA-Aβ3 was predominantly localized to the alpha cells in the periphery of the islet (*black arrows*) with less intense staining in the beta cell-rich islet core (*white arrows*). GABA-B was localized to the islet core. No differences in distribution were noted with diet or age (Reproduced from Durst et al. [55])

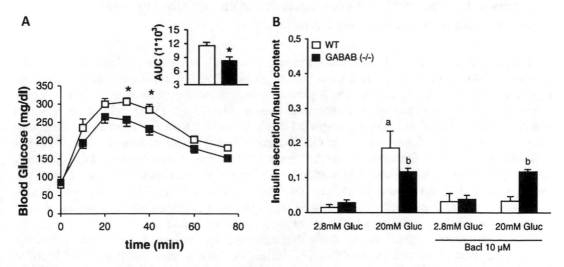

Fig. 38.3 Comparison of glucose tolerance and glucose-stimulated insulin release from islets in wild type and GABA-B −/− gene-knockout mice. (**a**) Blood glucose levels in wild type (WT, *open squares*) or GABA-B −/− knockout mice (*filled squares*) mice during a glucose tolerance test (GTT). Results were analyzed by two-way ANOVA with repeated measures design ($n − 16$ for each group): *$p < 0.03$ vs. wild type. Inset: area under the curve (AUC). *Open bars*, WT; *filled bars*, GABA-B −/−, *$p < 0.01$. (**b**) Glucose-stimulated insulin secretion in isolated islets from WT or GABA-B −/− mice in the presence or absence of the GABA-B agonist, baclofen (BACL). Results are expressed as insulin secretion/insulin content per incubation vial containing five islets each ($n − 4$ independent experiments). [a]$p < 0.01$ vs. 2.8 mM glucose in WT islets; [b]$p < 0.05$ vs. 2.8 mM glucose in GABA-B knockout islets. Baclofen inhibited glucose-stimulated insulin secretion in WT islets but had no effect on GABA-B −/− islets (Reproduced from Bonaventura et al. [44])

islet δ-cells utilizing GABA-A receptors [46] or the ability of insulin to negatively feedback within islets to reduce GABA synthesis [47].

Independently of effects on insulin secretion, GABA was also shown to increase β-cell proliferation, to prevent β-cell loss, and to normalize glucose tolerance in mice treated with multiple low-dose streptozotocin (STZ) to deplete β-cell mass [33] or partially pancreatectomy [48]. Similarly, GABA reduced insulitis, prevented β-cell apoptosis, and restored β-cell mass in the nonobese diabetic (NOD) mouse model of type 1 diabetes [33]. The ability of GABA to promote β-cell survival has been shown in rodents to be mediated by GABA-A receptors on β-cells, although these are much less abundant than the GABA-B receptors [33]. The trophic effects of GABA on β-cells also involve GABA-B receptor isoforms since deletion of the GABA-B receptor gene in mice disrupted pancreatic islet development with a reduction in islet number and an increased abundance of small, immature endocrine cell clusters [49]. This implies that any disruption to GABA synthesis or signaling during early development will have long-term implications for insulin availability. In isolated human islets, both GABA-A and GABA-B receptor types are responsible for the ability of GABA to promote β-cell proliferation [50, 51]. This may be relevant to the risk of development of type 2 diabetes which has been associated with a reduced expression of GABA-A receptors in human islets [52].

GABA release from the β-cells is also able to inhibit glucagon release from adjacent α-cells in rat pancreas [36], mouse islets, and perfused rat pancreas [53]. Glucose can indirectly alter GABA-A receptor gene expression within the α-cells [54] by inhibiting voltage-dependent calcium channels to prevent the rise in intracellular calcium following receptor stimulation. A lowering of calcium concentrations then releases a negative regulation of GABA-A receptor gene expression [54], resulting in an upregulation and leading to increased receptor trafficking to the α-cell membrane and an inhibition of glucagon secretion (Fig. 38.1).

Changes to the Pancreatic GABA Signaling Pathway During Fetal Programming of Adult Glucose Intolerance

We examined whether maternal nutritional imbalance in utero might result in persistent changes in the pancreatic GABA system that might contribute to an increased risk of diabetes in the offspring. L-glutamate levels, representing the GABA precursor, were reduced in pancreas at birth in offspring of rats given a LP diet throughout gestation until weaning [55]. In adult rats a prior exposure to LP diet in fetal and neonatal life caused changes in GABA-A subunit expression in pancreas when compared to animals that had received control diet. In adult offspring the abundance of GABA-Aβ3 subunit mRNA was much decreased in the LP group (Table 38.1). L-arginine-stimulated glucagon secretion and gene expression were increased in LP-fed rats, and this persists into adulthood. However, the expression of GABA-B receptor and GAD within islets was unaltered. These long-term changes to GABA-A receptor expression and glucagon secretion could contribute to the impaired glucose tolerance that develops in offspring of LP-fed mothers during adulthood [6].

Fetal programming of postnatal metabolic dysfunction could also be mediated via the pancreatic GABAergic pathways through the availability of taurine. Taurine is a nonessential amino acid derived from the metabolism of methionine and cysteine and is a normal dietary constituent [56, 57]. While present in most mammalian tissues, it is particularly enriched in the brain and pancreas [6]. In the pregnant rat given with LP diet, circulating levels of taurine were reduced in both maternal and fetal blood. Supplementation of the diet with taurine alone was able to reverse the long-term deficits in the offspring in islet vascularity, β-cell mass, and glucose- and amino acid-dependent insulin release [58–60]. Also, taurine addition to culture medium prevented IL-1 and TNFα-induced apoptosis in isolated islets [61]. Taurine is a potent GABA agonist and has acute effects through interaction with

Table 38.1 Messenger RNA expression measured with qPCR for GABA-Aα1, GABA-Aα4, GABA-Aβ1, GABA-Aβ2, GABA-Aβ3, and GABA-Aγ3 subunits, GABA-B1 and GABAB2, and GAD65 in islets isolated at 130 days age from rats that had previously received control of low-protein (LP)diet. Values represent mean ± SEM, relative to the reference gene HPRT and derived from 7 to 8 animals per group

Subunit	Control	LP
GABA-Aα1	5.6 ± 1.1	9.3 ± 1.2*
GABA-Aα4	2.6 ± 0.3	3.4 ± 0.4
GABA-Aβ1	2.5 ± 0.1	4.6 ± 0.2***
GABA-Aβ2	3.5 ± 0.2	6.1 ± 1.2*
GABA-Aβ3	12.4 ± 2.3	3.8 ± 0.3*
GABA-Aγ3	4.0 ± 0.2	5.4 ± 0.3*
GABA-B1	3.8 ± 0.3	4.4 ± 0.5
GABA-B2	1.6 ± 0.1s	1.7 ± 0.1
GAD65	4.3 ± 0.5	5.9 ± 0.6

Reproduced from Durst et al. [55]
Values represent mean ± SEM, relative to the reference gene HPRT and derived from 7 to 8 animals per group
*$p < 0.05$
***$p < 0.001$ vs. control

the GABA-A receptors to decrease insulin release and deplete cellular levels of GABA [62]. A depletion of intracellular GABA could subsequently restrict interactions with the GABA-B receptors.

An alternative pathway by which GABA may be involved in fetal programming of glucose intolerance involves the selection of pancreatic endocrine progenitors during pancreatic organogenesis and also during adaptive changes to β-cell mass deriving from progenitors postnatally. Pancreatic progenitors expressing the transcription factor Pdx1, but not yet insulin, also exhibit a high level of expression of GAD and GABA-A receptor subtypes from as early as E15.5 in mouse [63]. The ontogeny of expression of GAD and GABA-A receptors mirrored the development of functional β-cells suggesting that GABA signaling may be associated with endocrine lineage commitment. Changes in the pancreatic GABAergic system in development may respond to nutritional or other environmental changes in utero due to differential genetic or epigenetic modulation of gene expression. Two isoforms of GAD exist through the differential expression of two separate genes, GAD 65 and GAD67. A number of splice variants of GAD67 were identified in human fetal pancreas from as early as 14 weeks' gestation, which might differentially control GABA synthesis [64]. Additionally, epigenetic differences due to differential gene methylation exist in the neuronal production of GABA, representing a risk factor for schizophrenia, and in GAD activity in the cerebellum with an association to autism [65, 66].

Serotonin Synthesis Within the Pancreas

Serotonin is synthesized from tryptophan by two enzymes, tryptophan hydroxylase 1 (Tph1) and Tph2, both of which are present in β-cells [67]. This differs from other tissues where Tph2 is the dominant form in the central nervous system, while Tph1 is predominantly expressed in peripheral tissues. The expression of Tph1 is maximal in neonatal life in the rodent pancreas [67]. Also expressed is the transcription factor Pet1 whose expression is required for serotonin synthesis, being under the control of Nkx2.2 within the β-cells [67]. Pet1 directly activates the serotonin-synthesizing genes and also has insulin gene regulatory elements and facilitates the production of insulin and Glut2. Ablation of Pet1 in mice is associated with reduced insulin synthesis and glucose intolerance [67]. Pancreatic β-cells also express dopamine decarboxylase, which catalyzes the final stage of serotonin production and facilitates storage of serotonin precursor molecules, as well as the transporter molecule VMAT2 is responsible for packaging serotonin into secretory granules where it is co-released with insulin [68, 69]. Serotonin degradation is accomplished through the presence of monoamine oxidases A and B within β-cells.

Serotonin receptors are predominantly members of the G-protein-coupled receptor class and comprise at least seven subtypes (5-HTr1–7) [70]. 5-HTr3 differs in that it is a ligand-gated ion channel receptor. The 5-HTr1A, 5-HTr1D, and 5-HTr2A receptors are found on both β- and α-cells, while 5-HTr2B is only present on β-cells [71]. The HTr2B receptor is coupled to the $G_{\alpha q}$ G-protein subunit [72]. Other studies additionally identified 5-HTr3 on β-cells [73], although receptor abundance differentially changes during development and during pregnancy, as subsequently described.

Serotonin Action in the Pancreas

Serotonin synthesis and release from β-cells have been shown to be glucose dependent [71, 74]. However, transgenic mice lacking the *tph1*gene, or the *5-Htr2b* or *5-Htr3a* receptor genes, do not become glucose intolerant on a normal diet [75], but can become glucose intolerant in later adulthood with a primary lesion being a failure to release insulin- and serotonin-containing granules [76]. The morphology, number, and size of islets were not altered compared to wild-type animals. However, exposure of fetal rats to the serotonin reuptake inhibitor, sertraline hydrochloride, did reduce β-cell mass at birth through a decreased islet size and a reduced expression of key developmental transcription factors such as neurogenin3, Pdx1, and MafA [77]. The islet vasculature was also reduced along with the pancreatic expression of vascular endothelial growth factor (VEGF), suggesting that some of the effects on islet development may have been indirect. When *tph1* gene or *5-Htr2b* or *5-Htr3a* gene knockout mice were maintained on a high-fat diet for 6 weeks from 4 weeks of age, then *tph1*- and *5-Htr3a*-deficient animals showed impaired glucose tolerance, but not those lacking *5-Htr2b* [75]. Perifusion of isolated islets from *Tph1*- and *5-Htr3a*-deficient mice showed a lack of first phase insulin release, but there were no changes to islet morphology or transcription factor gene expression. These findings imply that in nonpregnant, adult mice serotonin action of the β-cells is mediated predominantly through the 5-HTr3a receptor.

Serotonin and Pancreatic Function During Pregnancy

Serotonin synthesis within the pancreas contributes to the two- to threefold increase in β-cell mass that occurs during pregnancy in both rodents and humans. This involves a reentry of normally nonproliferative β-cells back into the cell proliferation cycle, in addition to a recruitment and maturation of resident pancreatic endocrine progenitor cells [78, 79]. The latter process may be the predominant mechanism in human pregnancy [80]. A major hormonal driver for the increase in maternal β-cell mass is circulating placental lactogen, acting via the prolactin receptor [81]. Placental lactogen also increases local islet levels of serotonin, which directly increases both β-cell proliferation and glucose-stimulated insulin secretion during pregnancy. A primary action of placental lactogen is to increase the expression of Tph1 and Tph2 within β-cells, resulting in an increased synthesis, content, and exocytosis of serotonin [82] (Fig. 38.4). During pregnancy the ability of serotonin to modulate β-cell mass is mediated by the 5-HTr2b receptor in mid-gestation in mouse and 5-HTr1d in late gestation [83]. The expression levels of the 5-HTr2b receptor increase dramatically in pregnant mouse β-cells between E6 and E15, while 5-HTr1d expression is increased following E16 and postpartum [83]. Thus signaling via the 5-HTr1d receptor may represent an inhibitory growth signal to limit the increase in β-cell mass close to term and trigger the homeostatic apoptosis that occurs postpartum. However,

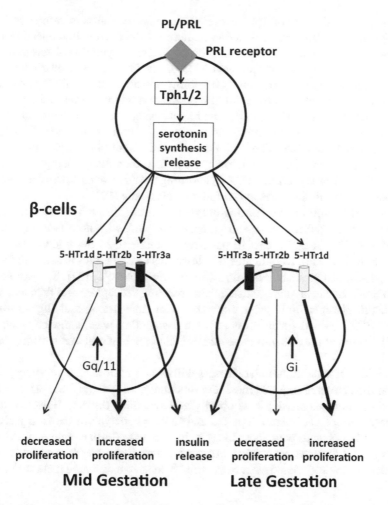

Fig. 38.4 Paracrine actions of serotonin on pancreatic β-cell proliferation and insulin release during pregnancy in a mouse model. Placental lactogen and prolactin signal through the prolactin receptor (*PRL*) to increase expression of the serotonin-synthesizing enzymes, Tph1 and Tph2. This results in the co-release of insulin and serotonin within insulin granules. Extracellular serotonin signals to adjacent β-cells via the 5-HT21d receptor to promote glucose-stimulated insulin release. In mid-gestation serotonin signaling via 5-HTr2b and the activation of the Gq/11 G-protein subunit promote β-cell replication. However, the expression of 5-HTr2b declines in late gestation to be replaced by 5-HTr3a, which inhibits further β-cell proliferation through the activation of the Gi subunit

the 5-HTr3a receptor is required for adequate glucose-stimulated insulin release (Fig. 38.4). Consequently, animals null for *5-HTr3a* show glucose intolerance during pregnancy despite undergoing the adaptation of β-cell mass [72].

Mechanisms by Which the Serotonin Axis Can Contribute Fetal Programming of Adult Glucose Intolerance

Two main tissue foci exist whereby serotonin availability or action might impact the development of normal metabolic homeostasis, resulting in an increased risk of adult metabolic disease. The first of these is serotonin synthesis and release from the placenta and the second the efficiency of the adaptive increase in β-cell mass within the maternal pancreas.

The placenta is an active site of Tph1 expression and the synthesis of serotonin from maternally derived tryptophan [84]. Nutritional restriction in utero is associated with reduced levels of both free and albumin-bound tryptophan in the mother, reduced placental synthesis of serotonin, and less tryptophan available for fetal tissue development [85]. Intrauterine growth restriction in the baboons caused by a 30% reduction in maternal food availability was associated with impaired development of serotonergic neurons in the fetus [86]. Serotonin production within the placenta was also reduced as a result of maternal stress [87]. Fetal nutritional imbalance or stress can also result in changes to the expression of the placental 5-HTr2a serotonin receptor, which mediates the actions of serotonin on placental growth and thereby fetal size [87]. Paquette and Marsit [88] showed that the *5-Htr2a* gene is subject to epigenetic control of expression and can be differentially methylated by DNA methyltransferase 1 (DNMT1), as is the gene (*slc6a4*) encoding the cellular serotonin transporter, SERT, that allows reuptake of serotonin from the intracellular environment [89].

Interference in the serotonin axis during pregnancy in rats through the administration of SSRIs resulted in changes to insulin release and glucose intolerance in the offspring, leading to type 2 diabetes. This was mediated, at least in part, by an increase in the underlying levels of tissue inflammation in the offspring as indicated by elevations in tissue tumor necrosis factor α (TNFα), interleukin-6 (IL-6), and monocyte chemotactic protein 1 (MCP1) [77]. The atypical antipsychosis drugs such as clozapine are antagonists for the serotonin receptors 5-HTr2a and 5-Htr1a, which are present in the placenta. Following treatment with such drugs, a change in the methylation status of the SERT gene was also observed. An association was found between the degree of placental methylation of the *5-Htr2a* gene and deficits in behavioral and learning outcomes in the offspring [90].

It is reasonable to assume that similar changes will occur in serotonin receptivity within the maternal pancreas to the detriment of β-cell mass and function, predisposing the mother to hyperglycemia and the offspring to an increased risk of obesity and metabolic disease. However, direct effects of these drugs may also impact the development and future phenotype of the fetal pancreas. Neonatal rats exposed to SSRIs in utero were more likely to have reduced birth weight and an increased risk of development of adult diabetes, associated with a reduction in pancreatic β-cell area at birth and an altered expression of transcription factors controlling β-cell neogenesis and maturation and a decreased survival of β-cells [79].

Conclusions

While a number of systemic and locally produced cytokines and adipokines, such as leptin and adiponectin, are well documented to alter β-cell function and survival, it is clear that the islets of Langerhans, and especially the β-cells, synthesize neurotransmitter molecules such as GABA and serotonin. These appear to have largely autocrine and paracrine actions within individual islets that include β-cell proliferation, survival, and glucose-stimulated insulin exocytosis. A key level of control appears to be a diverse expression of both GABA and serotonin receptor isotypes that are differentially expressed during development and during postnatal metabolic adaptations, such as pregnancy. An altered β-cell mass and phenotype that can persist throughout life are associated with offspring from compromised pregnancy resulting in intrauterine growth retardation. Both the paracrine GABA and serotonin axes within the islets are altered following such a prenatal experience and could contribute to the increased risk of type 2 diabetes seen in the offspring.

References

1. Barker DJ, Hales CN, Fall CH, et al. Type 2 (non-insulin-dependent) diabetes mellitus, hypertension and hyperlipidemia (syndrome X): relation to reduced fetal growth. Diabetologia. 1993;36:62–7.
2. Hill DJ. Nutritional programming of pancreatic β-cell plasticity. World J Diabetes. 2011;2:119–32.
3. Desai M, Crowther NJ, Lucas A, et al. Organ-selective growth in the offspring of protein-restricted mothers. Br J Nutr. 1996;76:591–603.
4. Fernandez-Twinn DS, Wayman A, Ekizoglou S, et al. Maternal protein restriction leads to hyperinsulinemia and reduced insulin-signaling protein expression in 21-mo-old female rat offspring. Am J Phys Regul Integr Comp Phys. 2005;288:R368–73.
5. Petrik J, Reusens B, Arany E, et al. A low protein diet alters the balance of islet cell replication and apoptosis in the fetal and neonatal rat and is associated with a reduced pancreatic expression of insulin-like growth factor-II. Endocrinology. 1999;140:4861–73.
6. Chamson-Reig A, Thyssen SM, Hill DJ, et al. Exposure of the pregnant rat to low protein diet causes impaired glucose homeostasis in the young adult offspring by different mechanisms in males and females. Exp Biol Med. 2009;234:1425–36.
7. Petrik J, Arany E, McDonald TJ, et al. Apoptosis in the pancreatic islet cells of the neonatal rat is associated with a reduced expression of insulin-like growth factor II that may act as a survival factor. Endocrinology. 1998;139:2994–3004.
8. Boujendar S, Arany E, Hill DJ, et al. Taurine supplementation of a low protein diet fed to rat dams normalizes the vascularization of the fetal endocrine pancreas. J Nutr. 2003;133:2820–5.
9. Cherif H, Reusens B, Ahn MT, et al. Effects of taurine on the insulin secretion of rat fetal islets from dams fed a low-protein diet. J Endocrinol. 1998;159:341–8.
10. Hill DJ, Beamish C, Hill TG. Mechanisms of plasticity of pancreatic β-cell mass. Curr Trends Endocrinol. 2014;7:57–79.
11. Wang DD, Kreigstein AR, Ben-Ari Y. GABA regulates stem cell proliferation before nervous system formation. Epilepsy Curr. 2008;8:137–9.
12. Manocha M, Khan WI. Serotonin and GI disorders: an update on clinical and experimental studies. Clin Trans Gastroenterol. 2012;3:e13.
13. Ebrahimkhani MR, Oakley F, Murphy LB, et al. Stimulating healthy tissue regeneration by targeting the 5-HT$_2$B receptor in chronic liver disease. Nat Med. 2011;17:1668–73.
14. Locker M, Bitard J, Collet C, et al. Stepwise control of osteogenic differentiation by 5-HT(2B) receptor signaling: nitric oxide production and phospholipase A2 activation. Cell Signal. 2006;18:628–39.
15. Ishida T, Kawashima S, Hirata K, et al. Nitric oxide is produced via 5-HT1B and 5-HT2B receptor activation in human coronary artery endothelial cells. Kobe J Med Sci. 1998;44:51–63.
16. Gerber JC, Hare TA. Gamma-aminobutyric acid in peripheral tissue, with emphasis on the endocrine pancreas: presence in two species and reduction by streptozotocin. Diabetes. 1979;28:1073–6.
17. Cavagnini F, Pinto M, Dubini A, et al. Effects of gamma aminobutyric acid (GABA) and muscimol on endocrine pancreatic function in man. Metabolism. 1982;31:73–7.
18. Gershon MD, Ross LL, et al. Location of sites of 5-hydroxytryptamine storage and metabolism by radioautography. J Physiol. 1966;186:477–92.
19. Okada Y, Taniguchi H, Schimada C. High concentration of GABA and high glutamate decarboxylase activity in rat pancreatic islets and human insulinoma. Science. 1976;194:620–2.
20. Wang C, Mao R, Van de Casteele M, et al. Glucagon-like peptide-1 stimulates GABA formation by pancreatic beta-cells at the level of glutamate decarboxylase. Am J Physiol Endocrinol Metab. 2007;294:E1201–6.
21. Wang C, Kerckhofs K, Van de Casteele M, et al. Glucose inhibits GABA release by pancreatic beta-cells through an increase in GABA shunt activity. Am J Physiol Endocrinol Metab. 2006;290:E494–9.
22. Chessler SD, Simonson WT, Sweet IR, et al. Expression of the vesicular inhibitory amino acid transporter in pancreatic islet cells: distribution of the transporter within rat islets. Diabetes. 2002;51:1763–71.
23. Gammelsaeter R, Froyland M, Aragon C, et al. Glycine, GABA and their transporters in pancreatic islets of Langerhans: evidence for a paracrine transmitter interplay. J Cell Sci. 2004;117:3749–58.
24. Saravia-Fernandez F, Faveeuw C, Blasquez-Bulant C, et al. Localization of gamma-aminobutyric acid and glutamic acid decarboxylase in the pancreas of the nonobese diabetic mouse. Endocrinology. 1996;137:3497–506.
25. Sorenson RL, Garry DG, Brelje TC. Structural and functional considerations of GABA in islets of Langerhans. Beta-cells and nerves. Diabetes. 1991;40:1365–74.
26. Satin LS, Kinard TA. Neurotransmitters and their receptors in the islets of Langerhans of the pancreas: what messages do acetylcholine, glutamate, and GABA transmit? Endocrine. 1998;8:213–23.
27. Braun M, Wendt A, Buschard K, et al. GABAB receptor activation inhibits exocytosis in rat pancreatic beta-cells by G-protein-dependent activation of calcineurin. J Physiol. 2001;559:397–409.

28. Brice NL, Varadi A, Ashcroft SJ, et al. Metabotropic glutamate and GABA(B) receptors contribute to the modulation of glucose-stimulated insulin secretion in pancreatic beta cells. Diabetologia. 2002;45:242–52.

29. Shi Y, Kanaani J, Menard-Rose V, et al. Increased expression of GAD65 and GABA in pancreatic beta-cells impairs first-phase insulin secretion. Am J Physiol Endocrinol Metab. 2000;279:E684–94.

30. Wang C, Mao R, Van de Casteele M, et al. Glucagon-like peptide-1 stimulates GABA formation by pancreatic beta cells at the level of glutamate decarboxylase. Am J Physiol Endocrinol Metab. 2007;292:E1201–6.

31. Michalik M, Erecińska M. GABA in pancreatic islets: metabolism and function. Biochem Pharmacol. 1992;44:1–9.

32. Caicedo A. Paracrine and autocrine interactions in the human islet: more than meets the eye. Semin Cell Dev Biol. 2013;24:11–21.

33. Soltani N, Qiu H, Aleksic M, et al. GABA exerts protective and regenerative effects on islet beta cells and reverse diabetes. Proc Natl Acad Sci U S A. 2011;108:11692–7.

34. Nayeem N, Green TP, Martin IL, et al. Quaternary structure of the native GABA-A receptor determined by electron microscopic image analysis. J Neurochem. 1994;62:815–8.

35. Tretter V, Ehya N, Fuchs K, et al. Stoichiometry and assembly of a recombinant GABAA receptor subtype. J Neurosci. 1997;17:2728–37.

36. Wendt A, Birnir B, Buschard K, et al. Glucose inhibition of glucagon secretion from rat alpha-cells is mediated by GABA released from neighboring beta-cells. Diabetes. 2004;53:1038–45.

37. Xu E, Kumar M, Zhang Y, et al. Intra-islet insulin suppresses glucagon release via GABA-GABAA receptor system. Cell Metab. 2006;3:47–58.

38. Bettler B, Kaupmann K, Mosbacher J, et al. Molecular structure and physiological functions of GABA(B) receptors. Physiol Rev. 2004;84:835–67.

39. Kaupmann K, Huggel K, Heid J, et al. Expression cloning of GABA B receptors uncovers similarity to metabotropic glutamate receptors. Nature. 1997;386:239–46.

40. Kaupmann K, Malitschek B, Schuler B, et al. GABA B receptor subtypes assemble into functional heteromeric complexes. Nature. 1998;396:683–7.

41. Kuner R, Kohr G, Grunewald S, et al. Role of heteromer formation in GABAB receptor function. Science. 1999;283:74–7.

42. White J, Wise A, Main M, et al. Heterodimerization is required for the formation of a functional GABAB receptor. Nature. 1998;396:679–82.

43. Marshall FH, Jones KA, Kaupmann K, et al. GABAB receptors – the first 7TM heterodimers. Trends Pharmacol Sci. 1999;20:396–9.

44. Bonaventura MM, Catalano PN, Chamson-Reig A, et al. GABA-B receptors and glucose homeostasis: evaluation in GABA-B receptor knock-out mice. Am J Physiol Endocrinol Metab. 2008;294:E157–67.

45. Faraji F, Ghasemi A, Motamedi F, et al. Time-dependent effect of GABA on glucose-stimulated insulin secretion from isolated islets in rat. Scand J Clin Lab Invest. 2011;71:462–6.

46. Braun M, Ramracheya R, Bengtsson M, et al. Gamma-aminobutyric acid (GABA) is an autocrine excitatory transmitter in human pancreatic beta-cells. Diabetes. 2010;59:1694–701.

47. Bansal P, Wang S, Liu S, et al. GABA coordinates with insulin in regulating secretory function in pancreatic INS-1 β-cells. PLoS One. 2011;6:e26225.

48. Wang Z, Purwana I, Zhao F, et al. β-cell proliferation is associated with increased A-type γ-aminobutyric acid receptor expression in pancreatectomized mice. Pancreas. 2013;42:545–8.

49. Crivello M, Bonaventura MM, Chamson-Reig A, et al. Postnatal development of the endocrine pancreas in mice lacking functional GABAB receptors. Am J Physiol Endocrinol Metab. 2013;304:E1064–76.

50. Tian J, Dang H, Chen Z, et al. γ-aminobutyric acid regulates both the survival and replication of human β-cells. Diabetes. 2013;62:3760–5.

51. Purwana I, Zheng J, Li X, et al. GABA promotes human β-cell proliferation and modulates glucose homeostasis. Diabetes. 2014;63:4197–41205.

52. Taneera J, Jin Z, Jin Y, et al. γ-aminobutyric acid (GABA) signalling in human pancreatic islets is altered in type 2 diabetes. Diabetologia. 2012;55:1985–94.

53. Gilon P, Bertrand G, Loubatieres-Mariani MM, et al. The influence of gamma-aminobutyric acid on hormone release by mouse and rat endocrine pancreas. Endocrinology. 1991;129:2521–9.

54. Bailey SJ, Ravier MA, Rutter GA. Glucose-dependent regulation of gamma- aminobutyric acid (GABA A) receptor expression in mouse pancreatic islet alpha-cells. Diabetes. 2007;56:320–7.

55. Durst MA, Lux-Lantos VA, Hardy DB, et al. Protein restriction during early life in rats alters pancreatic GABA$_a$ receptor subunit expression and glucagon secretion in adulthood. Can J Diabetes. 2012;36:101–8.

56. Huxtable RJ. Physiological actions of taurine. Physiol Rev. 1992;72:101–63.

57. Huxtable R, Fanconi F, Gironi A. The biology of taurine. Methods and mechanisms. New York: Plenum Press; 1987.

58. Chamson-Reig A, Thyssen S, Arany E, et al. Altered pancreatic morphology in the offspring of pregnant rats given reduced dietary protein is time and gender specific. J Endocrinol. 2006;191:83–92.

59. Serradas P, Goya L, Lacorne M, et al. Fetal insulin and insulin-like growth factor-2 production is impaired in the GK rat model of type 2 diabetes. Diabetes. 2002;51:392–7.

60. Boujender S, Reusens B, Merezak S, et al. Taurine supplementation to a low protein diet during foetal and early postnatal life restores normal proliferation and apoptosis of rat pancreatic islets. Diabetologia. 2002;45:856–66.
61. Merezak S, Hardikar AA, Yajnik CS, et al. Intrauterine low protein diet increases fetal ß cell sensitivity to NO and IL-1ß: the protective role of taurine. J Endocrinol. 2001;171:299–308.
62. Cuttitta CM, Guariglia SR, Idrissi AE, et al. Taurine's effects on the neuroendocrine functions of pancreatic β cells. Adv Exp Med Biol. 2013;775:299–310.
63. Feng MM, Xiang YY, Wang S, et al. An autocrine γ-aminobutyric acid signaling system exists in pancreatic β-cell progenitors of fetal and postnatal mice. Int J Physiol Pathophysiol Pharmacol. 2013;27:91–101.
64. Korpershoek E, Verwest AM, Ijzendoorn Y, et al. Expression of GAD67 and novel GAD67 splice variants during human fetal pancreas development: GAD67 expression in the fetal pancreas. Endocr Pathol. 2007;18:31–6.
65. Kozlenkov A, Wang M, Roussos P, et al. Substantial DNA methylation differences between two major neuronal subtypes in human brain. Nucleic Acids Res. 2015;44:2593.
66. Peedicayil J, Thangavelu P. Purkinje cell loss in autism may involve epigenetic changes in the gene encoding GAD. Med Hypotheses. 2008;71:978.
67. Ohta Y, Kosaka Y, Kishimoto N, et al. Convergence of the insulin and serotonin programs in the pancreatic β-cell. Diabetes. 2011;60:3208–16.
68. Borelli MI, Villar MJ, Orezzoli A, et al. Presence of DOPA decarboxylase and its localisation in adult rat pancreatic islet cells. Diabete Metab. 1997;23:161–3.
69. Sakano D, Shiraki N, Kikawa K, et al. VMAT2 identified as a regulator of late-stage β-cell differentiation. Nat Chem Biol. 2014;10:141–8.
70. El-Merahbi R, Loffler M, Mayer A, et al. The roles of peripheral serotonin in metabolic homeostasis. FEBS Lett. 2015;589:1728–34.
71. Bennet H, Mollet IG, Balhuizen A, et al. Serotonin (5-HT) receptor 2b activation augments glucose-stimulated insulin secretion in human and mouse islets of Langerhans. Diabetologia. 2016;59:744–54.
72. OHara-Imaizumi M, Kim H, Yoshida M, et al. Serotonin regulates glucose-stimulated insulin secretion from pancreatic beta cells during pregnancy. Proc Natl Acad Sci U S A. 2013;110:19420–5.
73. Amisten S, Salehi A, Rorsman P, et al. An atlas and functional analysis of G-protein coupled receptors in human islets of Langerhans. Pharmacol Ther. 2013;139:359–91.
74. Peschke E, Peschke D, Hammer T, et al. Influence of melatonin and serotonin on glucose-stimulated insulin release from perifused rat pancreatic islets in vitro. J Pineal Res. 1997;23:156–63.
75. Kim K, Oh C-H, Ohara-Imaizumi M, et al. Functional role of serotonin in insulin secretion in a diet-induced insulin-resistant state. Endocrinology. 2015;156:444–52.
76. Paulmann N, Grohmann M, Voigt JP, et al. Intracellular serotonin modulates insulin secretion from pancreatic beta-cells by protein serotonylation. PLoS Biol. 2009;7:e1000229.
77. De Long N, Gutgesall MK, Petrik JJ, et al. Fetal exposure to sertraline hydrochloride impairs pancreatic β-cell development. Endocrinology. 2015;156:1952–7.
78. Sorenson RL, Brelje TC. Adaptation of islets of Langerhans to pregnancy: beta-cell growth, enhanced insulin secretion and the role of lactogenic hormones. Horm Metab Res. 1997;29:301–7.
79. Abouna S, Old RW, Pelengaris S, et al. Non-β-cell progenitors of β-cells in pregnant mice. Organ. 2010;6:125–33.
80. Butler AE, Cao-Minh L, Galasso R, et al. Adaptive changes in pancreatic beta cell fractional area and beta cell turnover in human pregnancy. Diabetologia. 2010;53:2167–76.
81. Freemark M, Avril I, Fleenor D, et al. Targeted deletion of the PRL receptor: effects on islet development, insulin production, and glucose tolerance. Endocrinology. 2002;43:1378–85.
82. Schraenen A, Lemaire K, de Faudeur G, et al. Placental lactogens induce serotonin biosynthesis in a subset of mouse beta cells during pregnancy. Diabetologia. 2010;53:2589–99.
83. Kim H, Toyofuku Y, Lynn FC, et al. Serotonin regulates pancreatic beta cell mass during pregnancy. Nat Med. 2010;16:804–8.
84. Bonnin A, Goeden N, Chen K, et al. A transient placental source of serotonin for the fetal forebrain. Nature. 2011;472:347–50.
85. Sano M, Ferchaud-Roucher V, Kaeffer B, et al. Maternal and fetal tryptophan metabolism in gestating rats: effects of intrauterine growth restriction. Amino Acids. 2016;48:281–90.
86. Ye W, Xie L, Li C, Nathanielsz PW, et al. Impaired development of fetal serotonergic neurons in intrauterine growth restricted baboons. J Med Primatol. 2014;43:284–7.
87. St-Pierre J, Laurent L, King S et al. Effects of prenatal maternal stress on serotonin and fetal development. Placenta. 2015; S0143-4004(15)30094-1. doi: 10.1016/j.placenta.2015.11.013. [Epub ahead of print].
88. Paquette AG, Marsit CJ. The developmental basis of epigenetic regulation of HTR2A and psychiatric outcomes. J Cell Biochem. 2014;115:2065–72.
89. Philibert R, Madan A, Andersen A, et al. Serotonin transporter mRNA levels are associated with the methylation of an upstream CpG island. Am J Med Genet B Neuropsychiatr Genet. 2007;144B:101–5.
90. Holloway T, González-Maeso J. Epigenetic mechanisms of serotonin signaling. ACS Chem Neurosci. 2015;6:1099–109.

Chapter 39
Maternal Malnutrition, Glucocorticoids, and Fetal Programming: A Role for Placental 11β-Hydroxysteroid Dehydrogenase Type 2

Emily K. Chivers and Caitlin S. Wyrwoll

Key Points

- Frequently underlying the association between maternal malnutrition and developmental programming outcomes is increased placental and fetal exposure to glucocorticoids.
- Glucocorticoids are stress hormones which, while essential for fetal maturation in late gestation, are detrimental in excess as they restrict placental and fetal growth and development.
- Exposure of the fetus to glucocorticoids is tightly controlled by placental expression of the enzyme 11β-HSD2, which converts glucocorticoids to their inactive form.
- Direct manipulation of glucocorticoid parameters in animal models reveals that glucocorticoid excess restricts fetal growth and cause adverse health outcomes in later life.
- Glucocorticoid overexposure also adversely affects placental development and function, with marked changes in vascular development and nutrient transporters.
- In models of maternal malnutrition (obesity, restriction of food intake, low-protein diet), maternal and fetal glucocorticoids are frequently elevated while placental 11β-HSD2 is decreased, thus further enhancing fetal glucocorticoid exposure.

Keywords Placenta • Glucocorticoid • 11β-hydroxysteroid dehydrogenase type 2 • Developmental programming • Malnutrition • Low-protein diet

Abbreviations

11β-HSD2	11-β hydroxysteroid dehydrogenase type 2
CBG	Corticosteroid binding globulin
DOHAD	Developmental programming of adult health and disease
GLUT	Glucose transporter
HPA	Hypothalamic-pituitary-adrenal
LPD	Low-protein diet

E.K. Chivers, BSc • C.S. Wyrwoll, PhD (✉)
School of Human Sciences, The University of Western Australia, Crawley, WA, Australia
e-mail: 21126167@student.uwa.edu.au; caitlin.wyrwoll@uwa.edu.au

© Springer International Publishing AG 2017
R. Rajendram et al. (eds.), *Diet, Nutrition, and Fetal Programming*,
Nutrition and Health, DOI 10.1007/978-3-319-60289-9_39

PPAR   Peroxisome proliferator-activated receptor
SAME   Syndrome of apparent mineralocorticoid excess
VEGF   Vascular endothelial growth factor

Introduction

In the early 1990s, epidemiological studies revealed that low birth weight (a marker of adverse intra-uterine conditions) was associated with an increased susceptibility to hypertension, hyperlipidemia, and type 2 diabetes later in life [1, 2]. From these initial observations arose the theory of "develop-mental programming of adult health and disease" (DOHAD) whereby exposure of the fetus to adverse intrauterine conditions during critical periods of growth and development elicit modifications to struc-ture, physiology, and metabolism. These permanent alterations manifest in poor health outcomes in later life including cardiometabolic disease and neuropsychiatric disorders. Over recent decades there has been extensive support for the hypothesis, with investigations in both human and animal models linking poor intrauterine conditions and subsequent fetal growth restriction with cardiovascular dis-ease, the metabolic syndrome, and affective disorders.

While there are multiple factors that contribute to DOHAD, much of the attention in this field focuses on two key "programming" agents: maternal malnutrition and stress. Critically, however, malnutrition and stress are not mutually exclusive factors. Blockade of glucocorticoid synthesis has been shown to prevent the programming effects of maternal undernutrition in rats, indicating that these stress hormones partially mediate the effects of malnutrition on offspring [3]. Additional studies support this notion, demonstrating that malnutrition invokes a stress response in the mother and fetus [4, 5], and that stress may reduce food intake [6]. Furthermore, underlying these agents is a common mechanism of action, exposure of the developing fetus to excess glucocorticoids. While fetal matura-tion is fundamentally reliant upon glucocorticoids, inappropriate timing of glucocorticoid exposure or excessive exposure restricts fetal growth and causes permanent structural, functional, and behavioral changes with adverse consequences later in life. This chapter will focus on how fetal glucocorticoid exposure is regulated, with a particular emphasis on the role of the placenta, and how this is altered in maternal malnutrition.

What are Glucocorticoids?

Glucocorticoids are a class of steroid hormone which have many vital functions throughout the body. Cortisol and corticosterone (the major glucocorticoids in humans and rodents, respectively) influence many physiological processes including the regulation of blood pressure, fluid and electrolyte bal-ance, immune function, and metabolism of macronutrients [7, 8]. Importantly, glucocorticoids play a fundamental role in mediating the body's adaptive responses to physiological and psychological stressors. Production and release of glucocorticoids are controlled by the hypothalamic-pituitary-adrenal (HPA) axis. Corticotrophin-releasing hormone and vasopressin from the hypothalamus stimu-late the release of adrenocorticotrophic hormone from the anterior pituitary, which stimulates production and release of glucocorticoids from the cortical cells of the adrenal gland [9]. In humans, the amount of cortisol which is able to exert biological activity on tissues is limited by corticosteroid binding globulin (CBG). CBG is a glycoprotein which binds approximately 70% of circulating corti-sol. An additional 20% of total cortisol circulates bound to albumin, leaving only 10% free and meta-bolically active [10].

During pregnancy, activity of the HPA axis is markedly upregulated, and accordingly, free cortisol levels rise, peaking in the third trimester at triple nonpregnant levels [11]. CBG levels approximately double over the first 6 months of pregnancy which partially compensates for the increase in maternal cortisol levels that occur during gestation [12]. The upregulation of glucocorticoids enables the mother to meet the metabolic demands of pregnancy and plays an essential role for preparation of the fetus for extrauterine life [13]. Glucocorticoids shift cells from a proliferating state to a mature, differentiated state, and thus exposure of the fetus to glucocorticoids in the final part of gestation is critical in the preparation for life *ex utero*. Indeed, this is most notable in the lungs where glucocorticoids stimulate the production of pulmonary surfactant in the alveoli. This knowledge has been utilized for decades, with synthetic glucocorticoids administered to pregnant women threatening preterm labor in order to accelerate fetal lung maturation [14]. Glucocorticoids are also responsible for maturation of other fetal tissues including induction of gluconeogenesis in the liver [15, 16], neuronal and glial cell maturation in the brain [17], and adrenal gland development [16].

Fetal Glucocorticoid Exposure is (Normally) Tightly Regulated By 11β-HSD2

Glucocorticoids are lipophilic and therefore can readily pass through the placenta; however, fetal glucocorticoid levels remain up to tenfold lower than maternal levels during the majority of gestation [18]. How does this marked differential come about? It is largely due to the presence of the enzyme 11-β hydroxysteroid dehydrogenase type 2 (11β-HSD2) in the placenta which acts as a barrier to the transport of maternal glucocorticoids (Fig. 39.1). 11β-HSD2 catalyzes the conversion of cortisol and corticosterone into their inactive forms, cortisone and 11-dehydrocorticosterone, respectively (Fig. 39.2). In humans, 11β-HSD2 is highly expressed in the syncytiotrophoblast [19] at the interface between maternal and fetal circulations. Similar patterns of 11β-HSD2 expression are seen in a functionally analogous area of the rodent placenta (known as the labyrinth zone) [20, 21]. Expression of 11β-HSD2 decreases at the end of

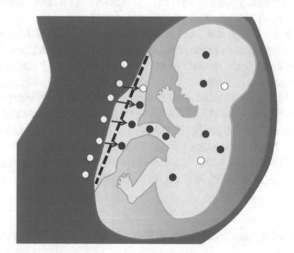

━ ━ ━ 11β-HSD2 barrier   ○ Active cortisol   ● Inactive cortisone

Fig. 39.1 Placental 11β-HSD2 prevents the much higher levels of active glucocorticoids in the maternal blood reaching the fetus. Normally, 11β-HSD2 oxidizes active cortisol to inactive cortisone. Thus, the major source of active glucocorticoid in the fetus is its own adrenal glands. In late gestation, 11β-HSD2 expression declines, enabling exposure of the fetus to maternal glucocorticoids and thus facilitating fetal tissue maturation

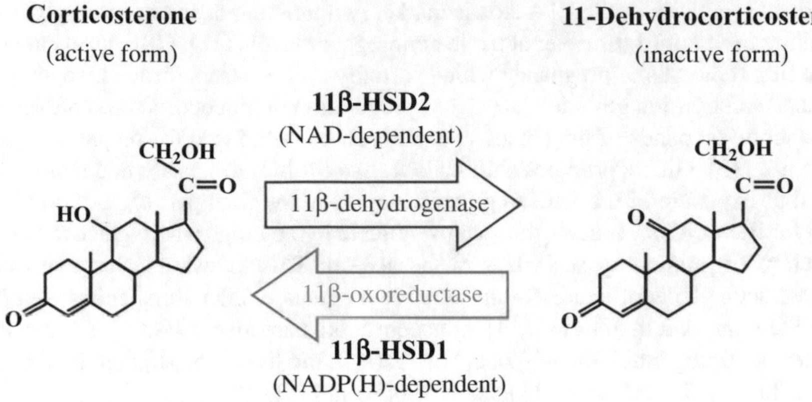

Corticosterone   **11-Dehydrocorticosterone**

(active form)   (inactive form)

11β-HSD2

(NAD-dependent)

11β-dehydrogenase

11β-oxoreductase

11β-HSD1

(NADP(H)-dependent)

Fig. 39.2 The enzymatic actions of 11β-hydroxysteroid dehydrogenase (*11β-HSD*) in interconversion of active and inactive glucocorticoid in rodents. Active glucocorticoid (*corticosterone*) is metabolized by 11β-HSD2 to its inactive form (*11-dehydrocorticosterone*) while regeneration can occur via 11β-HSD1

gestation, presumably to facilitate fetal organ maturation [20]. Additive to this, there is evidence that P-glycoprotein, a membrane protein that extrudes a wide range of substances from cells, also plays a marginal role in limiting the passage of glucocorticoids across the placenta [22, 23].

An additional layer of regulation of fetal glucocorticoid exposure is served by expression of 11β-HSD2 in fetal tissues. Expression of fetal 11β-HSD2 is initially widespread but later becomes specific to several fetal tissues including the brain, gut, kidney, and male reproductive organs [24, 25]. During early postnatal life, 11β-HSD2 continues to limit the glucocorticoid exposure of postnatally developing regions of the thalamus and cerebellum [26]. In adulthood 11β-HSD2 is localized to the kidneys and a few brain regions where it ensures the aldosterone specificity of the mineralocorticoid receptor (MR). This is vital for homeostasis of blood pressure and salt appetite [27], as demonstrated by inactivating mutations of 11β-HSD2 which cause the syndrome of apparent mineralocorticoid excess (SAME), a condition primarily characterized by hypertension and suppression of the renin-angiotensin-aldosterone axis [28].

Despite these layers of regulation, it is important to note that 11β-HSD2 does not completely shield the fetus from maternal glucocorticoids as premature exposure can restrict fetal growth and development. Ten to twenty percent of maternal glucocorticoids reach the fetus unaltered [29], and thus, increases in maternal glucocorticoid levels (caused by stressors) have the ability to increase fetal glucocorticoid exposure. Furthermore, alterations in 11β-HSD2 expression and/or activity can significantly alter fetal glucocorticoid exposure [30]. The efficiency of 11β-HSD2 varies between individuals and can also be reduced by dietary insults, inflammation, and hypoxia [13]. Additionally, reduced activity of placental 11β-HSD2 associates with low birth weight in humans [19, 31], although not in all studies [32]. Similarly, genetic ablation of 11β-HSD2 reduces fetal growth in a mouse model [33]. Taken together, these results highlight the crucial role of 11β-HSD2 in limiting fetal exposure to glucocorticoids.

What Happens When Placental 11β-HSD2 is Bypassed? Implications for Fetal Development…

One of the most notable effects of excess glucocorticoid exposure is fetal growth restriction and the underlying alteration in fetal organ development trajectories. The majority of epidemiological and experimental data suggests that increased exposure to exogenous or endogenous glucocorticoids causes fetal growth restriction; however, the evidence can appear mixed in part due to the many confounding factors involved in the studies. Antenatal glucocorticoid treatment (to stimulate fetal lung maturation) has been linked to reduced birth weight, higher blood pressure, and insulin resistance later in life [34–36]. Despite these observations, it is important to note that exogenous glucocorticoid exposure is only necessary in complicated pregnancies at risk of preterm birth so it is difficult to identify the effects of the treatment alone. As for endogenous glucocorticoid exposure, Bolten and colleagues [37] found that maternal cortisol levels were negatively correlated with weight and length at birth but, failed to show any significant relationship between mothers' perceived stress levels and cortisol level or size at birth. The strongest evidence linking excess endogenous glucocorticoid exposure and fetal growth restriction in humans comes from studies that examine placental 11β-HSD2 expression and activity. Fetal growth restriction is a characteristic of SAME, a condition caused by inactivating mutations in the 11β-HSD2 gene [38]. Placental 11β-HSD2 expression has also been found to be significantly lower in other cases of fetal growth restriction [31, 39]. Additionally, 11β-HSD2 activity correlates positively with birth weight in general [19, 40]. Heavy consumption of liquorice (which contains glycyrrhizin, a 11β-HSD2 inhibitor) has been linked to reduced gestation length although no effect on birth weight was observed [41]. It is clear that environmental insults are capable of increasing fetal glucocorticoid exposure by altering the placental glucocorticoid barrier.

While human studies have provided evidence for association between reduced placental 11β-HSD2, low birth weight, and later adverse health outcomes, animal models have been critical in establishing causation and mechanistic information. The most common model of glucocorticoid excess involves administering synthetic glucocorticoids, usually dexamethasone or betamethasone, to animals during pregnancy. Both drugs are poor substrates for 11β-HSD2 [42] and have been demonstrated to decrease the activity of the enzyme [43]; therefore, treatment with these substances results in high levels of placental and fetal glucocorticoid exposure. Cortisol or corticosterone can also be administered during pregnancy to increase "natural" glucocorticoid exposure [44, 45]. Excess glucocorticoid exposure can also be achieved by pharmacological inhibition (through administration of carbenoxolone) or genetic ablation of 11β-HSD2. Both of these models greatly increase fetal exposure to maternal glucocorticoids [46, 47]. Each glucocorticoid excess model reliably demonstrates pronounced and dose-dependent fetal growth restriction [33, 44, 46–52]. Additionally, offspring consistently exhibit signs of developmental programming, suffering from conditions such as hypertension [48, 53, 54], hyperglycaemia [46, 49], hyperleptinemia [54, 55], and anxiety [47].

...and Don't Forget the Placenta!

The significance of maternal glucocorticoid excess and placental 11β-HSD2 is frequently placed in the context of *fetal* glucocorticoid exposure and subsequent programming effects. Yet, optimal placental development and function are clearly essential for optimal fetal growth and development, so *what impact does glucocorticoid excess and modification of placental 11β-HSD2 have on the placenta itself?* Evidence is emerging that the placenta is a key mediator behind the fetal growth restriction observed in models of glucocorticoid excess. Reinforcing this notion are observations in sheep that maternal but *not fetal* administration of glucocorticoids is responsible for fetal growth restriction [56].

With regard to placental structure, excess glucocorticoid exposure is detrimental. Thus, placental weight (particularly the weight of the labyrinth zone) is significantly reduced in rodent models of glucocorticoid excess [33, 44, 51, 57, 58]. This decrease in weight appears to be caused by a decline in the complexity of feto-placental blood vessel development. Treatment with dexamethasone from day 13 of gestation onward significantly decreases the volume and density of the fetal vascular network and decreases the length and size of capillaries [51]. Dexamethasone has also been found to reduce branching complexity of fetal vascular networks in rats (Fig. 39.3, unpublished observations,

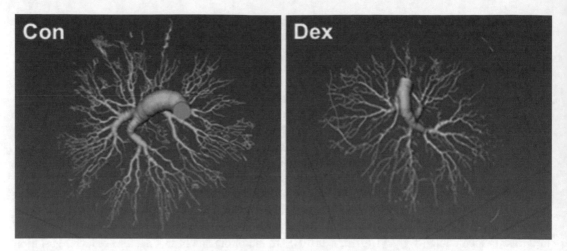

Fig. 39.3 Dexamethasone exposure reduces the complexity of the feto-placental vascular architecture. These micro-CT images were obtained from vascular casts of rat placentas that were either controls or exposed to dexamethasone (*Dex*) during pregnancy

Burrows and Wyrwoll). Similarly, mid- and late-gestation administration of corticosterone decreased fetal capillary volume in mice [44]. Comparable outcomes are seen in an 11β-HSD2 knockout model of glucocorticoid excess; Wyrwoll and colleagues [33] observed a dramatic decrease in the total volume and diameter of fetal capillaries in the labyrinth zone of 11β-HSD2-KO placentas. These changes are likely to decrease the efficiency of maternal-fetal nutrient transport, making the placenta unable to meet the high energy demands of the fetus. Importantly, the volume of the maternal blood space does not appear to be altered in either of these models indicating that glucocorticoids exert their effects predominantly on fetal tissues.

Accompanying these structural changes are a range of changes to gene expression in the placenta. In the dexamethasone model, the decrease in fetal blood vessel development was accompanied by a decrease in the expression of the genes encoding angiogenic vascular endothelial growth factor (VEGF)-A [51]. In a related study Hewitt and colleagues also found that dexamethasone treatment decreased expression of peroxisome proliferator-activated receptor (PPAR)-γ, which normally increases *Vegfa* [59]. Expression of *Vegfa* and *Pparγ* was also found to be reduced in 11β-HSD2 knockout placentas [33]. Thus, the observed reduction in fetal blood vessel development is likely caused by reductions in these angiogenic factors. Excess glucocorticoids exposure has complex effects on the transport of glucose and amino acids across the placenta. In models of glucocorticoid excess, transplacental transfer of these nutrients tends to decrease although the exact effects appear to be dependent on the route and timing of exposure [60]. In the 11β-HSD2 knockout model, system A amino acid transporter expression is increased at embryonic day 15, as is placental amino acid transport. This may represent a compensatory mechanism of the placenta to maintain fetal weight. By day 18, however, placental expression of the genes encoding glucose transporter (GLUT) 3 is reduced, and a corresponding decrease in fetal weight and plasma glucose levels is observed [33]. Similarly, overexposure to cortisol reduced placental glucose transport near term in an ovine model [45]. Late-gestation exposure to dexamethasone has produced contradictory results [57]. An increase in GLUT1 and GLUT3 expression was observed; however, blood glucose levels were reduced by as much as 49% in dexamethasone-treated fetuses and fetal growth restriction was evident [57]. Clearly, the action of glucocorticoids on placental function is complex and requires further clarification.

Maternal Malnutrition Alters Glucocorticoid-Related Parameters Including Placental 11β-HSD2

Rodent models of maternal malnutrition (over and undernutrition) during pregnancy provide important insights into the mechanisms underlying the perturbed fetal development and subsequent health outcomes. Animal models of maternal undernutrition generally involve restricting food intake or feeding dams a low-protein diet. A frequent observation in these models is alteration of glucocorticoid-related parameters such as maternal and fetal corticosterone and 11β-HSD2 expression [4, 5, 61–63]. This suggests that glucocorticoids, at least in part, mediate the effects of malnutrition on the fetus and placenta. Animal models have demonstrated that maternal overnutrition also has detrimental effects on the health outcomes of offspring.

Maternal Overnutrition

Unlike undernutrition, the effects of maternal overnutrition during pregnancy are a relatively new field of investigation. Animal models of maternal overnutrition usually involve dams consuming a high-fat diet; however, some studies use a high-sugar high-fat diet or a "cafeteria" diet (where rodents are fed human "junk foods"). In humans, maternal obesity usually increases offspring birth weight, although it is also a risk factor for being born small for gestational age [64]. Conversely, most studies in rodents have found that maternal overnutrition decreases birth weight [65–68] although some have found no change [69]. Changes to placental structure and function may underlie the growth restriction observed in these models. Decreases in labyrinth zone vascularity have been observed in some [70] but not in all studies [66, 71]. Hayes and colleagues [68] found that labyrinth zone vascularity increased but deficits in vessel maturity and tissue oxygenation were evident. In humans, maternal obesity has been associated with placental insufficiency and inflammation [71, 72]. As well as perturbing fetal and placental development, maternal overnutrition has substantial adverse effects on later-life health outcomes. Offspring of over-nourished mothers exhibit increased adiposity, hypertension, insulin resistance, hyperphagia, and decreased physical activity [65–68, 71, 73, 74]. While this list of conditions is similar to those programmed by excess exposure to glucocorticoids, it appears that the effects of overnutrition may involve other mechanisms. A recent study of obese women by Stirrat and colleagues [75] found that although the normal gestational increase in placental 11β-HSD2 activity was blunted, cortisol levels were lower throughout pregnancy indicating that excess exposure to glucocorticoids did not occur. In fact, the authors proposed that decreased maternal cortisol may actually be a mechanism underlying the increase in fetal weight observed in many obese pregnancies.

Restriction of Food Intake

Restricting food intake of pregnant rodents has detrimental consequences for fetal growth and later-life health outcomes which is caused, in part, by glucocorticoid-related changes in placental structure and function. In this model of malnutrition, dams are fed a fraction (usually 50%) of the amount of food consumed by control animals. This treatment consistently causes fetal growth restriction, and accordingly, birth weight is reduced [5, 76–78]. Alterations of placental structure and function are, again, key mechanisms underlying fetal growth restriction in this model. Fifty percent food restriction decreases placental weight in some studies [5, 63] but not in others [62]. Decreased placental weight is accompanied by lower expression of 11β-HSD2, increasing exposure of the fetus and placenta to glucocorticoids [5, 63]. Additionally, expression of the genes encoding GLUT 3 and amino acid trans-porters 1 and 2 are also reduced, resulting in decreased nutrient availability to the fetus. Together, these changes in placental function contribute to the observed fetal growth restriction.

It is unclear whether stress responses from the mother and the fetus also contribute to fetal growth restriction in this model. Maternal and fetal corticosterone levels increase in response to food restriction, suggesting increased exposure of the fetus to glucocorticoids [5, 62, 63]. Consistent with this, offspring exhibit signs of "programming" that are similar to those seen in models of glucocorticoid excess. Severe maternal intake restriction (30% of ad libitum) causes hyperphagia, hypertension, hyperinsulinemia, and hyperleptinemia in offspring 4-month-old offspring [78]. Similarly, pups of 50% intake-restricted mothers showed signs of increased susceptibility to developing insulin resistance and other symptoms of the metabolic syndrome [77]. On the other hand, only a weak, nonsignificant inverse relationship is seen between serum corticosterone levels and fetal and placental weight [63]. Further, food restriction-induced fetal and placental growth restriction has been observed in mothers who have had their adrenal glands removed [62]. Together, these results suggest that dysregulation of the placental glucocorticoid barrier and decreased nutrient supply to the fetus (caused by decreased transporter expression and nutrient unavailability) make the largest contribution to fetal growth restriction and subsequent programming in the intake-restriction model.

Low-Protein Diet

A maternal low-protein diet (LPD) is one of the most commonly used models of fetal growth restriction, particularly in rodents [79]. A balanced rodent diet contains around 20% protein. Rodents exposed to a low-protein diet receive between 5% and 10% protein depending on the study. Birth weight is consistently reduced in this model [79] but how a low-protein diet affects earlier patterns of fetal and placental development is less clear. Variation in results may be explained by methodological differences (including severity and duration of the dietary insult and the rodent species used) but overall, combining the results of multiple studies creates a roughly consistent picture.

It appears that the low-protein diet affects the fetus and placenta differently during different stages of gestation, as summarized in Table 39.1. Fetal growth restriction is evident as early as day 14.5 in the mouse [80], although some studies have reported no change until day 17.5 [4]. Interesting changes in placental structure and function underlie this pattern of fetal growth. Early in the last third of gestation, placental weight may actually increase in response to protein restriction, possibly as a compensatory mechanism to limit or delay fetal growth restriction [80, 81]. Consistent with this, the labyrinth zone of placentas was relatively smaller in protein-restricted rats (at day 18); however, the overall increase in placental size meant that the absolute size of the labyrinth zone was not different from control placentas [81]. While the placenta may be able to compensate initially, a decline in function is seen in the final days leading to parturition and fetal growth suffers accordingly. Placental weight is reduced at day 17.5 and 18.5 in protein-restricted mice [4, 80]. Nutrient transport is also impaired in the final days of gestation. Jansson and colleagues [82] found that protein restriction in rats caused a decline in SNAT 2 mRNA expression at day 15, decreased transport of amino acids at day 19, and reduced fetal and placental growth at day 21. This evidence suggests that a decline in the nutrient transport capacity of the placenta plays a key role in low-protein-induced fetal growth restriction.

Another factor that significantly affects the nutrient transport capacity of the placenta is labyrinth zone vascularity. How a low-protein diet affects placental vascularity is not well characterized, and contradictory findings have been reported in the few studies that have addressed this question. Rutland and colleagues [80] reported a decrease in labyrinthine blood vessel length near parturition in mice. On the other hand, Doherty and colleagues [81] found no differences in fetal capillary length, diameter, or surface area at day 18 of gestation in rats; however, this may be because they did not examine

Table 39.1 Summary of studies investigating the effect of low-protein diet on fetal weight, placental weight, and glucocorticoid parameters in rodent pregnancy

Study	Animal	% protein in diet	Day and (%) of gestation	Fetal weight	Placental weight	11β-HSD2 activity	Maternal cort	Fetal cort
Langley-Evans et al. (1996)	Rat	9%	20 (89)	↓	↑	↓		
Doherty et al. (2003)	Rat	8%	18 (80)	↓	↑			
Jansson et al. (2006)	Rat	4%	15 (65)	↔	↔			
			18 (78)	↔	↔			
			19 (83)	↔	↔			
			21 (91)	↓	↓			
Rutland et al. (2007)	Mouse	9%	14.5 (74)	↓	↑			
Cottrell et al. (2012)	Mouse	8%	14.5 (74)	↓	↓	↓	↑	↑
			15.5 (79)	↔	↔	↑	↔	↑
			16.5 (85)	↔	↓	↑	↔	↑
			17.5 (90)	↔	↓	↓	↔	↑

Studies are separated by species (rat and mouse) and the time point in gestation when the parameters are assessed
↔ indicates no change, ↑ an increase, and ↓ a decrease

placental vascularity close enough to term. The evidence above would suggest that at day 18 of rat gestation the placenta has not yet lost its ability to compensate for the protein deficiency.

Glucocorticoids have been implicated in LPD-induced fetal programming [3] but their role in LPD-induced fetal growth restriction remains unclear. Recent evidence has begun to examine this issue. Interestingly, it appears that the fetus' stress response to maternal protein restriction is the major driver behind the patterns of fetal and placental growth observed in this model [4]. Fetal corticosterone levels are increased from day 14.5 onward in response to the low-protein diet. While environmental insults reduce 11β-HSD2 expression, glucocorticoids themselves upregulate 11β-HSD2 expression [83]. Accordingly, 11β-HSD2 activity is higher in protein-restricted placentas than controls [4] from day 13.5 to day 15.5. Maternal corticosterone levels are not different from controls at this stage so the increase in 11β-HSD2 means that feto-placental exposure to maternal corticosterone should be lower in protein-restricted pregnancies compared to controls. It is proposed that the fetal HPA axis (prematurely activated because of the low-protein diet) assumes the primary role in determining the exposure of the fetus to glucocorticoids. Thus, the fetus appears to drive the early maturation (and subsequent growth restriction) of its own tissues in order to prepare for early birth and an adverse extrauterine environment [4]. Late in gestation, when the placentas adaptive capacity is exhausted, the protein restriction causes a decrease in 11β-HSD2 activity. This increases feto-placental exposure to maternal corticosterone. In the fetus, this increase likely amplifies the tissue maturation stimulus. In the placenta, the increased glucocorticoid exposure may underlie the observed decline in amino acid transporter expression [82] and labyrinthine vascularity [80], both of which contribute to fetal growth restriction.

Conclusions

Epidemiological data and animal models have identified excess glucocorticoid exposure as a key mechanism underlying fetal growth restriction (summarized in Fig. 39.4). Key factors that determine feto-placental glucocorticoid exposure include fetal and maternal corticosterone levels and placental activity of the protective enzyme 11β-HSD2. Glucocorticoid excess is known to disrupt placental

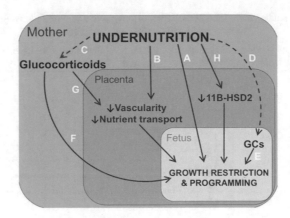

Fig. 39.4 A summary of the mechanisms underlying undernutrition-induced fetal growth restriction. Inadequate nutrient availability directly restricts fetal (*A*) and placental (*B*) growth and development. This nutrient deficit also causes a stress response in the mother (*C*) and fetus (*D*) which involves the release of glucocorticoids (*GCs*). Glucocorticoids exacerbate the effects of undernutrition as they themselves restrict fetal growth (*E, F*) and disrupt placental development (*G*). Undernutrition increases the vulnerability of the fetus and placenta to glucocorticoids as it also decreases placental expression of 11β-hydroxysteroid dehydrogenase type 2 (*11β-HSD2; H*)

development, resulting in fetal growth restriction and the programming of cardiometabolic and neuropsychiatric diseases. Poor maternal nutrition during pregnancy also causes profound changes in fetal and placental growth and is known to be linked to poor later-life health outcomes. Animal models have revealed that maternal undernutrition causes stress responses in the mother and fetus which involve increased secretion of glucocorticoids. This is accompanied by a decrease in placental 11β-HSD2 activity and results in excess fetal and placental glucocorticoid exposure. It is important to note that glucocorticoids are by no means solely responsible for the effects of maternal malnutrition on fetal growth and later-life health outcomes. Rather, malnutrition-induced fetal growth restriction appears to be exacerbated by the excess glucocorticoid exposure that occurs as a result of the mother and fetus' responses to this physiological stressor.

References

1. Barker DJP, Hales CN, Fall CHD, Osmond C, Phipps K, Clark PMS. Type 2 (non-insulin-dependent) diabetes mellitus, hypertension and hyperlipidaemia (syndrome X): relation to reduced fetal growth. Diabetologia. 1993;36(1):62–7.
2. Hales C, Barker D, Clark P, Cox L, Fall C, Osmond C, et al. Fetal and infant growth and impaired glucose tolerance at age 64. BMJ. 1991;303(6809):1019–22.
3. Langley-Evans SC. Hypertension induced by foetal exposure to a maternal low-protein diet, in the rat, is prevented by pharmacological blockade of maternal glucocorticoid synthesis. J Hypertens. 1997;15(5):537–44.
4. Cottrell EC, Holmes MC, Livingstone DE, Kenyon CJ, Seckl JR. Reconciling the nutritional and glucocorticoid hypotheses of fetal programming. FASEB J. 2012;26(5):1866–74.
5. Lesage J, Blondeau B, Grino M, Breant B, Dupouy J. Maternal undernutrition during late gestation induces fetal overexposure to glucocorticoids and intrauterine growth retardation, and disturbs the hypothalamo-pituitary adrenal axis in the newborn rat. Endocrinology. 2001;142(5):1692–702.
6. Martí O, Martí J, Armario A. Effects of chronic stress on food intake in rats: influence of stressor intensity and duration of daily exposure. Physiol Behav. 1994;55(4):747–53.
7. Baxter JD, Forsham PH. Tissue effects of glucocorticoids. Am J Med. 1972;53(5):573–89.
8. Young EA, Abelson J, Lightman SL. Cortisol pulsatility and its role in stress regulation and health. Front Neuroendocrinol. 2004;25(2):69–76.

9. Tsigos C, Chrousos GP. Hypothalamic–pituitary–adrenal axis, neuroendocrine factors and stress. J Psychosom Res. 2002;53(4):865–71.

10. Brien TG. Human corticosteroid binding globulin. Clin Endocrinol. 1981;14(2):193–212.

11. Jung C, Ho JT, Torpy DJ, Rogers A, Doogue M, Lewis JG, et al. A longitudinal study of plasma and urinary cortisol in pregnancy and postpartum. J Clin Endocrinol Metab. 2011;96(5):1533–40.

12. Doe RP, Fernandez RL, Seal US. Measurement of corticosteroid-binding globulin in man. J Clin Endocrinol Metab. 1964;24(10):1029–39.

13. Seckl JR, Holmes MC. Mechanisms of disease: glucocorticoids, their placental metabolism and fetal 'programming' of adult pathophysiology. Nat Clin Pract Endocrinol Metab. 2007;3(6):479–88.

14. Surbek D, Drack G, Irion O, Nelle M, Huang D, Hoesli I. Antenatal corticosteroids for fetal lung maturation in threatened preterm delivery: indications and administration. Arch Gynecol Obstet. 2012;286(2):277–81.

15. Cole TJ, Blendy JA, Monaghan AP, Krieglstein K, Schmid W, Aguzzi A, et al. Targeted disruption of the glucocorticoid receptor gene blocks adrenergic chromaffin cell development and severely retards lung maturation. Genes Dev. 1995;9(13):1608–21.

16. Cole TJ, Blendy JA, Monaghan AP, Schmid W, Aguzzi A, Schütz G. Molecular genetic analysis of glucocorticoid signaling during mouse development. Steroids. 1995;60(1):93–6.

17. Diaz R, Brown RW, Seckl JR. Distinct ontogeny of glucocorticoid and mineralocorticoid receptor and 11β-hydroxysteroid dehydrogenase types I and II mRNAs in the fetal rat brain suggest a complex control of glucocorticoid actions. J Neurosci. 1998;18(7):2570–80.

18. Edwards CRW, Benediktsson R, Lindsay RS, Seckl JR. Dysfunction of placental glucocorticoid barrier: link between fetal environment and adult hypertension? Lancet. 1993;341(8841):355–7.

19. Stewart PM, Rogerson FM, Mason J. Type 2 11 beta-hydroxysteroid dehydrogenase messenger ribonucleic acid and activity in human placenta and fetal membranes: its relationship to birth weight and putative role in fetal adrenal steroidogenesis. J Clin Endocrinol Metab. 1995;80(3):885–90.

20. Burton PJ, Smith RE, Krozowski ZS, Waddell B. Zonal distribution of 11 beta-hydroxysteroid dehydrogenase types 1 and 2 messenger ribonucleic acid expression in the rat placenta and decidua during late pregnancy. Biol Reprod. 1996;55(5):1023–8.

21. Brown R, Diaz R, Robson A, Kotelevtsev Y, Mullins J, Kaufman M, et al. The ontogeny of 11 beta-hydroxysteroid dehydrogenase type 2 and mineralocorticoid receptor gene expression reveal intricate control of glucocorticoid action in development. Endocrinology. 1996;137(2):794–7.

22. Mark PJ, Waddell BJ. P-glycoprotein restricts access of cortisol and dexamethasone to the glucocorticoid receptor in placental BeWo cells. Endocrinology. 2006;147(11):5147–52.

23. Sun M, Kingdom J, Baczyk D, Lye SJ, Matthews SG, Gibb W. Expression of the multidrug resistance P-glycoprotein, (ABCB1 glycoprotein) in the human placenta decreases with advancing gestation. Placenta. 2006;27(6–7):602–9.

24. Condon J, Gosden C, Gardener D, Nickson P, Hewison M, Howie AJ, et al. Expression of type 2 11β-hydroxysteroid dehydrogenase and corticosteroid hormone receptors in early human fetal life. J Clin Endocrinol Metab. 1998;83(12):4490–7.

25. Brown R, Chapman KE, Kotelevtsev Y, Yau JLW, Linsday RS, Brett L, et al. Cloning and production of antisera to human placental 11 β-hydroxysteroid dehydrogenase type 2. Biochem J. 1996;313(3):1007–17.

26. Robson AC, Leckie CM, Seckl JR, Holmes MC. 11β-hydroxysteroid dehydrogenase type 2 in the postnatal and adult rat brain. Mol Brain Res. 1998;61(1–2):1–10.

27. Evans LC, Ivy JR, Wyrwoll C, McNairn JA, Menzies RI, Christensen TH, et al. Conditional deletion of Hsd11b2 in the brain causes salt appetite and hypertension. Circulation. 2016;133(14):1360–70.

28. Stewart PM, Gupta A, Sheppard MC, Whorwood CB, Howie AJ, Milford DV, et al. Hypertension in the syndrome of apparent mineralocorticoid excess due to mutation of the 11β-hydroxysteroid dehydrogenase type 2 gene. Lancet. 1996;347(8994):88–91.

29. Benediktsson R, Calder AA, Edwards CR, Seckl JR. Placental 11β-hydroxysteroid dehydrogenase: a key regulator of fetal glucocorticoid exposure. Clin Endocrinol. 1997;46(2):161–6.

30. Reynolds RM. Glucocorticoid excess and the developmental origins of disease: two decades of testing the hypothesis – 2012 Curt Richter award winner. Psychoneuroendocrinology. 2013;38(1):1–11.

31. McTernan CL, Draper N, Nicholson H, Chalder SM, Driver P, Hewison M, et al. Reduced placental 11β-hydroxysteroid dehydrogenase type 2 mRNA levels in human pregnancies complicated by intrauterine growth restriction: an analysis of possible mechanisms. J Clin Endocrinol Metab. 2001;86(10):4979–83.

32. Rogerson FM, Kayes KM, White PC. Variation in placental type 2 11β-hydroxysteroid dehydrogenase activity is not related to birth weight or placental weight. Mol Cell Endocrinol. 1997;128(1–2):103–9.

33. Wyrwoll CS, Seckl JR, Holmes MC. Altered placental function of 11β-hydroxysteroid dehydrogenase 2 knockout mice. Endocrinology. 2009;150(3):1287–93.

34. Bloom SL, Sheffield JS, McIntire DD, Leveno KJ. Antenatal dexamethasone and decreased birth weight. Obstet Gynecol. 2001;97(4):485–90.

35. Dalziel SR, Walker NK, Parag V, Mantell C, Rea HH, Rodgers A, et al. Cardiovascular risk factors after antenatal exposure to betamethasone: 30-year follow-up of a randomised controlled trial. Lancet. 2005;365(9474):1856–62.
36. Doyle L, Ford G, Davis N, Callanan C. Antenatal corticosteroid therapy and blood pressure at 14 years of age in preterm children. Clin Sci. 2000;98(2):137–42.
37. Bolten MI, Wurmser H, Buske-Kirschbaum A, Papoušek M, Pirke K-M, Hellhammer D. Cortisol levels in pregnancy as a psychobiological predictor for birth weight. Arch Womens Ment Health. 2011;14(1):33–41.
38. Kitanaka S, Tanae A, Hibi I. Apparent mineralocorticoid excess due to 11β-hydroxysteroid dehydrogenase deficiency: a possible cause of intrauterine growth retardation. Clin Endocrinol (Oxf). 1996;44(3):353–9.
39. Shams M, Kilby M, Somerset D, Howie A, Gupta A, Wood P, et al. 11Beta-hydroxysteroid dehydrogenase type 2 in human pregnancy and reduced expression in intrauterine growth restriction. Hum Reprod. 1998;13(4):799–804.
40. Benediktsson R, Noble J, Calder A, Edwards C, Seckl J. 11β-hydroxysteroid dehydrogenase activity in intact dually perfused fresh human placenta predicts birth weight. J Endocrinol. 1995;144:161.
41. Strandberg TE, Järvenpää A-L, Vanhanen H, McKeigue PM. Birth outcome in relation to licorice consumption during pregnancy. Am J Epidemiol. 2001;153(11):1085–8.
42. Blanford AT, Pearson-Murphy BE. In vitro metabolism of prednisolone, dexamethasone, betamethasone, and cortisol by the human placenta. Am J Obstet Gynecol. 1977;127(3):264–7.
43. Vackova Z, Vagnerova K, Libra A, Miksik I, Pacha J, Staud F. Dexamethasone and betamethasone administration during pregnancy affects expression and function of 11β-hydroxysteroid dehydrogenase type 2 in the rat placenta. Reprod Toxicol. 2009;28(1):46–51.
44. Vaughan OR, Sferruzzi-Perri AN, Fowden AL. Maternal corticosterone regulates nutrient allocation to fetal growth in mice. J Physiol. 2012;590(21):5529–40.
45. Vaughan O, Fowden A. Preterm fetal cortisol overexposure alters placental glucose delivery nearer term. Placenta. 2014;35(9):A69–70.
46. Lindsay R, Lindsay R, Waddell B, Seckl J. Prenatal glucocorticoid exposure leads to offspring hyperglycaemia in the rat: studies with the 11 b-hydroxysteroid dehydrogenase inhibitor carbenoxolone. Diabetologia. 1996;39(11):1299–305.
47. Holmes MC, Abrahamsen CT, French KL, Paterson JM, Mullins JJ, Seckl JR. The mother or the fetus? 11β-hydroxysteroid dehydrogenase type 2 null mice provide evidence for direct fetal programming of behavior by endogenous glucocorticoids. J Neurosci. 2006;26(14):3840–4.
48. Benediktsson R, Lindsay R, Noble J, Seckl J, Edwards C. Glucocorticoid exposure in utero: new model for adult hypertension. Lancet. 1993;341(8841):339–41.
49. Nyirenda MJ, Lindsay RS, Kenyon CJ, Burchell A, Seckl JR. Glucocorticoid exposure in late gestation permanently programs rat hepatic phosphoenolpyruvate carboxykinase and glucocorticoid receptor expression and causes glucose intolerance in adult offspring. J Clin Investig. 1998;101(10):2174.
50. Ain R, Canham LN, Soares MJ. Dexamethasone-induced intrauterine growth restriction impacts the placental prolactin family, insulin-like growth factor-II and the Akt signaling pathway. J Endocrinol. 2005;185(2):253–63.
51. Hewitt DP, Mark PJ, Waddell BJ. Glucocorticoids prevent the normal increase in placental vascular endothelial growth factor expression and placental vascularity during late pregnancy in the rat. Endocrinology. 2006;147(12):5568–74.
52. Cuffe JSM, Dickinson H, Simmons DG, Moritz KM. Sex specific changes in placental growth and MAPK following short term maternal dexamethasone exposure in the mouse. Placenta. 2011;32(12):981–9.
53. Lindsay R, Lindsay RM, Edwards CRW, Seckl JR. Inhibition of 11β-hydroxysteroid dehydrogenase in pregnant rats and the programming of blood pressure in the offspring. Hypertension. 1996;27(6):1200–4.
54. Wyrwoll CS, Mark PJ, Mori TA, Puddey IB, Waddell BJ. Prevention of programmed hyperleptinemia and hypertension by postnatal dietary ω-3 fatty acids. Endocrinology. 2006;147(1):599–606.
55. Sugden MC, Langdown ML, Munns MJ, Holness MJ. Maternal glucocorticoid treatment modulates placental leptin and leptin receptor expression and materno-fetal leptin physiology during late pregnancy, and elicits hypertension associated with hyperleptinaemia in the early-growth-retarded adult offspring. Eur J Endocrinol. 2001;145(4):529–39.
56. Newnham JP, Evans SF, Godfrey M, Huang W, Ikegami M, Jobe A. Maternal, but not fetal, administration of corticosteroids restricts fetal growth. J Maternal-Fetal Med. 1999;8(3):81–7.
57. Langdown ML, Sugden MC. Enhanced placental GLUT1 and GLUT3 expression in dexamethasone-induced fetal growth retardation. Mol Cell Endocrinol. 2001;185(1–2):109–17.
58. Vaughan OR, Sferruzzi-Perri AN, Coan PM, Fowden AL. Adaptations in placental phenotype depend on route and timing of maternal dexamethasone administration in mice. Biol Reprod. 2013;89(4):80. 1–12.
59. Hewitt DP, Mark PJ, Waddell BJ. Placental expression of peroxisome proliferator-activated receptors in rat pregnancy and the effect of increased glucocorticoid exposure. Biol Reprod. 2006;74(1):23–8.
60. Fowden AL, Forhead AJ, Sferruzzi-Perri AN, Burton GJ, Vaughan OR. Review: endocrine regulation of placental phenotype. Placenta. 2015;36(Supplement 1):S50–9.

61. Langley-Evans SC, Phillips GJ, Benediktsson R, Gardner DS, Edwards CRW, Jackson AA, et al. Protein intake in pregnancy, placental glucocorticoid metabolism and the programming of hypertension in the rat. Placenta. 1996;17(2–3):169–72.
62. Lesage J, Hahn D, Leonhardt M, Blondeau B, Breant B, Dupouy J. Maternal undernutrition during late gestation-induced intrauterine growth restriction in the rat is associated with impaired placental GLUT3 expression, but does not correlate with endogenous corticosterone levels. J Endocrinol. 2002;174(1):37–43.
63. Belkacemi L, Jelks A, Chen C-H, Ross MG, Desai M. Altered placental development in undernourished rats: role of maternal glucocorticoids. Reprod Biol Endocrinol. 2011;9(1):1–11.
64. Grieger JA, Clifton VL. A review of the impact of dietary intakes in human pregnancy on infant birthweight. Forum Nutr. 2014;7(1):153–78.
65. Howie GJ, Sloboda DM, Kamal T, Vickers MH. Maternal nutritional history predicts obesity in adult offspring independent of postnatal diet. J Physiol. 2009;587(4):905–15.
66. Mark PJ, Sisala C, Connor K, Patel R, Lewis JL, Vickers MH, et al. A maternal high-fat diet in rat pregnancy reduces growth of the fetus and the placental junctional zone, but not placental labyrinth zone growth. J Dev Orig Health Dis. 2011;2(01):63–70.
67. Nivoit P, Morens C, Van Assche F, Jansen E, Poston L, Remacle C, et al. Established diet-induced obesity in female rats leads to offspring hyperphagia, adiposity and insulin resistance. Diabetologia. 2009;52(6):1133–42.
68. Hayes EK, Lechowicz A, Petrik JJ, Storozhuk Y, Paez-Parent S, Dai Q, et al. Adverse fetal and neonatal outcomes associated with a life-long high fat diet: role of altered development of the placental vasculature. PLoS One. 2012;7(3):e33370.
69. Akyol A, Langley-Evans SC, McMullen S. Obesity induced by cafeteria feeding and pregnancy outcome in the rat. Br J Nutr. 2009;102(11):1601–10.
70. Sferruzzi-Perri AN, Vaughan OR, Haro M, Cooper WN, Musial B, Charalambous M, et al. An obesogenic diet during mouse pregnancy modifies maternal nutrient partitioning and the fetal growth trajectory. FASEB J. 2013;27(10):3928–37.
71. Roberts KA, Riley SC, Reynolds RM, Barr S, Evans M, Statham A, et al. Placental structure and inflammation in pregnancies associated with obesity. Placenta. 2011;32(3):247–54.
72. Huang L, Liu J, Feng L, Chen Y, Zhang J, Wang W. Maternal prepregnancy obesity is associated with higher risk of placental pathological lesions. Placenta. 2014;35(8):563–9.
73. Khan IY, Dekou V, Douglas G, Jensen R, Hanson MA, Poston L, et al. A high-fat diet during rat pregnancy or suckling induces cardiovascular dysfunction in adult offspring. Am J Physiol Regul Integr Comp Physiol. 2005;288(1):R127–33.
74. Samuelsson A-M, Matthews PA, Argenton M, Christie MR, McConnell JM, Jansen EHJM, et al. Diet-induced obesity in female mice leads to offspring hyperphagia, adiposity, hypertension, and insulin resistance: a novel murine model of developmental programming. Hypertension. 2008;51(2):383–92.
75. Stirrat LI, O'Reilly JR, Barr SM, Andrew R, Riley SC, Howie AF, et al. Decreased maternal hypothalamic-pituitary-adrenal axis activity in very severely obese pregnancy: associations with birthweight and gestation at delivery. Psychoneuroendocrinology. 2016;63:135–43.
76. Garofano A, Czernichow P, Bréant B. In utero undernutrition impairs rat beta-cell development. Diabetologia. 1997;40(10):1231–4.
77. Hietaniemi M, Malo E, Jokela M, Santaniemi M, Ukkola O, Kesäniemi YA. The effect of energy restriction during pregnancy on obesity-related peptide hormones in rat offspring. Peptides. 2009;30(4):705–9.
78. Vickers MH, Breier BH, Cutfield WS, Hofman PL, Gluckman PD. Fetal origins of hyperphagia, obesity, and hypertension and postnatal amplification by hypercaloric nutrition. Am J Physiol Endocrinol Metab. 2000;279(1):E83–7.
79. Zohdi V, Lim K, Pearson JT, Black MJ. Developmental programming of cardiovascular disease following intrauterine growth restriction: findings utilising a rat model of maternal protein restriction. Forum Nutr. 2014;7(1):119–52.
80. Rutland CS, Latunde-Dada AO, Thorpe A, Plant R, Langley-Evans S, Leach L. Effect of gestational nutrition on vascular integrity in the murine placenta. Placenta. 2007;28(7):734–42.
81. Doherty C, Lewis R, Sharkey A, Burton G. Placental composition and surface area but not vascularization are altered by maternal protein restriction in the rat. Placenta. 2003;24(1):34–8.
82. Jansson N, Pettersson J, Haafiz A, Ericsson A, Palmberg I, Tranberg M, et al. Down-regulation of placental transport of amino acids precedes the development of intrauterine growth restriction in rats fed a low protein diet. J Physiol. 2006;576(3):935–46.
83. van Beek JP, Guan H, Julan L, Yang K. Glucocorticoids stimulate the expression of 11β-hydroxysteroid dehydrogenase type 2 in cultured human placental trophoblast cells. J Clin Endocrinol Metab. 2004;89(11):5614–21.

Chapter 40
High-Fat Diet and Foetal Programming: Use of P66Shc Knockouts and Implications for Human Kind

Alessandra Berry and Francesca Cirulli

Key Points

- Prenatal stress affects foetal programming leading to long-term detrimental effects for health.
- Maternal high-fat diet and/or obesity are metabolic stressors that can result in lifelong metabolic vulnerability in the offspring.
- The p66Shc gene modulates oxidative stress and insulin signalling.
- Knocking out the p66Shc gene in mice protects from the long-term effects of prenatal metabolic stress.
- The ultimate role of p66Shc in human health is highly dependent from environmental conditions and life stage.
- To maximize the effects, interventions strategies should be started as early as possible.

Keywords P66Shc • Mice • Humans • Oxidative stress • Fat accumulation • Insulin • Metabolic stress • Foetal programming • Ageing • Healthspan

Abbreviations

11β-HSD-1	11β-dehydrogenase-1
11β-HSD-2	11β-dehydrogenase-2
BMI	Body mass index
CAD	Coronary artery disease
HFD	High-fat diet
HPA	Hypothalamic-pituitary-adrenal
KO	Knockout
MetS	Metabolic syndrome
OS	Oxidative stress
PBMC	Peripheral blood mononuclear cells

A. Berry (✉) • F. Cirulli
Center for Behavioral Sciences and Mental Health, Istituto Superiore di Sanità,
Viale Regina Elena 299, I-00161 Rome, Italy
e-mail: alessandra.berry@iss.it

© Springer International Publishing AG 2017
R. Rajendram et al. (eds.), *Diet, Nutrition, and Fetal Programming*,
Nutrition and Health, DOI 10.1007/978-3-319-60289-9_40

557

ROS   Reactive oxygen species
T2D   Type 2 diabetes
WT   Wild type

Introduction

Obesity during pregnancy is a main risk factor for adverse health outcomes of both the mother and the offspring. The negative consequences of maternal obesity might become manifest early during development but also in the long run [1]. This condition has been associated with hyperinsulinemia and gestational diabetes and is likely to result in pre-eclampsia [2]. Moreover, it has been causally related to an excessively rapid foetal growth, perinatal morbidity, in addition to elevated levels of cord leptin and interleukin-6 and to an overall increased chance for the offspring to develop metabolic and cardiovascular pathologies later in life. Despite this evidence, still little is known about the mechanisms underlying these effects. Beyond the individual/genetic background, the intrauterine *milieu* has been advocated as the main effector accounting for a developmental origin of health outcome in a lifelong perspective ultimately affecting lifespan, as well as the quality of life during ageing (healthspan) [3, 4].

A developing mammal is an experience-seeking organism, characterized by an elevated degree of plasticity. Its development is a very dynamic process relying upon the continuous interactions between a detailed species-specific genetic program and the many experiences provided by the pre- and post-natal environment. These environmental triggers have the potential to shape a best-adapted phenotype acting as a forecast for the conditions the organism will face once adult (i.e. when the developmental program has been completed) [5]. To this regard, from an evolutionary perspective, the overall outcome of such a dynamic process is highly dependent upon the stability of the environmental conditions. Thus, if a mismatch occurs with respect to the *milieu* experienced by the developing and the adult organism, the ontogenetic adjustments aimed at finely tuning the individual to the environment might turn into embedded detrimental traces setting the stage for an increased vulnerability to later-life diseases. In line with this hypothesis, it has been suggested that a number of non-communicable diseases characterized by metabolic dysfunction might be the result of the effects of "thrifty genes" selected – and evolutionary conserved – to increase survival chances of individuals living in poor nutritional environments. Yet, the effects of these "thrifty genes" would turn out to be maladaptive when these individuals are exposed to abundant nutrition across their lives, eventually leading to the onset of metabolic diseases [6].

The pregnant dam perceives, elaborates and conveys external inputs of different nature to the foetus through the placenta. This organ, of both maternal and foetal origin, regulates the access of nutrients and of hormones at proper times during development and is able to modify its structure and function in response to changes in the maternal environment [7]. Psychological or metabolic stressors can disrupt placental function. This might acutely affect the development of foetal tissues and organs, as well as redirect developmental trajectories through epigenetic reprogramming, resulting in long-term effects [8, 9]. Ever increasing evidence points to oxidative stress (OS) as a common mediator linking maternal stress to placental dysfunctions, foetal programming and metabolic memory throughout life [10]. Oxidative stress derives from the unbalance between the production of pro-oxidants (mainly reactive oxygen species – ROS) and the antioxidant capacity of the body to detoxify. This condition associates to very different pathological manifestations, including those related to metabolic dysfunctions (e.g. obesity, type 2 diabetes (T2D), cardiovascular diseases as well as metabolic syndrome (MetS), inflammatory state) and can be also triggered by chronic consumption of high-fat diet (HFD). In general, OS may cause random damage to proteins, lipids and DNA. Moreover, being involved in the process of telomere shortening, it may promote the ageing of tissues and organs by affecting cellular senescence. Oxidative stress associated to maternal obesity might result in pathological conditions of the placenta, the embryo and the foetus [11, 12] also leading to epigenetic changes and altered gene expression in the foetus due to DNA damage [13]. However, the generation of ROS, within certain boundaries, is essential during the early gestation to promote cell proliferation and differentiation [14]. Thus, the redox homeostasis of the intrauterine *milieu* needs to be tightly regulated and changes to this environment may profoundly affect the developmental trajectories of the foetus, setting the stage for later-life vulnerability. Notwithstanding this evidence, environmental adversities may not act alone in determining the developmental origin of health and diseases as a growing body of literature suggests that modulators (genes) of lifespan exist and are conserved over large evolutionary distances.

In this context, the p66Shc has been described as a mammalian *gerontogene* involved in the regulation of OS and metabolism affecting health throughout life and during ageing [15]. Genetically modified mice lacking the p66Shc gene (p66Shc−/−) are long-lived and show an increased healthspan [16–19]. Moreover, prenatal exposure to HFD in the p66Shc−/− mouse results in a gender-specific resilience to both stressful and metabolic challenges [20]. Thus, the p66Shc gene appears as a very appealing *trait d'union* linking together foetal development and senescence through OS and metabolism.

This chapter will focus on the role of the p66Shc gene throughout mammalian life. It will describe the effects of this gene from early developmental stages to senescence. Evolutionary as well as mechanistic perspectives will be provided and implications for human kind discussed.

The P66Shc Gerontogene: Setting the Stage for Extended Healthspan

Almost two decades ago, Pelicci and colleagues reported the serendipitous discovery of the long-lived p66Shc−/− mouse [21]. These mutants show a 30% increase in longevity and are characterized by elevated resistance to OS, reduced triglyceride accumulation in the adipocytes, increased metabolic rate, decreased fat mass and resistance to diet-induced obesity [22].

P66Shc is one of the three isoforms encoded by the ShcA gene. This gene is almost ubiquitously expressed throughout the body showing tissue-specific changes in the levels of the p66Shc protein during development (see [15, 19] and references therein for complete a review). Each ShcA isoform harbours three identical functional domains; however, only p66Shc holds an additional N-terminal

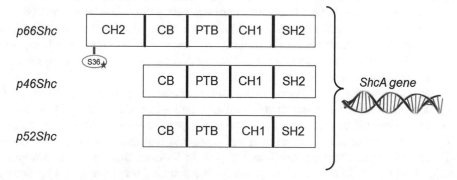

Fig. 40.1 Structure of the ShcA gene. P66Shc and p52Shc/p46Shc are encoded by two different m-RNAs. The p66Shc transcript has an alternative transcription initiation site from that of the p46Shc and p52Shc isoforms that are generated from an alternative splicing. Each of the three proteins holds an N-terminal phosphotyrosine-binding domain (*PTB*), a proline-rich domain (*CH1*) and a carboxy-terminal Src homology 2 (*SH2*) domain. The p66Shc is characterized by an additional N-terminal proline-rich domain (*CH2*) that becomes phosphorylated (*red star*) on a serine residual (*S36*) upon cellular stressors including metabolic and OS signals

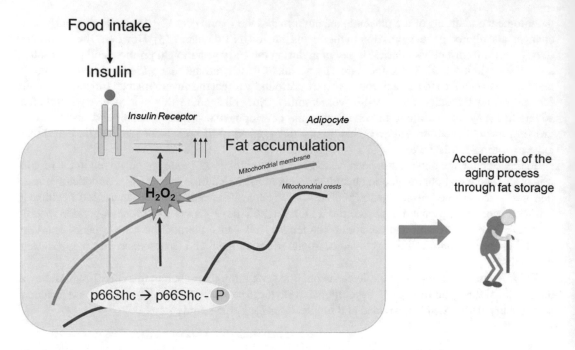

Fig. 40.2 Function of the p66Shc protein within the adipose tissue. Food intake stimulates insulin secretion that leads to the activation of p66Shc upon phosphorylation. The active form of p66Shc triggers the generation of H_2O_2 within the mitochondrion that, in turn, potentiates the insulin-mediated signalling pathway of fat accumulation within the adipocyte eventually promoting fat accumulation and the onset and/or precipitation of fat-related disorders

proline-rich domain (CH2) containing a serine phosphorylation site – Ser36 – that plays a key role in the specific signalling pathway triggered by cellular stress of different nature (e.g. OS and insulin; see below; Fig. 40.1). The main function of the p66Shc protein is to act specifically within the mitochondrion as a redox enzyme able to respond to OS insults by reinforcing this stress signal through the generation of H_2O_2 to trigger mitochondrial swelling and apoptosis [23]. Most intriguingly, within the adipose tissue, p66Shc generates H_2O_2 in response to insulin and, through this mechanism, it is able to reinforce the insulin-signalling cascade promoting fat accumulation [22]. To this regard, an interesting hypothesis is that this gene has been evolutionary conserved in the mammalian genome for its capacity to increase survival chances under harsh environmental conditions characterized by reduced food availability and/or low temperatures [24]. However, this 'thrifty function' might turn out to be detrimental when food is constantly available. Thus, in westernized lifestyles countries, p66Shc, by boosting intracellular OS, might promote fat deposition and the onset of metabolic-related pathologies accelerating in turn the ageing process (Fig. 40.2).

As previously mentioned, knocking out the p66Shc gene in mice overall results in an increased longevity and in an elevated resistance to both oxidative and metabolic insults [22]. A thorough phenotypic characterization of these mutants has revealed that p66Shc−/− mice show reduced central and peripheral levels of inflammatory markers upon immunogenic challenges, and these features are associated to a more efficient neuroendocrine function [18]. In addition, these mutants showed improved cognitive abilities [25], a reduced emotionality, and when reaching senescence, by improved physical performance and by increased neurogenesis within the hippocampus; this latter feature appeares as a gender-dependent trait that is more pronounced in females [16–18, 24, 25]. Thus, it clearly appears that the signalling cascades mediated by p66Shc activation may be located at the crossroad of pathways involved both in central and peripheral stress responses, as well as in the regulation of energy homeostasis [19]. Moreover, and most importantly, the p66Shc knockout (KO) mice are characterized not only by increased longevity but also by an increased healthspan [19].

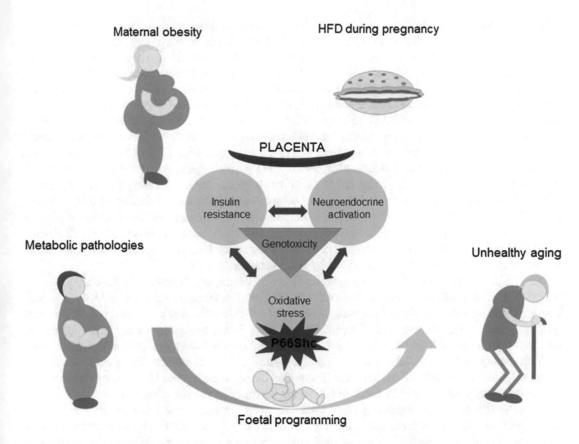

Fig. 40.3 The role of p66Shc in metabolic stress-mediated foetal programming. Coexisting mechanisms might underlie the detrimental effects of early programming triggered by prenatal metabolic stress (insulin resistance, glucocorticoid overexposure and OS). The mutual interaction among these players might result in genotoxic effects (e.g. telomere shortening, DNA methylation and oxidation) overall leading to increased vulnerability to chronic disease and unhealthy ageing. P66Shc might play a key role in mediating the effects of OS in early programming (Figure modified from Iozzo et al. [4])

High-Fat Diet Feeding During Pregnancy and Its Implications for the Mother and the Foetus: Lessons from the P66Shc Knockout Mouse

Preclinical and clinical data suggest that OS might play a pivotal role linking maternal metabolic stress to placental dysfunction, foetal programming and later-life vulnerability [10]. Despite the increasing evidence to support this field of research, still little is known about the possible underlying mechanisms.

Being involved in the modulation of fat metabolism and OS, the p66Shc gene might indeed play a role in the pathways linking metabolic maternal stress to foetal programming and later-life health outcome (Fig. 40.3) [4]. This issue was thoroughly investigated within the frame of the DORIAN study ("Developmental Origins of Healthy and Unhealthy Aging: the role of maternal obesity"). This large European project was aimed specifically at dissecting the prenatal determinants of healthspan and longevity by focussing on the mutual interaction among maternal cortisol, insulin resistance and OS, both in clinical and preclinical research.

We hypothesized that the lack of the p66Shc gene in mice might buffer the detrimental effects of a metabolic stress (HFD) during pregnancy, protecting both the mother and the offspring. To this aim

HFD (or a standard control diet) was administered during peri-conceptional time and throughout pregnancy to female p66Shc wild-type (WT) and KO mice until delivery. To focus specifically on foetal programming, HFD consumption was stopped just before parturition; for the same reason, the offspring was weaned onto standard diet. Since the effects of prenatal stress strongly interact with sex hormones, both male and female offspring were phenotyped from birth to adult age. The characterization of the metabolic, neuroendocrine and emotional profile of the adult offspring indicated that prenatal diet affects stress responses and metabolic features in a gender-dependent fashion, while knocking out the p66Shc gene attenuates such effects, acting as a protective factor. Overall, prenatal HFD resulted in reduced body weight at birth and in a greater catch-up, particularly in male subjects at adult age. The most striking effects of maternal HFD were observed in the female offspring that showed an increased body mass index (BMI) as well as higher leptin levels (compared to the prenatal standard diet-fed group); however, p66Shc−/− subjects were protected. Females of this genotype showed a better ability to cope with both metabolic and neuroendocrine stressors (enhanced glucose tolerance and insulin resistance, in addition to being protected from HFD-induced hypothalamic-pituitary-adrenal (HPA) axis hyperactivity) overall suggesting that the effects of a metabolically stressful environment might be finely tuned by sex hormones [20].

As partial confirmation of the role played by OS early during development, we have also recently observed that the administration of antioxidants (N-acetylcysteine) to C57Bl6 mice during peri-conceptional time and throughout pregnancy is able to buffer the effects of a maternal metabolic stress (HFD) on both the mother and the offspring. This piece of data is quite interesting since it appears to mimic the protective effects observed as a result of the lack of the p66Shc gene overall strengthening the link among maternal metabolic stress, foetal programing and OS/p66Shc (Berry et al. manuscript in preparation). A further interesting finding provided by our study is that HFD consumption before and during pregnancy results in detrimental effects not only in the offspring but also in the dams, affecting their reproductive success. In fact, we observed an increased maternal mortality during pregnancy, particularly around parturition, and the occurrence of aberrant maternal behaviours (increased cannibalistic episodes) immediately after delivery. In this context, it is interesting to note that, since HFD consumption did not lead to maternal obesity, all the observed effects (in both the offspring and in the dams) were purely due to maternal exposure to a metabolic stress [20]. Thus, extreme changes in the diet during pregnancy might indeed represent a powerful source of stress for the dams negatively affecting their ability to cope with demanding psychophysical conditions dealing with reproduction (pregnancy and delivery) and the care of the offspring.

Indeed, clinical data clearly indicate that a diet rich in fats is a physiological stressor for pregnant women [26]; preclinical studies suggest that HFD consumption during pregnancy might challenge the maternal HPA axis resulting in increased secretion of glucocorticoids stress hormones associated with amplified emotional reactivity [27]. In addition, the effects of HFD during pregnancy appear to overlap with those provided by psychophysical stress and to converge to similar consequences on foetal growth, neurodevelopment and metabolism [28]. In this regard, it is worth mentioning that foetal exposure to glucocorticoid hormones is a fundamental process for mammalian development that is efficiently regulated throughout pregnancy and that the placenta plays a key role in this process [7].

In a very recent study, we have dissected out the effects of HFD-feeding specifically focusing on the narrow time comprising the final stages of pregnancy in mice. Indeed, we provided evidence that maternal HFD increased levels of maternal corticosterone immediately before and after delivery. This was associated with a lower placental weight, reduced 11β-HSD-2 enzymatic activity and m-RNA expression of the 11β-HSD-1 gene in this organ, resulting in a disruption of the time window of foetal exposure to maternal glucocorticoids. In this regard, prenatal HFD resulted in reduced body/foetal weight at the end of pregnancy and in an extended pregnancy length, suggesting a possible attempt to allow further foetal growth [29].

From a behavioural point of view, HFD-fed dams showed a disorganized social and maternal behaviour at parturition. Most intriguingly maternal HFD consumption reduced c-Fos expression in the dams' olfactory bulbs suggesting a reduced neural activity in brain regions involved in olfactory processing and social recognition. In this context, the inappropriate behavioural patterns observed, such as cannibalism, could depend upon an inability to discriminate salient olfactory stimuli, such as those provided by the newborn pups [29]. These data are particularly interesting when considering that olfaction (and the associated neuronal system) can account for behavioural decisions related to food choice and consumption [30]. Moreover, food odours are essential to control for food intake [31]. Thus, changes in the activity of the olfactory system, as a result of early exposure to HFD, have the potential to impact negatively on food choices at adulthood, reinforcing inappropriate behaviours, such as the choice of poor quality food.

P66Shc Friend or Foe? Implications for Human Kind

Ever increasing evidence strongly suggests that the lack of p66Shc leads to undeniable beneficial effects. Indeed, this evidence is quite strong in animal models of metabolic and cardiovascular pathologies [32–34], and studies on human subjects mostly support the hypothesis of p66Shc being involved in the onset and/or precipitation of these pathological processes. As an example p66Shc gene expression was found to be increased in peripheral blood mononuclear cells (PBMC) of patients with coronary artery disease (CAD) [35, 36] and with T2D [37] in association with increased levels of OS markers. Moreover, Natalicchio recently reported increased levels of p66Shc and of p53 (a pro-apoptotic gene) in human pancreatic islet of donors with elevated BMI [32] supporting the link among obesity, lipotoxicity and the pathogenesis of T2D. Of note, Fadini and co-workers suggested that the p66Shc gene might be involved in the pathogenesis of MetS, a cluster of metabolic and cardiovascular conditions overall mimicking a precocious ageing process [38] strengthening the idea that the insulin-p66Shc-H_2O_2 axis might be a critical component in both healthspan and longevity conditions.

Despite this convincing evidence, studies on p66Shc human cohorts, particularly in relation with ageing and/or prenatal conditions, are still limited and somehow controversial. Research focusing on genetic variants in the p66Shc gene show that these are extremely rare, not associated to longevity (at least in the Japanese population) [39] and probably not even involved in the genetic susceptibility to CAD [40] though an association between the Met410Val polymorphism and longevity in humans might exist [41]. By contrast, results from studies aimed at investigating the role of epigenetic changes in relation to human ageing appear overall more solid, and preserved DNA methylation of genes involved in the regulation of metabolism has been suggested to be a potential mechanism underlying healthspan during ageing [42]. To this regard, it is worth to note that the DNA methylation in CpG islands is associated with gene silencing and that the p66Shc promoter contains a relatively high CG content [43]. Interestingly, recent data suggest a role for decreased DNA methylation of the p66Shc promoter in placental tissue from women delivering intrauterine growth restricted neonates, a condition that is often associated to the development of metabolic disorders via foetal programming in later life [44]. In addition, Kim and co-workers found that low-density lipoprotein (LDL) cholesterol upregulates human endothelial p66Shc expression via hypomethylation of its promoter, a finding that may have relevance in the development of endothelial dysfunctions and its consequences in adults/aged individuals who have been exposed to hypercholesterolemic environment in utero [45]. Notwithstanding the above-mentioned evidence, Pandolfi and co-workers found that fibroblasts from centenarians were characterized by the highest basal levels of p66Shc m-RNA and that these changes occurred in the absence of any modification of the p66Shc promoter methylation pattern [46]. In line with this finding, it has been recently proposed that the p66Shc-induced ROS formation might contribute to self-endogenous defences against mild ischemia and reperfusion injury [47].

Indeed, increasing evidence indicates that although excessive ROS might lead to the negative effects of OS on cellular homeostasis, low non-toxic levels of ROS can hold beneficial effects acting as second messengers in a broad range of intracellular signalling pathway dealing with cell proliferation and survival [48, 49]. This might promote health and longevity by delaying the progression or preventing the onset of chronic diseases. Thus, it is possible to hypothesize that low levels of ROS might set the conditions for a favourable environment aimed at improving systemic defences by inducing adaptive responses. This concept has been defined as mitochondrial hormesis or *mitohormesis* [50, 51]. To this regard, it is worth mentioning that both calorie restriction (the most robust, non-genetic intervention increasing healthspan and longevity in different species) [52] and physical exercise [53] might exert their positive effects on health through enhanced mitochondrial biogenesis. In addition, in the case of physical training, oxidative metabolism and increased generation of ROS have been also shown to play a key role [50, 51].

Taken together, evidence concerning the impact of p66Shc on human health appears more complex than expected, at least given the results of animal studies carried out in controlled experimental settings [24]. We propose that the issue of beneficial vs. toxic effects deriving from changes in the expression levels of p66Shc should be carefully considered in the context of the different metabolic needs characterizing different life stages and the availability of nutritional sources (see conclusions and Fig. 40.4 below).

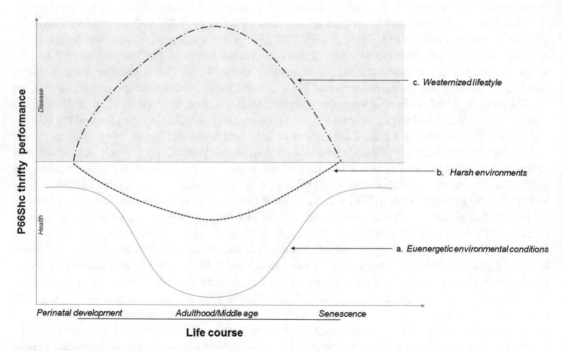

Fig. 40.4 Evolutionary overview of the p66Shc function and implications for human health. The p66Shc protein accumulates fat within the adipocyte through a mechanism involving OS signalling. This thrifty function plays a pivotal role during perinatal development as well as during senescence, when fat accumulation and the generation of ROS, within certain boundaries, might trigger main pro-survival signalling cascades. This optimal performance occurs only under 'euenergetic' conditions (*a. green solid line*) reaching its best under harsh environmental times when also adult-/middle-aged subjects benefit from improved energy storage (*b. red dashed line*) as shown by a smooth U-shaped curve. By contrast, p66Shc over-performs under westernized lifestyle conditions (characterized by excessive caloric intake) promoting the onset of metabolic disorders setting the stage for unhealthy ageing (*c. black dashed line*). This fuel-driven metabolic liability originates during perinatal life leading to the occurrence of overt metabolic pathologies during adulthood/middle age. Those subjects who will survive the burden of metabolic diseases during adult life will be characterized by unhealthy ageing

Conclusions

Extreme changes in the metabolic milieu before and during pregnancy, independently from maternal obesity, might represent a powerful source of stress affecting foetal programming with lifelong deleterious consequences on the healthspan and longevity of the offspring. A number of different and non-mutually exclusive mechanisms, including OS, might underlie the detrimental effects of early programming triggered by prenatal metabolic stress, leading to important trans-generational effects also mediated by epigenetic remodelling of selected genes. The p66Shc 'thrifty gerontogene' might play a key role in mediating the long-term trans-generational effects of maternal obesity and/or HFD by affecting insulin metabolism and redox balance throughout pregnancy. Indeed, we have recently provided evidence that p66Shc−/− mice are protected from the stressful and metabolic challenges following prenatal exposure to HFD. However, the role of p66Shc in human healthspan, in relation to prenatal life, is more complex than expected, and we propose that its function may vary according to the metabolic needs characterizing different life stages and also to the availability of nutritional sources (Fig. 40.4). Thus, in a 'euenergetic' nutritional status, p66Shc might play a pro-survival/pro-longevity role during life times characterized by an elevated energy demand such as early pre- and postnatal development as well as during senescence (Fig. 40.4a); adult organisms might also take advantage of this thrifty function in poor nutritional environments (Fig. 40.4b). By contrast, the p66Shc gene might over-perform when high caloric food is constantly available, leading to non-communicable metabolic disorders (Fig. 40.4c). In addition, it should be taken into account that, at the cellular level, the generation of ROS (H_2O_2 in this case) is also involved in mediating specific signalling pathways, leading to cell proliferation/differentiation vs. cell death; and thus a further synergistic level of action of the p66Shc gene might also rely upon these mechanisms.

Overall, an extensive and growing body of research demonstrates multiple linkages between prenatal life, metabolic stress and health outcomes at adulthood. Thus, knowledge of the biological mechanisms occurring during foetal development might help understanding/predicting individual variations in healthspan, including metabolic health [5]. To this regard, a life-course intergenerational approach to fight non-communicable metabolic disorders would be certainly worth pursuing starting from very early life stages rather than at middle-age, i.e. by the time the risk for individual vulnerability to metabolic and cardiovascular pathologies is the highest [54] (Fig. 40.5). This should include changes in the overall lifestyle, such as nutritional habits, as well as moderate physical exercise for the pregnant women. Antioxidant therapy is currently emerging as a promising strategy to counteract the fuel-mediated metabolic liability originating during prenatal life (antioxidant supplementation and/or a diet rich in antioxidants). However, to this regard, a note of caution should be raised since, while it might prevent some of the deleterious consequences of prenatal metabolic stress, we are becoming more and more aware that ROS might also play an important role in hormetic processes, thus a right balance in the overall oxidative status of the organisms should be achieved [50, 51].

Acknowledgements This work was supported by EU (FP7) Project DORIAN "Developmental Origin of Healthy and Unhealthy aging: the role of maternal obesity" (grant n. 278603) and ERA net-NEURON 'Poseidon'. The authors are grateful to Irene Pistella, Stella Falsini and Luigia Cancemi for their skilful help in retrieving and selecting bibliographic entries.

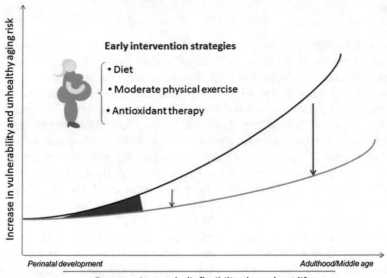

Fig. 40.5 Life-course intergenerational approach to fight non-communicable metabolic disorders. The ability of the organism to cope with stressful challenges decreases throughout life and is paralleled by the physiological decrease in metabolic flexibility characterizing adult/middle-aged subjects. Thus, an allostatic metabolic burden accumulates increasing the risk for the onset and progression of non-communicable metabolic diseases in late life stages. Yet, triggers to later-life vulnerability might be set in place during early life stages (maternal obesity or high-fat diet consumption during pregnancy) disrupting foetal programming. Early intervention (*purple* area within the *curves*) – which should include maternal diet, physical exercise and antioxidant therapies administration – has the potential to greatly reduce the disease risk later in life (*purple arrows*) in the face of a relatively modest precocious effort (Figure modified from Godfrey et al. [54])

References

1. Tenenbaum-Gavish K, Hod M. Impact of maternal obesity on fetal health. Fetal Diagn Ther. 2013;34(1):1–7.
2. Jeyabalan A. Epidemiology of preeclampsia: impact of obesity. Nutr Rev. 2013;71(Suppl 1):S18–25.
3. Barker DJ. In utero programming of chronic disease. Clin Sci (Lond). 1998;95(2):115–28.
4. Iozzo P, Holmes M, Schmidt MV, Cirulli F, Guzzardi MA, Berry A, et al. Developmental ORIgins of healthy and unhealthy AgeiNg: the role of maternal obesity – introduction to DORIAN. Obes Facts. 2014;7(2):130–51.
5. Bateson P, Barker D, Clutton-Brock T, Deb D, D'Udine B, Foley RA, et al. Developmental plasticity and human health. Nature. 2004;430(6998):419–21.
6. Neel JV. Diabetes mellitus: a "thrifty" genotype rendered detrimental by "progress"? Am J Hum Genet. 1962;14:353–62.
7. Harris A, Seckl J. Glucocorticoids, prenatal stress and the programming of disease. Horm Behav. 2011;59(3):279–89.
8. Dimasuay KG, Boeuf P, Powell TL, Jansson T. Placental responses to changes in the maternal environment determine fetal growth. Front Physiol. 2016;7:12.
9. Gluckman PD, Hanson MA. Developmental and epigenetic pathways to obesity: an evolutionary-developmental perspective. Int J Obes. 2008;32(Suppl 7):S62–71.
10. Perrone S, Santacroce A, Picardi A, Buonocore G. Fetal programming and early identification of newborns at high risk of free radical-mediated diseases. World J Clin Pediatr. 2016;5(2):172–81.
11. Hracsko Z, Orvos H, Novak Z, Pal A, Varga IS. Evaluation of oxidative stress markers in neonates with intra-uterine growth retardation. Redox Rep Commun Free Radic Res. 2008;13(1):11–6.
12. Shaker OG, Sadik NA. Pathogenesis of preeclampsia: implications of apoptotic markers and oxidative stress. Hum Exp Toxicol. 2013;32(11):1170–8.
13. Del Rio D, Stewart AJ, Pellegrini N. A review of recent studies on malondialdehyde as toxic molecule and biological marker of oxidative stress. Nutr Metab Cardiovasc Dis NMCD. 2005;15(4):316–28.
14. Dennery PA. Effects of oxidative stress on embryonic development. Birth Defects Res C Embryo Today. 2007;81(3):155–62.

15. Trinei M, Berniakovich I, Beltrami E, Migliaccio E, Fassina A, Pelicci P, et al. P66Shc signals to age. Aging. 2009;1(6):503–10.
16. Berry A, Amrein I, Notzli S, Lazic SE, Bellisario V, Giorgio M, et al. Sustained hippocampal neurogenesis in females is amplified in P66(Shc-/-) mice: an animal model of healthy aging. Hippocampus. 2012;22(12):2249–59.
17. Berry A, Capone F, Giorgio M, Pelicci PG, de Kloet ER, Alleva E, et al. Deletion of the life span determinant p66Shc prevents age-dependent increases in emotionality and pain sensitivity in mice. Exp Gerontol. 2007;42(1–2):37–45.
18. Berry A, Carnevale D, Giorgio M, Pelicci PG, de Kloet ER, Alleva E, et al. Greater resistance to inflammation at adulthood could contribute to extended life span of p66(Shc-/-) mice. Exp Gerontol. 2010;45(5):343–50.
19. Berry A, Cirulli F. The p66(Shc) gene paves the way for healthspan: evolutionary and mechanistic perspectives. Neurosci Biobehav Rev. 2013;37(5):790–802.
20. Bellisario V, Berry A, Capoccia S, Raggi C, Panetta P, Branchi I, et al. Gender-dependent resiliency to stressful and metabolic challenges following prenatal exposure to high-fat diet in the p66(Shc-/-) mouse. Front Behav Neurosci. 2014;8:285.
21. Migliaccio E, Giorgio M, Mele S, Pelicci G, Reboldi P, Pandolfi PP, et al. The p66shc adaptor protein controls oxidative stress response and life span in mammals. Nature. 1999;402(6759):309–13.
22. Berniakovich I, Trinei M, Stendardo M, Migliaccio E, Minucci S, Bernardi P, et al. p66Shc- generated oxidative signal promotes fat accumulation. J Biol Chem. 2008;283(49):34283–93.
23. Giorgio M, Migliaccio E, Orsini F, Paolucci D, Moroni M, Contursi C, et al. Electron transfer between cytochrome c and p66Shc generates reactive oxygen species that trigger mitochondrial apoptosis. Cell. 2005;122(2):221–33.
24. Giorgio M, Berry A, Berniakovich I, Poletaeva I, Trinei M, Stendardo M, et al. The p66Shc knocked out mice are short lived under natural condition. Aging Cell. 2012;11(1):162–8.
25. Berry A, Greco A, Giorgio M, Pelicci PG, de Kloet R, Alleva E, et al. Deletion of the lifespan determinant p66(Shc) improves performance in a spatial memory task, decreases levels of oxidative stress markers in the hippocampus and increases levels of the neurotrophin BDNF in adult mice. Exp Gerontol. 2008;43(3):200–8.
26. Reynolds RM, Labad J, Buss C, Ghaemmaghami P, Raikkonen K. Transmitting biological effects of stress in utero: implications for mother and offspring. Psychoneuroendocrinology. 2013;38(9):1843–9.
27. Tannenbaum BM, Brindley DN, Tannenbaum GS, Dallman MF, McArthur MD, Meaney MJ. High-fat feeding alters both basal and stress-induced hypothalamic-pituitary-adrenal activity in the rat. Am J Phys. 1997;273(6 Pt 1):E1168–77.
28. Zeltser LM, Leibel RL. Roles of the placenta in fetal brain development. Proc Natl Acad Sci U S A. 2011;108(38):15667–8.
29. Bellisario V, Panetta P, Balsevich G, Baumann V, Noble J, Raggi C, et al. Maternal high-fat diet acts as a stressor increasing maternal glucocorticoids' signaling to the fetus and disrupting maternal behavior and brain activation in C57BL/6J mice. Psychoneuroendocrinology. 2015;60:138–50.
30. Thiebaud N, Johnson MC, Butler JL, Bell GA, Ferguson KL, Fadool AR, et al. Hyperlipidemic diet causes loss of olfactory sensory neurons, reduces olfactory discrimination, and disrupts odor-reversal learning. J Neurosci Off J Soc Neurosci. 2014;34(20):6970–84.
31. Rolls ET. Taste, olfactory, and food texture processing in the brain, and the control of food intake. Physiol Behav. 2005;85(1):45–56.
32. Natalicchio A, Tortosa F, Labarbuta R, Biondi G, Marrano N, Carchia E, et al. The p66(Shc) redox adaptor protein is induced by saturated fatty acids and mediates lipotoxicity-induced apoptosis in pancreatic beta cells. Diabetologia. 2015;58(6):1260–71.
33. Paneni F, Cosentino F. p66 Shc as the engine of vascular aging. Curr Vasc Pharmacol. 2012;10(6):697–9.
34. Paneni F, Costantino S, Cosentino F. p66(Shc)-induced redox changes drive endothelial insulin resistance. Atherosclerosis. 2014;236(2):426–9.
35. Franzeck FC, Hof D, Spescha RD, Hasun M, Akhmedov A, Steffel J, et al. Expression of the aging gene p66Shc is increased in peripheral blood monocytes of patients with acute coronary syndrome but not with stable coronary artery disease. Atherosclerosis. 2012;220(1):282–6.
36. Noda Y, Yamagishi S, Matsui T, Ueda S, Jinnouchi Y, Hirai Y, et al. The p66shc gene expression in peripheral blood monocytes is increased in patients with coronary artery disease. Clin Cardiol. 2010;33(9):548–52.
37. Pagnin E, Fadini G, de Toni R, Tiengo A, Calo L, Avogaro A. Diabetes induces p66shc gene expression in human peripheral blood mononuclear cells: relationship to oxidative stress. J Clin Endocrinol Metab. 2005;90(2):1130–6.
38. Fadini GP, Ceolotto G, Pagnin E, de Kreutzenberg S, Avogaro A. At the crossroads of longevity and metabolism: the metabolic syndrome and lifespan determinant pathways. Aging Cell. 2011;10(1):10–7.
39. Kamei H, Adati N, Arai Y, Yamamura K, Takayama M, Nakazawa S, et al. Association analysis of the SHC1 gene locus with longevity in the Japanese population. J Mol Med. 2003;81(11):724–8.
40. Sentinelli F, Romeo S, Barbetti F, Berni A, Filippi E, Fanelli M, et al. Search for genetic variants in the p66Shc longevity gene by PCR-single strand conformational polymorphism in patients with early-onset cardiovascular disease. BMC Genet. 2006;7:14.

41. Mooijaart SP, van Heemst D, Schreuder J, van Gerwen S, Beekman M, Brandt BW, et al. Variation in the SHC1 gene and longevity in humans. Exp Gerontol. 2004;39(2):263–8.
42. Gentilini D, Mari D, Castaldi D, Remondini D, Ogliari G, Ostan R, et al. Role of epigenetics in human aging and longevity: genome-wide DNA methylation profile in centenarians and centenarians' offspring. Age. 2013;35(5):1961–73.
43. Ventura A, Luzi L, Pacini S, Baldari CT, Pelicci PG. The p66Shc longevity gene is silenced through epigenetic modifications of an alternative promoter. J Biol Chem. 2002;277(25):22370–6.
44. Tzschoppe A, Doerr H, Rascher W, Goecke T, Beckmann M, Schild R, et al. DNA methylation of the p66Shc promoter is decreased in placental tissue from women delivering intrauterine growth restricted neonates. Prenat Diagn. 2013;33(5):484–91.
45. Kim YR, Kim CS, Naqvi A, Kumar A, Kumar S, Hoffman TA, et al. Epigenetic upregulation of p66shc mediates low-density lipoprotein cholesterol-induced endothelial cell dysfunction. Am J Physiol Heart Circ Physiol. 2012;303(2):H189–96.
46. Pandolfi S, Bonafe M, Di Tella L, Tiberi L, Salvioli S, Monti D, et al. p66(shc) is highly expressed in fibroblasts from centenarians. Mech Ageing Dev. 2005;126(8):839–44.
47. Di Lisa F, Giorgio M, Ferdinandy P, Schulz R. New aspects of p66Shc in ischemia reperfusion injury and cardiovascular diseases. Br J Pharmacol. 2017;174(12):1690–1703.
48. Park SG, Kim JH, Xia Y, Sung JH. Generation of reactive oxygen species in adipose-derived stem cells: friend or foe? Expert Opin Ther Targets. 2011;15(11):1297–306.
49. Finkel T, Holbrook NJ. Oxidants, oxidative stress and the biology of ageing. Nature. 2000;408(6809):239–47.
50. Merry TL, Ristow M. Mitohormesis in exercise training. Free Radic Biol Med. 2015;98:123.
51. Ristow M, Schmeisser K. Mitohormesis: promoting health and lifespan by increased levels of reactive oxygen species (ROS). Dose-response Publ Intern Hormesis Soc. 2014;12(2):288–341.
52. Lopez-Lluch G, Hunt N, Jones B, Zhu M, Jamieson H, Hilmer S, et al. Calorie restriction induces mitochondrial biogenesis and bioenergetic efficiency. Proc Natl Acad Sci U S A. 2006;103(6):1768–73.
53. Radak Z, Chung HY, Goto S. Exercise and hormesis: oxidative stress-related adaptation for successful aging. Biogerontology. 2005;6(1):71–5.
54. Godfrey KM, Gluckman PD, Hanson MA. Developmental origins of metabolic disease: life course and intergenerational perspectives. Trends Endocrinol Metab TEM. 2010;21(4):199–205.

Chapter 41
Fetal Programming of Telomere Biology: Role of Maternal Nutrition, Obstetric Risk Factors, and Suboptimal Birth Outcomes

Sonja Entringer, Karin de Punder, Glenn Verner, and Pathik D. Wadhwa

Key Points

- Suboptimal intrauterine conditions have been linked to a wide variety of adverse effects later in life. Telomere biology is a candidate underlying mechanism by which maternal health, nutrition, and obstetric risk conditions can be transduced into long-term health effects in offspring.
- Animal and human studies point to the importance of the initial setting of the telomere system in development and progression of disease, aging, and mortality, and show that these effects persist across the life span.
- The initial programming of telomere homeostasis appears to be plastic and influenced by the intrauterine environment. Known genetic factors explain only a small amount of observed interindividual variability, and maternal-offspring correlation in telomere length is significantly higher than paternal-offspring correlation.

Note: Portions of this chapter have previously been published in the following of our own papers and are cited herein.
Entringer S, Wadhwa PD. Developmental programming of telomere biology: role of stress and stress biology. In: Stress and developmental programming of health and disease: beyond phenomenology. New York: Nova Science Publishers; 2014. p. 633–650
Entringer S, Buss C, Wadhwa PD. Prenatal stress and developmental programming of human health and disease risk: concepts and integration of empirical findings. Curr Opin Endocrinol Diabetes Obes. 2010;17:507–16.
Entringer S, Buss C, Swanson JM, Cooper DM, Wing DA, Waffarn F, Wadhwa PD. Fetal programming of body composition, obesity, and metabolic function: the role of intrauterine stress and stress biology. J Nutr Metab. 2012;2012:632548.
Entringer S, Buss C, Wadhwa PD. Prenatal stress, telomere biology, and fetal programming of health and disease risk. Sci Signal. 2012;5:pt12.

S. Entringer, PhD (✉)
Department of Medical Psychology, Charité – Universitätsmedizin Berlin, corporate member of Freie Universität Berlin, Humboldt-Universität zu Berlin, and Berlin Institute of Health (BIH), Institute of Medical Psychology, Berlin, Germany

Department of Pediatrics, Development, Health and Disease Research Program University of California, Irvine, School of Medicine, Irvine, CA, USA
e-mail: sonja.entringer@charite.de

K. de Punder, MSc
Charité – Universitätsmedizin Berlin, corporate member of Freie Universität Berlin, Humboldt-Universität zu Berlin, and Berlin Institute of Health (BIH), Institute of Medical Psychology, Laramie, WY, USA

© Springer International Publishing AG 2017
R. Rajendram et al. (eds.), *Diet, Nutrition, and Fetal Programming*, Nutrition and Health, DOI 10.1007/978-3-319-60289-9_41

- Maternal (mal)nutrition, obstetric risk conditions, and maternal stress and lifestyle have been shown to be associated with fetal telomere length.
- Stress hormones, oxidative stress, and inflammatory agents are biological pathways which may link adverse conditions during pregnancy to fetal telomere length. Epigenetic regulation also appears to be very important in controlling the telomere system.

Keywords Telomere • Developmental programming • Pregnancy • Nutrition • Obstetric complications • Birth outcomes

Abbreviations

CBMC   Cord blood mononuclear cells
CRP   C-reactive protein
FGR   Fetal growth restriction
GDM   Gestational diabetes mellitus
IL-6   Interleukin-6
IUGR   Intrauterine growth restriction
LBW   Low birth weight
LGA   Large for gestational age
NCD   Noncommunicable disorder
SES   Socioeconomic status
SGA   Small for gestational age
TA   Telomerase activity
TL   Telomere length
TNF-α   Tumor necrosis factor α
VLBW   Very low birth weight

Introduction

The origins of many, if not all, the of conditions that constitute a major burden of disease and also exhibit health disparities can be traced back to developmental processes in fetal life. The likelihood of developing any complex, common, noncommunicable disorder (NCD) is a function of both cumulative risk exposure (e.g., excess caloric intake, stressful life events) and susceptibility to these exposures, as reflected in the wide interindividual variation in the biological responses to any given risk exposure [1–3]. Contrary to the belief that individual susceptibility is determined primarily by genetic (DNA sequence) variation,

G. Verner, MSc
Charité – Universitätsmedizin Berlin, corporate member of Freie Universität Berlin, Humboldt-Universität zu Berlin, and Berlin Institute of Health (BIH), Institute of Medical Psychology, Berlin, Germany

École des Hautes Études en Santé Publique, Paris, France

P.D. Wadhwa, MD
Departments of Psychiatry & Human Behavior, Obstetrics & Gynecology, Pediatrics, Epidemiology, Development, Health and Disease Research Program, University of California, Irvine, School of Medicine, Irvine, CA, USA

susceptibility to NCDs is determined by dynamic interplay between genetics and environment, particularly during intrauterine life [1, 4–6]. Development is a plastic, context-dependent process, wherein a range of different phenotypes can be expressed from a given genotype. The fetus seeks, receives, and responds to, or is acted upon by, the intrauterine environment during sensitive periods, resulting in structural and functional changes. Some of these changes may, either independently or through interactions with subsequent developmental processes and environments, have major consequences for health and disease susceptibility [1, 6, 7]. These concepts have variously been referred to as the fetal or developmental programming of health and disease risk [4, 8–10]. Except in extreme cases, fetal programming does not, per se, "cause" disease, but instead determines propensity for disease(s) in later life by shaping responsivity to endogenous and exogenous conditions [10]. For example, exposure to excess maternal glucocorticoids during pregnancy (which may result from under- or overnutrition, infection, or stress) has been shown to alter the developing fetal brain and peripheral systems, with long-term consequences for the offspring's future risk of developing obesity and/or cardiometabolic disorders [11–16].

The majority of studies on the mechanisms underlying these effects are focused on processes that are specific to organs, phenotypes, or disorders of interest (e.g., mechanisms within the brain, adipocyte, pancreas, liver, etc.). However, it's possible that something else of importance is being overlooked. The observation that adverse intrauterine conditions simultaneously influence a diverse set of disease risk-related phenotypes, coupled with the fact that the majority of these phenotypes are implicated in increased risk of common age-related disorders, raises the possibility that intrauterine adversity may also additionally (not instead) exert effects via some common underlying mechanism and that such a mechanism may involve cellular aging-related molecular processes. Telomere biology represents a candidate outcome of particular interest in this context, because; first, this system is among the most salient antecedent cellular phenotypes for risk of common age-related disorders implicated in health disparities; second, the initial setting of the system appears to account for the largest attributable effects on long-term health and disease-related outcomes; and third, initial setting appears to be plastic and substantially impacted by developmental conditions during intrauterine and early postnatal life.

We have recently reviewed the role of maternal stress and stress biology in fetal programming of the telomere system [17]. This chapter will focus on the role of maternal nutrition and obstetric complications during pregnancy in programming the telomere biology system in a manner that may alter cellular function, aging, and disease susceptibility over the life span.

The Importance of Telomere Biology for Disease Risk and Aging

Telomere biology is a highly evolutionarily-conserved system that plays a central role in maintaining the integrity of the genome and cell. Telomere biology refers to the structure and function of two entities—telomeres, noncoding double-stranded repeats of guanine-rich tandem DNA sequences and shelterin protein structures that cap the ends of linear chromosomes [18, 19], and telomerase, the reverse transcriptase enzyme that adds telomeric DNA to telomeres [20].

Telomeres

Telomeres protect chromosomes from mistaken recognition by the DNA damage-repair system as DNA breaks. Because DNA polymerase is unable to fully replicate the 3′ end of the DNA strand, telomeres lose approximately 30–150 bp with each cell division. Eventually, telomeres reach a critical short length, resulting in decreased recruitment of shelterin proteins to form the protective internal nucleotide loops, which, in turn, leads to cellular senescence. Once cells become senescent, they exhibit a variety of genetic and morphological changes that result in loss of tissue function. This is how telomere attrition relates not only to longevity but also to the progression of common chronic diseases.

Telomerase

Conventional DNA polymerase machinery is unable to fully replicate the ends of linear chromosomes. The enzyme telomerase utilizes its own template to add short TG-rich repeats to chromosome ends, thus reversing their gradual erosion at each round of replication [21]. Typically, telomerase activity (TA) is diminished or absent in most adult somatic cells, with the exception being cells with a strong potential for division, such as certain types of stem cells and active lymphocytes [22]. The selective reduction of telomerase expression makes senescence inevitable by placing an upper bound on cellular life span [23]. Telomerase not only maintains telomere length but also preserves healthy cell function. Loss of telomerase affects chromatin configuration and impairs the DNA damage response. Telomerase also promotes proliferation of resting stem cells and directly modulates crucial developmental signaling pathways [24]. Finally, through telomere capping and maintenance, telomerase plays a particularly important role in cellular proliferation capacity and survival under conditions of cellular stress. Telomerase also performs an extranuclear role by co-localizing with mitochondria to protect mitochondrial DNA, decrease oxidative stress, and improve energy production and cellular function [25–28]. Thus, if telomere shortening represents the clock ticking forward on cells' limited life span, telomerase can reverse or slow this clock [29], making the two an intricately interdependent, dynamic system. A very substantial body of research has established that shortened telomeres and reduced telomerase expression are linked to several age-related diseases [30–33] and earlier mortality [34, 35].

Consequences of Telomere Shortening

As somatic cells divide, telomeres eventually reach a critical short length, resulting in decreased ability to recruit shelterin proteins, thus leading to cellular senescence or apoptosis [36]. Loss of telomere function causes chromosomal fusion, activation of DNA damage checkpoint responses, genome instability, and impaired stem cell function. After cells become senescent, they produce inflammatory mediators [37] that also affect neighboring cells, leading to further damage within organs and tissues that accumulates over the life course. Thus, as individuals age, they acquire more senescent cells, accompanied by various age-related pathologies (e.g., arteriosclerosis). This is how a reduction of telomere length (TL) and a steeper telomere attrition rate relate not only to longevity but also to earlier onset and more rapid progression of common chronic diseases. Moreover, recent important discoveries suggest that the integrity of telomeres affects not only the replicative capacity of the cell but also underlies other changes that enforce a self-perpetuating pathway of global epigenetic changes affecting the integrity of overall chromatin structure (DNA folding) that protects against senescence and cellular aging [38–41].

Consequences of Dysregulation of Telomerase Expression Capacity

In addition to maintenance of TL, telomerase plays a central role in preserving healthy cell function by promoting the proliferation of resting stem cells, modulating signaling pathways during embryogenesis and adult tissue homeostasis [42], and protecting cellular proliferation capacity and survival under conditions of cellular stress. Telomerase also plays a key extranuclear function: it localizes to mitochondria, where it protects mitochondrial DNA, increases mitochondrial membrane potential, and decreases mitochondrial superoxide production, thus decreasing oxidative stress and improving mitochondrial efficiency and cellular function [27, 43]. Thereby, a diminished capacity to express telomerase leads to more rapid telomere attrition over time, impaired DNA damage responses, and impaired cellular energetic function.

Importance of the Initial Setting of the Telomere System

The initial (newborn) setting of TL and telomerase expression capacity represent critically important aspects of an individual's telomere system [44]. TL at any given age during life is a joint function of (a) the initial (newborn) TL, and (b) telomere attrition rate over time (which, in turn, is a function of number of cell divisions (growth, age), the effects of exposures that produce TL shortening (e.g., oxidative stress), and the counteracting effects of the activity of the enzyme telomerase) [44]. Birds are a particularly well-suited and commonly used animal model to study telomere dynamics over the life span and across generations. Findings from avian studies suggest that TL and telomere attrition rates in early life are (i) far better predictors of realized life span than TL and attrition rates in later life, and (ii) their effects persist over and above those for risk exposures in later life [45–47]. Thus far, there are no human studies that have prospectively tracked TL from birth until old age. However, a human study that prospectively assessed TL across different adult populations over a 12-year period found almost no within-individual rank change in TL from baseline to follow-up and concluded that the relationship of TL with pathology and longevity appears to originate in the initial (early life) setting of TL [48]. Another recent human study in newborns demonstrated that compared to newborns with normal TL, newborns with reduced TL at birth exhibited greater DNA damage at baseline and also upon exposure to mitomycin C challenge (a common genotoxic agent) [49]. Thus, there is strong plausibility for the hypothesis that a reduction in the initial (newborn) setting of TL and telomerase expression capacity confers greater susceptibility for earlier onset and faster progression of age-related disorders that manifest in later life.

Determinants of the Initial Setting of TL

The assumption that initial setting of TL is largely under genetic control has been challenged for the following reasons: first, although the heritability of TL is high, (a) known genetic variants across all studies to date collectively account for only a small proportion of variation in TL (e.g. [50, 51]), and (b) the mother-offspring correlation in TL is substantially larger than the father-offspring correlation, regardless of the sex of the offspring. These findings, in conjunction with the understanding that heritability may overestimate genetic effects (because it includes maternal intrauterine effects), lead to a hypothesis that favors a major role for maternal effects in the initial setting of TL. Second, several experimental and observational studies in animals and humans demonstrate that adverse intrauterine conditions such as stress, dietary manipulations, and obstetric complications are associated with shorter TL at birth and in adult life and provide biological plausibility for this hypothesis [52, 53]. Thus, it appears that the initial setting and regulation of telomere homeostasis, including chromosomal telomere length and both the telomeric and extra-telomeric activities of telomerase, may be plastic and receptive to the influence of intrauterine or other early postnatal life conditions (see below). Also, telomere homeostasis in various cell types, including the germ line, stem cells, and proliferating as well as postmitotic tissue may serve as a fundamental integrator and regulator of processes underlying cell genomic integrity, function, aging, and senescence over the life span. This may have major implications for health and disease susceptibility for complex common disorders. We have advanced the hypothesis that context- and time-inappropriate exposures to physiological stresses during the embryonic, fetal, and early postnatal periods of development may alter or program the telomere biology system in a manner that accelerates cellular dysfunction, aging, and disease susceptibility over the life span [17, 52].

Nutrition During Pregnancy and Programming of Offspring Telomere System

Recent studies in animals and humans suggest that adverse or suboptimal conditions in intrauterine life are associated with shorter offspring TL and altered expression of TA in various tissues [52], thereby supporting the notion that TL may in part be programmed in utero. The role of maternal nutrition during pregnancy in programming various disease risk phenotypes in offspring is well established. In this section, we summarize available data from animal and human studies (Tables 41.1 and 41.2, respectively) reporting on the consequences of maternal (mal)nutrition on the offspring telomere biology system.

Malnutrition During Pregnancy and Offspring TL

Although calorie restriction after the third month of life increased life span in mice [64], energy restriction during gestation seems to have opposite effects on cellular aging. Experimental studies in rodents showed that protein restriction in utero combined with rapid postnatal catch-up growth (recuperated phenotype) were associated with increased oxidative stress, decreased antioxidant defense mechanisms, and accelerated telomere shortening across different tissues [53, 55–57] in the offspring, and that these effects even persisted in tissues of the reproductive tracts of second-generation offspring [54]. Importantly, post-weaning supplementation with coenzyme Q10, a key component of the electron transport chain and a potent antioxidant, attenuated telomere shortening in leukocytes and aortic cells of recuperated animals [58, 59], indicating that therapeutic interventions can be effective in counteracting the detrimental effects of suboptimal intrauterine conditions on cellular aging (Table 41.1). The recuperated rodent model described above reflects the so-called thrifty phenotype, characterized by low birth weight (LBW) and adaptations in metabolic activity advantageous for the immediate survival of the organism in continued conditions of poor postnatal nutrition but detrimental in an affluent postnatal environment [65].

In humans, the consequences of suboptimal intrauterine nutrition and its long-term health effects were studied in individuals conceived during the Dutch "Hunger Winter," a 5-month period of severe famine in the Netherlands at the end of World War II. Results from the Dutch Famine Birth Cohort Study show that individuals exposed to famine during early gestation are more susceptible to age-related diseases compared to individuals conceived before or after the famine. However, no differences were observed in leukocyte TL and the number of short telomeres at the age of 68 [60]. In contrast, increased telomere shortening was observed in survivors of the siege of Leningrad. Exposure to famine in intrauterine life and later childhood was associated with a higher prevalence of hypertension and shorter leukocyte TL [61]. Compared to the Dutch "Hunger Winter," the famine in Leningrad continued for a longer period of time, and food supplies did not return to adequate levels as rapidly as in the Netherlands, which might explain the observed differences between the two studies (Table 41.2).

Table 41.1 Nutrition during pregnancy and subsequent telomere length in offspring (animal studies)

Author, year	Sample size	Tissue	Species	Age	% Female	Assay	Prenatal exposure	Association of exposure with outcome
Protein restriction								
Aiken et al. 2013 [53]	N = 40 (N = 10 per group; 2 different experimental groups, tested at two different ages)	Oviduct and somatic ovarian tissue	Rats	3 and 6 months (cross-sectional)	N/A	Southern blot	Gestational protein restriction/fetal growth restriction (FGR)	Fewer long telomeres and more short telomeres in exposed animals
Aiken et al. 2015 [54]	N = 32 (N = 8 per group; 2 different experimental groups, tested at two different ages)	Ovarian	Rats	3 and 6 months (cross-sectional)	N/A	Southern blot	Grand maternal gestational protein restriction	Fewer long telomeres and more short telomeres in exposed animals only at 6 months of age
Jennings et al. 1999 [55]	N = 34 (N = 18 experimental group, N = 16 control group)	Liver, kidney, brain	Rats	3–33 days and 13 months	0 (male only)	Southern blot	Gestational protein restriction/FGR	Shorter life span and shorter kidney telomeres in exposed animals; no effect on liver or brain TL (postnatal growth retardation was associated with longer telomeres in the kidney)
Tarry-Adkins et al. 2008 [56]	N = 48 (N = 8 per group; 3 different experimental groups, tested at two different ages)	Aortic cells	Rats	3 and 12 months (cross-sectional)	0 (male only)	Southern blot	Gestational protein restriction/FGR vs. postnatal protein restriction/growth restriction vs. controls	Fewer long telomeres and more very short telomeres in exposed animals
Tarry-Adkins et al. 2009 [57]	N = 16 (N = 8 experimental group and N = 8 controls)	Islet cells	Rats	3 months	0 (male only)	Southern blot	Gestational protein restriction/ FGR	Shorter islet telomeres in exposed animals
Tarry-Adkins et al. 2013 [58]	N = 48 (N = 6 per group; 4 different experimental groups, tested at two different ages)	Aortic cells	Rats	3 and 12 months (cross-sectional)	0 (male only)	Southern blot	Gestational protein restriction/FGR and coenzyme Q10 supplementation	Fewer long telomeres and more short telomeres in exposed animals, coenzyme Q10 supplementation ameliorated telomere shortening
Tarry-Adkins et al. 2014 [59]	N = 48 (N = 6 per group; 4 different experimental groups, tested at two different ages)	Aortic cells, leukocytes	Rats	3 and 12 months (cross-sectional)	0 (male only)	Southern blot	Gestational protein restriction/FGR and coenzyme Q10 supplementation	At 12 months fewer long telomeres and more short telomeres in exposed animals, coenzyme Q10 supplementation slowed down telomere shortening, leukocyte Q10 levels correlated with aortic TL

Table 41.2 Nutrition during pregnancy and subsequent telomere length in offspring (human studies)

Author, year	Sample size	Tissue	Age	% Female	Assay	Prenatal exposure	Adjusted for	Association of exposure with outcome
Famine								
de Rooij et al. 2015 [60]	N = 131 (N = 41 exposed to famine during early gestation; N = 45 born before famine (control); N = 45 conceived after famine (control))	Leukocytes	67.6	Born before famine, 40; conceived during famine, 49; conceived after famine, 53	FISH	Famine	Age, sex, SES at birth, current employment, alcohol consumption, history of cancer, self-reported health status	No association
Rotar et al. 2015 [61]	N = 305 (N = 210 childhood exposed group; N = 50 new-born/infant exposed group; N = 45 intrauterine exposed group; N = 51 controls)	Leukocytes	70.7 (women), 70.5 (men)	73	qPCR	Famine	Age, income, education, marital status, smoking, alcohol consumption	Shorter TL in exposed group compared to controls, subjects exposed when newborn/infant longer TL compared to those exposed during childhood or intrauterine
Maternal nutrient state								
Entringer et al. 2015 [62]	119 mother-newborn dyads	CBMC	1st trimester, birth	Newborns: 45	qPCR	Maternal serum folate levels	SES, race/ethnicity, maternal prepregnancy BMI, maternal age, obstetric complications, infant sex, length of gestation, birth weight	10 ng/ml increase in maternal total folate was associated with a 5.8% increase in median TL
Sinkey et al. 2015 [63]	77 mother-newborn dyads	CBMC	Birth	N/A	qPCR	Homocysteine	Maternal age, gestational age, parity, maternal BMI, maternal smoking, red blood cell folate, vitamin B12 levels, birth weight, head circumference at birth, marital status, race/ethnicity, type of insurance	No association between homocysteine and TL, association between folate and TL and between smoking and TL

Maternal Nutrient State and Offspring TL

Associations between dietary behaviors and the telomere system have been described in cross-sectional studies in human adults. For example, the Mediterranean diet, which is related to lower levels of inflammation and oxidative stress, has been associated with longer TL and increased TA [66–69]. In addition, studies reported positive associations between the dietary intake and supplementation of several vitamins, antioxidants, fiber, and leukocyte TL, while high-fat intake (except for n-3 polyunsaturated fatty acids), the consumption of processed and red meat and sweetened carbonated beverages inversely related to TL (extensively reviewed by Freitas-Simoes et al. [70]).

Until recently, no human data was available regarding the associations between specific maternal nutrient states during pregnancy and offspring telomere biology. Therefore, as a first step toward addressing this question, we conducted a prospective longitudinal study focused on the effect of maternal folate state during early pregnancy on newborn TL [62]. In the developing fetus, folate is crucial in the contexts of DNA synthesis, cell proliferation, and neural tube development, and, in addition, folate plays a critical role in the maintenance of DNA integrity and DNA methylation, both important determinants of TL [71, 72]. Since the fetus is completely dependent on maternal folate supplies [73], we hypothesized that lower maternal folate concentrations are associated with shorter telomeres in newborns. In our study population, consisting of 119 mother-infant dyads, maternal folate plasma levels in the first trimester of pregnancy were related to newborn cord blood TL. After adjusting for established determinants of newborn TL, a 10 ng/ml increase in maternal total folate was associated with a 5.8% increase in median TL (Fig. 41.1a, b). Recently, these findings were replicated in an independent study cohort in which an association was observed between folate concentrations and newborn TL, both assessed in cord blood [63] (Table 41.2).

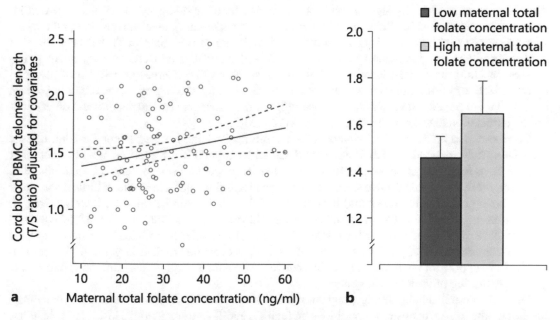

Fig. 41.1 (a) Scatterplot depicting the association between maternal plasma folate concentrations and newborn cord blood mononuclear cell (CMBC) telomere length (T/S ratio). Newborn CMBC telomere length was residualized (adjusted) for maternal socioeconomic status, race/ethnicity, prepregnancy BMI, length of gestation, birth weight, infant sex, and obstetric complications. (b) Mean adjusted cord blood PMBC telomere length (T/S ratio, ± standard error of the mean (SEM)) for newborns of mothers who fall in the lowest quartile (low maternal total folate concentration) vs. newborns of mothers in the highest folate quartile (high maternal total folate concentration) (Adapted from Entringer et al. [62])

Taken together, these results suggest programming effects of maternal nutrition during pregnancy on the telomere biology system of offspring. In addition, because newborn TL is an important determinant of telomere biology-related processes and subsequent health and disease outcomes later in life, these data indicate the potential benefit of nutrition-related therapeutic interventions already during pregnancy in the prevention of age-related diseases.

Obstetric Complications During Pregnancy, Suboptimal Birth Outcomes, and Offspring Telomere Biology

Obstetric complications during pregnancy and suboptimal birth outcomes such as LBW and preterm birth are associated with increased risk for morbidity and early mortality. A growing body of research seeks to link these adverse prenatal exposures and suboptimal birth outcomes to subsequent TL or TA in the offspring. Fetal growth, weight, and maturity are frequently studied exposures, and current studies in this area are presented in Table 41.3a (fetal growth and weight) and Table 41.3b (preterm birth). Placental insufficieny leading to impaired fetal growth, of which the most severe form is intrauterine growth restriction (IUGR)(fetal growth below the tenth percentile) is a risk factor for many newborn and adult health disorders [92] and may impact telomere homeostasis [77]. A decrease in mean TL has been reported among IUGR newborns [77, 87], and other studies have noted a parallel decrease in TA [75, 79, 82] and lower expression of telomerase components [76, 77] in pregnancies complicated with IUGR. Placentas of infants born small for gestational age (SGA) have also been observed to have reduced TA compared to controls and shorter placental TL [78]. Other studies, however, have found no association between SGA and TL in cord blood [74, 78] or have even observed an increase in TL among a cohort of young men born SGA [83]. Paradoxically, this paper reported that these men also showed early signs of vascular aging, and the authors suggested that the increased TL observed in this context (of SGA) may be the result of compensatory mechanisms due to the initial settings of telomere homeostasis in a deprived fetal environment [83]. Shorter TL has been found in babies born large for gestational age (LGA) as well [86]. TL generally decreases as pregnancy progresses, reaching its shortest length in the third trimester and likely serves as a signal of placental maturity [89], offering a potential explanation of this finding. Results regarding the effect of preterm birth on TL are mixed, with some studies observing shorter TL in preterm infants [91] and others finding no association between preterm birth and TL [88, 90].

LBW can also be the result of adverse fetal conditions [84] and is a risk factor for adult disease [80]. One study reported that LBW was associated with shorter TL at 5 years of age [84], but other cohorts have found no association between very low birth weight (VLBW) and TL in adults [80]. However, these were retrospective studies lacking data regarding telomere length at birth. Thus, other factors acting over the lifetime could have obscured the relationship between birth weight and TL [80]. Differences in TL and TA have also been studied in growth-discordant twins [81, 85, 86] (defined as a 20–25% difference in the birth weights of twins) [81]. Smaller twins have been shown to have both shorter telomeres [85] and lower levels of TA [81] as compared to their larger co-twins, providing further support for the hypothesized link between suboptimal intrauterine conditions and subsequent functioning of the telomere system.

Obstetric complications during pregnancy are associated with several adverse fetal outcomes. Studies on the impact of obstetric conditions on fetal TL and TA are summarized in Table 41.3c. It has been hypothesized that TL may be affected by perinatal complications, including rupture of the fetal membranes, which can lead to premature birth or stillbirth [95, 103]. Rupture of the fetal membranes is significantly associated with shorter TL, and this association is not seen with premature birth alone [103]. TL is even shorter among stillbirths than spontaneous preterm births [95]. Maternal diabetes is an obstetric risk condition of increasing prevalence and concern. Biron-Shental et al. [93] hypothesized that poorly controlled maternal diabetes may exert an effect via increased senescence in the

Table 41.3a Fetal growth and birth weight and telomere biology

Author, year	Sample size	Tissue	Age	% Female	Assay	Prenatal exposure	Adjusted for	Association of exposure with outcome
Fetal growth and weight								
Akkad et al. 2006 [74]	$N = 72$ ($N = 34$ small-for-gestational-age; $N = 38$ appropriate for gestational age)	CBMC	Birth	N/A	Southern blot	Impaired fetal growth	None	No association between size for gestational age and TL
Biron-Shental et al. 2010 [75]	$N = 57$ ($N = 14$ intrauterine growth restricted (IUGR); $N = 14$ preeclampsia; $N = 9$ IUGR+preeclampsia; $N = 20$ controls)	Placenta	Birth	N/A	FISH for TL; immunohistochemistry for TA	IUGR; preeclampsia; IUGR+preeclampsia	None	TL shorter and TA lower in all exposed groups compared to control group; increased telomere aggregate formation in preeclampsia but not IUGR
Biron-Shental et al. 2011 [76]	$N = 10$ ($N = 5$ IUGR; $N = 5$ controls)	Trophoblasts	Birth	N/A	FISH for estimating TERC gene copy number	IUGR	None	Lower TERC gene copy number in IUGR trophoblasts
Biron-Shental et al. 2014 [77]	$N = 30$ (15 healthy, 15 IUGR)	Placenta	Birth	N/A	FISH for estimating TERT gene copy number	IUGR	Maternal age, maternal BMI, gestational week at delivery, birth weight, mode of delivery	Decreased TERT, increased trophoblasts with senescence-associated heterochromatin foci, higher % of trophoblasts with telomere capture in exposed group
Davy et al. 2009 [78]	$N = 65$ ($N = 32$ FGR; $N = 36$ controls)	CBMC, placenta	Birth	N/A	Southern blot for TL; TRAP for TA	FGR	None	TL shorter in placenta but not in CBMC of exposed group; reduced TA in placental of exposed group
Izutsu et al. 1998 [79]	$N = 35$ ($N = 10$ IUGR; $N = 25$ normal pregnancies)	Placenta	Birth	N/A	TRAP	IUGR	None	Lower TA in IUGR group (TA detected in 72% of the samples from normal pregnancies and in only 10% of the IUGR placentas)

(continued)

Table 41.3a (continued)

Author, year	Sample size	Tissue	Age	% Female	Assay	Prenatal exposure	Adjusted for	Association of exposure with outcome
Kajantie et al. 2012 [80]	Three cohorts: (1) N = 1894	Leukocytes	(1) 56–69 years	(1) 53.3	qPCR	VLBW <1500 g	Age at study, gender, smoking status, BMI, length of gestation, weight, length, head circ., maternal BMI, age at delivery, parity, smoking during pregnancy, maternal hypertensive disorders during pregnancy, father's occupational status, highest educational level of either parent	(1) Shorter TL with age, smoking, younger age of mother, lower occupational status of father, higher maternal BMI (2) No association with VLBW preterm birth (3) Lower childhood SES associated with shorter TL
	(2) N = 334; N = 164 born preterm at VLBW, 170 controls		(2) 18–27 years	(2) 57.9 among preterm, 60 among controls				
	(3) N = 248 twins		(3) 23–31 years	(3) 46				
Kim et al. 2006 [81]	N = 20 pairs of twins (N = 11 growth discordant, N = 9 control)	Placental trophoblasts	Birth	N/A	ELISA and immunoblot	Growth discordant twins	Maternal age, week of gestation at delivery, parity, chorionisity	Higher TA in larger twin, no correlation between TA and degree of growth discordance
Kudo et al., 2000 [82]	N = 75 (N = 31 from chorionic villi (group A); N = 32 placental tissue samples from fetuses without IUGR (group B); N = 12 placental tissue samples from fetuses with asymmetric IUGR) (group C)	Chorionic villi and placenta	Group A: first trimester; Group B: second and third trimester; Group C: 26–39 weeks	N/A	TRAP	IUGR	None	TA detected in 20/32 placenta without IUGR (62.5%), no TA detected in 12 placentas exposed to IUGR
Laganovic et al. 2014 [83]	N = 114	Leukocytes	20–23 years	0	qPCR	SGA	Age, BMI, blood pressure, birth parameters, sex, maternal parity	Longer TL, early signs of vascular aging in exposed group
Raqib et al. 2007 [84]	N = 132 (N = 66 LBW, N = 66 normal birth weight)	Leukocytes	5 years	52 in LBW group; 38 in normal birth weight group	Southern blot	LBW	N/A	Shorter TL in LBW group

Author, year	Sample size	Tissue	Age	% Female	Assay	Prenatal exposure	Adjusted for	Association of exposure with outcome
Strohmaier et al. 2015 [85]	N = 1207 pairs of twins	CBMC	Mean age at DNA extraction for AUS group=14 mean age at DNA extraction for ND group = 36	53.4	qPCR	LBW discordant MZ twin	IQ, anxiety/depression	Shorter TL in lower birth weight twin
Tellechea et al. 2015 [86]	N = 69 (N = 45 appropriate weight for gestational age, N = 12 SGA, N = 12 LGA)	Leukocytes	Birth	N/A	qPCR	Small and large for gestational age OBFC1 and CTC1 genetic variants	Birth weight adjusted for gestational age, head circumference, length, Apgar score, leptin, plasma homocysteine, maternal age, physical activity, smoking level, pregestational BMI, weight gain during pregnancy, DABP, SABP	LTL significantly shorter in LGA as compared with SGA, significantly inversely correlated with maternal history of hypertension in previous pregnancies
Toutain et al. 2013 [87]	N = 52 (24 IUGR subjects, 28 controls)	Placenta	18–37 weeks of amenorrhea	N/A	FISH, qPCR	IUGR	Maternal age, gestational age, number of pregnancies, number of children, pregnancy term, birth weight, clinical signs of preeclampsia	Shorter TL in exposed group

Table 41.3b Preterm birth and telomere biology

Author, year	Sample size	Tissue	Age	% Female	Assay	Prenatal exposure	Adjusted for	Association of exposure with outcome
Preterm birth								
Friedrich et al. 2001 [88]	N = 36 (N = 15 preterm infants, N = 11 full-term infants)	CBMC	Birth	51 in preterm sample; not specified for control sample	Southern blot	Preterm birth	None	No association between TL and preterm birth
Gielen et al. 2014 [89]	N = 329	Placenta	Birth, parental questionnaires	54	qPCR	Gestational age	Sex, birth order, placental characteristics (including zygosity and chorion type), parity, maternal and paternal age, diabetes, hypertension, smoking, alcohol use, SES	Shorter TL with greater gestational age; smaller correlation coefficient when SES or diabetes considered, larger coefficient when parity considered; shorter placental TL among primiparous mothers, longer among diabetic mothers, and inversely correlated with SES
Hadchouel et al. 2015 [90]	N = 274 (N = 236 preterm; N = 38 full term)	Saliva	22–32 weeks of gestation (preterm); 33–34 and 39–40 weeks of gestation (controls) spirometry measure in adolescence, mean age = 14.9 years	51.5	qPCR	Preterm birth	Spirometric indices, birth weight, sex, BPD and postnatal sepsis, smoking during pregnancy, ethnicity, gestational age at birth, perinatal events	Female sex associated with longer TL, positive correlation between TL and abnormal airflow in individuals born extremely preterm
Smeets et al. 2015 [91]	N = 470 (N = 186 born preterm; N = 284 born at term)	Leukocytes	18–24 years	56.6	qPCR	Preterm birth	Gender, size at birth, age, height, weight, smoking, SES	Shorter TL in exposed group

Table 41.3c Obstetric risk factors and perinatal complications and telomere biology

Author, year	Sample size	Tissue	Age	% Female	Assay	Prenatal exposure	Adjusted for	Association of exposure with outcome
Obstetric risk factors								
Biron-Shental et al. 2015 [93]	$N = 32$ (16 mothers with uncontrolled diabetes; $N = 16$ controls)	Placenta and CBMC	Birth	N/A	FISH	Poorly controlled diabetes	Gestational age	Higher % of trophoblasts with short telomeres, increased signs of senescence in exposed group
Cross et al. 2010 [94]	$N = 319$ ($N = 26$ type 1 diabetes; $N = 20$ type 2 diabetes; $N = 71$ GDM, $N = 202$ control subjects)	CBMC	Birth	Control offspring, 42.2; diabetes offspring, 38.5	TL, FACS; TA, PCR-ELISA	Diabetes during pregnancy (type 1 diabetes, type 2 diabetes, GDM)	Maternal age, gestational age	No association of diabetes during pregnancy with TL; higher TA in type 1 and GDM
Ferrari et al. 2015 [95]	$N = 100$ ($N = 42$ unexplained stillbirths, $N = 43$ term births; $N = 15$ preterm births)	Placenta	Birth/delivery	58	qPCR	Stillbirth	Birth weight, gestational age	Twofold decrease in TL in stillbirths, TL shorter among stillbirths than spontaneous preterm births
Geifman-Holtzman et al. 2010 [96]	$N = 61$ ($N = 32$ preeclamptic; $N = 29$ controls)	Placenta	Birth	100	qPCR	Hypertensive disorders of pregnancy	Age, BMI, blood pressure, race, obstetrics history, smoking, previous hypertension or preeclampsia, clinical diagnosis at time of delivery, birth weight, mode of delivery	Elevated TERT mRNA levels, increased TERT with increasing BMI, lower TERT in preterm than full-term newborns
Li et al. 2014 [97]	$N = 73$ mothers and their newborns ($N = 26$ mothers with GDM, $N = 47$ controls)	CMBC	Birth	38.5 GDM, 57.4 controls	PCR-ELISA	GDM	Maternal age, parity, gravidity, height, prepregnancy weight, pregnancy weight gain, family history of delivering, LBW, gestational age at birth, birth weight and weight ratio, delivery method, fasting plasma glucose	Ratio of mitochondrial/nucleic TERT elevated in diabetic mothers and positively correlated with oxidative stress markers in newborn cord blood

(continued)

Table 41.3c (continued)

Author, year	Sample size	Tissue	Age	% Female	Assay	Prenatal exposure	Adjusted for	Association of exposure with outcome
Okuda et al. 2002 [98]	$N = 168$	CBMC	Birth	49	Southern blot	Hypertension, preeclampsia during pregnancy, pregestational diabetes	None	No association between TL and any of the obstetric risk conditions
Shalev et al. 2014 [99]	$N = 829$	Leukocytes	38 years	48	qPCR	Perinatal complications	Family history, social risk, childhood social adversity, cognitive health, mental health, vascular health, physical health, smoking, hypertension, gender	Shorter TL and greater perceived age in exposed group
Sukenik-Halevy et al. 2009 [100]	$N = 22$ ($N = 11$ preeclampsia; $N = 11$ controls)	Placenta	Birth	N/A	FISH	Preeclampsia	None	More telomere aggregate formation in exposed group
Sukenik-Halevy, 2016 [101]	$N = 23$ (9 preeclampsia, 14 control)	Placenta, CBMC	Birth	N/A	FISH for TERC gene copy number and telomere capture, FISH for TL	Preeclampsia	Maternal age and BMI, parity, gestational age at birth, birth weight	No differences in CBMC, higher % of cells with senescence-associated heterochromatin foci, abnormal TERC copy number, and increased telomere capture in preeclampsia trophoblasts
Xu et al. 2014 [102]	$N = 82$ GDM $N = 65$ normal pregnancies $N = 45$ preeclampsia $N = 15$ gestational hypertension	Leukocytes	Birth	47.3	qPCR	GDM, preeclampsia	Maternal age, gestational age at delivery, birth weight, fetal gender	Shorter TL in newborns from GDM pregnancies, no association between newborn TL and maternal preeclampsia

placenta, resulting in shorter telomeres and changes in other cellular markers. Indeed, they found that pregnancies complicated with diabetes exhibited a higher percentage of trophoblasts with shortened telomeres. Xu et al. [102] also demonstrated a connection between gestational diabetes (GDM) and leukocyte TL at birth. GDM also seems to lead to an upregulation of telomerase in mitochondria as a compensatory response to the damage caused by oxidative stress [97]. However, several studies have failed to find an association between maternal diabetes and cord blood mononuclear cell (CBMC) TL [94, 98]. Maternal hypertension and its more serious form, preeclampsia, are important maternal obstetric complications that confer serious risks for mother and baby. Hypertensive disorders of pregnancy have been shown to lead to increased expression of TERT (catalytic protein domain of telomerase) mRNA in the placenta [96]. They have also been linked to signs of telomere dysfunction in the placenta, such as telomere aggregate formation [100], abnormal TERC (RNA component of telomerase) copy number, and increased telomere capture [101]. However, associations between maternal hypertension or preeclampsia and TL in fetal cord blood have not been reported [98]. In a study that followed individuals from birth through adulthood, exposure to maternal or perinatal complications was linked with shorter leukocyte TL at 38 years of age [99].

As discussed previously [17, 52], maternal stress may also be an important mechanism by which intrauterine conditions have long-term effects on fetal telomere biology and therefore may confer a lifetime impact on health. Studies on this topic are presented in Table 41.3d. We and others have demonstrated that maternal psychosocial stress during pregnancy is linked to leukocyte TL at birth [104, 106]. Furthermore, severe life events occurring during pregnancy are linked with leukocyte TL in the offspring as young adults [105]. Poor sleep quality may be another means by which maternal obstetric complications are passed on to the fetus, as researchers have found an association between sleep apnea and daytime sleepiness in mothers and shorter TL in the cord blood of their newborns [107].

Biological Pathways Linking Adverse Conditions During Pregnancy and Telomere Biology

Different interrelated biological pathways link adverse exposures during pregnancy with offspring telomere biology. Here we discuss the influence of three groups of biological mediators on telomere biology-related processes: stress hormones, inflammatory agents, and oxidative stress.

Stress Hormones

Several in vitro and in vivo studies have established the influence of stress hormones on the telomere system. For example, treatment of stimulated human T-cells with cortisol in vitro decreased cell proliferation, TA, and TERT mRNA levels [108], while noradrenaline induced TERT expression and TA in an ovarian tumor cell line [109]. In chicken embryos, corticosterone injections produced higher levels of reactive oxygen metabolites and an overrepresentation of short telomeres [110]. In humans, elevated levels of stress hormones, larger acute stress-induced cortisol responses, and dysregulation of diurnal cortisol have been linked to shorter TL [111–113]. In addition, leukocyte TA responds to acute stress [114] and is influenced by stress-reducing therapies [115]. Chronic stress exposure induces higher levels of oxidative stress and inflammation [116]. Additionally, prolonged periods of psychological stress might also render individuals more susceptible to virus reactivation and continuous virus exposure, which induces senescence of specific T cells [117, 118].

Table 41.3d Maternal stress and sleep during pregnancy and offspring telomere length

Author, year	Sample size	Tissue	Age	% Female	Assay	Prenatal exposure	Adjusted for	Association of exposure with outcome
Maternal stress and lifestyle								
Entringer et al. 2011 [104]	$N = 94$ ($N = 45$ prenatally stressed and $N = 49$ controls)	Leukocytes	25	Prenatal stress group: 84; control group: 71	qPCR	Prenatal stress (severe life events during pregnancy)	Age, BMI, sex, birth weight percentile, postnatal/early-life adversity, current chronic stress, depressive symptom levels	Shorter TL in exposed group, prenatal stress significantly associated with TL
Entringer et al. 2013 [105]	$N = 27$	Leukocytes	Birth/delivery	52	qPCR	Maternal psychosocial stress	Gestational age at birth, weight, sex, antepartum obstetric complications	TL inversely associated to pregancy-specific stress
Marchetto et al. 2016 [106]	$N = 24$	CBMC	Birth	N/A	Southern blot	Maternal psychological stress	Maternal age, gestational age at birth, birth weight	Shorter TL in high-stress group as opposed to low-stress group
Salihu et al. 2015 [107]	$N = 67$	CBMC	Birth	N/A	qPCR	Maternal sleep apnea and daytime sleepiness	Maternal age, gestational age, number of previous pregnancies, maternal BMI, birth weight, head circumference at birth, marital status, race/ethnicity, type of insurance, smoking status	Shorter TL among newborns of women with high risk of sleep apnea

Oxidative Stress

Stress and many unhealthy behaviors, such as smoking, alcohol consumption, and a high-fat diet, increase oxidative stress levels (summarized in [116, 119]). Oxidative stress accelerates telomere shortening, decreases TA, and induces senescence (or apoptosis) via DNA damage-induced activation of the p53 pathway [26, 120, 121]. Due to a high content of guanine residues, telomeres are highly sensitive to oxidative damage, which is further indicated by studies showing that an oxidative stress imbalance [122] (ratio of oxidative stress to antioxidants) and various other markers of oxidative stress are associated with shorter TL [66, 123, 124]. Conversely, higher circulating concentrations of anti-oxidative micronutrients are related to longer telomeres [125–127], suggesting that antioxidants can decelerate TL attrition. Oxidative stress has been reported to induce the nuclear export of TERT to the cytosol and into the mitochondria, thereby decreasing nuclear and total TA [120].

Inflammatory Agents

Many, if not all, age-related diseases are associated with higher levels of pro-inflammatory cytokines (including interleukin (IL)-6 and tumor necrosis factor (TNF)- α). Several studies have demonstrated that markers of inflammation such as C-reactive protein (CRP), IL-6, and TNF- α are linked to TL shortening [66, 128–131] and T-cell senescence [37]. In leukocytes, TA and nuclear translocation of telomerase is induced by a NF-κB signaling pathway in response to TNF-α [132]. It has also been shown that TERT regulates the expression of a subset of NF-κB-dependent genes [133, 134]. Ghosh et al. [134] observed TERT binding to the NF-κB p65 subunit and its recruitment to a subset of NF-κB promoters such as those of IL-6 and TNF-α, suggesting that telomerase can provide a feed forward loop for the immune system by stimulating NF-κB-dependent gene expression.

Mechanisms of Programming of TL

Although a link between developmental processes in early life and changes in telomere biology has been established (as reviewed above), little is known about potential mechanisms by which these effects are mediated. As discussed by us previously [17], epigenetic modifications have been considered the context of fetal programming as a process whereby developmental exposures can affect fetal gene expression and subsequent disease risk (e.g., [10]). The telomere system is under tight epigenetic control. There is evidence that chromatin modifications are important regulators of mammalian telomeres. Subtelomeric regions are enriched in epigenetic marks that are characteristic of heterochromatin, and the abrogation of master epigenetic regulators, such as histone methyltransferases and DNA methyltransferases, correlates with loss of TL control (reviewed in [71]). Specifically, the regulation of TL is dependent on the level of methylation of the histones H3 and H4 associated with subtelomeric regions. The methylation of these histones decreases access to telomere sequences and thus reduces TA [71]. Hence, proteins that play a role in regulation of these methylations, such as DNA methyltransferase, have an impact on TL. DNA methyltransferase is a key candidate mechanism by which early-life conditions (e.g., nutrition [135], stress [136]) produce stable, long-term epigenetic alternations. In addition, several studies have suggested that epigenetic modulation of the core promoter region of the TERT gene that regulates TA is involved in regulating telomere maintenance (see [137]). Examining how these epigenetic mechanisms can potentially be modified by early stress biology-related factors in animal and human models is a priority for future studies.

Conclusion

Based on the conceptual framework and empirical findings presented here, we suggest it is important to consider the potential role of intrauterine factors to arrive at a better understanding of the developmental programming of the telomere biology system and, beyond this, aging-related diseases and aging itself. Telomere biology is an important determinant of health throughout the life span, and the above-discussed evidence demonstrates the potentially important role of prenatal conditions in the newborn setting of the telomere system. Questions remain regarding the molecular mechanism(s) underlying the effect of intrauterine conditions on telomere homeostasis and potential interactions with other biological processes.

Insofar as the newborn setting of TL is an important determinant of subsequent telomere biology-related processes and health outcomes, the findings summarized in this chapter add evidence to the growing awareness that age-related complex, common disorders may have their foundations very early in life and, secondly, point to potentially modifiable factors for possible clinical intervention with implications for primary prevention. Prenatal programming of the telomere system could be an important means by which health disparities are propagated intergenerationally, influencing the health of individuals and their offspring even before their birth. However, conversely, improving maternal health can also have long-lasting effects, throughout the newborn's life span and on to future generations. Ensuring appropriate prenatal care, both physical and psychological, is thus an essential public health goal with far-reaching impacts.

References

1. Entringer S, Buss C, Swanson JM, et al. Fetal programming of body composition, obesity, and metabolic function: the role of intrauterine stress and stress biology. J Nutr Metab. 2012;2012:632548.
2. Entringer S, Buss C, Wadhwa PD. Prenatal stress and developmental programming of human health and disease risk: concepts and integration of empirical findings. Curr Opin Endocrinol Diabetes Obes. 2010;17(6):507–16.
3. Swanson JM, Entringer S, Buss C, Wadhwa PD. Developmental origins of health and disease: environmental exposures. Semin Reprod Med. 2009;27(5):391–402.
4. Gluckman PD, Hanson MA. Living with the past: evolution, development, and patterns of disease. Science. 2004;305(5691):1733–6.
5. Gluckman PD, Hanson MA. The developmental origins of health and disease, Early life origins of health and disease. New York: Springer; 2006.
6. Wadhwa PD, Buss C, Entringer S, Swanson JM. Developmental origins of health and disease: brief history of the approach and current focus on epigenetic mechanisms. Semin Reprod Med. 2009;27(5):358–68.
7. McDade TW, Hoke M, Borja JB, Adair LS, Kuzawa C. Do environments in infancy moderate the association between stress and inflammation in adulthood? Initial evidence from a birth cohort in the Philippines. Brain Behav Immun. 2013;31:23–30.
8. Adair LS. Long-term consequences of nutrition and growth in early childhood and possible preventive interventions. Nestle Nutr Inst Workshop Ser. 2014;78:111–20.
9. Gluckman PD, Low FM, Buklijas T, Hanson MA, Beedle AS. How evolutionary principles improve the understanding of human health and disease. Evol Appl. 2011;4(2):249–63.
10. Hanson M, Godfrey KM, Lillycrop KA, Burdge GC, Gluckman PD. Developmental plasticity and developmental origins of non-communicable disease: theoretical considerations and epigenetic mechanisms. Prog Biophys Mol Biol. 2011;106(1):272–80.
11. Breier B, Vickers M, Ikenasio B, Chan K, Wong W. Fetal programming of appetite and obesity. Mol Cell Endocrinol. 2001;185(1):73–9.
12. Cripps R, Martin-gronert M, Ozanne S. Fetal and perinatal programming of appetite. Clin Sci. 2005;109(1):1–12.
13. Portha B, Chavey A, Movassat J. Early-life origins of type 2 diabetes: fetal programming of the beta-cell mass. Exp Diabetes Res. 2011;2011:16 pages. doi:10.1155/2011/105076.
14. Rees W, McNeil C, Maloney C. The roles of PPARs in the fetal origins of metabolic health and disease. PPAR Res. 2008;2008(Article ID 459030):8.

15. Desai M, Ross MG. Fetal programming of adipose tissue: effects of IUGR and maternal obesity/high fat diet. Paper presented at: Seminars in reproductive medicine. Thieme Medical Publishers; 2011.
16. Catalano PM, Presley L, Minium J, Hauguel-de Mouzon S. Fetuses of obese mothers develop insulin resistance in utero. Diabetes Care. 2009;32(6):1076–80.
17. Entringer S, Wadhwa PD. Developmental programming of telomere biology: role of stress and stress biology. In: Stress and developmental programming of health and disease: beyond phenomenology. New York: Nova Science Publishers; 2014. p. 633–50.
18. Blackburn EH, Gall JG. A tandemly repeated sequence at the termini of the extrachromosomal ribosomal RNA genes in Tetrahymena. J Mol Biol. 1978;120(1):33–53.
19. Moyzis RK, Buckingham JM, Cram LS, et al. A highly conserved repetitive DNA sequence, (TTAGGG)n, present at the telomeres of human chromosomes. Proc Natl Acad Sci U S A. 1988;85(18):6622–6.
20. Blackburn EH, Greider CW, Henderson E, Lee MS, Shampay J, Shippen-Lentz D. Recognition and elongation of telomeres by telomerase. Genome. 1989;31(2):553–60.
21. Shore D, Bianchi A. Telomere length regulation: coupling DNA end processing to feedback regulation of telomerase. EMBO J. 2009;28(16):2309–22.
22. Forsyth NR, Wright WE, Shay JW. Telomerase and differentiation in multicellular organisms: turn it off, turn it on, and turn it off again. Differ Res Biol Divers. 2002;69(4–5):188–97.
23. Aubert G, Lansdorp PM. Telomeres and aging. Physiol Rev. 2008;88(2):557–79.
24. Madonna R, De Caterina R, Willerson JT, Geng YJ. Biologic function and clinical potential of telomerase and associated proteins in cardiovascular tissue repair and regeneration. Eur Heart J. 2011;32(10):1190–6.
25. Ahmed S, Passos JF, Birket MJ, et al. Telomerase does not counteract telomere shortening but protects mitochondrial function under oxidative stress. J Cell Sci. 2008;121(Pt 7):1046–53.
26. Saretzki G. Telomerase, mitochondria and oxidative stress. Exp Gerontol. 2009;44(8):485–92.
27. Sahin E, Colla S, Liesa M, et al. Telomere dysfunction induces metabolic and mitochondrial compromise. Nature. 2011;470(7334):359–65.
28. Jaskelioff M, Muller FL, Paik JH, et al. Telomerase reactivation reverses tissue degeneration in aged telomerase-deficient mice. Nature. 2011;469(7328):102–6.
29. Chan SW, Blackburn EH. Telomerase and ATM/Tel1p protect telomeres from nonhomologous end joining. Mol Cell. 2003;11(5):1379–87.
30. Haycock PC, Heydon EE, Kaptoge S, Butterworth AS, Thompson A, Willeit P. Leucocyte telomere length and risk of cardiovascular disease: systematic review and meta-analysis. BMJ. 2014;349:g4227.
31. Zhao J, Miao K, Wang H, Ding H, Wang DW. Association between telomere length and type 2 diabetes mellitus: a meta-analysis. PLoS One. 2013;8(11):e79993.
32. Ma H, Zhou Z, Wei S, et al. Shortened telomere length is associated with increased risk of cancer: a meta-analysis. PLoS One. 2011;6(6):e20466.
33. Armanios M, Blackburn EH. The telomere syndromes. Nat Rev Genet. 2012;13(10):693–704.
34. Cawthon RM, Smith KR, O'Brien E, Sivatchenko A, Kerber RA. Association between telomere length in blood and mortality in people aged 60 years or older. Lancet. 2003;361(9355):393–5.
35. Kimura M, Hjelmborg JV, Gardner JP, et al. Telomere length and mortality: a study of leukocytes in elderly Danish twins. Am J Epidemiol. 2008;167(7):799–806.
36. Stewart SA, Weinberg RA. Telomeres: cancer to human aging. Annu Rev Cell Dev Biol. 2006;22:531–57.
37. Effros RB. Kleemeier award lecture 2008 – the canary in the coal mine: telomeres and human healthspan. J Gerontol A Biol Sci Med Sci. 2009;64(5):511–5.
38. Karlseder J. Chromosome end protection becomes even more complex. Nat Struct Mol Biol. 2009;16(12):1205–6.
39. Cesare AJ, Kaul Z, Cohen SB, et al. Spontaneous occurrence of telomeric DNA damage response in the absence of chromosome fusions. Nat Struct Mol Biol. 2009;16(12):1244–51.
40. O'Sullivan RJ, Kubicek S, Schreiber SL, Karlseder J. Reduced histone biosynthesis and chromatin changes arising from a damage signal at telomeres. Nat Struct Mol Biol. 2010;17(10):1218–25.
41. Alabert C, Groth A. Chromatin replication and epigenome maintenance. Nat Rev Mol Cell Biol. 2012;13(3):153–67.
42. Sharpless NE, DePinho RA. How stem cells age and why this makes us grow old. Nat Rev Mol Cell Biol. 2007;8(9):703–13.
43. Sahin E, Depinho RA. Linking functional decline of telomeres, mitochondria and stem cells during ageing. Nature. 2010;464(7288):520–8.
44. Aviv A. The epidemiology of human telomeres: faults and promises. J Gerontol A Biol Sci Med Sci. 2008;63(9):979–83.
45. Heidinger BJ, Blount JD, Boner W, Griffiths K, Metcalfe NB, Monaghan P. Telomere length in early life predicts lifespan. Proc Natl Acad Sci U S A. 2012;109(5):1743–8.
46. Bateson M, Brilot BO, Gillespie R, Monaghan P, Nettle D. Developmental telomere attrition predicts impulsive decision-making in adult starlings. Proc Biol Sci. 2015;282(1799):20142140.

47. Asghar M, Hasselquist D, Hansson B, Zehtindjiev P, Westerdahl H, Bensch S. Chronic infection. Hidden costs of infection: chronic malaria accelerates telomere degradation and senescence in wild birds. Science. 2015;347(6220):436–8.
48. Benetos A, Kark JD, Susser E, et al. Tracking and fixed ranking of leukocyte telomere length across the adult life course. Aging Cell. 2013;12(4):615–21.
49. Moreno-Palomo J, Creus A, Marcos R, Hernandez A. Genomic instability in newborn with short telomeres. PLoS One. 2014;9(3):e91753.
50. Prescott J, Kraft P, Chasman DI, et al. Genome-wide association study of relative telomere length. PLoS One. 2011;6(5):e19635.
51. Codd V, Nelson CP, Albrecht E, et al. Identification of seven loci affecting mean telomere length and their association with disease. Nat Genet. 2013;45(4):422–7. 427e421–422
52. Entringer S, Buss C, Wadhwa PD. Prenatal stress, telomere biology, and fetal programming of health and disease risk. Sci Signal. 2012;5(248):12.
53. Aiken CE, Tarry-Adkins JL, Ozanne SE. Suboptimal nutrition in utero causes DNA damage and accelerated aging of the female reproductive tract. FASEB J: Off Publ Fed Am Soc Exp Biology. 2013;27(10):3959–65.
54. Aiken CE, Tarry-Adkins JL, Ozanne SE. Transgenerational developmental programming of ovarian reserve. Sci Rep. 2015;5:16175.
55. Jennings BJ, Ozanne SE, Dorling MW, Hales CN. Early growth determines longevity in male rats and may be related to telomere shortening in the kidney. FEBS Lett. 1999;448(1):4–8.
56. Tarry-Adkins JL, Martin-Gronert MS, Chen JH, Cripps RL, Ozanne SE. Maternal diet influences DNA damage, aortic telomere length, oxidative stress, and antioxidant defense capacity in rats. FASEB J: Off Publ Fed Am Soc Exp Biology. 2008;22(6):2037–44.
57. Tarry-Adkins JL, Chen JH, Smith NS, Jones RH, Cherif H, Ozanne SE. Poor maternal nutrition followed by accelerated postnatal growth leads to telomere shortening and increased markers of cell senescence in rat islets. FASEB J: Off Publ Fed Am Soc Exp Biology. 2009;23(5):1521–8.
58. Tarry-Adkins JL, Blackmore HL, Martin-Gronert MS, et al. Coenzyme Q10 prevents accelerated cardiac aging in a rat model of poor maternal nutrition and accelerated postnatal growth. Mol Metab. 2013;2(4):480–90.
59. Tarry-Adkins JL, Fernandez-Twinn DS, Chen JH, et al. Nutritional programming of coenzyme Q: potential for prevention and intervention? FASEB J: Off Publ Fed Am Soc Exp Biology. 2014;28(12):5398–405.
60. de Rooij SR, van Pelt AM, Ozanne SE, et al. Prenatal undernutrition and leukocyte telomere length in late adulthood: the Dutch famine birth cohort study. Am J Clin Nutr. 2015;102(3):655–60.
61. Rotar O, Moguchaia E, Boyarinova M, et al. Seventy years after the siege of Leningrad: does early life famine still affect cardiovascular risk and aging? J Hypertens. 2015;33(9):1772–1779; discussion 1779.
62. Entringer S, Epel ES, Lin J, et al. Maternal folate concentration in early pregnancy and newborn telomere length. Ann Nutr Metab. 2015;66(4):202–8.
63. Sinkey RG, Salihu HM, King LM, et al. Homocysteine levels are not related to telomere length in cord blood leukocytes of newborns. Am J Perinatol. 2016 May;33(6):552–9. doi:10.1055/s-0035-1570318. Epub 2015 Dec 21
64. Vera E, Bernardes de Jesus B, Foronda M, Flores JM, Blasco MA. Telomerase reverse transcriptase synergizes with calorie restriction to increase health span and extend mouse longevity. PLoS One. 2013;8(1):e53760.
65. Barnes SK, Ozanne SE. Pathways linking the early environment to long-term health and lifespan. Prog Biophys Mol Biol. 2011;106(1):323–36.
66. Boccardi V, Esposito A, Rizzo MR, Marfella R, Barbieri M, Paolisso G. Mediterranean diet, telomere maintenance and health status among elderly. PLoS One. 2013;8(4):e62781.
67. Crous-Bou M, Fung TT, Prescott J, et al. Mediterranean diet and telomere length in Nurses' Health Study: population based cohort study. BMJ. 2014;349:g6674.
68. Garcia-Calzon S, Martinez-Gonzalez MA, Razquin C, et al. Pro12Ala polymorphism of the PPARgamma2 gene interacts with a mediterranean diet to prevent telomere shortening in the PREDIMED-NAVARRA randomized trial. Circ Cardiovasc Genet. 2015;8(1):91–9.
69. Gu Y, Honig LS, Schupf N, et al. Mediterranean diet and leukocyte telomere length in a multi-ethnic elderly population. Age. 2015;37(2):24.
70. Freitas-Simoes TM, Ros E, Sala-Vila A. Nutrients, foods, dietary patterns and telomere length: update of epidemiological studies and randomized trials. Metab Clin Exp. 2016;65(4):406–15.
71. Blasco MA. The epigenetic regulation of mammalian telomeres. Nat Rev Genet. 2007;8(4):299–309.
72. Moores CJ, Fenech M, O'Callaghan NJ. Telomere dynamics: the influence of folate and DNA methylation. Ann N Y Acad Sci. 2011;1229:76–88.
73. Antony AC. In utero physiology: role of folic acid in nutrient delivery and fetal development. Am J Clin Nutr. 2007;85(2):598S–603S.
74. Akkad A, Hastings R, Konje JC, Bell SC, Thurston H, Williams B. Telomere length in small-for-gestational-age babies. BJOG. 2006;113(3):318–23.

75. Biron-Shental T, Sukenik Halevy R, Goldberg-Bittman L, Kidron D, Fejgin MD, Amiel A. Telomeres are shorter in placental trophoblasts of pregnancies complicated with intrauterine growth restriction (IUGR). Early Hum Dev. 2010;86(7):451–6.
76. Biron-Shental T, Kidron D, Sukenik-Halevy R, et al. TERC telomerase subunit gene copy number in placentas from pregnancies complicated with intrauterine growth restriction. Early Hum Dev. 2011;87(2):73–5.
77. Biron-Shental T, Sukenik-Halevy R, Sharon Y, Laish I, Fejgin MD, Amiel A. Telomere shortening in intra uterine growth restriction placentas. Early Hum Dev. 2014;90(9):465–9.
78. Davy P, Nagata M, Bullard P, Fogelson NS, Allsopp R. Fetal growth restriction is associated with accelerated telomere shortening and increased expression of cell senescence markers in the placenta. Placenta. 2009;30(6):539–42.
79. Izutsu T, Kudo T, Sato T, et al. Telomerase activity in human chorionic villi and placenta determined by TRAP and in situ TRAP assay. Placenta. 1998;19(8):613–8.
80. Kajantie E, Pietiläinen KH, Wehkalampi K, et al. No association between body size at birth and leucocyte telomere length in adult life—evidence from three cohort studies. Int J Epidemiol. 2012;41(5):1400–8.
81. Kim SY, Lee SP, Lee JS, Yoon SJ, Jun G, Hwang YJ. Telomerase and apoptosis in the placental trophoblasts of growth discordant twins. Yonsei Med J. 2006;47(5):698–705.
82. Kudo T, Izutsu T, Sato T. Telomerase activity and apoptosis as indicators of ageing in placenta with and without intrauterine growth retardation. Placenta. 2000;21(5–6):493–500.
83. Laganovic M, Bendix L, Rubelj I, et al. Reduced telomere length is not associated with early signs of vascular aging in young men born after intrauterine growth restriction: a paradox? J Hypertens. 2014;32(8):1613–20.
84. Raqib R, Alam DS, Sarker P, et al. Low birth weight is associated with altered immune function in rural Bangladeshi children: a birth cohort study. Am J Clin Nutr. 2007;85(3):845–52.
85. Strohmaier J, van Dongen J, Willemsen G, et al. Low birth weight in MZ twins discordant for birth weight is associated with shorter telomere length and lower IQ, but not anxiety/depression in later life. Twin Res Hum Genet: Off J Int Soc Twin Stud. 2015;18(2):198–209.
86. Tellechea M, Gianotti TF, Alvarinas J, Gonzalez CD, Sookoian S, Pirola CJ. Telomere length in the two extremes of abnormal fetal growth and the programming effect of maternal arterial hypertension. Sci Rep. 2015;5:7869.
87. Toutain J, Prochazkova-Carlotti M, Cappellen D, et al. Reduced placental telomere length during pregnancies complicated by intrauterine growth restriction. PLoS One. 2013;8(1):e54013.
88. Friedrich U, Schwab M, Griese EU, Fritz P, Klotz U. Telomeres in neonates: new insights in fetal hematopoiesis. Pediatr Res. 2001;49(2):252–6.
89. Gielen M, Hageman G, Pachen D, Derom C, Vlietinck R, Zeegers MP. Placental telomere length decreases with gestational age and is influenced by parity: a study of third trimester live-born twins. Placenta. 2014;35(10):791–6.
90. Hadchouel A, Marchand-Martin L, Franco-Montoya ML, et al. Salivary telomere length and lung function in adolescents born very preterm: a prospective multicenter study. PLoS One. 2015;10(9):e0136123.
91. Smeets CCJ, Codd V, Samani NJ, Hokken-Koelega ACS. Leukocyte telomere length in young adults born preterm: support for accelerated biological ageing. PLoS One. 2015;10(11):e0143951.
92. Hallows SE, Regnault TRH, Betts DH. The long and short of it: the role of telomeres in fetal origins of adult disease. J Pregnancy. 2012;2012:638476.
93. Biron-Shental T, Sukenik-Halevy R, Naboani H, Liberman M, Kats R, Amiel A. Telomeres are shorter in placentas from pregnancies with uncontrolled diabetes. Placenta. 2015;36(2):199–203.
94. Cross JA, Temple RC, Hughes JC, et al. Cord blood telomere length, telomerase activity and inflammatory markers in pregnancies in women with diabetes or gestational diabetes. Diabet Med J British Diabet Assoc. 2010;27(11):1264–70.
95. Ferrari F, Facchinetti F, Saade G, Menon R. Placental telomere shortening in stillbirth: a sign of premature senescence? Journal Matern-Fetal neonatal Med: Off J Eur Assoc Perinatal Med, Fed Asia Oceania Perinatal Soc, Int Soc Perinatal Obstet. 2016;29(8):1283–8.
96. Geifman-Holtzman O, Xiong Y, Holtzman EJ, Hoffman B, Gaughan J, Liebermann DA. Increased placental telomerase mRNA in hypertensive disorders of pregnancy. Hypertens Pregnancy: Off J Int Soc Study Hypertens Pregnancy. 2010;29(4):434–45.
97. Li P, Tong Y, Yang H, et al. Mitochondrial translocation of human telomerase reverse transcriptase in cord blood mononuclear cells of newborns with gestational diabetes mellitus mothers. Diabetes Res Clin Pract. 2014;103(2):310–8.
98. Okuda K, Bardeguez A, Gardner JP, et al. Telomere length in the newborn. Pediatr Res. 2002;52(3):377–81.
99. Shalev I, Caspi A, Ambler A, et al. Perinatal complications and aging indicators by midlife. Pediatrics. 2014;134(5):e1315–23.
100. Sukenik-Halevy R, Fejgin M, Kidron D, et al. Telomere aggregate formation in placenta specimens of pregnancies complicated with pre-eclampsia. Cancer Genet Cytogenet. 2009;195(1):27–30.
101. Sukenik-Halevy R, Amiel A, Kidron D, Liberman M, Ganor-Paz Y, Biron-Shental T. Telomere homeostasis in trophoblasts and in cord blood cells from pregnancies complicated with preeclampsia. Am J Obstet Gynecol. 2016;214(2):283.e281–7.

102. Xu J, Ye J, Wu Y, et al. Reduced fetal telomere length in gestational diabetes. PLoS One. 2014;9(1):e86161.

103. Menon R, Yu J, Basanta-Henry P, et al. Short fetal leukocyte telomere length and preterm prelabor rupture of the membranes. PLoS One. 2012;7(2):e31136.

104. Entringer S, Epel ES, Kumsta R, et al. Stress exposure in intrauterine life is associated with shorter telomere length in young adulthood. Proc Natl Acad Sci U S A. 2011;108(33):E513–8.

105. Entringer S, Epel ES, Lin J, et al. Maternal psychosocial stress during pregnancy is associated with newborn leukocyte telomere length. Am J Obstet Gynecol.. 2013;208(2):134.e131–7.

106. Marchetto NM, Glynn RA, Ferry ML, et al. Prenatal stress and newborn telomere length. Am J Obstet Gynecol. 2016;215:94.e1.

107. Salihu HM, King L, Patel P, et al. Association between maternal symptoms of sleep disordered breathing and fetal telomere length. Sleep. 2015;38(4):559–66.

108. Choi J, Fauce SR, Effros RB. Reduced telomerase activity in human T lymphocytes exposed to cortisol. Brain Behav Immun. 2008;22(4):600–5.

109. Choi MJ, Cho KH, Lee S, et al. hTERT mediates norepinephrine-induced Slug expression and ovarian cancer aggressiveness. Oncogene. 2015;34(26):3402–12.

110. Haussmann MF, Longenecker AS, Marchetto NM, Juliano SA, Bowden RM. Embryonic exposure to corticosterone modifies the juvenile stress response, oxidative stress and telomere length. Proc Biol Sci/R Soc. 2012;279(1732):1447–56.

111. Epel ES, Lin J, Wilhelm FH, et al. Cell aging in relation to stress arousal and cardiovascular disease risk factors. Psychoneuroendocrinology. 2006;31(3):277–87.

112. Parks CG, Miller DB, McCanlies EC, et al. Telomere length, current perceived stress, and urinary stress hormones in women. Cancer Epidemiol, Biomark Prev Publ Am Assoc Cancer Res, Am Soc Prev Oncol. 2009;18(2):551–60.

113. Tomiyama AJ, O'Donovan A, Lin J, et al. Does cellular aging relate to patterns of allostasis? An examination of basal and stress reactive HPA axis activity and telomere length. Physiol Behav. 2012;106(1):40–5.

114. Epel ES, Lin J, Dhabhar FS, et al. Dynamics of telomerase activity in response to acute psychological stress. Brain Behav Immun. 2010;24(4):531–9.

115. Schutte NS, Malouff JM. The relationship between perceived stress and telomere length: a meta-analysis. Stress Health: J Int Soc Investig Stress. 2014;32:313.

116. Epel ES. Psychological and metabolic stress: a recipe for accelerated cellular aging? Hormones. 2009;8(1):7–22.

117. Akbar AN, Vukmanovic-Stejic M. Telomerase in T lymphocytes: use it and lose it? J Immunol. 2007;178(11):6689–94.

118. Glaser R, Kiecolt-Glaser JK. Stress-induced immune dysfunction: implications for health. Nat Rev Immunol. 2005;5(3):243–51.

119. Lin J, Epel E, Blackburn E. Telomeres and lifestyle factors: roles in cellular aging. Mutat Res. 2012;730(1–2):85–9.

120. Haendeler J, Hoffmann J, Diehl JF, et al. Antioxidants inhibit nuclear export of telomerase reverse transcriptase and delay replicative senescence of endothelial cells. Circ Res. 2004;94(6):768–75.

121. von Zglinicki T. Oxidative stress shortens telomeres. Trends Biochem Sci. 2002;27(7):339–44.

122. Epel ES, Blackburn EH, Lin J, et al. Accelerated telomere shortening in response to life stress. Proc Natl Acad Sci U S A. 2004;101(49):17312–5.

123. Gonzalez-Guardia L, Yubero-Serrano EM, Rangel-Zuniga O, et al. Influence of endothelial dysfunction on telomere length in subjects with metabolic syndrome: LIPGENE study. Age. 2014;36(4):9681.

124. Ma D, Zhu W, Hu S, Yu X, Yang Y. Association between oxidative stress and telomere length in type 1 and type 2 diabetic patients. J Endocrinol Investig. 2013;36(11):1032–7.

125. Min KB, Min JY. Association between leukocyte telomere length and serum carotenoid in US adults. Eur J Nutr. 2016;56:1045.

126. Sen A, Marsche G, Freudenberger P, et al. Association between higher plasma lutein, zeaxanthin, and vitamin C concentrations and longer telomere length: results of the Austrian Stroke Prevention Study. J Am Geriatr Soc. 2014;62(2):222–9.

127. Garcia-Calzon S, Moleres A, Martinez-Gonzalez MA, et al. Dietary total antioxidant capacity is associated with leukocyte telomere length in a children and adolescent population. Clin Nutr. 2015;34(4):694–9.

128. Carrero JJ, Stenvinkel P, Fellstrom B, et al. Telomere attrition is associated with inflammation, low fetuin-A levels and high mortality in prevalent haemodialysis patients. J Intern Med. 2008;263(3):302–12.

129. Fitzpatrick AL, Kronmal RA, Gardner JP, et al. Leukocyte telomere length and cardiovascular disease in the cardiovascular health study. Am J Epidemiol. 2007;165(1):14–21.

130. Garcia-Calzon S, Zalba G, Ruiz-Canela M, et al. Dietary inflammatory index and telomere length in subjects with a high cardiovascular disease risk from the PREDIMED-NAVARRA study: cross-sectional and longitudinal analyses over 5 y. Am J Clin Nutr. 2015;102(4):897–904.

131. Wong JY, De Vivo I, Lin X, Fang SC, Christiani DC. The relationship between inflammatory biomarkers and telomere length in an occupational prospective cohort study. PLoS One. 2014;9(1):e87348.

132. Akiyama M, Yamada O, Hideshima T, et al. TNFalpha induces rapid activation and nuclear translocation of telomerase in human lymphocytes. Biochem Biophys Res Commun. 2004;316(2):528–32.
133. Ding D, Xi P, Zhou J, Wang M, Cong YS. Human telomerase reverse transcriptase regulates MMP expression independently of telomerase activity via NF-kappaB-dependent transcription. FASEB J: Off Publ Fed Am Soc Exp Biology. 2013;27(11):4375–83.
134. Ghosh A, Saginc G, Leow SC, et al. Telomerase directly regulates NF-kappaB-dependent transcription. Nat Cell Biol. 2012;14(12):1270–81.
135. Burdge GC, Lillycrop KA. Nutrition, epigenetics, and developmental plasticity: implications for understanding human disease. Annu Rev Nutr. 2011;30:315–39.
136. Weaver IC, Cervoni N, Champagne FA, et al. Epigenetic programming by maternal behavior. Nat Neurosci. 2004;7(8):847–54.
137. Daniel M, Peek GW, Tollefsbol TO. Regulation of the human catalytic subunit of telomerase (hTERT). Gene. 2012;498(2):135–46.

Part VIII
Resources

Chapter 42
Current Research and Recommended Resources on Fetal Nutrition

Rajkumar Rajendram, Vinood B. Patel, and Victor R. Preedy

Key Points

- Occasionally the developing fetus is subjected to nutritional imbalances due to under- or overnutrition of the mother or placental insufficiencies. Other stresses may also arise in utero which will subject the fetus to metabolic burdens.
- These impositions can lead to a spectrum of effects such as smaller birth weights, postnatal developmental disorders and adverse outcome in adult life. The latter includes increased risk of lifelong conditions such as cardiovascular disease, diabetes mellitus and the metabolic syndrome.
- As a consequence of suboptimal fetal nutrition (either directly or indirectly), a variety of organs are also affected such as the liver, bone, central nervous and endocrine systems.
- The fetal origins hypothesis is based on epidemiological studies of fetal and adult morbidity and mortality.
- The theories surrounding the concept of fetal programming have driven investigation on the developmental origin of health and disease (DOHaD).
- It is difficult to keep up to date with developments in fetal nutrition and subsequent effects such as programming.
- This chapter lists the most up-to-date resources on the regulatory bodies, journals, books, professional bodies and websites that are relevant to an evidence-based approach to fetal nutrition and its subsequent effects.

Keywords Pregnancy • Fetal programming • Evidence • Resources • Books • Journals • Regulatory bodies • Professional societies

R. Rajendram, AKC BSc. (hons) MBBS (dist) EDIC FRCP Edin (✉)
Department of Internal Medicine, King Abdulaziz Medical City, Riyadh, Ministry of National Guard Health Affairs, Saudi Arabia

King's College London, Department of Nutrition and Dietetics, Nutritional Sciences Division, School of Biomedical & Health Sciences, London, UK
e-mail: rajkumarrajendram@doctors.org.uk

V.B. Patel
University of Westminster, Faculty of Science & Technology, Department of Biomedical Sciences, London, UK

V.R. Preedy
Department of Nutrition and Dietetics, Nutritional Sciences Division,
School of Biomedical & Health Sciences, King's College London, London, UK

© Springer International Publishing AG 2017
R. Rajendram et al. (eds.), *Diet, Nutrition, and Fetal Programming*,
Nutrition and Health, DOI 10.1007/978-3-319-60289-9_42

Abbreviations

DOHaD   Developmental origin of health and disease

Introduction

Occasionally the developing fetus is subjected to nutritional imbalances due to under- or overnutrition of the mother or placental insufficiencies. Other stresses may also arise in utero which will subject the fetus to metabolic impositions leading to a spectrum of effects such as smaller birth weights, postnatal developmental disorders affecting the infant and adverse outcome in adult life. With regard to the latter, fetal programming associates conditions in utero with increased risk of lifelong diseases such as cardiovascular disease, diabetes mellitus and the metabolic syndrome. However, it is also important to consider that as a consequence of suboptimal fetal nutrition (either directly or indirectly), a variety of organs are affected such as the liver, bone, central nervous and endocrine systems which are covered in the various chapters of this book.

The concept of fetal programming is based on the fetal origins hypothesis which suggests that the conditions to which the fetus is exposed in utero can have long-term effects on adult health [1]. At critical times in fetal development, the effects of environmental stimuli on structure and organ function may persist into adulthood [1]. This is consistent with theories on developmental plasticity; genes can express different ranges of physiological or morphological states in response to the environmental conditions during fetal development [1].

The scientific basis for fetal programming and the developmental origin of health and disease (DOHaD) was born from epidemiological studies of fetal and adult morbidity and mortality [1–4]. In the 1970s, Forsdahl associated increased risk of death from coronary heart disease with prosperity after poverty during adolescence [2]. Forsdahl suggested that the nutritional deficit may have caused permanent damage [2]. In 1986, Barker and colleagues correlated increased risk of coronary heart disease in adults with an adverse intrauterine environment, as suggested by low birth weight [3] Further investigations correlated low birth weight with impaired glucose tolerance, type 2 diabetes, hypertension and the metabolic syndrome [4]. Collectively, these studies formed the basis for the Forsdahl-Barker hypothesis [1].

The Forsdahl-Barker hypothesis associated conditions in utero with increased risk of lifelong diseases including cardiovascular disease, type-2 diabetes, hypertension, hypercholesterolaemia, obesity and the metabolic syndrome [1, 4]. Although this raised the intriguing possibility that disease prevention strategies could be initiated whilst the fetus is still in utero; the Forsdahl-Barker hypothesis was initially met with significant scepticism.

The main criticism was that low birth weight should not be considered as an independent risk factor because many of the environmental confounding variables could be attributed to the chronic diseases themselves [1]. Subsequent research studies attempted to adjust for these factors and provided more convincing results with fewer confounders [1, 4].

Nearly half a century has passed since Forsdahl's initial epidemiological studies of infant and adult mortality laid the foundations for the concept of fetal programming. Within this relatively short period, the Forsdahl-Barker hypothesis has become more widely accepted as the fetal origins hypothesis and the concept of fetal programming have given birth to the field of science that now focuses on DOHaD.

The investigations and interventions relevant to DOHaD have become more and more complicated as the understanding of fetal nutrition has increased. It is now nearly impossible even for experienced scientists and clinicians to remain up-to-date. For those new to the field, it is difficult to know which of the myriad of available sources are reliable. To assist colleagues who are interested in learning

Table 42.1 Regulatory bodies and organisations

Australia Health Practitioners Regulation Agency (AHRPA)   www.ahpra.gov.au
Center for Disease Control and Prevention   www.cdc.gov
European Food Safety Authority   www.efsa.europa.eu
Food Standards Australia New Zealand   www.foodstandards.gov.au
Medicines and Healthcare products Regulatory Agency (MHRA)   mhra.gov.uk
National Institutes of Health   www.nlm.nih.gov
National Institute for Health and Care Excellence   www.nice.org.uk
Public Health Agency (Belfast)   www.publichealth.hscni.net
Public Health Agency of Canada and Canadian Institute for Health Information   www.phac-aspc.gc.ca/
United States Food and Drug Administration   www.fda.gov
United States Preventive Services Task Force (USPSTF)   www.uspreventiveservicestaskforce.org
World Health Organization   www.who.int

Legend: This table lists the regulatory bodies and organisations involved with various aspects of fetal nutrition, physiology, programming and health. Some of these are international (such as the World Health Organization) and regional (such as the European Food Safety Authority) whilst others are national (such as the Australia Health Practitioners Regulation Agency)

more about fetal programming, we have therefore produced tables containing reliable, up-to-date resources in this chapter. The experts who assisted with the compilation of these tables of resources are acknowledged below.

Tables 42.1, 42.2, 42.3, 42.4 and 42.5 list the most up-to-date information on the regulatory bodies (Table 42.1), professional bodies (Table 42.2), journals (Table 42.3), books (Table 42.4) and websites (Table 42.5) that are most relevant to an evidence-based study of fetal nutrition, physiology, programming and health.

Acknowledgements We would like to thank the following authors for contributing to the development of this resource: Baba Usman A, Berry A, Boer P, Chatzi L, Correia M, Edwards M, Hardy D, Hill D, Kim YJ, Lo J, Marc I, Mattos S, Musumeci G, Nielsen MO, Prabhakaran P, Preissl H, Silveira P, Skilton M, Souza Torsoni A, Taylor R, Weisz G and Yiallourou S.

Table 42.2 Professional societies and organisations

American College of Human Genetics
www.acmg.net
American Society of Human Genetics
www.ashg.org
American College of Obstetrics and Gynecology
www.acog.org
American Society of Nutrition
www.nutrition.org/
Australian Epigenetics Alliance
epialliance.org.au
Australasian Sleep Association (ASA)
www.sleep.org.au
Centre for Fetal Programming (CFP)
www.cfp-research.com
Children's Health Research Institute (CHRI)
www.chri.org
Clinical Epigenetics Society
www.clinical-epigenetics-society.org
Epigenetics Society
epigeneticssocietyint.com
European Association for the Study of Obesity
easo.org
Federation of European Nutrition Societies
www.fensnutrition.eu
Human Genetics Society of Australasia
www.hgsa.org.au
International Human Epigenome Consortium
ihec-epigenomes.org
International Society for Developmental Origins of Health and Disease
dohadsoc.org
Liggins Institute, New Zealand
www.liggins.auckland.ac.nz/en.html
North American Spine Society
www.spine.org
Obesity Society
www.obesity.org
Perinatal Research Society
www.perinatalresearchsociety.org
Perinatal Society for Australia and New Zealand (PSANZ)
www.psanz.com.au
Royal Australian College of Surgeons
www.surgeons.org
Society for Reproductive Investigation
www.sri-online.org
Society for Study of Ingestive Behavior (SSIB)
www.ssib.org/web
Spine Society of Australia
spinesociety.org.au
The Nutrition Society
www.nutritionsociety.org

Legend: This table lists the professional societies involved in fetal nutrition, physiology, programming and health

Table 42.3 Journals covering fetal nutrition and programming

Plos One
Journal of Developmental Origins of Health and Disease
Journal of Animal Science
American Journal of Obstetrics and Gynecology
Endocrinology
American Journal of Physiology Regulatory Integrative and Comparative Physiology
Journal of Nutritional Biochemistry
Placenta
Epigenetics
Nutrients
Biology of Reproduction
Acta Physiologica
FASEB Journal
Journal of Endocrinology
Reproduction Fertility and Development
Psychoneuroendocrinology
Advances in Experimental Medicine and Biology
American Journal of Physiology Endocrinology and Metabolism
American Journal of Physiology Renal Physiology
Physiological Reports
Reproductive Sciences
Scientific Reports
Acta Obstetricia et Gynecologica Scandinavica
Diabetologia
European Journal of Nutrition

Legend: This table lists the top 25 journals publishing original research and review articles related to fetal nutrition and programming. The list was generated from SCOPUS (www.scopus.com) using general descriptors "fetal programming" and "fetal nutrition". The journals are listed in descending order of the total number of articles published in the past 5 years. Of course, different indexing terms or different databases will produce different lists so this is a general guide only. Note also that the coverage includes both human and non-human studies

Table 42.4 Relevant books and other publications

Bock GR, Whelan J, *The Childhood Environment and Adult Disease*. Wiley, UK, 1991
Burton GJ, Barker DJP, Moffett A, *The placenta and human developmental programming*, Cambridge University Press, New York, 2011
Gillman MW, Poston L, *Maternal Obesity*, Cambridge University Press, UK, 2012
Gluckman P, Hanson M, *Mismatch: The lifestyle diseases timebomb*, Oxford University Press, UK, 2008
Gluckman P, Hanson M, *The Fetal Matrix*, Cambridge University Press, UK, 2005
Gluckman P, Hanson M, *Developmental origins of health and disease*, Cambridge University Press, UK, 2006
Khu D, Ben Shlomo Y, *A Life Course Approach to Chronic Disease Epidemiology*, Oxford University Press, UK, 1997
Kundu TK, *Epigenetics: Development and Disease*, Springer, USA, 2013
Lechtig A, Klein RE, Dobbing J, *Maternal Nutrition in Pregnancy – Eating for Two?* Academic Press, UK, 1981
Newnham JP. Ross MG., *Early Life Origins of Human Health and Disease*, Karger, Germany, 2009
Ovesen PG, Jensen DM, *Maternal Obesity and Pregnancy*, Springer, USA, 2012
Parmelee A, Stern E, Development of States in Infants. In: Clemente C, Purpura D, Mayer F (editors). *Sleep and the Maturing Nervous System*. Academic Press, USA, 1972
Pinstrup-Andersen P, *The African Food System and Human Health and Nutrition: a conceptual and empirical overview*, Cornell University Press, Ithaca, 2010
Sandler B, *The African Cookbook*. Carol Publishing Group, USA, 1993
Tollefsbol T, *Medical Epigenetics*, Elsevier USA, 2016

Legend: This table lists books on fetal nutrition, physiology, programming and health

Table 42.5 Relevant internet resources

American Association of Clinical Endocrinologists Obesity Guidelines www.aace.com/publications/guidelines
Asia Pacific Nutrigenomics and Nutrigenetics Organisation 2016 Biennial Conference (APNNO 2016) www.apnno.com/#!biennial-conference/cx3
Centre for Genetics Education www.genetics.edu.au
DORIAN – Developmental Origins of healthy and unhealthy aging: the role of maternal obesity cordis.europa.eu/result/rcn/150415_en.html
Endocrinology Society Education and Clinical Practice www.endocrine.org/education-and-practice-management/clinical-practice-guidelines
Evidence Analysis Library www.andeal.org
Genetic science learning centre (University of Utah Health Sciences) learn.genetics.utah.edu
International Fetal and Newborn Growth Consortium for the 21st Century (INTERGROWTH-21st) intergrowth21.tghn.org
Medscape www.medscape.com
Obesity Society Clinical Resources www.obesity.org/publications/clinical-resources
Online Mendelian Inheritance in Man www.omim.org
Pathway Commons www.pathwaycommons.org
Centre for Maternal and Child Enquiries (CMACE) www.publichealth.hscni.net/publications/maternal-obesity-uk-findings-national-project
Pubmed www.ncbi.nlm.nih.gov/pubmed
US Food and Drug Administration Foodborne Illness Contaminants www.fda.gov/Food/FoodborneIllnessContaminants/Metals/ucm393070.htm
US National Nutrient Database for Standard Reference www.ars.usda.gov/nutrientdata
World Health Organization Child Health www.who.int/topics/child_health/en/
World Health Organization Hypertension www.who.int/cardiovascular_diseases/publications/global_brief_hypertension/en/
1st International Conference on Food Bioactives & Health Conference www.fbhc2016.com
6th World Sustainability Forum sciforum.net/conference/wsf-6
16th International Nutrition & Diagnostics Conference www.indc.cz/en

Legend: This table lists some internet resources on fetal nutrition, physiology, programming and health

References

1. Barker DJ. The origins of the developmental origins theory. J Intern Med. 2007;261:412–7.
2. Forsdahl A. Are poor living conditions in childhood and adolescence an important risk factor for arteriosclerotic heart disease? Br J Prev Soc Med. 1977;31:91–5.
3. Barker DJ, Osmond C. Infant mortality, childhood nutrition, and ischaemic heart disease in England and Wales. Lancet. 1986;1(8489):1077–81.
4. Barker DJP, Hales CN, Fall CHD, Osmond C, Phipps K, Clark PMS. Type 2 (non-insulin-dependent) diabetes mellitus, hypertension and hyperlipidaemia (syndrome X): relation to reduced fetal growth. Diabetologia. 1993;36:62–7.

Index

A

Abdominal obesity, 93
Abnormal birth weight, 505
    biochemical components and processes, 505
    HBW (*see* High birth weight (HBW))
    health consequences, 506, 507
    LBW (*see* Low birth weight (LBW))
    mother and offspring, 506, 507
    risk factors, 507, 508
Abnormal nutritional exposure, foetal development,
    96, 97
Acculturation, 391
ACTH levels, 82
ACTH response, 219
Adequate for gestational age (AGA), 433
ADHD, 24–25
Adipocyte development
    foetal predisposition, visceral adiposity, 97–99
Adipocyte fatty acid-binding protein (A-FABP), 511
Adipogenesis, 98, 332, 333, 361
Adipogenic transcription factors, 98
Adipokines, 100
Adiponectin, 361
Adipose tissue, 361
Adipose tissue adipogenesis, 98
Adipose tissue macrophages (ATM), 101
Adipose-tissue resident macrophages, 100
Adolescent behaviour, 217
Adolescent lambs, 96
Adrenocorticotrophic hormone (ACTH), 18, 148,
    151, 215
Adrenocorticotropin-releasing hormone (ACTH)
    injection, 217
Adult blood pressure, 510
Adult brain and behavior
    BDNF, 20
    chronic illnesses, 20
    CPT, 19
    DNA sequences, 16, 17
    DNMTs, 16
    histones, 17
    HPA axis, 18
    limbic system, 17
    PS, 19, 20
    TSST, 19

Adult glucose intolerance, 534, 535, 537, 538
    fetal programming
        pancreatic GABA signaling pathway, 534, 535
        serotonin axis, 537–538
Adult height, 510
Adult human brain
    insulin sensitivity, 68
Adult-onset disease, 126
Adverse metabolic outcomes, 111–114
Africa's hunger problems, 389
African perspectives, 388–391
    maternal nutrition and BW babies
        diet play, 388
        Financial Security, 389–391
        food and energy consumption, 388, 389
        human catastrophe, 389–391
        quantity and quality of food eaten, 388
        Starvation, 389–391
        urbanization, 389–390
Ageing, 558, 560, 561, 563
Aging Kidney, 139
Agouti gene, 361
Akt, 520
Akt pathway, 521
Alcohol
    inappropriate nutrient intakes, 405, 406
    usage, 405
Allergic diseases in childhood
    and fish, 250–256
ALSPAC cohort, 250
Amygdala, 217
Anabolic hormones, 83
Andhra Pradesh Children and Parents Study (APCAPS),
    380–381
Aneuploid embryos, 364
Angelman syndrome, 360
AngII receptors, 138
Angiogenic vascular endothelial growth factor
    (VEGF)-A, 548
Angiotensin receptors, 136–138
Animal Models, 444
Antenatal glucocorticoid treatment, 547
Anthropometric measurements, 242
Antibodies, 366
Antidiuretic hormone (ADH), 133

© Springer International Publishing AG 2017
R. Rajendram et al. (eds.), *Diet, Nutrition, and Fetal Programming*,
Nutrition and Health, DOI 10.1007/978-3-319-60289-9

Antiphospholipid syndrome, 60
Anxiety, 214, 218, 221, 362
Anxiety-like behaviour, 217, 219
Appropriate weight for gestational age (AGA), 494
Area under the curve (AUC), 266
Arginine-vasopressin (AVP), 18, 138
Arterial blood pressure, 137
Arterial hypertension, 132, 135–137, 139, 141
ASD, 24–25
Asthma, 242, 246, 254
Atherogenic, 361
Atlantic Diabetes in Pregnancy (Atlantic-DIP) study, 399
Atypical antipsychosis drugs, 538
Autoimmune, 364
Autoimmune diseases, 60
Autonomous nervous system (ANS), 521, 523
Avon Longitudinal Study of Parents and Children
        (ALSPAC), 236, 243, 360

B
Baby's birthweight (BW) in Africa
    acculturation, 391
    anthropology, 391
    embryology of maternal nutrition, 388
    and factors affecting maternal nutrition, 387
    food quality, 387
    food safety, 387
    food security, 387
    ICESCR, 386
    macronutrients, 386
    micronutrients, 386
Bacterial infection, 363
Barker hypothesis, 358
Base excision repair (BER), 37
Beckwith-Wiedemann syndrome, 360, 363
Before birth *vs.* suckling period, 231
Behavioral endocrinologists, 147
Benzodiazepines, 530
Beta-cell dysfunction, 518
β-cells, 530, 531, 534–538
Biased ascertainment, 364
Biological samples, 508
Biomarkers, 510–512
    abnormal birth weight
        adult blood pressure, 510
        A-FABP, 511
        classification of pregnant women, 511
        epidemiological studies, 510
        hypothesis linking, 511
        IGF-I, 510
        macrosomia, 510
        MMPs, 510
        multiplex protein array assay, 510
        proteomics markers, 510
        type 2 diabetes, 510
        types, 511, 512
    adult height, 510
    bioinformatics tools, 508
    biological samples, 508

definition, 505
foetal programming, 505, 510
foetus development, 505
gene mapping, 508
genetic and environmental factors, 505
genomics, 508
high-throughput analytical methods, 508
holistic approach, 510
LC, 509
macrosomia, 507
maternal diseases influencing birth weight, 511, 513
metabolites, 509
metabolomics, 508, 509
metabonomics, 508
MS, 509
NGS, 508
omics cascade, 508, 509
omics technologies, 509
protein quantification, 509
proteomics, 508
system biology, 510
top-down and bottom-up proteomics, 508, 509
and transcriptomics, 508
trypsin, 509
Birth rate, 364
Birth weight, 242, 243, 246, 296, 297, 299–301, 358,
        359, 361–363
    biological mechanisms, 50, 51
    biomarkers, maternal diseases influencing, 511–513
    classification, 433, 434
    complex interactions, numerous factors, 435
    excessive, 507
    exercise, 50, 51
    and foetal development, 507
    gestational age, 434
    interpretation, 432
    HBW (*see* High birth weight (HBW))
    LBW (*see* Low birth weight (LBW))
    neonatal mortality, 434
    physical activity, 45–49
    physical fitness, 44, 45
    risk, 49
Birth weight ratio (BWR), 456
Birth weight standard deviation score (BWSDS) groups, 415
Bisphenol, 361
Blood pressure (BP)
    autonomic nervous system, 280
    cardiovascular and cerebrovascular diseases, 280
    diastolic, 280, 281
    life course, 288
    n-3 PUFA, 283, 284
    offspring, 283, 287–290
    physiological control, 280
    programmed hypertension, 280
    systolic, 280, 281
Blood-brain barrier (BBB), 5
Body mass index (BMI), 93, 246, 249, 372, 412
Bone mesenchymal stem cells (BMSCs), 347
Brain development, 36–38, 146, 147
    epigenetics, 35

methyl donor nutrient (*see* Methyl donor nutrients)
nutrition, 33
SNPs, 33
superior longitudinal fasciculus, 31
uncinate fasciculus, 31
Brain insulin resistance, 68
Brain insulin sensitivity
developmental programming, 69
in animals, 69
Brain-derived neurotrophic factor (BDNF), 20, 218

C
Caesarean delivery, 506
Cafeteria diet, 215, 229–231
Caffeine
developmental toxicity, 341, 342
epigenetic modifications, 347
foetal-originated metabolic disease, 347, 348
foetus, 344
glucocorticoids, 344, 345
HPA axis, 344
metabolic diseases, 342
methylxanthine alkaloid, 340
placenta effect, 343, 344
StAR, 343
Caloric density, 390
Caloric intake, 395–400
excessive (*see* Excessive caloric intake)
Caloric restriction, 444–445
Capillary electrophoresis (CE), 509
Carcinogenesis, 361
Cardiometabolic
risk factors, 374, 377, 380
Cardiovascular
risk factors, 377, 380
Cardiovascular disease (CVD), 92, 94, 108, 122, 530
β-adrenergic pathways, 123
adult-onset disease, 126
endothelial dysfunction, 125
epidemiological studies, 123
etiology, 122
fetal growth restriction, 125
fetal metabolic programming, 123
heart growth and development, 124
hyperperfusion, 123
IUGR, 125
maternal low-protein diet, 125
maternal protein restriction, 125
nutritional restriction, 123
postnatal environmental, 122
risk factors, 122
sarcomere, 125
Catabolic hormones, 83
Catch-Up Growth, 126
Celiac disease, 60
Cell mass, 388
Cell-signaling, 521
Cellular hypertrophy, 58
Central America, 360

Central nervous insulin sensitivity, 75
Central nervous system (CNS), 137, 146, 518
Cereals, 387
Childhood bacterial infection, 363
Childhood leukaemia and astrocytoma, 506
Childhood obesity, 246, 248, 249
and fish
BMI, 246
child growth and adiposity, 246, 248
contamination, 246
harmonized and pooled individual data, 246
human trials, 246
in vitro and animal studies, 246
intrauterine life, 246
MI, 246, 249
n-3 LCPUFA, 246
overweight, 246
PIAMA birth cohort study, 246
fish intake during pregnancy, 246–249
Chinese adult population, 93
Chromosome 11, 363
Chronic disease
development, 381
risk factors, 379
Chronic kidney disease (CKD), 132
Chronic stress, 214
Cigarette smoking, 359, 360
Circadian rhythms, 488, 492, 494–497
Circumventricular organ (CVO) neurons, 138
Classical × customized growth criteria, 436–437
Classical growth curves, 435
Clozapine, 538
Cluster of differentiation 68 (CD 68), 101
Cognition, 302, 303
Cognitive ability, 359
Cold pressor test (CPT), 19
Congenic, 364, 365
Congenic strains of laboratory animals, 363
Congenital abnormalities, 359
Congenital anomalies (CA), 416–417
Conscripts, 359
Copy number variations, 363, 365
Cord blood mononuclear cell (CBMC), 585
Coronary artery disease (CAD), 563
Coronary heart disease, 126, 242
Cort levels, 217, 218
Corticosteroid binding globulin (CBG), 544
Corticosterone, 215
Corticotrophin-releasing hormone, 544
Corticotropin-releasing hormone (CRH), 6, 18, 148, 215, 217, 345
Cortisol, 82, 83, 85, 87, 362
CpG sites, 101
Critical period
development, 374
foetal programming, 374
Cross-fostering study, 231
Customised growth criteria, 432, 436
Cysteine dioxygenase (CDO), 320
Cysteine-phosphate-guanine (CpG), 111

D
Danish National Birth Cohort (DNBC), 243, 250
Darwinian, 365, 366
Deacetylation, 358, 363
Demethylation, 216
Dendritic cells, 364
Dental disease, 363
Developmental Origins of Health and Disease (DOHaD),
        7, 132, 214, 333, 373, 411, 518, 598
Dexamethasone (DEX), 150, 151, 547, 548
Diabetes, 92, 359–361
Diabetes mellitus (DM), 412
Diastolic BP (DBP), 280
Differentially methylated regions (DMRs), 525
Dihydrofolate (DHF), 36
Dioxins, 242
DNA methylation, 111, 116, 219, 422, 424, 448
    BER, 37
    histone modification, 35
    IAP, 35
    Igf2 gene, 523
    MECPs, 34
DNA methyltransferases (DNMTs), 16, 220
Docosahexaenoic acid (DHA), 242, 249, 262, 404, 458
Dopamine, 234, 235
Dopamine active transporters (DAT), 234, 235
Dutch famine, 60, 359

E
Early fetal loss, 364
Early life programming, 214
Echocardiographic analysis, 125
Ectopic fat accumulation, 99
Eicosapentaenoic acid (EPA), 242, 262, 404
Electrospray ionization-liquid chromatography-tandem
            mass spectrometry (ESI-LC-MS/MS)
            techniques, 512
Embryonic loss, 364
Embryonic or cell deaths, 362
Embryonic survival, 364
Endocrine disruptors, 361
Endocrine pancreas, 519
    development, 530
    functional deficiencies, 530
    GABA signaling pathway, 531–533
    neurotransmitters, 530
    programming, 87
Endocrine pancreatic cells, 519
Endocrine programming
    fetal growth, 85
    fetal nutrient supply, 83
    hormones, 83
    IGFs, 83
    insulin, 83
    intrauterine, 83
    leptin, 84, 85
    thyroid hormones, 83, 84
Endoplasmic reticulum (ER) stress, 113, 114, 116
Energy consumption, 361

Energy-rich foods, 92
Environmental compounds, 361
Environmental influences, 361, 363, 365
Environmental Protection Agency, 242
Epididymal white adipose tissue, 94
Epigenesis *vs.* Mutation in Genes, 363–365
Epigenetic mark, 362
Epigenetic mechanisms, 359
    maternal programming in offspring, 219, 220
Epigenetic programming, 56
Epigenetics, 111, 113, 114, 116, 359–365
    brain development, 35
    CpG, 34
    DNA methylation, 34, 35
    and fetal programming, 523, 524
    FGR, 62, 63
    maternal diet, 35, 36
    methionine/homocysteine metabolic pathway, 34
Epigenome, 262, 266, 275
Epigenomics
    dysregulation of nuclear receptors, 297
    gene expression, 295
    mechanisms, 296, 302, 303
Epigenotype, 362, 363, 365
Equilibrated-homeostatic environment, 519
ER latencies, 72
Essential fatty acids (EFA), 262
Ethics committees, 366
Euglycaemic–hyperinsulinaemic clamp, 68
European Food Safety Authority (EFSA), 242, 404
Evolution, 366
Evolutionary bottlenecks, 358
Evolutionary process, 365
Excessive birth weight, 507
Excessive caloric intake
    GDM, 399–400
    GWG, 396–398
    pre-conception weight/maternal obesity, 395
Excessive nutrient supply, 228
Exendin-4 (Ex-4), 116
Exercise, 50, 51

F
Famine, 358–360, 364
Fat accumulation, 560
Fat deposition, 232, 233, 235
    foetal predisposition, visceral adiposity, 99, 100
    and prenatal undernutrition, 93
Fat distribution
    and prenatal undernutrition, 93–94
Fat mass, 232
    and Offspring Growth, 230
Fatty acid catabolism, 361
Fatty acid oxidation, 361
Fatty acids, 262
Feeding behavior, 459–461
    DHA, 458
    food preferences (*see* Food preferences)
    homeostasis, 454

IUGR, 456, 459
LMPT, 458
low birth weight, 457
metabolic syndrome, 455
n-3 PUFAs, 458
Fertility, 358, 364
Fetal brain
activity in humans, 71–72
development, 69
fMEG, 69–71
human maternal metabolism, 69
insulin resistance, 74
and maternal metabolism, 71–73
Fetal corticosterone, 551
Fetal epigenome, 362
Fetal evoked responses (ER), 69–71
Fetal glucocorticoid, 545–547
Fetal growth, 358, 363
and preterm birth, 242, 244
Fetal growth restriction (FGR), 57, 489–494
assessment, 56, 57
assessment and determinants
ultrasound evaluation, 57
cardiovascular consequences, 488
cellular hyperplasia and encompasses, 58
cellular hypertrophy, 58
concomitant hyperplasia and hypertrophy, 58
definition, 56, 488
determinants, 57, 58
epigenetic modifications, 62
external intervention and maternal
exposures, 58
health outcomes in childhood and adult life, 56
in utero and transgenerational effect, periconceptional
maternal environment, 58, 59
inflammation, 61
intrauterine, 56
intrauterine growth trajectories, 58
live-born infants, 56
maternal determinants, 58–60
maternal factors, 58
mortality and morbidity, 56
neurodevelopmental impairment, 488
one-carbon metabolism and molecular biological
processes, 56
oxidative stress, 61, 62
sleep and development (see Sleep)
trimester growth, 58
ultrasound evaluation, 56
Fetal growth restriction retarded cardiomyocyte
maturation, 124
Fetal magnetoencephalography (FMEG)
direct non-invasive measurement, fetal neuronal
activity, 69, 70
fetal evoked responses (ER), 69–71
fetal heart dynamics, 69
fetal neuronal activity in utero, 70
non-invasive technique, 69
oddball paradigms, 69
single-channel MEG system, 70
SQUIDs, 70
ultrasound measurements, 70
Fetal metabolic programming and epigenetic
modifications
epigenetics and noncoding sequences, 268, 269
ncRNAs, 269, 270
small noncoding RNAs and epigenetic consequences,
270–274
Fetal mortality, 364
Fetal nutrient, 444
Fetal nutrient supply, 83
Fetal nutrition
internet resources, 602
journals, 601
professional societies and organisations, 600
regulatory bodies and organisations, 599
Fetal nutritional imbalance or stress, 538
Fetal origins hypothesis, 147
Fetal outcomes in Republic of Ireland, 394
Fetal postprandial evoked response (ER) latency, 72, 73
Fetal programming, 358–360
Fetal programming, 4, 5, 9, 69, 75, 122, 530, 534, 535,
537, 538
adult glucose intolerance
pancreatic GABA signaling pathway, 534, 535
serotonin axis, 537–538
adult obesity, 166
behavioral endocrinologists and neuroscientists, 147
behavioral outcomes, 148, 149
caesarean birth, 192–194
cardiovascular disease, 186
and epigenetics, 523–525
ethnicity, 187–190
GABA (see GABA signaling pathway)
HHPA axis, 148
hippocampal neuron changes, 153
hypothesis, 147, 151
postnatal metabolic dysfunction, 534
preterm birth and low birth weight, 190–192
psychiatric outcomes, 148
psychological and psychiatric outcomes, 151
rodent dietary studies, 447
serotonin (see Serotonin)
type 2 diabetes, 186
Fetal starvation, 362
Feto-placental circulation, 57
Fibrogenesis, 332, 333
Financial Security, 389–391
Fish intake during pregnancy
allergic diseases in childhood, 250–256
and childhood obesity, 246, 248
consumption, 242
EFSA, 242
exposure to pollutants, 242
fetal growth and preterm birth
ALSPAC, 243
and birth weight, 247
anthropometric measurements, 242
birth weight, 246
definition, 242

Fish intake during pregnancy (*cont.*)
 DNBC, 243
 Europe-wide study, 243
 gestation length and birth weight, 242
 growth-restricted fetuses, 242
 MeHg, 243
 MoBa, 243
 n-3 LCPUFAs, 243
 n-3 LCUFAs, 242, 243
 organic pollutants, 243
 prospective studies, 244, 245
 neurodevelopment in childhood, 249–253
 nutritional stress or stimulus, 242
 rich source, 242
Fish oil intake, pregnancy
 dietary fatty acids, 263, 264
 insulin sensitivity, 264, 265
 programmed effects, metabolic function, 266, 267
 small noncoding RNAs and epigenetic consequences, 270–274
Fish oil supplements, pregnancy
 benefits, 265
 control diets, 266
 degree of oxidation, 265
 efficacy, 265
 gene function responses, 262
 insulin sensitivity, 275
Fitness, 44–45
 birth weight (*see* Birth weight)
 physical activity, 44
Foetal adipose tissue, 96
Foetal and suckling periods
 junk food diets, 231, 232
Foetal metabolic programming, 92
Foetal predisposition, 96–101
 visceral adiposity
  adipocyte development and growth, 97–99
  epigenetic regulation, 100–101
  fat deposition patterns, 99, 100
  inflammatory responses, 100–101
  timing of abnormal nutritional exposure, 96, 97
Foetal programming, 96–101, 135, 140, 141, 358, 360
 critical period, 374
 biomarkers, 505, 510
 maternal metabolic stress, 561
 metabolic stress-mediated, 561
 and nutritional status, 372–374
 p66Shc gene, 561, 562
 stress affecting, 565
 thrifty phenotype hypothesis, 505
Foetal supply line, 388
Foetal-derived shift in fat deposition, 99
Foetus development
 biomarkers, 505
Folate, 296, 297, 299–302, 361
 and dietary patterns, 401
 folic acid, 400–402
 HSE, 400
 macro and micronutrient intakes, 401
 mean daily energy, 401

micronutrient supplementation in pregnancy in Ireland, 400
 natural sources, 400
 NTDs, 400
Folic acid, 396, 400–402
Food and Agriculture Organization, 387
Food deprivation, 519–521
Food insecurity, 390
Food preference, 231, 235
 animal model, 461
 BWR, 456
 couch potato syndrome, 460
 DA and opioid systems, 463, 464
 homeostatic control system, 461
 HPA, 459
 internal and external influences, 465, 466
 IUGR, 456, 457, 460–463
 junk food diets, 234, 235
 moderators, 464
 n-3 PUFAs, 465
 NAcc, 463
 SGA, 456
 TH, 461
 VLBW, 457
Food quality, 387
Food safety, 387
Food security
 definition, 387
Forsdahl-Barker hypothesis, 598
Framingham Offspring Birth History Study, 506
Free fatty acid (FFA), 72, 74, 75

G
GABA receptor, 530–534
GABA signaling pathway
 endocrine pancreas
  autocrine fashion, 531
  GABA receptor, 531–534
  GAD, 531
  glucagon-like polypeptide 1 (GLP-1), 531
  insulin secretion, 534
  islet β-cells, 531
  islets of Langerhans, 531
  in pancreatic islets, 532
  transaminase and GABA transporter proteins, 531
  β-cell, 534
  β-cells, 531, 534
 fetal programming
  adult glucose intolerance, 534, 535
 GABA receptor, 530
 hippocampus, 530
 in non-neural tissues, 530
 inhibitory neurotransmitter, 530
 insulin secretion, 531
 peripheral tissue growth and development, 530
Gametogenesis, 333, 334
Gas chromatography (GC), 509
Gene mapping, 508
Gene-encoding glucose transporter (GLUT) 3, 548

Generation time, 366
Genesis changes, 149, 150
Genetic contributors to metabolic syndrome, 365
Genetic drift, 359
Genetic selection, 364
Genome sequences, 364, 365
Genomic DNA, 358, 363, 365
Genomic mutations, 363–365
Genomic sequence alterations, 362
Genomics, 508, 510, 513
Genotype frequencies, 364
Genotypes, 364, 366
Germ cells, 365, 366
Germline, 362
Gestation, 216, 218, 221, 522
Gestational age, 434–436
Gestational diabetes, 524
Gestational diabetes mellitus (GDM), 72, 75, 187, 188, 507
    definition, 399
    genetic background, 511
    interventions to reduce in Ireland, 399
    metabolomics, 512
    non-invasive biomarkers, 511
    policy and clinical guidelines, 400
    prevalence, 399
    prognostic biomarkers, 512
    protein biomarkers, 512
    proteomics biomarkers, 511
Gestational HFD, 218
Gestational hypertension, 187, 189
Gestational nutrient restriction, 101
Gestational programming animal models, 135
Gestational protein restriction, 133, 134
    CA3 pyramidal neurons, 153
    CRF/ACTH, 152
    hippocampus, 153
Gestational weight gain (GWG)
    in American population, 397
    data collection, 397
    independent researchers, 397
    interventions to prevent in Ireland, 398
    IOM guidelines, 397
    in Ireland, 397
    and negative infant outcomes, 396
    and negative maternal outcomes, 396
    policy and clinical guidelines, 398
    prevalence, 397
    SCOPE study, 398
    self-reported pre-pregnancy weight, 398
Gestational/lactational HFD effects, 218
Gliomas, 506
Global hypomethylation, 220
Global protein detection, 508
Glucagon-like peptide-1 (Glp-1), 116
Glucagon-like polypeptide 1 (GLP-1), 531
Glucocorticoid receptor (GR), 148, 215
Glucocorticoid receptor (GR) mRNA ratio, 82
Glucocorticoids (GCs), 18, 82, 83, 87, 151, 153, 362
    adverse conditions in pregnancy, 86
    alter gene expression, 86

11β-HSD2, 545
    CBG, 544
    corticosterone, 547
    cortisol levels, 85
    definition, 544
    developmental effects of glucocorticoid on visceral
        tissues, 86
    epigenetic effects, 86
    epigenetic modifications, 346
    fetal growth restriction, 546, 547
    fetal, 544–546
    glucose and amino acids, 548
    HPA axis, 345, 346, 544
    IGF1, 346, 347
    in fetal endocrine function, 86
    knockout model, 11β-HSD2, 548
    lipid metabolic pathways, 342
    LPD-induced fetal programming, 551
    maternal malnutrition, 549
    mechanism of action, 86
    physiological processes, 86
    placenta, 545
    placental barrier, 344
    placental effects, 86
    programming effects, maternal undernutrition, 544
    regulatory effects, 86
    rodent models, 547
    shift cells, 545
    synthetic, 545, 547
    undernutrition, 552
Glucose intolerance, 359
Glucose transporter 4 (GLUT4), 520
Glutamate decarboxylase (GAD), 531
Gotype, 364
G-protein-coupled receptor, 536
GR expression, 218, 221
GR gene expression, 217
Great Leap Forward, 360, 362, 364
Growth-regulatory imprinted genes, 86
Growth-restricted fetuses, 242
Growth-restricted infants, 99
GUI (Growing Up in Ireland), 405
Gut flora, 363

H
HAPO criteria, 400
HDL, 361
Head circumference, 360
Health Service Executive (HSE), 396, 400
Healthspan, 559–561, 563–565
Heart development, 124
Heat shock factor protein 1 (HSF1), 302
Hematological disorders, 60
Hepatic dysfunction, 108
Hepatic gene expression, 111
Hepatic metabolism, 201, 207
Hepatoblastoma, 506
Hepatocellular carcinoma (HCC), 203
Hepatocyte nuclear factor 4-α (HNF-4α), 524

Heterogeneous syndrome, 507
Hexose-6-phosphate dehydrogenase (H6PDH), 179
High birth weight (HBW)
    and adolescent BMI, 506
    caesarean delivery, 506
    childhood leukaemia and astrocytoma, 506
    colon and rectal cancer, 506
    diseases in adulthood, 506
    and hypertension exists, 506
    and LBW, 507, 508
    nutritional status, 374, 375
    population-based study, 506
High blood pressure (BP), 280
High fat diet (HFD)
    adaptations, 214
    BMI, 562
    c-Fos expression, 563
    consumption, 221, 222
    epigenetic mechanisms, 219, 220
    fat metabolism, 561
    foetal programing, 562
    genetic models, 23
    glucocorticoid hormones, 562
    HPA axis, 214, 215, 562
    insulin resistance, 562
    maternal care, 23
    maternal corticosterone, 562
    maternal obesity effects, 217
    metabolic stress, 561, 562
    neuropsychological disorders, 214
    non-human animal models, 22
    obesity, 214
    on mothers
        energy in milk production, 216
        environmental factors, 216
        gestation and lactation, 216
        glucose levels, 216
        inflammation, 217
        locomotor activity, 216
        lower c-fos expression, 216
        maternal obesity, 216
        milk composition, 216
        ND, 217
        obese dams, 216
        pregestational exposure, 216
        pup cannibalism, 216
        weigh-suckle-weigh test, 217
        weight loss during lactation, 216
    OS, 561
    p66Shc gene, 561
    psychosocial stress, 214
    reduced body weight, 562
    rodent models, 214, 221, 222
    timing, development and effects, 218, 219
    types, 215
High-throughput analytical methods
    biomarkers, 508
Hippocampal formation, 150
Hippocampal gyrus, 151–152
Hippocampal neurons, 361

Hippocampus, 217
Hippocampus and memory, 151–153
Hippocampus of HFD, 218
Histone deacetylase (HDAC), 35, 302
Histone modification, 424
Histones, 358, 362, 363
Holistic approach, 510
Homeostatic model assessment (HOMA) of insulin
        resistance, 266, 313
Hormone, 83
    and maternal nutrition, 85
    secretion, 149
Hormone replacement therapy (HRT), 472
Hormones act, 82
Household Dietary Diversity Score (HDDS), 387
Household Food Insecurity Access Prevalence
        (HFIAP), 387
Household Food Insecurity Access Scale (HFIAS), 387
Household food security, 387, 390
HPA axis, 87
HSE Obesity and Pregnancy Clinical Practice
        Guidelines, 403
5-HTr1d receptor, 536
Human brain, 68
    adult (see Adult human brain)
Human catastrophe, 389–391
Human embryo, 366
Hunger Winter, 359, 362
Hyderabad Nutrition Trial, 375–376
Hyderabad Nutrition Trial Follow-Up, 377, 378
11β-hydroxysteroid dehydrogenase system
        (11β-HSDs), 344
11β-hydroxysteroid dehydrogenase type 1
        (11ß-HSD1), 179
11β-hydroxysteroid dehydrogenase type 2 (11β-HSD 2),
        83, 216, 510, 545
    fetal glucocorticoid, 546, 547
    feto-placental exposure, 551
    glucocorticoid, 545, 546
    knockout model, 548
    placental, 546, 547
    protein-restricted placentas, 551
    SAME, 546
25–hydroxyvitamin D (25(OH)D), 402
Hypercholesterolemia, 506
Hyperinsulinaemia, 361
Hyperserotonemia, 332, 333
Hypertension, 123, 124, 126
Hypertensive disorders, 163
Hypertrophic adipose expansion, 102
Hypothalamic-pituitary-adrenal (HPA) axis, 4, 6, 7, 82,
        83, 123, 179, 341, 448, 459, 544
    and behavioural dysfunction, 215
    and behavioural outcomes, 221
    GC receptors, 21
    HFD, 22
    hyperactivated, 214
    in lactating HFD dams, 217
    limbic system, 20
    and stress-related behaviours, 217

Hypothalamic-pituitary-adrenal activity, 362
Hypoxia, 111, 113, 117, 136
Hypoxia-inducible factor-1 (HIF-1), 98

I
IGF1 signalling, 362
Immune function
    BMI and obesity prevalence, 9
    inflammatory cytokines, 8
    somatic illnesses, 9
Immunological processes, 361
Immunological tolerance, 364
Impaired hepatic function, 109
Implantations, 364
Imprinting, 358, 360, 363, 366
Imprinting defect, 363
Inappropriate nutrient intakes
    alcohol, 405, 406
    folate, 400–402
    iron, 401, 403, 404
    Long Chain Omega 3-PUFA (EPA and DHA), 404
    vitamin D, 402–403
Induce oxidative stress in neurons, 218
Infant stress physiology, 6, 7
Infertility, 364
Inflammation, 361
    FGR, 61
Inflammatory agents, 587
Inflammatory processes, 361
Inflammatory response, 136
Inflammatory responses and epigenetic regulation, 100
Inner cell mass, 388
Institute of medicine (IOM), 397
Insulin, 83, 359, 361
Insulin- and serotonin-containing granules, 536
Insulin growth factor 1 (IGF-1), 109
Insulin receptor substrate-1 (IRS-1), 521
Insulin resistance, 361, 377, 378, 530, 561, 562
Insulin secretion, 534
Insulin sensitivity, 264, 266, 267, 270, 274
    definition, 68
    developmental programming, 69
    fMEG, 69
    human brain, 75
    and maternal metabolism, 71
    mechanisms, 74, 75
Insulin-like growth factor 1 (IGF-I), 233, 510
Insulin-like growth factors (IGFs), 82–84, 87, 329
Insulin-p66Shc-H$_2$O$_2$ axis, 563
Insulin-target tissues, 530
Integrated Child Development Services (ICDS), 375, 376, 381
Interference, 538
Intergenerational cycle of obesity, 228
International Association for Food Protection, 387
International Association of Diabetes and Pregnancy Study Groups (IADPSG), 399
International Covenant on Economic, Social and Cultural Rights (ICESCR), 386

International Food Information Council, 387
Intracisternal A-type particle (IAP), 35, 361
Intrauterine and suckling phases
    sensitive periods of life, metabolic programming, 518–522
Intrauterine development
    regulatory signals, 85–87
Intrauterine environment, 364, 366
Intrauterine growth curves
    classical, 435
    customised, 436
Intrauterine growth restriction (IUGR), 83, 92, 93, 109, 507, 512, 513, 538
    adverse intrauterine environment, 146
    associated lipid peroxidation, 116
    carbohydrates, 457
    chronic diseases, 459
    echocardiographic analysis, 125
    feeding preferences, 461–463
    fetal liver development, 109
    gestational malnutrition, 122
    idiopathic, 109
    maternal diabetes model, 116
    maternal dietary-induced, 110
    maternal undernourishment, 110
    MPR model, 110
    offspring, 116
    placental insufficiency/maternal malnutrition, 109
    placental insufficiency-induced, 109
Intrauterine growth retardation (IUGR), 347, 358, 364
    caffeine ingestion (*see* Caffeine)
    metabolic diseases, 340
Intrauterine hyperglycemia, 524
Intrauterine life, 246
Intrauterine nutrition
    calcification paradox, 482
    mesenchymal-cartilaginous tissue, 477
    musculo-skeletal diseases, 478
    osteoporosis development, 478–481
    vitamin K-anticoagulant antagonism, 481–483
Intrauterine programming, 82, 83, 87
IOM guidelines, 397
Irish College of General Practitioners (ICGP), 396
Irish Health Service Executive (HSE), 396
Iron
    inappropriate nutrient intakes, 401, 403, 404
Ischemic heart disease (IHD), 329, 505
Islet vasculature, 536
Islets of Langerhans, 530, 531, 538

J
Japan
    BMI, 412
    congenital anomalies status, 416–417
    environmental factor, fetal development
        air pollution and neurodevelopmental diseases, 424
        methyl mercury and polychlorinated biphenyls, 423
        polychlorinated biphenyls and environmental hormones, 423

Japan (*cont.*)
  epigenetics studies, 424
  female nutritional status, 416, 418
  LBW infants and adult diseases, 412, 415, 420
  male nutritional status, 417
  maternal nutritional status, pregnancy, 418, 419, 421
  nutritional factors on fetal
    fatty acids and lipids, 422, 423
    folic acid, 422
    trace elements and micronutrients, 423
    vitamins and related elements, 422
  nutritional status and outcomes, 413–415
  obesity, 412
  vital statistics, birth and young women, 415
Junk food diets
  advantages, 229
  biological mechanisms, 228
  clinical studies, 235–236
  definition, 229
  disadvantages, 229
  excessive nutrient supply, 228
  fat deposition, 232, 233
  foetal and suckling periods, 231, 232
  food preferences, 231, 234, 235
  growth and fat mass, 230
  intergenerational cycle, 228
  intergenerational cycle of obesity, 228
  maternal overnutrition, 228
  metabolic programming, 228
  organs and physiological systems, 228
  physical activity, 228
  pregnancy and neonatal outcomes, 230
  sex differences, 235

L
Laboratory animals, 363, 365
Lactation, 216–218, 506, 521, 522
  maternal n-3 PUFA, 287–290
Langerhans, 522
Large birth weight, 442, 443
Late and moderately preterm children
    LMPT), 458
LC-MS, 512
Legumes, 387
Leptin, 82–87, 219, 361
L-glutamate levels, 534
Life-Course Studies in India
  APCAPS, 380–381
Limbic system, 22
  gestational over-nutrition, 22, 23
  gestational under-nutrition, 21
  HFD (*see* High fat diet (HFD))
  high-fat consumption, 22, 23
  HPA-axis and metabolic disruption, 23, 24
Linseed oil (LO), 271
Lipogenesis, 98
Liquid chromatography (LC), 509
Live birth, 364
Locomotor activity, 216

Long-chain polyunsaturated fatty acids (LCPUFA),
    262–264, 266, 267, 281, 404
Long-term hepatic function, 109, 110
Long-term metabolic dysfunction, 114–116
Low birth weight (LBW), 359
  and adult depression, 506
  adult disease, 506
  colon cancer, 506
  and HBW, 507, 508
  hypercholesterolemia, 506
  and IHD, 505
  infants, 411, 412, 415, 417, 420, 423
  maternal under-nutrition, 387
  meta-regression analysis, 506
  nutritional status, 374, 375
  in organ development, 506
  palatable foods, 456
  placental pathology, 507
  and pre-term delivery, 510
  risk factors, 507
  and small for gestational age (SGA), 507
  and type 2 diabetes, 506
  VLBW, 506
Low glycaemic index dietary, 399
Low-density lipoprotein (LDL), 422, 563
Low-protein diet (LPD), 94, 124, 445
  fetal growth restriction, 550, 551
  fetal weight, placental weight, and glucocorticoid
      parameters, 551
  glucocorticoids, 551
  nutrient transport capacity, 550
Low-protein or low-calorie dietary regimen, 519

M
mAChRs, 523
Macro- *vs.* micronutrients
  MMA levels, 376
  Mumbai SARAS Kids Study, 377
  Pune Intervention Study, 377
Macronutrients, 386
  BW in Africa, 386
Macrosomia, 386, 507, 510
Magnetic resonance imaging (MRI), 141
Magnetoencephalographic study, 68
Malnutrition, 330, 359–363, 366
  glucocorticoid-related parameters, 549
  placental 11β-HSD2, 549
Malprogramming effects, 521
Mammalian target of rapamycin (mTOR), 521
Mass spectrometry (MS), 509
Maternal determinants, FGR
  alcohol, cigarettes and illicit drugs, 60
  autoimmune diseases, 60
  celiac disease, 60
  chronic maternal hypoxemia, 60
  etiology, 58
  external and internal factors, 58
  hematological disorders, 60
  maternal risk factors, 58, 59

maternal undernutrition, 60
metabolism and health status, 60
nutrition and nutrient absorption, 60
overnutrition, 60
placental function, 58
SGA newborn, 60
Maternal diet
epigenetics, 35, 36
Maternal dietary protein restriction, 124
Maternal HFD. See HFD
Maternal high-fat feeding, 445, 446
Maternal iron restriction, 446
Maternal low-protein diet, 112–114
Maternal LP diet, 530
Maternal malnutrition, 362, 364
Maternal metabolism
and fetal brain, 71, 73
and insulin sensitivity, 71–72
Maternal nutrient restriction (MNR) model, 110
Maternal nutrition, 372, 395, 400, 421, 424
and fetal outcomes, 394
excessive caloric intake (see Excessive caloric intake)
framework, 394, 395
inappropriate nutrient intakes (see Inappropriate
    nutrient intakes)
outcomes, research and strategies, 394
status (see Nutritional status)
Maternal nutritional factors, 386
BW (see Babies' birthweight (BW) in Africa)
Maternal nutritional status, 411
Maternal obesity (MO)
animal models, 174, 175
blood metabolites and hormones, 176, 177
gestational diabetes, 172
HPA axis and stress-related behaviours, 217–218
insulin resistance, 175, 176
mid-gestation fetal vs. adult offspring, 181
multigenerational vs. transgenerational impacts, 173
NHP, 182
ovine model, 172
puberty, 173
rodents, 181, 182
tissue and organ structure
    11ß-HSD1, 179
    fetal pancreatic β-cells, 180
    H6PDH, 179
    HPA, 179
    melanocortin system, 180
    NAFLD, 179
    overnutrition, 178
    WAT, 179
Maternal overnutrition, 60, 549
Maternal protein restriction (MPR) model, 110, 111,
    124, 125
aging kidney, 139, 140
and brain, 146
glucocorticoid, 151
hypertension development, 135, 137, 138
kidney programming, 133
nephrogenesis, 134–140

nephrons, 133
offspring, 146
postnatal nTS angiotensin receptors, 138
pregnancy and breastfeeding, 153
renal tissue renin and angiotensin II levels, 136
Maternal risk factors, 58, 59
Maternal starvation, 358, 359, 361, 362, 366
Maternal undernutrition, 60, 109. See also Prenatal
    undernutrition
direct mechanisms, 111–113
hypoxia, 111
indirect mechanisms, 113, 114
IUGR (see Intrauterine growth restriction (IUGR))
MNR model, 110
MPR model, 110, 111
uterine ligation, 109–110
Matrix metalloproteinases (MMPs), 510
Matrix-assisted laser desorption/ionization-time-of-
    flight-mass spectrometry
    (MALDI-TOF-MS), 512
Mean arterial pressure (MAP), 283
MECP2, 362
Medial solitary tract nucleus (nTS), 138
Melanocortin receptor antagonist, 361
Melanocortin system, 180
Memory, 361, 362
Menstrual cycle, 364
Mesenchymal metanephron (MM), 134
Messenger RNA (mRNA), 268
Metabolic bone syndrome, 473
Metabolic dysfunctions, 558
Metabolic malprogramming, 520
Metabolic programming
CNS, 518
DOHaD, 518
epigenetics and fetal programming, 523–525
nutritional insults, 522–523
pancreatic beta cells, 523–525
pancreatic islets, 518
prenatal and postnatal nutritional insults, 518
sensitive periods of life, 518–522
T2D, 518
thrifty phenotype hypothesis, 518
Metabolic stress, 558, 561, 562, 565
Metabolic syndrome, 92, 358–364, 366
abnormal feeding behavior and altered endocrine
    status, 445
animal models, 444
definition, 440
DNA methylation, 297
epidemiological studies, 440
epigenome influence, age-related outcomes, 301
fetal programming, 448
fetal undernutrition, 441
gestational age infants, 443
gestational malnutrition, birth weight and adult
    metabolic diseases, 442
liver and heart, 297
nutritional deficiency, 441
over-nutrition, obesity and diabetes, 442, 443

Metabolic syndrome (*cont.*)
    post-natal nutrition and risk development, 443, 444
    rodent models, 445
Metabolic syndrome pattern, 519
Metabolomics, 508–513
Metabonomics, 508
Methyl donor deficiency (MDD), 294–296, 298
Methyl donor nutrients
    choline and betaine, 37
    folate, 36, 37
    methionine, 38
    supplements, 36
    vitamins B_2, B_6 and B_{12}, 38
Methyl donors, 297
    choline, 295
    deficiency, 297
    dietary, 301–303
    epidemiological facts, 297–299
    experimental facts, 299
    maternal status, 299
    status, pregnancy, 299, 302, 303
Methylated region (DMR), 300, 301
Methylation, 358, 360–366
Methyl-CpG-binding proteins (MECPs), 34, 35
Methylenetetrahydrofolate reductase (MTHFR), 295
Methylmalonic acid (MMA) levels, 376
Methylmercury (MeHg), 242, 243, 249, 250, 257
Methylome, 300, 301, 304, 366
Microalbuminuria, 360
Micronutrients, 230, 386
Microorganisms, 363
MicroRNAs (miRNAs), 111, 113, 114, 126, 262, 267,
      269, 270, 360, 362, 363
    epigenetics, 200, 204, 209
    fatty acid metabolism, 207
    fatty liver, 200
    foetal hypothesis, 200
    glucose intolerance and insulin resistance, 209
    hepatic lipid metabolism, 201
    HFD, 204, 205
    inflammation-related proteins, 206
    lactation, 203
    lipid homeostasis, 208
    miR-122, 204
    miR-370, 206
    NAFLD, 203
    ncRNA, 201
Mid pregnancy, 360
Mineralocorticoid (MR), 153
Mineralocorticoid receptors (MRs), 82, 149, 217, 218, 546
Missing genotypes, 365
Mitochondria, 361
Molecular evidence, 361, 365
Molecular mechanisms, 358, 362
Molecular Studies, 360–362
Monozygotic, 365
Monozygotic human twins, 363
Monozygotic twins, 363, 365
Months of Adequate Household Food Provision Indicator
    (MAHFP), 387
Mood disorders, 19, 22

Morphogenesis, 519
Morris water maze (MWM) test, 153
Mortality, 358–360, 363, 364
Mosaic, 360
Mosaicism, 363, 365
Mosaicism for mutations, 363
Mother-infant pair, 388
mRNA expression, 98, 99, 233
mtDNA-encoded COX I, 316
Multiple pregnancies, 364
Multiplex protein array assay, 510
Mumbai SARAS Kids Study, 377
Muscarinic acetylcholine receptor (mAChR), 522
Musculo-skeletal pathology
    bone metabolism, 474
    early life starvation, 474, 475
    fracture risk, 476
    Garvan nomogram, 474
    transgenerational effect, 476
Myelination, 361
Myocardial hypertrophy, 125
Myogenesis, 332, 333, 478
Mysore Birth Cohort, 377, 378

N
n-3 long-chain polyunsaturated fatty acids (LCPUFAs),
      242, 243, 246, 249, 250, 458
Nasal insulin, 68
National Adult Nutrition Survey (NANS), 401
National Family Health Survey (NFHS), 372
National Food Security Bill 2013, 381
National Institute of Nutrition (NIN), 376
National Maternity Hospital, Dublin, 397
National Nutrition Policy of 1993, 381
Nauru, 360
Neonatal body composition, 49
Neoplasms, 360
Nephrogenesis, 134, 139
Nephron number, 141
Neural Tube Defects (NTDs), 400
Neurodevelopment, 9, 10
Neurodevelopment in childhood
    ALSPAC cohort, 250
    brain and cognitive development, 249
    DHA, 249
    DNBC, 250
    MeHg, 249, 250
    n-3 LCPUFAs, 249, 250
    prospective studies, 250–253
    second-trimester fish intake, 250
Neurohumoral and Kidney Dysfunction, 135–139
Neuronal plasticity, 361
Neuropsychiatric disorders
    ADHD and ASD, 24–25
    anxiety and depression, 25, 26
    cognitive impairments, 24
    schizophrenia, 26
New Delhi Birth Cohort (NDBC), 378, 379
Next-generation sequencing (NGS), 508
Non-adipose tissues, 99

Non-alcoholic fatty liver disease (NAFLD), 301
Non-alcoholic steatohepatitis (NASH), 203, 303
Noncoding RNAs (ncRNAs), 201, 268–270, 358, 359
Noncommunicable disorder (NCD), 570
Nonhuman primates (NHP)
    HFD, 175
    insulin resistance, 176
Nonpenetrance, 363
Non-rapid eye movement (NREM), 489
Normal glucose tolerant (NGT), 72
Norwegian research, 359
Novelty-suppressed feeding test (NSFT), 25
Nuclear factor 4 (NF-4), 298
Nuclear factor Y (NF-Y), 265
Nuclear factor κB (NFκB), 218
Nuclear magnetic resonance (NMR), 509
Nuclear receptors (NRs), 116, 298
Nucleosomes, 358
Nucleus accumbens (NAcc), 234, 463
Nutrient intakes, 400–405
    inappropriate (see Inappropriate nutrient intakes)
Nutrient restriction, 446
Nutrition
    brain development, 33
    cognitive development, 31
    foetal brain development, 30
    maternal nutrient state and offspring TL, 577, 578
    neurological processes, 31, 32
    pregnancy and offspring TL, 574
Nutritional deficiency, 441
Nutritional factors and infant growth in Japan, 422, 423
Nutritional insults
    pancreatic islet, 522–523
Nutritional restriction in utero, 538
Nutritional scarcity, 93
Nutritional status, 375–381
    and foetal programming, 372, 374
    HBW, 374, 375
    India
        Hyderabad Nutrition Trial, 375–376
        Life-Course Studies, 380–381
        macro- vs. micronutrients, 376–377
        NDBC, 378, 379
        PMNS, 376
        Prospective Studies, 378
        Retrospective Studies, 377, 378
        Vellore Birth Cohort, 380
    Japan, 418–421
    LBW, 374, 375
    of Indian women, 372, 373
    policies, 381, 382
    and prevalence of obesity across migration, 372, 373
    risk factors, 372
Nutritional stress or stimulus, 242

O
Obesity, 359, 364, 365
    abdominal, 93
    adult disease risk, 166, 167
    anesthetic complications, 163

    and associated disorders, 92
    BMI, 159, 160
    definition, 92
    development, 92, 94
    disparity, 161
    epidemic, 160
    epidemiological and animal studies, 92
    fetal and neonatal period, 166
    gestational weight gain, 164, 165
    hypertensive disorders, 163–164
    and metabolic disorders, 92
    peripartum risks, 163
    preeclampsia, 163–164
    pregestational and gestational diabetes, 163
    pre-pregnancy, 161, 162
    prevalence, 159
    trends, 160, 161
    visceral, 92
    weight/maternal, 395–396
Obesity-induced hyperplasia, 94
Obesity-induced metabolic disorders, 94
Obesity-induced metabolic syndrome, 94
Obesity-induced subcutaneous fat deposition, 99
Oddball paradigms, 69
Olive oil (OO), 266, 267, 271
Omega-3 polyunsaturated fatty acids (ω-3 PUFA)
    anti-hypertensive actions, 281–283
    beneficial effects, 281
    intake and offspring BP, outcomes, 285, 286
    lactation and offspring BP, 287–290
    LCPUFAs, 281
    offspring BP, 283
    pregnancy and offspring BP, 284–287
Omics cascade, 508, 509
Omics techniques, 510
Omics technologies, 508–510, 513
One-carbon metabolisms (1-CM)
    DNA methylation, 300
    markers and methyl donor status, 297–299, 302, 303
    metabolic and nutritional factors, 294
    network of pathways, 294–296
Ontogenesis, 134
Ontogeny, 132
Operative birth/caesarean section, 506
Opioid, 234
Oral glucose tolerance test (OGTT), 71, 400
Organization for Economic Co-operation and
        Development (OECD), 412
Osteogenesis, 478
Osteopenia, 472, 474–476, 480
Osteoporosis, 473, 477–483
    atherogenesis, 473
    bone quality, 483, 484
    intrauterine nutrition (see Intrauterine nutrition)
    musculo-skeletal pathology (see Musculo-skeletal
        pathology)
    postnatal compensatory growth, 483, 484
    prophylaxis, 472
    treatment, 472
Outer cell mass, 388
Ovulations, 364

Oxidative damage, 218
Oxidative stress (OS), 61, 218, 448, 558, 587

P
P66Shc
    DNA methylation, 563
    gene expression, 563
    gerontogene, 559, 560
    human health, 564
    human healthspan, 565
    induced ROS formation, 563
    Met410Val polymorphism, 563
    mitochondrial hormesis, 564
    OS and metabolism, 559
    PBMC, 563
    ROS, 564
    WT and KO, 562
Palm oil (PO), 271
Pancreas
    endocrine, 531–534
    serotonin synthesis, 535–537
Pancreatic and duodenal homeobox factor 1 (Pdx1),
        519, 525
Pancreatic beta cells
    critical stage, 523
    epigenetic, 523
    epigenome pathways, 525
    and fetal programming, 523–525
    functional disability, 523
    gene targets, 524
    glucose-induced insulin secretion, 521
    high-fat diet program, 525
    HNF-4α, 524
    Igf2 and H19, 524
    insulin secretion, 523
    intrauterine hyperglycemia, 524
    mAChRs, 523
    maternal environment and nutrition, 523, 524
    metabolic networks, 525
    metabolic programming, 523, 524
    methylation pattern, DMRs, 525
    Pdx1, 525
    physiological ability, 522
    T2D, 523, 525
    weak ability, 523
Pancreatic islet
    GABA signaling pathway, 531, 532
    nutritional insults malprogram
        acetylcholine-responsiveness, 523
        ANS, 523
        insulin, 522
        Langerhans, 518, 522
        mAChRs, 523
        metabolic malprogramming effects, 523
        physiological ability, pancreatic beta cells, 522
        prediabetic obese mice, 522
        transcription factors, 523
        undernourishment, 522
Pancreatic progenitors, 535

Paraventicular nucleus (PVN), 138, 215, 217
Partial least square discriminant analysis (PLS-DA), 511
Patent ductus arteriosus (PDA), 416
Paternal diet, 16–26
    brain and behavior (*see* Adult brain and behavior)
    limbic system function (*see* Limbic system)
    neuropsychiatric disorder (*see* Neuropsychiatric
        disorders)
Pedersen Hypothesis, 74
Peripheral blood mononuclear cells (PBMC), 563
Perirenal fat, 96
Perirenal-abdominal adipose tissue, 96
Peroxisome proliferator-activated receptor alpha
        (PPARα), 361
Peroxisome proliferator-activated receptor gamma
        (PPARγ), 233, 548
Peroxisomes, 361
Phosphatidylinositol-3 kinase (PI3-K), 520
Physical activity
    birth weight, 49
    infant body composition, 49, 50
    long term impact, 50
Phytoestrogens, 361
Placenta, 545, 547–549
Placental 11β-HSD2, 545
Placental function, 56, 58, 60, 62–64
Placental insufficiency, 364
Placental insufficiency-induced IUGR, 109
Placental lactogen, 536
Placental malaria, 388
Plastic liver intervening, 114–116
Point mutations, 365, 366
Policy
    and clinical guidelines, GDM, 400
    and clinical practice guidelines, maternal obesity
        management, 396
    Malnutrition India, 381, 382
Political incentives and bias, 366
Polychlorinated biphenyls (PCBs), 242, 423
Polycystic ovary syndrome, 361
Polymorphisms, 361, 511
Polyunsaturated fatty acids (PUFA), 262
Poor nutrition, 506
Postnatal catch-up growth, 113
Postnatal day (PND), 217
Postnatal diet
    visceral adiposity, 94–96
Postnatal malnutrition, 363
Postnatal weight gain, 506
Posttranslational histone modifications, 111
Post-translational modifications (PTMs), 508
Postzygotic mutations, 363, 364, 366
Poverty and food insecurity in Africa, 390
Prader-Willi syndrome, 360
PRAMS (Pregnancy Risk Assessment Monitoring
        System), 405
Pre- and postnatal development
    adipogenesis, 332, 333
    B vitamins, 331
    DOHaD, 328

embryo-fetal development, 326, 327
embryo-fetal programming, 335
endogenous and/or exogenous factors, 326
fetal programming, 328
fibrogenesis, 332, 333
folate, 331
gametogenesis and reproductive function, 333, 334
genetic and environmental factors, 330
IGFs, 329
immune response, 331
malnutrition, 330
micronutrients supplementation, 326, 327
molecular mechanisms, 334
myogenesis, 332, 333
tryptophan, 331
Preadolescence, 359, 360
"Predictive adaptive response" hypothesis, 109
Preeclampsia (PE), 163, 187, 189, 402, 512
Pre-existing diabetes mellitus, 400
Pregestational and gestational diabetes, 163
Pregnancy, 242–246, 262, 358–360, 363, 364
    complications, 187–190
    fatty acid supplementation, 265
    fish intake (*see* Fish intake during pregnancy)
    fish oil intake (*see* Fish oil intake, pregnancy)
    fish-based diet, 266
    oxidative stress, 266
Pregnancy Risk Assessment Monitoring System
        (PRAMS), 160
Pregnancy-induced hypertension, 446
Prenatal stress
    child neurodevelopment, 9, 10
    diet and nutrition, 4, 6
    immune function, 8, 9
    infant growth and metabolism, 7, 8
    infant stress physiology, 6, 7
    psychosocial stress, 6
Prenatal undernutrition
    and fat deposition in young offspring, 93
    and fat distribution in adult offspring, 93
    with postnatal diet on visceral adiposity, 94–96
Pre-pregnancy BMI, 397
Preterm birth
    and fetal growth, 242–246
Prevention and Incidence of Asthma and Mite Allergy
        (PIAMA) birth cohort study, 246
Profibrogenic markers, 110
Programmed effects, maternal fish oil intake, 266, 267
Programmed hypertension
    effective strategies, 280
    maternal nutritional interventions, 281
    pathophysiology, 280
    prevention, 280–281
Pro-inflammatory, 361
Pro-inflammatory transcription factor, 218
Proopiomelanocortin (POMC), 82, 216, 220
Protein kinase B (PKB), 114, 520
Protein quantification, 509
Proteomics, 508–513
Proteomics markers, 510

Psychosocial stress, 214
Public health concern. *See* Maternal nutrition in Ireland
Pune Intervention Study, 377
Pune Maternal Nutrition Study (PMNS), 376
Pup cannibalism, 216

R
Rapid eye movement (REM), 489
Reactive oxygen species (ROS), 448
Recommended dietary allowance (RDA), 377
Reduced nephron number, 133–135
Renal disorders, 94
Renal tubular progressive dysfunction, 139
Renin-angiotensin system (RAS), 136
Reproductive function, 333, 334
Respiratory disease, 363
Restricting food intake, pregnant rodents, 549
Retinoblastoma, 506
Retrotransposon, 361
Rett syndrome, 362
Reverse transcription, 365
Reward pathways, 228, 234–236
Ribosomal RNA (rRNA) molecules, 268
RNA Regulation, 363–365
Rodent models, 446
    maternal HFD, 214–215
    as translational models, 221, 222
ROLO study, 398, 399

S
S-adenosylmethionine (SAM), 295
Satiety hormone, 75
Schizophrenia, 359, 362
Screening for pregnancy endpoints (SCOPE) study,
        398, 405
Sedentary lifestyles, 92
Selection, 365, 366
Selection of cells, 365
Selective advantage, 364
Selective serotonin reuptake inhibitors (SSRIs), 530, 538
Sensitive periods of life
    metabolic programming
        cell-signaling, 521
        critical phase, 518
        endocrine pancreas, 519
        food deprivation, 519–521
        gestation, 522
        healthy and functioning endocrine pancreas, 519
        insulin production/secretion, 522
        lactation, 521, 522
        mAChR, 522
        maternal undernutrition in critical phase, 519, 521
        metabolic syndrome pattern, 519
        morphogenesis, 519
        Pdx1, 519
        pregnancy and lactation, 519
        progression of pregnancy, 519
        T2D, 518

Serotonin
    action in pancreas, 536
    axis, fetal programming of adult glucose intolerance,
        537
    5-HT2b receptors, 531
    in non-neural tissues, 530
    neuronal activity, 530
    pancreatic β-cells, 531
    and pancreatic function during pregnancy, 536, 537
    peripheral tissue growth and development, 530
    receptors, 536
    SSRIs, 530
    synthesis within pancreas, 535–536
Serotonin availability, 537
Serotonin receptors, 530, 536, 538
Serotonin-specific receptors, 153
Serum 25(OH)D, 402, 403
Sex differences, junk food diets, 235
Sickle cell disease, 60
Single cells, 364, 366
Single nucleotide polymorphisms (SNPs), 33
Single-channel MEG system, 70
siRNA, 365
Sleep
    active sleep (AS), 493
    AGA, 494
    children and adults, 489
    fetal life, 490, 492
    FGR
        fetus, 495
        long-term effects, 496, 497
    function, 489
    infancy
        active sleep (AS), 492–493
        architecture, 493
        EEG patterns, 494
        quiet sleep (QS), 492
        sleep-wake cycling, 494
    NREM, 489
    preterm birth
        circadian rhythms, 494–495
        long-term effects, 496, 497
    quiet sleep (QS), 493
    REM, 489
Small birth weight, 441
Small for gestational age (SGA), 56, 93, 109, 415, 433,
        507, 578
    feeding and eating disorders, 457
Small RNA molecules, 365
Social class, 364
Socioeconomic factors, 363
Somatic, 359, 362, 365, 366
Somatic mosaicism, 363–365
Somatic mutation, 363, 365
Somatic recombination, 366
Soy oil (SO), 271
Sperm transfer RNA-derived small RNAs (stRNAs),
        269–270
Stable isotope labelling/label-free approach, 509
Starvation, 358, 360–365, 389, 390
Steroidogenic acute regulatory protein (StAR), 343

Sterol regulatory element binding protein-1 (SREBP-1), 265
Stochastic, 361
Stress hormones, 585
Stress-related behavior. *See also* Adult brain and
        behavior
    and HPA axis, 217–218
Stress-related gene expression, 218
Subcutaneous expandability, 99
Suboptimal nutrition, 94
Suckling and foetal periods
    junk food diets, 231, 232
Superconducting Quantum Interference Devices
        (SQUIDs), 70
Supplementation, 400–404, 407
Suprachiasmatic nucleus (SCN), 492
Surface-enhanced laser desorption/ionization-time-of-
        flight-mass spectrometry
        (SELDI-TOF-MS), 512
Surviving embryos, 364
Symbiotic bacteria, 363
Synapse formation, 361
Syncytiotrophoblast (STB), 311
Syndrome of apparent mineralocorticoid excess
        (SAME), 546
Systolic blood pressure, 93, 136
Systolic BP (SBP), 280

T
T2D, 518, 521, 523, 525
Taurine, 316
    adiponectin, 320
    CDO, 320
    endocrine pancreas, 315, 316
    pyridoxal 5′-phosphate, 311
    STB, 311
    T1D (*see* Type 1 diabetes (T1D))
    T2D (*see* Type 2 diabetes (T2D))
    TauT, 312
    utero effects, 312–315
Taurine transporter (TauT), 311, 312
Telomerase, 572
Telomerase activity (TA), 572
Telomere biology system
    disease risk and aging
        dysregulation, expression capacity, 572–573
        telomerase, 572
        telomere shortening, 572
    inflammatory agents, 587
    initial setting, 573
    malnutrition, pregnancy and offspring TL, 574–576
    maternal nutrient state and Offspring TL, 577, 578
    obstetric complication
        fetal growth and birth weight, 579–581
        fetal TL and TA, 578, 583, 584
        maternal stress, 585
        maternal stress and sleep, 586
        pregnancy, 578, 585
        preterm birth, TL, 578
        SGA, 578
        suboptimal birth outcomes, 578

oxidative stress, 587
    preterm birth, 582
    stress hormones, 585
Telomere homeostasis, 578
Telomere length (TL)
    initial setting, 573
    maternal stress and sleep, 586
    preterm births, 578
    programming mechanisms, 587
Tetrahydrofolate (THF), 36
Thermogenesis, 361
Thiazolidinedione drugs, 361
Thrifty genotype, 358, 362, 364, 366
Thrifty genotype hypothesis, 358, 366
Thrifty phenotype, 359, 374
Thrifty phenotype hypothesis, 359, 441, 505, 518
Thyroid hormones, 82–84, 86, 87
Timing of HFD Exposure, 218, 219
Tissue inhibitor of metalloprotease 2 (TIMP-2), 125
Toll-like receptor (TLR4), 101
Transcription, 361, 365
Transcriptome sequencing, 366
Transcriptomics, 508, 510, 513
Transfer of organisms, 362
Transfer RNA (tRNA), 268
Transgenerational effects, 366
Transgenerational epigenetics, 366
Transgenerational studies, 446–448
Translational models, 221, 222
Transposons, 361
Trier social stress test (TSST), 19
Triglycerides, 361
Trimester growth, 58
Trypsin, 509
Tryptophan, 331, 535
Two-dimensional difference gel electrophoresis
        (2D-DIGE), 512
Type 1 angiotensin II receptor (AT_1), 153
Type 1 diabetes (T1D), 316, 317
Type 2 diabetes (T2D), 68, 242, 314, 316, 320, 361, 400,
        506, 510, 530
Tyrosine-hydroxylase (TH), 461

U

UBE3A gene, 360
UK biobank data, 506
Undernutrition, 93–94
    endocrine hormones, 82
    endocrine pancreas, 87
    endocrine programming, 83–85
    environmental factors, 82
    genetic factors, 82
    glucocorticoids, 82, 85–87
    Hormones act, 82
    HPA axis, 82, 83, 87
    prenatal (*see* Prenatal undernutrition)
    reduction, 87
    in utero and nutritional status, 87
Undernutrition-induced fetal growth restriction, 552
Unfolded protein response (UPR), 113

Unhealthy diet, 92
United Nations Multiple Micronutrient Preparation
        (UNIMAP), 377
Urbanization
    in Africa, 389
Ureteral bud (UB), 134
US Food and Drug Administration (FDA), 242
Uterine ligation, 109–111, 113

V

Van Gieson stained subcutaneous adipose tissue, 94, 95
Vascular diseases, 364
Vascular endothelial growth factor (VEGF), 98, 536
Vascular endothelial growth factor-A (VEGF-A), 313
Ventral tegmental area (VTA), 234
Very low birth weight (VLBW), 457, 506, 578
Visceral adipose tissues, 100
Visceral adiposity
    foetal predisposition
        adipocyte development and growth, 97–99
        epigenetic regulation, 100–101
        fat deposition patterns, 99, 100
        inflammatory responses, 100–101
        timing of abnormal nutritional exposure, 96, 97
    prenatal undernutrition with postnatal diet, 94–96
Visceral obesity, 92
Vitamin B12, 295–297, 302
Vitamin D, 402–403

W

Waist circumference, 93
Weigh-suckle-weigh test, 217
Weight/maternal obesity
    after delivery and sociodemographic characteristics, 396
    diverse range of health problems, 395
    interventions to reduce in Ireland, 396
    Ireland-based study, 395
    management, 396
    outcomes, 395
    policy and clinical practice guidelines, 396
    prevalence, 395
    public health and economic importance, 395
    weight at first antenatal visit, 395
White adipose tissue (WAT), 179
Whole genome sequencing, 362–364, 366
Whole-genome miRNAs (miRNome), 271
World Food Programme, 387
World Health Organization (WHO), 399, 505
World Resources Institute, 387
Worms, 365
Wound healing, 361

X

Xenobiotics, 365

Z

Zeta of protein kinase C (PKC ζ), 520

Printed in the United States
By Bookmasters